Healthcare Management

4th edition

Healthcare Management

4th edition

Edited by Simon Moralee, Manbinder Sidhu, Judith Smith and Kieran Walshe

Mc Graw Hill

Open University Press

Open University Press
McGraw Hill
Unit 4
Foundation Park
Roxborough Way
Maidenhead
SL6 3UD

email: emea_uk_ireland@mheducation.com
world wide web: www.mheducation.co.uk

Executive Editor: Sam Crowe
Editorial Assistant: Hannah Church
Content Product Manager: Graham Jones

A catalogue record of this book is available from the British Library

ISBN-13: 9780335252596
ISBN-10: 0335252591
eISBN-13: 9780335252602

Typeset by Transforma Pvt. Ltd., Chennai, India

010268   ACL   2025

Praise for this book

"The 4th edition of Healthcare Management *continues to provide a comprehensive overview of healthcare management necessary for any student of the subject to understand the nature of the challenges theory may face in delivering healthcare services. This edition acknowledges the significance shifts that have occurred since the third editions and indeed while writing this edition. Covid 19 changed the game introducing the need for fast, accurate and values driven decision making at time of crisis often while managing the understandable anxieties of both colleagues and communities. Attempting to understand the healthcare environments, not just in the UK but across the world, introduces the true nature of healthcare as a complex adaptive system in which small changes can have disproportionate effects thus requiring healthcare managers to 'see the system' while understanding the contribution that they and their organisation needs to make in order to meet the growing demands and expectations of the public. This edition comes highly commended by me, it's an excellent reference and companion to developing the experience and expertise necessary to function in today's Healthcare environment"*
Lord Victor O Adebowale MA CBE, Chair NHS confederation,
Leadership coach, Executive Chairman, Visionable

"A welcome update, given the even more acute challenges we face in healthcare and policy since the last edition, with new and timely chapters, edited by one of the leading groups in healthcare management and policy. We will be using it as a text in our Masters courses, and our researchers will use chapters as background on the latest research."
Professor John Øvretveit, Medical Management Center,
Karolinska Medical University, Sweden

*"*Healthcare Management, 4th Edition *is a vital resource for anyone engaged in the complex task of managing and improving healthcare systems. Covering a wide range of critical topics—from governance and policy to quality improvement, sustainability, and workforce challenges—this edition provides timely, evidence-based insights for healthcare leaders. Its emphasis on integrating research, data, and management strategies makes it an invaluable guide for those committed to advancing healthcare performance and delivering high-quality, equitable care."*
Dionne S. Kringos, PhD, Associate Professor in Health Systems & Services Research,
Amsterdam UMC, University of Amsterdam, NL

"I am delighted to endorse Healthcare Management, 4th Edition. *This latest edition masterfully addresses the pressing challenges in healthcare management,*

from governance and financing to sustainability and creating supportive work-place cultures. With contributions from leading experts, it offers both theoretical insights and practical applications, making it a valuable guide for anyone navigating today's highly complex healthcare landscape. Its interdisciplinary approach and inclusion of global perspectives ensure relevance across diverse healthcare systems, making it an indispensable resource for professionals, policymakers, and students alike."

Dr Thomas West, Lecturer in Healthcare Leadership and
Management and Programme Co-Director Masters in
Healthcare Management, Bristol Business School,
University of Bristol, UK

Dedications

We dedicate this book to four people – we each chose someone who has inspired us in our careers by their work to improve healthcare policy, management and leadership and to make a real difference to patient care in the NHS.

Nicole Andrews was a Birmingham-based sociology scholar with a particular focus on health and illness relative to addressing inequity of care. With warmth, humour and compassion, she became a voice for the hard-to-reach and marginalized, always advocating for those who are silenced. Her expertise and dedication to addressing inequality touched many lives. She had courage, kindness and a relentless pursuit for achieving a fairer society for all. She was a wonderful colleague and a great source of advice, support and guidance. [Manni]

Peter Spurgeon has been actively involved in healthcare management research and practice for over 40 years. At one time Director of the Health Services Management Centre at the University of Birmingham and more recently as founding Director of the Institute of Clinical Leadership at the University of Warwick, he has been at the forefront of developing understanding of medical leadership in the UK and abroad. An insightful, kind and warm person, he has been a great research supervisor and advisor to me over the past 20 years of my career, as well as a dedicated supporter and mentor of many others. [Simon]

Rosemary Stewart of Templeton College Oxford was an applied academic who devoted her long career to the study of management and organizations, and in particular management in the NHS. Her studies focused on what it was really like to be an NHS manager or leader, including the demands, constraints and choices associated with the role. Rosemary's lecture given (with Professor Sue Dopson) at the Health Services Management Centre, University of Birmingham when I was an NHS management trainee, inspired me to want to research the career paths, roles and impact of senior NHS managers, something that I fulfilled in my later PhD studies into the role and experience of women chief executives in the NHS, and as I moved from NHS management into health services and management research. [Judith]

John Yates was an MTS trainee and NHS manager in the 1970s and became an academic at the University of Birmingham from the 1980s onwards – he pioneered the development of the first NHS performance indicators; led the first real waiting list initiatives; and researched the relationships between private practice and the NHS in areas like heart, hip and eye surgery. He was absolutely fearless in speaking truth to power to politicians and the great and the good. His work on reducing waiting times for elective surgery changed many patients' lives for the better. He was kind, down to earth, generous with his time and a great mentor to me and many others. [Kieran]

Table of contents

List of figures x

List of tables xii

List of boxes xiii

List of editors and contributors xvi

1 Introduction: the current and future challenges of healthcare management 1
Judith Smith, Simon Moralee, Manbinder Sidhu and Kieran Walshe

2 Governance and leadership in healthcare 11
Naomi Chambers

3 Quality improvement in healthcare 36
Joy Furnival

4 Public health and global inequalities 58
Peymané Adab

5 Equality, diversity and inclusion 83
Sandie Dunne

6 Research and evaluation 113
Tara Lamont and Gareth Hooper

7 The politics of healthcare and the health policy process 133
Ruth Thorlby and Mark Exworthy

8 Global health: governance in a new geopolitical era 157
Scott L. Greer and Matthias Wismar

9 Healthcare financing 179
Suzanne Robinson

10 The economics of healthcare 206
Richard Lewis and Matthew Bell

11 Setting and managing priorities for healthcare 227
Iestyn Williams and Chris Q. Smith

12 Climate change and sustainability 250
Chris Naylor and Hayley Pinto

13 Primary care 276
Manbinder Sidhu and Judith Smith

14 Acute care 303
Nigel Edwards and Louella Vaughan

15 Integrated care 332
Robin Miller and Viktoria Stein

16 Mental health 352
Sarah-Jane Fenton and Sarah Carr

17 Adult social care 377
Emily Burn and Catherine Needham

18 Informatics for healthcare systems   401
    Paul Taylor
19 Healthcare innovation   420
    Robert J. Romanelli and Sonja Marjanovic
20 The healthcare workforce   450
    Billy Palmer
21 Service user perspectives, experiences and involvement   470
    Jo Ellins and Tina Coldham
22 Measuring and managing healthcare performance   496
    Arne Wolters
23 Conclusions: future challenges for healthcare managers   520
    Simon Moralee and Manbinder Sidhu

Index   529

List of figures

2.1 Interconnectedness of roles, behaviours and outcomes of the full-service diligent and dynamic healthcare board — 22

5.1 Equality vs equity — 86

5.2 Four dimensions for assessing inequalities — 97

6.1 General logic model — 123

8.1 Top contributors to WHO — 160

9.1 Healthcare triangle — 181

9.2 Different forms of revenue generation methods — 182

9.3 Total health spending estimates on healthcare in 2022 across OECD countries — 190

9.4 Public health funding as a percentage of total healthcare expenditure, 2021 — 192

9.5 Primary care health services spending as a share of health expenditure 2021 — 193

9.6 Annual real growth rate in per capita health expenditure and GDP, OECD, 2006–22 — 194

12.1 Mechanisms that show how climate action can improve health and reduce social inequality — 253

12.2 Sources of greenhouse gas emissions attributable to the NHS in England — 255

12.3 Five principles of sustainable healthcare – driver diagram — 258

12.4 The sustainable value equation — 262

12.5 Strategies to increase engagement in sustainability — 265

14.1 Mean length of stay by age cohort — 308

16.1 Example of how stigma forms, operates, and is perpetuated resulting in active discrimination against individuals — 356

16.2 Treatment in relation to the spectrum of mental health — 359

17.1 The Care Diamond — 378

18.1 A mathematical model of an epidemic showing how the proportions of individuals that are susceptible, infectious or recovered change over time — 409

18.2 A control chart showing mean turnaround times for pathology tests over a 28- day period (Taylor, 2006). The data show the spread of the points around a mean, drawn in grey. The dark horizontal lines indicate the upper and lower control lines. Two data points, days 7 and 8, are above the upper control limit and suggest special cause variation. — 411

19.1 Healthcare innovation pathway — 423

19.2 Key influences on the development and implementation of innovations — 432

20.1 Size of health workforce relative to the population — 452

20.2 Key considerations in workforce planning — 453

20.3 Remuneration of specialist medical practitioners relative to average earnings, 2022 — 461

20.4 Breakdown of staff employed in hospitals, by profession grouping — 462

20.5 Some key findings from independent reviews of NHS leadership in England   464
21.1 Arnstein's Ladder of Participation   474
22.1 Average length of stay (in days) for inpatients in Germany, over time   501
22.2 Average length of stay (in days) for inpatients in selected OECD countries, over time   508
22.3 Average length of stay (in days) for inpatients in selected OECD countries, over time   508
22.4 Process map for developing new performance metrics   514

List of tables

2.1 A realist framework for healthcare boards 21
3.1 Definitions of healthcare quality 37
3.2 Categories of performance improvement 38
3.3 Quality improvement approaches 40
3.4 Core challenges to organizing for quality 48
4.1 Examples of groups affected by health inequalities, how they are affected and implications for health managers 61
6.1 Example logic model to reduce falls 123
6.2 Quantitative study designs for evaluation 126
7.1 Medical organizations in five countries (Freeman 2000; European Observatory, 2012; Busse and Blümel 2014; Chevreul et al., 2010; Rand Europe 2009) 140
7.2 Examples of countries' mix of control of their health system 145
8.1 Terminology in global health 159
9.1 Countries grouped by similar funding systems 183
9.2 Total expenditure on health as a percentage of GDP in selected OECD countries, 1970–2022 191
14.1 Acute beds per 1000 population 313
15.1 Dimensions of integration 334
19.1 Key implications of innovation systems and sociotechnical perspectives for decision-making about innovation 427
19.2 Key implications of health services and implementation science perspectives for decision-making about innovation (IOF, CFIR and NASSS) 429
20.1 Countries with significant proportion of doctors who were foreign-trained 456
21.1 Different levels and types of involvement 475
21.2 UK Public Involvement Standards 481
21.3 Potential criteria for evaluating success in involvement 487
22.1 Six domains of care quality that provide a good framework for a comprehensive set of performance metrics 499
22.2 Different users of performance metrics and their use purposes 503
22.3 Handle with care: seven principles to take into account when using performance metrics 515

List of boxes

2.1 Eight enduring international challenges for healthcare governance 12
2.2 Management of the COVID-19 pandemic in five high-income countries 15
2.3 Case study – example of a failing board: Mid Staffordshire NHS Foundation Trust in England 21
3.1 Lean healthcare 44
3.2 Summary 49
4.1 Some definitions of public health and inequalities 59
4.2 Examples of within-country inequalities 67
4.3 Some resources that summarize tools and interventions for addressing health inequalities for health managers 73
5.1 UK Equality Act (2010) (UK legislation) 85
5.2 Key points to note regarding power and privilege 87
5.3 White privilege 87
5.4 Social construction 89
5.5 Power (Batliwala, 2010; Veneklasen and Miller, 2002) 89
5.6 Key terms associated with race and racism 91
5.7 Key terms related to sex and gender 93
5.8 LGBTQIA+ What do the acronyms mean? (Cherry, 2023) 94
5.9 Case Study – the UK gender pay gap in the NHS (NHS England, 2023b) 96
5.10 Indigenous health strategies to tackle inequality in Australia, New Zealand and Canada 98
5.11 EDI implications for healthcare managers (Kline, 2022): The UK Messenger Review into Healthcare Leadership (Messenger and Pollard, 2022) 102
5.12 Positive action and positive discrimination 103
6.1 Case study – early evaluation of telehealth and telecare 115
6.2 Case study – evidence on twelve-hour nursing shifts 119
6.3 Case study – inequalities in mortality and morbidity in UK maternity services 124
7.1 The politics of health or healthcare? 134
7.2 Functions of governance 137
7.3 The role of professional organizations in the United Kingdom 139
8.1 What are countries? 157
8.2 The pandemic treaty 162
8.3 Comparative health data 167
8.4 COVID-19 vaccines and vaccine diplomacy 171
8.5 Global health and the health workforce 172
9.1 Defining terms 180
9.2 General taxation advantages and disadvantages 184
9.3 Typical features of social health insurance systems 185
10.1 Economic concepts used to analyse healthcare systems 207
10.2 Costs and prices in healthcare 209

10.3 Prices and value in healthcare 210
10.4 Consumers and patients 211
10.5 DRGs 215
11.1 The seven forms of rationing 229
11.2 Ethical standpoints and principles to consider in priority setting 232
11.3 Deliberative involvement methods 235
11.4 Case study – community involvement in priority setting in Tanzania 236
11.5 The four conditions of Accountability for Reasonableness (A4R) 237
11.6 Case study from Argentina 239
12.1 Four reasons to prioritize sustainability 251
12.2 Newcastle University Hospitals NHS Foundation Trust: Embedding
sustainability at organizational level 255
12.3 Remote monitoring hub in Northwest England 259
12.4 Saving lives with solar 260
12.5 Sustainable quality improvement in HIV care 263
12.6 Communicating effectively about climate change 264
12.7 Spreading and scaling good practice in the Royal National Orthopaedic Hospital 266
12.8 The Greener NHS programme in England 269
13.1 Key characteristics of primary care networks: A model of the organization of
primary healthcare in England 279
13.2 Categorization of core activities in primary care 280
13.3 Starfield's four Cs as an organizing framework 281
13.4 Example of a super-partnership in the UK 285
13.5 Community Health Centre Botermarkt 286
13.6 Tu Ora Compass Health, Aoetearoa New Zealand 288
13.7 Danish health clusters 289
13.8 Different models of vertical integration in England: Wolverhampton and Somerset 292
14.1 Hospital levels 304
14.2 Standalone planned treatment hospitals 305
14.3 National reconfigurations of acute care 316
15.1 Examples of definitions of integrated care 333
15.2 Community Health Centres, Canada 339
15.3 Wigan Deal, UK (Naylor and Wellings, 2019) 342
16.1 An outline of key concepts 354
16.2 Case study – service organization change in England for children and young
people 361
16.3 Case study – service architecture in Colombia for children and young people 362
17.1 Case study – Royal Commission, Australia 383
17.2 Case study – social care in Germany 384
17.3 An example of a strengths-based approach to social care 385
17.4 Different interventions included in the term 'care technology' 387
17.5 Social care policy reform in Japan and Germany 389
17.6 The 21st Century Public Servant 391
18.1 Case study – using AI in breast cancer screening 402
18.2 Case study – linked data sets 407

18.3 Case study – mathematical modelling and the pandemic response   408
18.4 Case study – bias and fairness in AI   414
19.1 Examples of funding sources for research, innovation development and
          adoption in the UK   432
19.2 Examples of initiatives to support a workforce engaged with innovation in the UK   435
19.3 Examples of programmes related to information and evidence in the UK   436
19.4 Examples of programmes related to relationships and networking   437
19.5 Examples of sources of information about capital and infrastructure funding
          in the UK   438
19.6 Service user engagement and involvement with research and innovation   439
19.7 Sleepio: a digital health technology approach to treating insomnia   440
19.8 Cascade model for genetic testing of familial hypercholesterolemia: an
          example of a diagnostic service innovation   442
19.9 NHS Blood donor chair – an example of a low-tech innovation   443
20.1 Case studies – turning off the taps on training numbers   455
20.2 Case study – outsourced training   457
20.3 Case study – Retention Direct Support Programme in England   458
21.1 Levels of involvement   474
21.2 What matters most to people when using health services?   476
21.3 Veterans Affairs Whole Health Coaching Programme   479
21.4 Patient participation in the Federal Joint Committee in Germany   483
21.5 Health Education England Education and Training Framework for Person-
          Centred Approaches   484
21.6 Eight characteristics of person-centred organizations   485
21.7 Five dimensions of accessible and inclusive involvement   488
22.1 The value of trends over time, and how to interpret them, considering average
          length of stay for inpatients in Germany   500
22.2 The proliferation of quality metrics and dashboards   505
22.3 International comparison of average length of stay   507
22.4 Case study – evaluating the named, accountable GP policy for patients aged
          75 and over   511
23.1 Major challenges facing healthcare managers   521

List of editors and contributors

Co-editors: Simon Moralee, Manbinder Sidhu, Judith Smith, Kieran Walshe

Peymané Adab, Professor of Chronic Disease Epidemiology and Public Health, University of Birmingham

Matthew Bell OBE, Director, Frontier Economics Ltd

Emily Burn, Research Fellow, Centre for Care, University of Birmingham

Sarah Carr, Visiting Senior Research Fellow, Department of Health Service and Population Research, Institute of Psychiatry, Psychology and Neuroscience, King's College London

Naomi Chambers, Professor of Healthcare Management, Alliance Manchester Business School, The University of Manchester

Tina Coldham BEM, Participation Involvement & Engagement Advisor, National Institute for Health & Social Care Research (NIHR)

Sandie Dunne, Executive Coach, Leadership, Diversity & Inclusion and Organisational Development Consultant, and Associate Professor, Health Services Management Centre, University of Birmingham

Nigel Edwards, Senior Associate, Nuffield Trust and Honorary Professor, University of Birmingham

Jo Ellins, Senior Fellow, Health Services Management Centre, University of Birmingham

Mark Exworthy, Professor of Health Policy and Management, Health Services Management Centre, University of Birmingham

Sarah-Jane Fenton, Associate Professor, Mental Health Policy, Health Services Management Centre, University of Birmingham

Joy Furnival, Deputy Director of Strategic Insight, Care Quality Commission

Scott Greer, Professor of Health Management and Policy and Global Public Health, University of Michigan, and Senior Expert Advisor, Health Governance, European Observatory on Health Systems and Policies

Gareth Hooper, Impact Evaluation Analytics Manager, The Strategy Unit

Tara Lamont, Fellowships Senior Advisor, The Healthcare Improvement Studies (THIS) Institute, University of Cambridge, and Senior Scientific Advisor, NIHR Health Services and Delivery Research Programme, University of Southampton

Richard Lewis, Senior Associate, Frontier Economics Ltd.

Sonja Marjanovic, Director of Healthcare Innovation, Industry and Policy, RAND Europe

Robin Miller, Professor of Collaborative Learning in Health and Social Care, Department of Social Work and Social Care, University of Birmingham

Simon Moralee, Senior Lecturer/Associate Professor, and Head of the Health Management Group, Alliance Manchester Business School, The University of Manchester

Chris Naylor, Senior Policy Fellow, The King's Fund and Policy Lead, Centre for Sustainable Healthcare

Catherine Needham, Professor of Public Policy and Public Management, Health Services Management Centre, University of Birmingham

Billy Palmer, Senior Fellow, Nuffield Trust

Hayley Pinto, Education and Training Lead, Centre for Sustainable Healthcare

Suzanne Robinson, Chair and Director of Deakin Health Economics, Institute for Health Transformation, Deakin University

Rob Romanelli, Senior Research Leader, Health and Wellbeing, RAND Europe

Manbinder Sidhu, Associate Professor and Co-Director, NIHR BRACE Rapid Evaluation Centre, Health Services Management Centre, University of Birmingham

Chris Q Smith, Assistant Professor, Sociology and Social Policy, Department of Social Policy, Sociology and Criminology, University of Birmingham

Judith Smith, Professor of Health Policy and Management, Health Services Management Centre, University of Birmingham, and Director of Health Services Research, Birmingham Health Partners.

Viktoria Stein, Co-Founder and Co-CEO, VM Partners Integrating Health and Care, and Assistant Professor, Leiden University Medical Center

Paul Taylor, Professor of Health Informatics, University College London

Ruth Thorlby, Assistant Director of Policy, The Health Foundation

Louella Vaughan, Consultant Physician, Barts Health NHS Trust

Kieran Walshe, Professor of Health Policy and Management, Alliance Manchester Business School, The University of Manchester

Iestyn Williams, Professor of Health Policy and Management, Health Services Management Centre, University of Birmingham

Matthias Wismar, Programme Manager, European Observatory on Health Systems and Policies

Arne Wolters, Head of Improvement Analytics, Cumbria, Northumberland, Tyne and Wear NHS Foundation Trust and Implementation Lead, NIHR Applied Research Collaboration, North East and North Cumbria

NB. Biographies taken from institution webpages or LinkedIn where accessible and checked with contributors in March 2025

Introduction: the current and future challenges of healthcare management

Judith Smith, Simon Moralee, Manbinder Sidhu and Kieran Walshe

Introduction

When we introduced the third edition of this textbook in 2016, we noted among other things that:

> In short, the social, political and economic context in which healthcare organizations have to exist is often a hostile, fast-changing and pressured environment.
>
> (Walshe and Smith, 2016: 4)

Little did we, nor anyone else, know what hostile, fast-changing and pressured challenges lay ahead of the world's population, its healthcare organizations, and their staff, managers and policymakers. The COVID-19 global pandemic presented unprecedented challenges to healthcare managers in all nations where they were faced with making rapid decisions, including how to continue to deliver vital primary, secondary, mental health and other healthcare services in a safe manner, support social care for those living with disabilities and/or frailty, provide treatments for people with COVID-19, ensure effective public health protection, and set priorities for the use of scarce healthcare resources. This was arguably one of the most complex, acute and global healthcare management issues of all time. Yet global health events are always with us or lie not so far head, including the many and profound consequences of climate change; the potential and risks of using artificial intelligence (AI) in healthcare; the rising threat of antimicrobial resistance; possible new pandemics; and geopolitical turmoil, in part a result of climate change and associated patterns of migration.

In this fourth edition of *Healthcare Management*, we have sought to update and extend what we understand to have been the most important and useful material in the third edition. We have added new chapters, revised others and thought carefully about what evidence-based insights are most sought by busy, hard-pressed healthcare managers in many nations. For example, we have this time included chapters on climate change and sustainability in healthcare; equality, diversity and inclusion; and innovation in healthcare.

Regular users of this textbook will note a change to the editorial team. There are four editors this time, Professor Kieran Walshe and Professor Judith Smith, as for the three prior editions, along with two new editors: Dr Simon Moralee and Dr Manbinder Sidhu. The reason for this is to ensure a clear succession plan for the textbook beyond the time when Kieran and Judith, in due course, step back and hand over the reins. We wish to ensure that the textbook remains a core part of the strong and long-standing research and teaching collaboration between the Health Management Group at the University of Manchester and the Health Services Management Centre at the University of Birmingham, UK. On this occasion we have worked to share the experience and learning gained by Judith and Kieran from editing previous editions of the textbook, while drawing on the challenge, expertise and novel insights brought by Simon and Manbinder. It has been hugely rewarding to work as a team of four this time and Kieran and Judith know that they are handing on this excellent and highly valued textbook to the next generation of healthcare management experts within the Manchester–Birmingham collaboration.

Aim of the book

The aim of this fourth edition of our textbook is, as with prior editions, to inform and support the learning and development of practising managers in healthcare organizations and health systems, and those undertaking postgraduate study on programmes concerned with health policy, health management and related areas. These two groups continue to overlap as many managers undertake a master's degree or other accredited academic programme as part of their intellectual and career development, and we are firm believers in the power of the interaction between academic and experiential learning that this brings.

No one learns to be a manager just from being in a classroom, or from reading a book. Management is inevitably learned by doing, by experiencing the challenges and opportunities of leadership (Mintzberg, 2004) and working with others to find solutions to very complex and often contested problems. The best and most successful managers are evidence-based and reflective practitioners – profoundly aware of their own behaviours, attitudes and actions and their impact on others and on the organization, and able to analyse and review critically their own practice and set it in a wider context, framed by appropriate theories, models and concepts (Edmonstone, 2021; Chambers, 2023). The future leaders of our healthcare organizations and systems therefore need to be able to integrate theory and practice and have the adaptability and flexibility that come from really understanding the nature of management and leadership. The experience of the COVID-19 pandemic revealed the vital need for evidence to inform health policy and management, as well as other aspects of healthcare practice. For example, how best to protect and support staff working in high-risk and intense settings; how to procure personal protective and other equipment rapidly and yet with appropriate governance in place; how to design rapidly new care pathways in and across different sectors of health and social care; and how to try to assure that health inequalities be addressed and not ignored as rapid changes to the organization and delivery of care were made.

This chapter sets the context for the book, by first describing the challenges of the political and social environment in which healthcare systems and organizations exist and how that environment is continuing to change. It then describes some of the particular challenges of those organizations – some of the characteristics and dynamics that make healthcare organizations so interesting and yet so difficult to manage and lead. Then the chapter explains the structure of the book and how we anticipate that it might be used, both in support of formal programmes of study and by managers who want simply to develop and expand their own understanding and awareness.

Healthcare systems, politics and society

In most developed countries, the healthcare sector represents one of the largest industries – bigger generally than education, agriculture, IT, tourism or telecommunications, and a crucial component of wider economic performance. In countries that are members of the Organisation for Economic Co-operation and Development (OECD), around 1 worker in 10 is employed in the healthcare sector – as doctors, nurses, scientists, therapists, cleaners, cooks, engineers, administrators, clerks, finance controllers – and, of course, as managers (OECD, 2023). This means that almost everyone has a relative or knows someone who works in healthcare, and the healthcare workforce can be a politically powerful group with considerable influence over public opinion, something that became particularly evident during the COVID-19 pandemic. Furthermore, almost everyone uses health services or will do as they age, has members of their family or friends who are significant healthcare users, and everyone has a view to express about their local or national healthcare system.

In many countries, the history of the healthcare system is intertwined with the development of communities and social structures. Religious groups, charities, voluntary organizations, trade unions and local municipalities have all played important roles in building the healthcare organizations and systems we have today, and people in those communities often feel connected in a visceral manner to 'their' hospitals, community clinics, ambulance service, and other parts of the healthcare system. They raise funds to support new facilities or equipment and volunteer to work in a wide range of roles that augment or support the employed healthcare workforce. That connection with the community also comes to the fore when anyone – especially government – suggests changing or reconfiguring healthcare provision. Proposals to close much-loved community hospitals, reorganize district hospital services or change maternity services are often professionally or politically driven – frequently by a laudable policy imperative to make health services more effective, safe and efficient. But when evidence of clinical effectiveness and technocratic appraisals of service options collide with popular sentiment and public opinion, what matters is usually not 'what works' but what people want and how they might vote in municipal or national elections.

Indeed, for many local and national politicians, health policy and the healthcare system offer not only opportunities to shine in the eyes of the electorate when things are going well, but also threats to future electoral success when there are problems with healthcare funding or service provision and people look for someone to hold to account, as is explored in detail in Chapter 7 on the politics of healthcare and the health policy process. Constituents bring to politicians in their local offices concerns about healthcare services, and politicians are keenly aware of the attitudes and beliefs of the public about their local health service. While they will readily gain political benefit from the opening of a new facility, or the expansion of clinical services, they will equally happily secure benefit by criticizing the plans of 'faceless bureaucrats' in the local healthcare organization for unpopular changes in healthcare services and argue that there are too many managers and 'pen-pushers'.

Finally, for the press, TV, radio, online and social media, both locally and nationally, the healthcare system is an endless source of news stories, debates and current affairs topics. From patient safety to COVID-19, from 'dental deserts' to hospital closures, from waiting lists to celebrity illnesses and possible new uses of AI to 'transform' health services, the healthcare system is news across broadcast and online media and in all social media formats. For many people, social media platforms, like TikTok, may often be a much more ready source of health information than most media used by national and local healthcare organizations. Indeed, healthcare organizations and their leaders can use this level of media availability and interest to their advantage, to raise public awareness of health issues and try to communicate evidence-based messages with the community. They can however also find themselves on the receiving end of intense and hostile media scrutiny when things go wrong, and in a world of ever-expanding social media forms and outlets, assuring the quality and accuracy of health information – and countering misinformation – is a huge healthcare management challenge.

In other words, healthcare organizations exist in a turbulent political and social environment in which their actions and behaviour are highly visible and much scrutinized. Leadership and management take place in this 'goldfish bowl', where their performance and process can be just as important as their outcomes. But as if that were not enough, in every developed country the healthcare system is subject to four inexorable and challenging social trends:

1 the demographic shift;
2 the pace of technological innovation, including AI;
3 rapidly changing user and consumer expectations across generations; and
4 financial pressures within a context of emerging from a global pandemic, climate change and major economic downturns.

The demographic challenge we now face is that people are living longer, and the numbers of elderly and very elderly people are rising fast – and those people make much heavier use of the healthcare system. People may live longer, but they cost more to keep alive, they are more likely to have complex, chronic health conditions, and their last few years of life tend to require significant support (Sussex et al., 2024). A further dimension to this demographic challenge is the rising incidence of chronic disease in the wider population of developed countries. The World Health Organization (WHO) suggests that this is a direct result of risk factors such as tobacco use, physical inactivity and unhealthy diets (Costa Santos et al., 2022; Global Health Observatory, 2023).

The second challenge is related to the first in that it reflects an increasing ability to cure illnesses, control chronic disease and thus extend life – the pace of technological innovation. Most obviously in pharmaceuticals, but also in surgery, diagnostics, telehealth, precision medicine and other areas, we keep finding new ways to cure or manage disease. Sometimes that means new treatments that are more effective (and usually more expensive) than the existing ones. But it also means new therapies for diseases or problems that we simply could not treat before. Furthermore, the rise of genomic medicine means that treatments tailored to the individual are now very much a reality and are starting to bring about significant changes to the ways in which disease is anticipated, prevented and treated. This will in turn impact on how health services are planned, delivered and managed.

The third challenge is changing user and consumer expectations: people typically want more from health and social care services compared to previous generations. They are not content to be passive recipients of healthcare, prescribed and dispensed by providers at the convenience of professionals. Accustomed to an ever-widening choice and sovereignty in decisions in other areas of life such as banking, travel and education – and accessible through a smartphone or other device – they expect to be consulted, informed and involved by healthcare providers in any decisions that affect their health. They are better informed, more articulate and more likely to know about and demand new and expensive treatments. In a similar vein, people will be able to compare different providers, treatments and forms of care using publicly available data and reviews and this will add further to the shift in the balance of knowledge and power between providers and patients.

The first three challenges are in large measure responsible for the fourth – rising costs (Mintzberg, 2017). Each of them contributes to the constant pressure for more healthcare funding, a pressure which for very many countries is currently more acute as a result of the global pandemic and its aftermath. For many nations, the risks and costs associated with extreme weather events, climate change and global events, like pandemics, are also adding to economic pressures and the need for health protection and treatments: however much governments or others increase their spending on healthcare, it never seems to be enough. In a time of major economic pressures resulting from a global pandemic and other factors, this challenge is made more acute by real-term reductions in the resources available for healthcare in many countries, and hence a focus on setting priorities or rationing availability of services (see Chapters 9–11).

In short, the social, political and economic context in which healthcare organizations exist is too often a hostile, fast-changing and pressured environment. Managers and leaders strive to balance competing, shifting and irreconcilable demands from a wide range of stakeholders – and do so while under close public (and increasingly online) scrutiny. The task of leadership and management in healthcare organizations – defining the mission of the organization, setting out a clear and consistent vision, guiding and incentivizing the organization towards its objectives, and ensuring safe and high-quality care – is made much more challenging by the social, economic and political context in which they work.

Healthcare organizations and healthcare management

Organizations are the product of their environment and context, and many of the distinctive characteristics and behaviours of healthcare organizations result from some of the social, political and economic factors outlined above. However, some also result from the nature of the enterprise – healthcare itself. The uniquely personal nature of health services, the special vulnerability and need for support and advocacy of patients, the complexity of the care process, and the advanced nature of the technologies used all contribute to the special challenges of management in healthcare organizations.

We should, however, be cautious that this does not lead us to be parochial or narrow-minded in our understanding of what we do, or of what we can learn from other sectors and settings. Healthcare systems and organizations have a strong tendency to exceptionalism, something that needs to be challenged on a regular basis. Healthcare organizations are large, complex, professionally dominated entities providing a wide range of highly tailored and personalized services to large numbers of often vulnerable users. But those characteristics are shared in various degrees by local authorities, police and emergency services, universities, schools, public transport networks, law firms and other organizations. Healthcare is nevertheless distinctive, and four important areas of difference deserve some further consideration: the place of professionals; the role of patients; the nature of the healthcare process; and healthcare as a public good.

The place of professionals

For managers entering healthcare organizations from other sectors – whether from other public services, commercial for-profit companies or the voluntary sector – one of the first striking differences they notice is the absence of clear, hierarchical structures for command and control, and the powerful nature of professional status, knowledge and control. Healthcare organizations are professional bureaucracies (Mintzberg, 1979) in which more or less all the intellectual, creative and social capital exists in the frontline workers – clinicians of all professions, but particularly doctors. Like law firms and universities, it makes no sense to try to manage these talented, highly intelligent individuals in ways that are reductionist, or which run counter to their highly professionalized self-image and culture. This does not mean that they should not be managed – far from it, for the high-risk nature of healthcare means that careful attention to the quality and safety of care, and monitoring, supporting and governing professionals' role in this, is vital. The management challenge with healthcare professionals is that the processes and content of management and leadership need to take account of and indeed embrace the professional culture while assuring appropriate transparency and governance. Tasks largely get done not through instruction or direction, but by negotiation, persuasion, peer influence and agreement. Leaders need to make skilful use of the values, language and apparatus of the profession to achieve their objectives and learn to lead without needing to be 'in charge'.

The role of patients

The people who use healthcare services, whether you call them patients, service users or consumers, are not like the consumers of many other public or commercial services. There is a huge asymmetry of power and information in the relationship between a patient and a healthcare provider. Even the most highly educated, confident, social media-savvy patient cannot acquire the detailed knowledge, expertise, judgement and wisdom that come with many years of clinical training and practice. At some level, patients have to be able to trust that healthcare providers are competent and take their advice on important decisions about their health. No amount of performance measurement, league tables, audit or regulation can substitute for this trust.

When people become patients and use healthcare services, they are often at their most vulnerable and are less able to act independently and assertively than would normally be the case. They may be emotionally fragile following an unwelcome diagnosis of disease and weakened by the experience of illness or the effects of treatment. We are not likely to feel as well-placed as usual to exercise choice or to assert our right to self-determination. This means that healthcare organizations, and those who manage them, have a special responsibility to compensate for the unavoidable asymmetry of power and information in their relationships with patients, by providing mechanisms and systems to protect, empower and advocate for patients, seek and act on their views and experiences, listen carefully to and understand their concerns, and work constantly to make services more patient centred. Furthermore, as patients, we are not generally paying at the point of care, so assumptions about consumer behaviour do not apply. This is complex management work, for taking this strongly patient-centred approach will at times run counter to professional and organizational established practice (see Chapter 21: Service user perspectives, experiences and involvement).

The nature of the healthcare process

Despite all the high-technology medicine, complicated equipment and advanced pharmaceuticals and diagnostics available today, the healthcare process itself is still too often organized very much as it was a hundred years ago. It is a craft model of production in which individual health professionals ply their trade, providing their distinctive contribution to any patient's treatment when called upon. Fundamentally, it is an often unmanaged and undocumented process. Usually, there is no written timetable or plan showing how the patient should move through the system, and no one person acts as 'the manager of the process', steering and co-ordinating the care that the patient receives and assuring quality and efficiency. This model has endured because of its flexibility. The patient care process can be adapted endlessly or tailored to the needs of individual patients, the circumstances of their disease and their response to treatment.

Modern healthcare is increasingly complex, with multiple handovers of patients within and across departments, organizations and sectors of health and social care. The very many patients who live with several complex health conditions find themselves transferred from one health professional to another, with shifts between primary, secondary and social care often proving to be particularly delayed, fractured or poorly documented (this is explored in depth in Chapter 15: Integrated care). As lengths of hospital stays get shorter (for those for whom there are safe and appropriate places to be discharged to), patients are more frail and living with multiple complex conditions, and the risks and side-effects of many new healthcare interventions (the flip side of their much greater effectiveness) all mean that the traditional craft model of healthcare is increasingly seen as unreliable and prone to error and unexplained variation. More and more healthcare organizations use care pathways, treatment plans, clinical guidelines and electronic records to bring some structure and explicitness to the healthcare process. Gradually, the healthcare process is being made more transparent, exposed for discussion debate and challenge, and standardized or routinized in ways that make the delivery of healthcare more consistent, efficient and safer.

Healthcare as a public good

There is one other important feature of healthcare organizations. Whether they are government-owned, independent not-for-profits, or commercial healthcare providers, they all share to some degree a sense of social mission or purpose concerned with the public good (Abdalla et al., 2020; Galea, 2021). The professional values and culture of healthcare are deeply embedded, and most people working in healthcare organizations have both an altruistic belief in the social value of the work they do and a set of more self-interested motivations to do with reward, recognition and advancement. Similarly, healthcare organizations – even commercial, for-profit entities – sometimes do things that do not make sense in business terms but reflect their social mission, while at the same time they respond to financial incentives and behave entrepreneurially. The healthcare management challenge, at both the individual and organizational level, is to make proper use of both sets of motivations and not lose sight of the powerful and pervasive beneficial effects that can result from understanding and playing to the social mission.

About this fourth edition and how to use the book

The third edition of this book received very positive and encouraging feedback from the outset, particularly in relation to the balance between academic rigour and practical application of concepts and ideas, and its international focus. When given the opportunity to prepare a fourth edition, there were a number of key areas where we wished to focus our attention, these being:

- concentrating on core content relevant to healthcare management, with a particular focus on how this applies in relation to major societal challenges, such as emerging from the COVID-19 pandemic, addressing climate change, and tackling deep-seated inequalities of care, inclusion and healthcare organization;
- continuing to be genuinely international in approach; and
- designing and presenting content in ways that support structured management learning, application and further study.

We have therefore made further significant revisions for this fourth edition. First of all, in relation to the structure of the book, this time we present 21 chapters (in addition to the introduction and conclusions) organized in a manner that reflects the challenges of:

- managing complex healthcare services and organizations;
- addressing major issues that are at once societal and organizational;
- exploring the role and nature of management within specific sectors of health and social care; and

- concluding with the vital topics of patient and user perspective, measuring outcomes; and examining innovations that hold promise for the future.

In addressing the need for the book to remain clearly international in its focus, we have again included a chapter on the internationalization of health systems, this time with a particular focus on global health governance (Chapter 8: Global health: governance in a new geopolitical era). All chapter authors were encouraged strongly to draw on a wide range of international material and case studies, and this they have done, with many examples of research and practice from across the world.

In terms of adopting a design that supports structured learning, as with the third edition, each chapter has a common framework that places a strong emphasis on separating out core ideas and content from their application in one or more case studies. There are self-test learning activities throughout each chapter which are often designed to encourage the reader to go out into their own organization to gather information and discuss issues with colleagues. In addition, authors provide a set of key online sources for further reading and application.

All the chapters have been rewritten and edited to a significant degree, reflecting both the pace of change within the world of healthcare and our collective desire as an editorial team to ensure that the book is constantly improved to remain highly relevant and useful to healthcare managers and leaders. We hope that you will appreciate the changes we have made and find the book to be as helpful and thoughtful as ever.

This textbook is a collective endeavour, with over 30 contributors to the 21 chapters it contains, many drawn from among our current and former colleagues and recognized experts in their chosen fields. We are as appreciative as we hope you will be of the time, effort and skill they have invested in designing and planning the learning in their specialist areas.

It is great to get feedback on this book. With previous editions, we have met people who have used the book throughout an academic course or development programme, and we are always pleased when we hear that someone has used the book to support their learning and helped them to develop as a manager and leader. Others tell us of how specific chapters have informed their understanding of key challenges facing them in their healthcare management work, where a concise account of the topic, evidence base and possible solutions has proved invaluable. Equally, we welcome comments on and ideas for improvement, and we can promise they will be considered when Simon Moralee and Manbinder Sidhu start to think about a future edition of the book. Whether you use it primarily for your own interest and development or more intensively as part of a postgraduate programme of study, we would like your feedback. Please email either Simon or Manbinder at simon.moralee@manchester.ac.uk or m.s.sidhu@bham.ac.uk.

References and further reading

Abdalla, S.M., Maani, N., Ettman, C.K. and Galea, S. (2020) Claiming health as a public good in the post-COVID-19 era, *Development (Rome)*, 63 (2–4): 200–204. https://doi.org/10.1057/s41301-020-00255-z. Epub 2020 Nov 10. PMID: 33192033; PMCID: PMC7653666.

Chambers, N. (ed.) (2023) *Research Handbook on Leadership in Healthcare*. Cheltenham: Edward Elgar.

Costa Santos, A., Willumsen, J., Meheus, F., Ilbawa, A. and Bull, F.C. (2022) The cost of inaction on physical inactivity to public health-care systems: a population-attributable fraction analysis, *The Lancet*, 11 (1): E32–E39. https://doi.org/10.1016/S2214-109X(22)00464-8.

Edmonstone, J. (2021) *Organisation Development in Healthcare: A Critical Appraisal for Practitioners*. Abingdon: Routledge.

Galea, S. (2021) Health as a public good, in S.Galea, *The Contagion Next Time* (New York, 2022; online edn. Oxford Academic, 18 November 2021). https://doi.org/10.1093/oso/9780197576427.001.0001.

Global Health Observatory (2023) Noncommunicable diseases: Risk factors. World Health Organization [https://www.who.int/data/gho/data/themes/topics/noncommunicable-diseases-risk-factors; accessed 12 July 2024].

Mintzberg, H. (1979) *The Structuring of Organizations: A Synthesis of the Research*. University of Illinois at Urbana-Champaign's Academy for Entrepreneurial Leadership Historical Research Reference in Entrepreneurship [https://ssrn.com/abstract=1496182; accessed 12 July 2024].

Mintzberg, H. (2004) *Managers Not MBAs*. London: Prentice Hall.

Mintzberg, H. (2017) *Managing the Myths of Health Care: Bridging the Separations between Care, Cure, Control, and Community*. Oakland: Berrett-Koehler.

OECD (2023) *Health at a Glance 2023: OECD Indicators*. OECD Publishing, Paris. https://doi.org/10.1787/7a7afb35-en.

Sussex, J., Smith, J. and Wu, F.M. (2024) Service innovations for people with multiple long-term conditions: reflections of a rapid evaluation team, *Health and Social Care Delivery Research*, 12 (15).

Walshe, K. and Smith, J. (eds) (2016) *Healthcare Management* (3rd edn.). London: McGraw-Hill Education/Open University Press.

Governance and leadership in healthcare

Naomi Chambers

Introduction

This chapter begins by outlining the complexity of challenges in healthcare, and thus the importance of good governance in securing affordable, sustainable and safe services.

Different approaches to healthcare governance are covered in the following sections, including, at the country and system level, the use of hierarchies, markets and networks, and various mechanisms of accountability and oversight. A case study of the differing experiences of five countries in their political oversight of the COVID-19 pandemic is included.

Institution level governance is then scrutinized, especially healthcare board governance, including debates about the different structures and purposes of healthcare boards, and board practices, behaviours and dynamics. Leadership is a fundamental aspect of the enactment of good governance. Evolving paradigms in healthcare leadership as a result of changing demands in healthcare delivery and broader societal influences are presented. In healthcare, much is now known about the importance of leadership in making a positive difference to patient experience, clinical quality of care and outcomes, and to staff morale (Fulop and Ramsay, 2019; West and Bailey, 2023).

This chapter then points to the fundamental problem of variation in quality of leadership, some of the reasons why this prevails, and the impacts. The distinctive characteristics of desirable leadership in the healthcare setting are elucidated, for example, the qualities of leadership for patient safety (covered in more detail in Chapter 3 of this volume), leadership for compassionate care (see also Chapter 21 on the service user perspective), the implications of leading in a healthcare professional bureaucracy (see also Chapter 21 on workforce), leading in systems and for integrated care (see also Chapter 15). This chapter concludes with a call to action to improve the quality of leadership in ways that will benefit staff engagement, and thus the experiences of patients and the sustainability of services.

Challenges for healthcare governance

There is a raft of enduring governance challenges facing all healthcare systems, which have been well rehearsed by a number of publications, including Blank and Burau (2013), OECD (2023), and the World Health Organization (WHO, 2023). These challenges largely predate, sometimes by decades, and have been significantly exacerbated by, the COVID-19 pandemic. The issues are similar to those in other public sector or social welfare programmes (education, housing, out-of-work benefits and so on), but it can be argued that there are a greater number and complexity of strands coming together in health that make the successful endeavour here seemingly intractable. Eight strands are identified (see Box 2.1) that have to be handled by leaders contemporaneously. These are the sometimes conflicting and critical problems identified by Grint (2010) and which need 'clumsy' rather than elegant solutions.

Box 2.1   Eight enduring international challenges for healthcare governance

1   Financial pressure
2   Workforce shortage
3   Quality and safety of care
4   National and local politics
5   Consumer demands
6   Power of the professions
7   Complexity of the health system
8   Technological advances

Since the global economic downturn in 2008, and given the rate of technological advances in healthcare, top of the list of challenges has to be the affordability of care. Comprehensive controls and prioritization tools are therefore essential. Second, changing demographics with sharp rises in numbers in the over 65s and in the over 85s age groups contribute to a global scarcity in workforce that is predicted to increase to 18 million health workers by 2030 (Refsum and Britnell, 2023). In some countries, the age distribution is increasingly skewed to the older end, which means more burden on the shrinking working-age population to create wealth and to care for their elders. Third is the question of quality and safety in patient care. This demands accurate data, excellent systems of tracking and monitoring, and sophisticated influencing abilities over highly qualified professionals. Even in countries such as the UK, which boasts a national health service stretching back to 1948 and an elaborate professional regulation infrastructure, inquiries into failures of care, which first started in the 1960s, continue today, without the basic lessons being learnt and applied. These governance failures are replicated worldwide (Walshe and Shortell, 2004).

Fourth is the confounding factor of politics in healthcare, which nationally drives successive top-down reorganizations and restructurings (Klein, 1998), and which locally 'interferes with' evidence-based reconfigurations of services. Political astuteness in manoeuvring around this is called for (Waring et al., 2022). Fifth is increasing consumer demands and steadily increasing dissatisfaction with services, requiring a response that is both economic, for example, through the construction and implementation of technical prioritization tools, and socio-emotional, for example, through ensuring the design and delivery of services that are 'patient-centred'. Sixth is the power of the professionals, particularly doctors, who deliver the services and who can sabotage attempts to make changes if they make no sense to them (Goodwin, 2006). The only realistic way forward is through co-ownership, management by influence and distributed forms of leadership (Badaracco, 2001). Seventh, there is a growing acknowledgement that health services are managed more effectively in health systems that cross institutional boundaries than within single organizations (Pratt et al., 1999), which requires consideration of multi-form and multi-level governance and collaborative forms of leadership. Finally, technological advances are a financial challenge, as mentioned earlier, but also a significant opportunity requiring courageous system leadership: the Human Genome Project (International Human Genome Sequencing Consortium, 2004) and artificial intelligence, for example, now enable the personalizing of diagnostics and treatments for a range of conditions to the individual in ways that were recently unimaginable; and implementation of e-health strategies enables disruptive innovation in the way in which services and associated information systems are designed and delivered.

It should be emphasized that there are enduring themes in stakeholder power in the governance of all types of health systems (for example, whether social health insurance operated or tax-funded, privately provided or government run). These include the complementary or conflicting roles of healthcare professionals, politicians, civil servants, professional managers and citizens, all contributing to a crowded scene, which will now be explored.

System-level governance

A number of different elucidations of the term governance exist, all of which revolve around the notion of control, using different mechanisms. Within a political science paradigm, Pierre and Peters (2000) argue that, at a state level, governance revolves around the capacity of government to make and implement policy – in other words, to guide society. This is increasingly viewed as a 'steering' rather than a 'rowing' function (Osborne and Gaebler, 1993).

Within healthcare, Davies et al. (2005) examine markets, hierarchies and networks as the main contrasting forms of governance, relating these to different incentives and hence to different outcomes. Newman (2005) notes that each mode of governance has its own form of leader: for example, an administrative leader in a bureaucracy, a competitive leader in a market, and a putatively transformational one in a network.

Smith et al. (2012) argue that the main components of system governance are priority setting, performance monitoring and accountability arrangements. Expanding this perspective, Greer and Wismar in this volume (Chapter 8: Global health: governance in a new geopolitical era) refers to the multipolarity of the aims and goals of global health governance and outlines the very different governance practices in different areas of the world.

In particular, the politics involved in the oversight of healthcare services comes sharply into focus during crises. Box 2.2 contrasts the main features in five high-income countries, listed in descending order of the size of the population, of the political choices made and the governance mechanisms used to manage the biggest health crisis of a generation, the COVID-19 pandemic of 2020–2023. All countries struggled with the challenges created by the pandemic, but their responses reflected different cultures, leadership and governance. A threat on the scale of COVID-19 requires a degree of centralization of leadership, but how central government is organized, and how it works with devolved administrations, local politicians, community leaders and local healthcare leaders with expertise to contribute becomes germane (Ham, 2023: 479).

The experiences of the five countries outlined signal the relevance of the cultural and political contexts, especially in terms of how easy it is for rules to be enforced, and the extent of the room for manoeuvre for country level leaders in devolved systems. The experiences also demonstrate the consequences of political choices that were made about prioritizing the economy over the safety of citizens, and about choosing to ignore or to draw upon scientific knowledge and the expertise of other health experts.

Institution-level governance

Mirroring the intent of system level governance, at the institution level, governance is concerned with setting direction for an organization, and about exercising control. This is evidenced both by the architecture of governance (organization structures and so on) and by the enactment of governance, including the exercise of leadership, which there is more of later in this chapter.

The term 'governance' has only relatively recently gained currency as a distinct entity within the study of the management of organizations. The development of the debate around governance can be largely traced to incidents relating to the high-profile organization failures of the early 1990s (Maxwell, Polly Peck, Barings Bank), the US corporate scandals (Enron, WorldCom) a few years later and those which continued into this century, such as Equity Life, Parmalat, banking failures (that heralded the global economic recession of 2008–9) and more recent Silicon Valley failures, such as Theranos. The problem is international (Kakabadse and Kakabadse, 2008; Charan et al., 2014). The responses to these events have provided much of the impetus for clarifying concepts of 'good' governance and have also framed the discussions around the management of corporate risk.

At an institution level, the OECD (2015: 11) defines corporate governance as '. . . the structure through which the objectives of the company are set, and the means of attaining those objectives and monitoring performance are determined'. The Langlands review of governance for public services in the UK outlined the following as the function of governance: 'to ensure that an organisation or partnership fulfils its overall purpose, achieves its intended outcomes for citizens and service users, and operates in an effective, efficient and ethical manner' (Independent Commission for Good Governance in Public Services, 2004: 7).

Box 2.2 Management of the COVID-19 pandemic in five high-income countries

Country	United States of America (USA)	United Kingdom (UK)	United Arab Emirates (UAE)	Singapore	New Zealand
Population	334 million	67.6 million	9.8 million	5.4 million	5.3 million
Deaths from Covid-19	1,191,065	232,112	2,349	1,933	5,293
Response	- Defined by division of power between US state governments and federal government. - Much of the policy and technology was driven by individual state decisions. - Palpable tension between desire to re-open economy to mitigate financial hardship and efforts to contain spread of virus and reduce health impacts (Bergquist et al., 2020).	- Late awakening to severity of situation – Followed by highly centralized command and control approach that mirrors centralized nature of healthcare policy decision-making in the UK.	- UAE has transformed from an obscure desert nation to a wealthy, multicultural society. - Typical Middle Eastern leadership style emphasizes status and lengthy consensus building. - Ottoman hierarchical systems of government are also entrenched. -Evidence of a departure from the usual low charismatic style of leadership seen in other countries in the region.	- Singapore learned valuable lessons from handling severe acute respiratory syndrome and H1N1 outbreaks in 2003 and 2009. -Response to COVID-19 also underpinned by strong Confucian value of personal learning, collectivism and long-term orientation, and a culture of following strict rules imposed by government for the greater good.	- One of New Zealand's leading characteristics is its geographical remoteness from other countries. -Led by prime minister, and with high levels of community co-operation, the government chose to shut its borders for a lengthy period and focused on an elimination strategy before vaccines became widely available.

Country	United States of America (USA)	United Kingdom (UK)	United Arab Emirates (UAE)	Singapore	New Zealand
Main criticisms	- Early on, US president provided overly optimistic assumptions about scale and severity of virus and ignored the emerging scientific knowledge about how to treat the virus and contain the spread. - Pandemic impact reverberated throughout health system in every state, as healthcare use fell and deaths from drug overdoses and treatable causes rose (Commonwealth Fund, 2022).	- Poor emergency planning - No spare capacity in health and social systems to cope with surges in demand for care - Discharging of elderly patients with COVID-19 from hospitals into care homes, leading to high levels of mortality in the residential care sector - Delays in implementing restrictions at start and in subsequent waves. - Over-centralized decision making by the prime minister. - Delays in testing - Vacillations in policy making, e.g. mask wearing, social distancing, restrictions on gatherings. - Poor collaboration with local agencies and local partners (Ham, 2023).	-Overall preparedness only ranked at 56th out of 195 countries in the Global Health Security Index (Abbas et al., 2021)	- Initial implementation of home recovery programme, to avoid overwhelming hospitals not initially a success, causing confusion for population (Csiszar et al., 2023).	- Known problems in healthcare system infrastructure led to lack of preparedness (Cumming, 2022). - Initial strategy was fine, but it has been argued that execution lacked adaptability and agility, and implementation was also poor because it was politicized (Gorman and Horn, 2023).

Country	United States of America (USA)	United Kingdom (UK)	United Arab Emirates (UAE)	Singapore	New Zealand
Main achievements	- Efforts made by the states that ran the strongest healthcare system. The toll varied significantly state by state with those with the strongest health systems having lower rates of preventable deaths and healthier populations. (Commonwealth Fund, 2022).	-Speedy development and approval of a safe vaccine. - Roll-out of vaccination programme, drawing on teamwork within NHS at all levels and use of private sector, voluntary organizations and army (Ham, 2023).	- Capital city, Abu Dhabi, seen as safest city during the pandemic (Deep Knowledge Analytics Global, 2021). - Government response to pandemic was aggressive, decisive and comprehensive, from mass testing facilities, enforcing compliance with lockdowns, establishment of field hospitals, street cleaning and a vigorous vaccination programme. - Continuous co-ordination, collaboration and communication across agencies was a feature of the modus operandi (Csiszar et al., 2023).	- Decisive actions taken by Multi-Ministry Taskforce using collective multi-agency leadership, incl. experts from academia, healthcare, engineering and information technology companies. - Government created opportunities for citizens to take part in 'Emerging Stronger' conversations for new normal post-pandemic to build an inclusive and more humanistic vision for the future (Csiszar et al., 2023).	- Focal points were public health protection, following the science, and the use of the precautionary principle in the face of uncertainty. - 'Going hard and early' considered the right approach for these circumstances (Cumming, 2022). - Life expectancy actually rose during first 18 months of the pandemic (Baker and Wilson, 2022).

At the apex of corporate governance is usually the board. There are various board structures and other governance models in use in health services. There are non-executive boards, executive boards, two-tier boards and unitary boards. And there are models for different health service purposes: for insurers, commissioners, providers and partnerships (cross public sector and public/private). Board membership is achieved through different processes of nomination, appointment and election, and can be paid or unpaid. Many authors argue that board composition does and should vary according to circumstances (Chambers, 2013; Chambers et al., 2020; Aly et al., 2022).

As well as national, geographical, cultural, market, sectoral and service differences, the following are often mentioned as key variables: organization life cycle (start-up, mature, decline), stability compared with transformation or crisis, and degree of professionalization of the workforce. Institutional boards vary widely, according to political input (*Eurohealth*, 2013). For example, public hospitals in New Zealand are governed by an elected District Health Board, and healthcare organizations in Sweden are run by elected County Councils. This kind of participative mechanism no longer exists in France, although the local mayor used to chair the hospital board before the advent of New Public Management reforms in 2009 (Simonet, 2023). In Germany, the principle of co-determination ensures that in their dual board arrangement for healthcare insurance companies and providers, trade unions' representatives are at the centre of decision-making (Chambers et al., 2013).

While public ownership is predominant in the European hospital sector, there have been changes in recent years in hospital governance and in the level of autonomy that management and supervisory boards can exercise. England, France and Italy, for example, have all taken different approaches to implementing hospital governance changes over the past couple of decades (see Chambers et al., 2016).

Board structures

Taking the case of England in more detail, since 1990, local boards in the English NHS have been derived in structure from the Anglo-Saxon private sector unitary board model that predominates in UK and US business (Ferlie et al., 1996; Garratt, 1997). The unitary board typically comprises a chair, chief executive, executive directors and a majority of appointed independent (or non-executive) directors. All members of the board bear collective responsibility for the performance of the enterprise. Meanwhile, NHS Foundation Trusts, first established in 2004, are independent public benefit corporations modelled on co-operative and mutual traditions, which by 2022 totalled 215, including ten ambulance organizations (Kings Fund, 2023). Some Foundation Trusts are responsible for more than one hospital. Foundation Trusts have two boards – a board of governors (of up to about fifty people) constructed of individuals elected from local community membership, and a board of directors (around eleven people) made up of a chair and non-executive directors appointed by the governors, and a chief executive and executive directors, appointed by the chair and approved by the governors. This whole structure resembles the Anglo-Saxon unitary board model we have seen previously adopted by the English NHS, but nested within a two-tier European or Senate model, commonly found in the Netherlands, France and Germany.

The Senate model comprises a lower-tier operational board that deals with management and strategic issues and an upper-tier supervisory board that ratifies certain decisions taken by the operational board, sets the direction and represents the different interests in the company, particularly those of shareholders and employees (Johnson et al., 2005). This model can be seen, for example, in public hospitals in the Belgian system, which have a four-part governance structure comprising a constituent authority, hospital board, executive committee and medical council (Eeckloo et al., 2004).

From the US perspective, Pointer (1999) outlines four types of boards commonly found within US healthcare. Parent boards govern freestanding, independently owned institutions; subsidiary boards are local boards of large enterprises; advisory boards provide steer and guidance without a formal corporate governance role; and affiliate organization boards serve their members' interests.

Within the four countries of the UK, with the advent of devolution, there have been deepening policy differences (for example, in the role of the market) and an increasing divergence in the structures for managing health services. The Welsh board model is stakeholder-based with up to 25 members on each board, resembling the English NHS pre-1990. Scotland has an integrated health model and a unified board structure with strong local authority representation.

Purpose of boards

What are boards for? There is a common view that boards are there to set strategy and goals, to set the organization norms of behaviour and to monitor the performance of the organization against those goals. Beyond that, much of the territory is deeply contested. Boards were developed as a result of the growing commercial complexity of business and the gradual separation of ownership from control. Boards represented the interests of absent owners or shareholders (the principals), and management became the agents of the board (Pointer, 1999). The earliest theory about boards was agency theory based on the notion that the shareholders' and managers' interests are likely to be different and that the behaviours of both sets of actors are characterized by self-interested opportunism (Berle and Means, 1932).

Other theories developed later and are summarized in detail in a literature review (Chambers et al., 2017). These include managerial hegemony (according to which the managers rather than the owners make the key decisions), stewardship theory (in which managers and owners share a common agenda and interests), resource dependency theory (in which the main role of the board is to maximize benefits of external dependencies), and stakeholder theory (according to which board members represent the different interests of members and communities with a stake in the organization).

Board behaviour can be related to the (sometimes unconscious) orientation of individual board members towards these different theories. Agency theory is connected to a challenging and defensive set of behaviours in the boardroom. Stewardship theory puts a premium on a high trust and collaborative style of working, with the potential disadvantage of low challenge and groupthink. In a stakeholder model, board members tend to be most engaged when articulating the interests of 'their' constituency or special interests. A resource dependency model, with members appointed for their external connections and political and social capital, can result in a 'trophy' board with inadequate grip on the business. With managerial hegemony, the board is disempowered by a chief executive and management team who control the agenda and predetermine the outcome of meetings – with the board reduced to 'rubber-stamping.'

None of these models are of themselves, in all circumstances, right or wrong, but dysfunctional boards can occur, whatever their composition and structure, when there is a conflict between members about what the fundamental *raison d'être* of the board is, or where there is a disjuncture between the prevailing circumstances and challenges, and the characteristics, disposition and activities of that board.

Related to this are theories about the sources and use of board power, including the power of the chief executive (Herman, 1981), the discretionary effort and skill exercised by non-executive board members (Pettigrew and McNulty, 1995), and the increased role of the board in periods of crisis or transition (Lorsch and MacIver, 1989), which can be followed by 'coasting' according to stress/inertia theory (Jas and Skelcher, 2005). These ideas suggest that board members have enormous discretion, whatever the governance arrangements, about how they deploy their power and skill for the benefit of the organization and for the benefit of patients.

The above summary suggests that simplistic theories of how boards *should* work are unlikely to fit all circumstances. In particular, a binary view is inadequate for the task, such as proposing that either agency or stewardship is preferable for institution governance, in the same way as neither principal-agent governance nor network governance theories adequately sum up the way forward for good state governance. Utilizing a realist approach (Pawson, 2006), the likely organization performance outcomes from particular board theories-in-use and mechanisms deployed in different contexts are posited in Table 2.1.

Board practices

How do boards operate in practice? An understanding of the inner workings of boards is helped by considering separately three elements: composition (board structure), focus (what the board does) and dynamics (the behavioural dimension). In addition, there are some important distinguishing characteristics of boards in the public, non-profit and healthcare sectors (Chambers et al., 2017). Here, social performance (public value) as well as financial performance is a core purpose. The main mission of a healthcare organization is to serve patients. Mid Staffordshire NHS Foundation Trust in the UK is an example of an organization that lost sight of this purpose (see Box 2.3).

Table 2.1 A realist framework for healthcare boards

Theory	Contextual assumptions	Mechanism	Intended outcome
Agency	Low trust, high challenge and low appetite for risk	Control through intense internal and external and regulatory performance monitoring	Minimization of risk and good patient safety record
Stewardship	High trust, less challenge and greater appetite for risk	Board support for management in a collective leadership endeavour	Service improvement and excellence in performance
Resource dependency	Importance of social capital of the organization; collaboration seen as more productive than competition	Institution boundary spanning and close dialogue with other healthcare providers	Improved external reputation and relationships
Stakeholder	Importance of representation; risk is shared by many	Collaboration and consensus building	Sustainable organization with high levels of staff engagement and good long-term prospects

Source: adapted from Chambers et al. (2013).

Box 2.3　Case study – example of a failing board: Mid Staffordshire NHS Foundation Trust in England

The Mid Staffordshire NHS Trust scandal was about poor care and a high mortality rate and first came to light in 2007. Press reports suggested that substandard care led to the unnecessary deaths of up to 1200 patients between 2005 and 2008. An investigation, followed by two inquiries, found significant evidence of neglect of patients. Compensation was paid to families and a number of healthcare professionals have subsequently been struck off professional registers (Francis, 2010; Francis, 2013).

Robert Francis KC, who chaired the second public inquiry, made clear the culpability of the trust board in his letter to the Secretary of State for Health: '. . . the story . . . told is first and foremost of appalling suffering of many patients. This was primarily caused by a serious failure on the part of a provider Trust Board. It did not listen sufficiently to its patients and staff or ensure the correction of deficiencies brought to the Trust's attention. Above all, it failed to tackle an insidious negative culture involving a tolerance of poor standards and a disengagement from managerial and leadership responsibilities' (Francis, 2013).

Non-profit board members tend to invest more of their time and are more predisposed to 'managerial work' than their for-profit counterparts. But accountabilities on public boards may be blurred as a result of the influence of political patronage and the subversion of formal authority. Finally, as has been signalled earlier in this chapter, healthcare governance of individual organizations is increasingly embedded within a complex superordinate and subordinate governance network, which stretches across organizations that are interdependent in a healthcare system (Chambers et al., 2017).

Choosing the appropriate mechanisms (whether they be around board composition, board focus or board behaviours) to achieve the desired outcomes appears to be important according to the particular situation. For stable organizations, increased monitoring and a strengthened rein on a powerful chief executive officer (CEO), if they have been in position for some time, may be indicated (in accordance with agency theory), in contrast to a focus on boundary spanning and on the external environment (in accordance with resource dependency theory) in circumstances of turbulence, threat and reputation issues. A framework for understanding how full-service, dynamic and diligent healthcare boards can be guided to choose to operate depending on circumstances in order to produce specific outcomes is depicted in Figure 2.1.

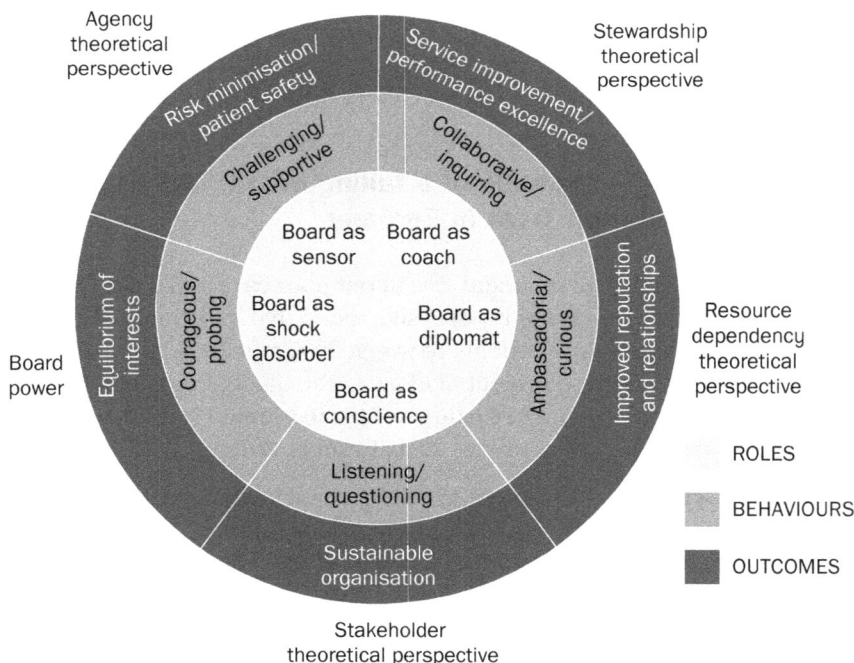

Figure 2.1 Interconnectedness of roles, behaviours and outcomes of the full-service diligent and dynamic healthcare board
Source: Adapted from Chambers et al. (2020).

A number of reports published following the Francis Inquiry in the UK offer advice for boards. These all emphasize the need for boards to focus on hearing the patient voice, gaining assurance on patient safety and clinical quality of services using accurate and timely data, ensuring board-level involvement of clinicians in decision-making, and improving and learning from staff engagement. The classic Good Governance Standard for Public Services (2004) remains a valuable touchstone for assessing the degree to which public bodies are fit for purpose (see Learning activity 2.1).

Learning activity 2.1

Answer the following questions to find out how far your organization meets the tests of the Good Governance Standard for Public Services (adapted from the Independent Commission on Good Governance in Public Services, 2004).

1   Good governance means focusing on the organization's purpose and on outcomes for citizens and service users.
    - What is this organization for?
    - What is being done to improve services?
    - Can I easily find out about the organization's funding and how it spends its money?
2   Good governance means performing effectively in clearly defined functions and roles.
    - Who is in charge of the organization?
    - How are they elected or appointed?
    - At the top of the organization, who is responsible for what?
3   Good governance means promoting values for the whole organization and demonstrating the values of good governance through behaviour.
    - According to the organization, what values guide its work?
    - What standards of behaviour should I expect from the organization?
    - Do the senior people put into practice the 'Nolan' principles for people in public life (selflessness, integrity, objectivity, accountability, openness, honesty and leadership)? (Nolan, 1994)
4   Good governance means taking informed transparent decisions and managing risk.
    - Who is responsible for what kinds of decisions?
    - Can I easily find out what decisions have been taken and the reasons for them?
    - Does the organization publish a clear annual statement on the effectiveness of its risk management system?
5   Good governance means developing the capacity and capability of the governing body to be effective.

Continued

Learning activity 2.1   *Continued*

- How does the organization encourage people to get involved in running it?
- What support does it provide for people to get involved?
- How does the organization make sure that all those running it are doing a good job?

6   Good governance means engaging stakeholders and making accountability real.

- Are there opportunities for me and other people to make our views known?
- How can I go about asking the people in charge about their plans and decisions?
- Can I easily find out how to complain and who to contact with suggestions for changes?

Depending on what your answers are, make time to speak to executive and non-executive directors to investigate further the governance processes and structures in your organization.

Approaches to accountability: structures, processes and impacts

How can governments and the public be assured that good practices are being followed to ensure that the triple aims of quality of patient care, population health improvement and efficiency in the use of resources are being followed?

Learning activity 2.2 offers an opportunity for individual citizens, including healthcare staff, to assess the effectiveness of their own local governance arrangements.

Learning activity 2.2

Board observation exercise to assess board effectiveness.

Ask to attend a board meeting at your local hospital or other healthcare provider, commissioner or insurer and, if possible, obtain the board papers (agenda, minutes, other documents) in advance. Some board meetings are held in public and therefore permission to attend is not required.

- Note the focus of discussion, decisions and the behaviours at the board meeting.
- Locate your observations in the framework for understanding the work of boards in Table 2.1.
- What are the strengths and weaknesses of this board?
- What do your findings indicate about the characteristics of this board, this organization and its leadership?

We have already touched on the different forms of governance and oversight regimes in our reference to the debate about hierarchies, markets and networks (Davies et al., 2005). Mechanisms of accountability are now discussed in terms of theory and in practice.

Governments introducing quasi-markets in healthcare in a hollowed-out state still wish to avoid uncontrolled market forces that could adversely affect these politically sensitive services. A solution is to construct accountability arrangements that keep a degree of state control over increasingly independent healthcare providers (Sheaff et al., 2015). A framework to understand healthcare purchasing or commissioning has been proposed that supplements the markets–hierarchy–networks trichotomy of governance structures with a more nuanced, specific account (Sheaff et al., 2015), which introduces six modes of power. First, managerial performance is associated with the normative cycle of assessing health needs, developing a service specification, procurement and the monitoring of performance. Second, negotiated order involves managing conflicts through relational contracting and making use of social capital already accumulated in relationships between key stakeholders. Third, discursive control, which can include soft coercion, rests on the use of prevailing ideologies about either what is considered 'important' or 'right' (for example, driving down waiting times for care) or what is considered to be evidence-based, using a clinical scientific paradigm. Fourth is the use of financial incentives and penalties, which draw on the influence of resource dependencies on the behaviour of healthcare providers. Fifth is the use of or the threat of provider competition, which, when prices are fixed, arguably, improves the quality of hospital care. Sixth is juridical governance, which concerns the use of contracts and the legal system for enforcement (Sheaff et al., 2015: 8–13).

The findings from case study research in three countries (England, Germany, Italy) found that the first three of these modes were widely reported to be in use but that managerial performance of providers was more effective in Germany because they had more complete contracts (deterring less off-contract work) and because of the right of insurers to inspect medical records to check whether treatments were necessary and had been correctly invoiced. Negotiated order in the case of England included micro-commissioning and often protracted discussions over detail to achieve agreed outcomes between purchaser and provider. Discursive control was the third medium of power widely cited and with significant impact: in England this was particularly associated with national policy diktats and local loyalties to local healthcare organizations. By contrast, juridical governance – the holding to account through the use of the contract mechanism – was used only exceptionally in all three countries (Sheaff et al., 2015: 88–9). Neither the use of provider competition nor the use of financial incentives, although frequently referenced by case study informants, were reported to be particularly effective in controlling or holding providers to account.

Actions have consequences. Accountability also includes the possibility of the imposition of sanctions if a standard is not met. Synthesizing from an extensive literature review, which identified sixty governance attributes, Greer et al. (2016) posit five health system governance categories of which the foremost is accountability; as the authors state: 'Accountability has a number of virtues that make it popular, perhaps foundational, in discussions of good governance. Without it, all kinds of incompetence, shirking, bloat and malversation are possible' (2016: 34). Good accountability includes the appropriate use of discretion to minimize bureaucratic rigidity. Effective accountability also means clarity about who is accountable to whom and mechanisms that are workable, avoiding the trap of entanglement in a web of accountability (Tuohy, 2003).

The changing and distinctive features of healthcare leadership

If governance and accountability are about setting direction and exercising control, leadership is the human enactment of this process of steering and controlling organizations and the individuals within them. Competing theories of leadership are the subject of intense academic scrutiny and a voluminous literature (see, for example, Bass and Bass, 2008; Storey et al., 2010; Northouse, 2021; Chambers, 2023). One of the characteristics of this literature is the extent to which evidence relating to each of the theories is contested and 'old' paradigms are rejected in favour of 'new' ones. This translates for managers into frames of reference around leadership that are constantly changing.

Healthcare system leadership

In addition to flux around the dominant narratives pertaining to leadership in general, there are challenges peculiar to complex public healthcare systems, especially reconciling quality and safety with financial and efficiency pressures, both individualizing and standardizing the healthcare offer, and managing the politics, including the power of the professions.

A body of theory gaining momentum in the public sector is predicated on the notion that the study of leadership based on the individual may be outmoded. Within organizations, there is a growing need for *distributed* leadership – exercised by the many rather than by a few – to tackle challenges, manage change and drive improvement in today's fast-paced times, and in acknowledgement that solo heroic leadership may have had its day (Badaracco, 2001). Second, with the growth of system management and network governance, there is a push for inter-organizational collaboration, or leadership that is *shared* across organizations (Brookes and Grint, 2010). Collective leadership, a combination of distributed and shared approaches, is argued by these authors to be the foundation of New Public Leadership (NPL). This builds on some of the concepts of New Public Management (NPM), such as continuous improvement and performance management, with a shift in emphasis away from measuring targets to incorporate the idea of public value, from Moore's (1995) work and from the notion of collaborative advantage (Brookes, 2010).

How do notions of public leadership apply in the healthcare sector? The concept of networks, collaborations, partnerships and integrated care organizations that plan, commission or purchase, and deliver health services now abounds. These 'chains of care' extend across health service institutions (e.g. hospitals and primary healthcare), across professions (e.g., clinical networks) and across sectors (e.g. joint commissioning units for health and social care). Different forms of chains of care can be found in government-operated health systems, such as the UK, in countries with social health insurance, such as the Netherlands, and in pro-market outliers, such as the United States. Operating in all such systems, Goodwin (2006) has proposed four main interconnected variables from his research that resonate strongly with the public leadership discourse. These include the quality of the leadership team as perceived by others (this would be an example of distributed leadership); the history and current strength of inter-organizational relations; the development of alliances; and the extent of power sharing across organizations (these last three being examples of shared leadership).

Given the increasing prominence in later iterations of theories of new public management that are given to networked governance and to performance management of programmes rather than institutions, this emerging public leadership discourse has a distinctive attraction, although empirical evidence to underpin the theory remains sparse (Brookes, 2010). In addition, the concept of system leadership remains under-theorized, with the distinctive features of this kind of leadership, which makes it stand apart from qualities of other kinds of leaders, so far not well understood, and with a paucity of empirical evidence (Kaehne et al., 2022). This is important since the embedding of integrated care as a principle of health and care practices and processes, which is the focus of Chapter 15 of this volume, can only be enabled by effective system leadership.

A situational approach to leadership

We have argued that the cultural context for healthcare leadership in many countries in the Global North has thus shifted from traditional bureaucracy (leaders were administrators or hospital secretaries) to managerialism (leaders were executives in a unified system) to a quasi-marketized or networked system (leaders are executives of either purchasing, competing, contracting or provider healthcare organizations). Furthermore, if we apply the theory that leadership is situational, it follows that different styles and characteristics are appropriate in different parts of healthcare systems (for example, in primary care, mental health, hospital care, planning and provision) and in different countries. Taking primary care, the current scale and scope of which is outlined in Chapter 13 of this book, Chambers and Colin-Thome (2009) have argued that, because of the context, doctors who thrive in primary care in general are likely to be people who prefer working in networks rather than hierarchies, show clinical and managerial entrepreneurial spirit, are tolerant of ambiguity and uncertainty, are inherently optimistic, are personally resilient and can see both the 'big picture' and be concerned with detail. It would not be difficult, by extension, to argue that hospital work may suit leaders with different preferences, since the hierarchical element is likely to be relatively stronger.

The unique feature of healthcare leadership is the role of clinicians in management. There is growing evidence of an association between involvement in the management of clinicians, from the board to the front line, and improvements in organization performance (Bohmer, 2012; Chambers et al., 2013; Veronesi et al., 2014; Savage et al., 2020). Doctors have considerable 'soft' power. The social construction of leadership (Grint, 2005) can be seen in how the medical elite is formed and sustained. This elite draws on sources of reward, position, referent and expert power (see French and Raven, 1959) and, through the medium of the consultation, continuously re-enact this power and reinforce followership in patients, junior colleagues and other professions ancillary to medicine. But for clinicians, the transition from clinical practice to a managerial role can be difficult. They can experience a profound clash between their professional and managerial identities and have to find ways of reconciling conflicting loyalties and ideologies, such as around the needs of individual patients versus population groups and what change can be implemented on the basis of evidence versus realpolitik (Walshe and Chambers, 2010).

The role of leaders is to some extent prescribed by the structures that are in place. These change over time. Since the Second World War, the Netherlands, which operates a compulsory social health insurance funded system, has had three reorganizations, and is currently operating in a quasi-marketized system in which there is competition among purchasers as well as providers. In England, by contrast, which has endured reorganization more than most countries, seven major reorganizations have affected governance structures since 1948 (in 1972, 1984, 1990, 2001, 2006, 2012 and 2022). This has consequences for the enactment of leadership in circumstances of uncertainty and policy churn.

Themes and patterns in the quality of healthcare leadership

Restructuring facilitates and accelerates the turnover of leaders, which leads to the loss of experienced and high-performing as well as under-performing leaders. A positive association between length of tenure of CEOs and better organization performance has been identified in a number of studies, although the extant literature is limited and somewhat contradictory (Simsek, 2007; Ballardini and Fabbri, 2011; Pryce and Chambers, 2011). A study of long serving CEOs in the NHS in England found personal characteristics that relate to high levels of emotional intelligence. They were adaptable to change and retained self-confidence and resilience during periods of organizational flux, combined with an ability to examine their feelings and motives (Chambers and Exworthy, 2021). By contrast, a study in Tuscany in Italy found no significant correlation between organization performance with length of tenure of the general managers (equivalent to CEOs). More important in this study, were the strengths of managerial competencies, particularly those linked to the information-sharing process developed into the organizations, including benchmarking of performance results (Vainieri et al., 2019). This focus on information sharing links to the work of Fulop and Ramsay (2019), who argue that it is the way in which health leaders operate that impacts positively on clinical quality improvement efforts. In particular, these leaders support system-wide clinical staff engagement in improvement activity and, where necessary, challenge professional interests and resistance. They are outward facing, learn from others and manage external influences. Leadership for quality improvement is explored in more detail in Chapter 4 of this volume. Drawing upon these themes, Learning activity 2.3 offers an opportunity for readers to identify and reflect on their own leadership qualities and areas for development based on a theoretically informed model in use in the NHS in England.

Learning activity 2.3

The Healthcare Leadership Model in England.

This model is intended to help to develop leaders in healthcare at all levels and in all settings. There are nine dimensions with five levels of performance against each (insufficient, essential, proficient, strong and exemplary) and a low/high performance rating of each depending on job role. It is free to complete online (following registration) as a personal assessment tool and generates an individual personal report on strengths and areas for development.

The nine dimensions are:

1   Inspiring shared purpose
2   Leading with care
3   Evaluating information
4   Connecting our service
5   Sharing the vision
6   Engaging the team
7   Holding to account
8   Developing capability
9   Influencing for results.

Exercise: Complete the free online assessment tool and access the report that the tool generates personally for you.

- What are your strengths?
- What are your development needs as a healthcare leader?
- How do these results relate to the importance of particular leadership dimensions in your current job role?
- What actions are you going to take to be a better leader?
- Who will you share this with?

See http://www.leadershipacademy.nhs.uk/resources/healthcare-leadership-model/

Notwithstanding the existence of 'good' leadership, its characteristics and its impacts in the healthcare setting, there is increasing evidence of the prevalence of poorer leadership, and the impacts of variations in the quality of leadership on health outcomes. West and Bailey (2023) argue that too often the focus is on surface-level enactments of leadership to improve quality, access and cost-effectiveness, neglecting features of organization cultures and subcultures that can drive and sustain potentially destructive leadership behaviours. These authors also report links between poorer staff well-being and engagement, lack of clarity about goals and effective teamworking, with lower rates of patient satisfaction, patient safety failures and compassionate care (West and Bailey, 2023).

Internationally, there is growing evidence that changing organization culture in healthcare is deeply problematic and tricky. Poorer performing organizations tend to remain so for lengthy periods. Evidence emerged, for example, in the Veterans Health Association in the US of high death rates during surgery in the 1980s and despite a significant quality improvement and transformation programme in the 1990s, a further scandal erupted in 2014 of lengthy waiting times and unspent budgets (Chambers, 2023). In South Australia, the inquiry into the Oakden facility found that unacceptable care persisted for over a decade without the knowledge and intervention on the part of authorities who had responsibility to act. Simply closing the facility was deemed a wholly inadequate way to 'fix the problem' (ICAC, 2018). In the UK, despite over 50 years of public inquiries into failures of care, similar themes recur over time, all related to poor culture (Powell and Walshe, 2019).

Conclusion

What does this analysis mean for healthcare managers and what they need to know and what evidence they need to pay attention to? Hospitals and other healthcare providers offer healthcare on a day-to-day basis as well as delivering policy objectives. They face crises and experience serendipity. They may operate in either a context of intense competition or a monopoly. We have argued earlier that there is no one simple model of how their boards *should* operate but there is evidence about what works in different circumstances, and there are consequences in terms of outcomes in their choice of *modus operandi*. The embeddedness of healthcare governance across networks and the coming of community-based models of care does suggest that a stakeholder model of governance, with an effort to build long-term collaborations and consensus, and to improve patient experience and staff engagement, is needed. Current healthcare governance forms are arguably more suited to the institutional level and may be less fit for purpose as we move to more out-of-hospital care and to system and programme, rather than institution, accountability. These differing and changing organizational, strategic and cultural contexts call for sophistication in leadership repertoires in the healthcare setting.

There remains the sticky question of persistent variation in the quality of leadership. Services facing similar challenges and with similar levels of resources result in different outcomes, depending on the quality of leadership. We do not yet know enough about why this is. Underlying this question is also a concern about the robustness of the moral and ethical underpinnings of leadership practice in the healthcare domain. The future sustainability of healthcare systems will depend on grasping the paradox of leadership, which is both technology enabled and also humane, with a more dispersed distribution of power across a more diversified workforce and with more fully engaged patients and communities.

Learning resources

Comparative healthcare systems performance: These two sites illuminate differences in country healthcare system performance and offer a valuable starting point for insights into the impacts of varying governance arrangements [https://www.oecd.org/health/health-at-a-glance/];

[https://www.commonwealthfund.org/series/mirror-mirror-comparing-health-systems-across-countries].

Good Governance Guide: A set of resources on governance in the international context, including the application of governance principles to government itself [http://www.goodgovernance.org.au/about-good-governance/what-is-good-governance/].

UK Corporate Governance Code: Includes guidance and reports on board effectiveness and related areas produced by the Financial Reporting Council [https://www.frc.org.uk/library/standards-codes-policy/corporate-governance/uk-corporate-governance-code/].

Personal values: This site provides free information about the importance of understanding personal values and how these connect to leadership behaviours [https://www.discoveryourvalues.com/free-personal-values-assessment].

Leadership for equality, diversity and inclusion: There are various online tests to find out your personal unconscious biases will affect how you practise inclusive leadership. This one is developed by Harvard University [https://www.implicit.harvard.edu/implicit/takeatest.html].

References

Abbas, Z., Ahamed, F., Ganesan, S., Warren, K. and Koshy, A. (2021) COVID-19 crisis management: lessons from the United Arab Emirates leaders, *Frontiers in Public Health* [www.frontiersin.org/journals/public-health/articles/10.3389/fpubh.2021.724494; accessed 22 March 2024].

Aly, D., Abdelqader, M., Darwish, T.K. and Scott, K. (2022) The impact of healthcare board characteristics on NHS trust performance, *Public Money & Management*, 43 (6): 594–601. https://doi.org/10.1080/09540962.2021.2022272.

Badaracco, J. (2001) We don't need another hero, *Harvard Business Review*, September, 111–16.

Baker, M. and Wilson, N. (2022) New Zealand's Covid strategy. *The Guardian*, 5 April 2022 [https://www.theguardian.com/world/commentisfree/2022/apr/05/new-zealands-covid-strategy-was-one-of-the-worlds-most-successful-what-can-we-learn-from-it; accessed 4 December 2024].

Ballardini, E. and Fabbri, D. (2011) Top executives turnover, politics and performance of healthcare providers: evidence from the Italian NHS. *Pavia* 19–20 Settembre, in Vainieri, M., Ferrè, F., Giacomelli, G. and Nuti, S. Explaining performance in health care: How and when top management competencies make the difference, *Health Care Management Review*, 2019 Oct/Dec; 44 (4): 306–317. doi: 10.1097/HMR.0000000000000164. PMID: 28448307; PMCID: PMC6749958.

Bass, B. and Bass, R. (2008) *Bass and Stogdill's Handbook of Leadership.* New York: Simon & Schuster.

Bergquist, S., Otten, T. and Sarich, N. (2020) COVID-19 pandemic in the United States, *Health Policy and Technology*, Dec; 9 (4): 623–638. doi: 10.1016/j.hlpt.2020.08.007. Epub 2020 Aug 27. PMID: 32874854; PMCID: PMC7451131.

Berle, A.A. and Means, G.C. (1932) *The Modern Corporation and Private Property.* New Brunswick, NJ: Transaction Publishers.

Blank, R. and Burau, V. (2013) *Comparative Health Policy.* Basingstoke: Palgrave Macmillan.

Bohmer, R. (2012) *The Instrumental Value of Medical Leadership.* London: The King's Fund.

Brookes, S. (2010) Reform, realisation and restoration: public leadership and innovation in government, in S. Brookes and K. Grint (eds) *A New Public Leadership Challenge?* Basingstoke: Palgrave Macmillan.

Brookes, S. and Grint, K. (2010) *The New Public Leadership Challenge.* Basingstoke: Palgrave Macmillan.

Chambers, N. (ed.) (2023) *Research Handbook on Leadership in Healthcare.* Cheltenham: Edward Elgar Publishing.

Chambers, N. and Colin-Thome, D. (2009) Doctors managing in primary care: an international focus, *Journal of Management and Marketing in Healthcare*, 2 (1): 28–43.

Chambers, N. and Exworthy, M. (2021) Personal and organizational ambidexterity during policy turbulence: the case of long serving chief executives in the National Health Service in England, in R. Kislov, D. Burns, B. Mork and K. Montgomery (eds) *Managing Healthcare Organizations in Challenging Policy Contexts.* Basingstoke: Palgrave Macmillan.

Chambers, N. and Gregory, B. (2013) What German businesses could teach FT Governors, *Health Service Journal* 29 May 2013 [https://www.hsj.co.uk/leadership/what-german-businesses-can-teach-ft-governors/5058711.article; accessed 24 March 2024].

Chambers, N., Harvey, G. and Mannion, R. (2017) Who should serve on health care boards? What should they do and how should they behave? A fresh look at the literature and the evidence, *Cogent Business & Management*, 4 (1).

Chambers, N., Joachim, M., and Mannion, R. (2016) Hospital governance: Policy capacity and reform in England, France and Italy, in S. Greer, M. Wismar, and J. Figueras (eds) *Strengthening Health System Governance: Better Policies, Stronger Performance.* Maidenhead: Open University Press.

Chambers, N., Harvey, G., Mannion, R., Bond, J. and Marshall, J. (2013) Towards a framework for enhancing the performance of NHS boards: a synthesis of the evidence about board governance, board effectiveness and board development, *Health Services and Delivery Research*, 1 (6).

Chambers, N., Smith, J., Proudlove, N., Thorlby, R., Kendrick, H. and Mannion, R. (2020) Roles and behaviours of diligent and dynamic healthcare boards, *Health Services Management Research* 33 (2): 96–108. Reproduced under the CC BY 4.0 Attribution 4.0 International Deed License: creativecommons.org/licenses/by/4.0/.

Charan, R., Carey, D. and Useem, M. (2014) *Boards that Lead: When to Take Charge, When to Partner, and When to Stay Out of the Way.* Boston, MA: Harvard Business Review Press.

Commonwealth Fund (2022) Scorecard on state health system performance: How did states do during the COVID-19 pandemic? [https://www.commonwealthfund.org/publications/scorecard/2022/jun/2022-scorecard-state-health-system-performance; accessed 7 January 2024].

Csiszar, J., Otani, A., Dawood, F. and Goh, Z. (2023) Cross-cultural leadership, in N. Chambers (ed.) *Research Handbook on Leadership in Healthcare.* Cheltenham: Edward Elgar Publishing.

Cumming, J. (2022) Going hard and early: Aotearoa New Zealand's response to Covid-19, *Health Economics, Policy and Law* (2022) Jan; 17 (1): 107–119. doi: 10.1017/S174413312100013X. Epub 2021 Mar 5. PMID: 33663626; PMCID: PMC8007940.

Davies, C., Anand, P., Artigas, L., Holloway, J., McConway, K., Newman, J., et al. (2005) *Links between Governance, Incentives and Outcomes: A Review of the Literature.* London: National Co-ordinating Centre for NHS Service Delivery and Organisation R&D.

Deep Knowledge Analytics Global (2021) [https://www.dka.global/covid-city-ranking-q2; accessed 4 December 2024].

Eeckloo, K., Van Herck, G., Van Hulle, C. and Vleugels, A. (2004) From corporate governance to hospital governance: authority, transparency and accountability of Belgian non-profit hospitals boards and management, *Health Policy*, 68: 1–15.

Eurohealth (2013) Governing public hospitals, *Eurohealth*, 19 (1).

Ferlie, E., Ashburner, L., Fitzgerald, L. and Pettigrew, A. (1996) *The New Public Management in Action*. Oxford: Oxford University Press.

Francis, R. (2010) *Independent Inquiry into Care Provided by Mid Staffordshire NHS Foundation Trust*. London: The Stationery Office.

Francis, R. (2013) Letter to the Secretary of State. In *Report of the Mid Staffordshire NHS Foundation Trust Public Inquiry*. London: The Stationery Office.

French, J. and Raven, B. (1959) The bases of social power, in D. Cartwright and A. Zander (eds) *Group Dynamics*. New York: Harper & Row.

Fulop, N. and Ramsay, A. (2019) How organizations contribute to improving the quality of healthcare, *BMJ*, 365: l1773 [accessed 2 April 2024].

Garratt, B. (1997) *The Fish Rots from the Head*. London: HarperCollins.

Gorman, D. and Horn, M. (2023) Lifting the lid: a critical analysis of the COVID-19 pandemic in New Zealand, 20 April 2023 [https://www.nzinitiative.org.nz/reports-and-media/reports/lifting-the-lid-a-critical-analysis-of-the-covid-19-pandemic-management-in-new-zealand/; accessed 22 March 2024].

Goodwin, N. (2006) *Leadership in Health Care: A European Perspective*. London: Routledge.

Greer, S., Wismar, M. and Figueras, J. (eds) (2016) *Strengthening Health System Governance: Better Policies, Stronger Performance*. Maidenhead: Open University Press.

Grint, K. (2005) *Leadership: The Heterarchy Principle*. Basingstoke: Palgrave Macmillan.

Grint, K. (2010) *Wicked Problems and Clumsy Solutions: The Role of Leadership in the New Public Leadership Challenge*. Basingstoke: Palgrave Macmillan.

Ham, C. (2023) Leadership and governance of the response to COVID-19 in the United Kingdom in Research Handbook on Leadership, in N. Chambers (ed.) *Healthcare*, 457–492. Cheltenham, UK: Edward Elgar Publishing.

Herman, E.S. (1981) *Corporate Control, Corporate Power*. Cambridge: Cambridge University Press.

ICAC (2018) Oakden: A shameful chapter in South Australia's history [https://www.icac.sa.gov.au/__data/assets/pdf_file/0008/370727/ICAC_Report_Oakden.pdf; accessed 3 April 2024].

Independent Commission on Good Governance in Public Services (2004) *The Good Governance Standard for Public Services* (The Langlands Review). London: OPM and CIPFA.

International Human Genome Sequencing Consortium (2004) Finishing the euchromatic sequence of the human genome, *Nature*, 431: 931–945.

Jas, P. and Skelcher, C. (2005) Performance decline and turnaround in public organizations: a theoretical and empirical analysis, *British Journal of Management*, 16 (3): 195–210.

Johnson, G., Scholes, K., and Whittington, R. (2005) *Exploring Corporate Strategy*. Harlow: Pearson Education.

Kaehne, A., Feather, J., Chambers, N., Mahon, A., Zubairu, K., Moen, C., et al. (2022) *Rapid Review on System Leadership in Health Care: System Leadership: What do we know and what do we need to find out?* Edge Hill University [https://research.edgehill.ac.uk/ws/

portalfiles/portal/49690310/Rapid_Review_System_Leadership_EHU_UoM_May_2022_Final_Report.pdf; accessed 1 April 2024].

Kakabadse, A. and Kakabadse, N. (2008) *Leading the Board: The Six Disciplines of World-class Chairmen*. Basingstoke: Palgrave Macmillan.

Kings Fund (2023) Key facts and figures about the NHS [https://www.kingsfund.org.uk/insight-and-analysis/data-and-charts/key-facts-figures-nhs; accessed 27 March 2024].

Klein, R. (1998) Why Britain is reorganizing its National Health Service – yet again, *Health Affairs*, 17 (4): 111–125.

Lorsch, J.W. and MacIver, E. (1989) *Pawns or Potentates: The Reality of America's Corporate Boards*. Boston, MA: Harvard Business School Press.

Moore, M. (1995) *Creating Public Value: Strategic Management in Government*. Cambridge, MA: Harvard University Press.

Newman, J. (2005) Enter the transformational leader: network governance and the micro-politics of modernization, *Sociology*, 39 (4): 735–753.

Northouse, P.G. (2021) *Leadership: Theory and Practice* (9th edn.). Thousand Oaks, CA: Sage.

OECD (2015) G20/OECD Principles of Corporate Governance. Paris: OECD. http://dx.doi.org/10.1787/9789264236882-en.

OECD (2023) *Health at a Glance*. Paris: OECD.

Osborne, D. and Gaebler, T. (1993) *Reinventing Government: How the Entrepreneurial Spirit is Transforming the Public Sector*. Reading, MA: Addison-Wesley.

Pawson, R. (2006) *Evidence-based Policy: A Realist Perspective*. London: Sage.

Pettigrew, A. and McNulty, T. (1995) Power and influence in and around the boardroom, *Human Relations*, 48 (8): 845–873.

Pierre, J. and Peters, B.G. (2000) *Governance, Politics and the State*. Basingstoke: Macmillan.

Pointer, D. (1999) *Board Work: Governing Health Care Organizations*. San Francisco, CA: Jossey-Bass.

Powell, M. and Walshe, K. (2019) 50 years of NHS inquiries: Why they matter and what can we learn from them [https://www.health.org.uk/news-and-comment/blogs/50-years-of-nhs-inquiries; accessed 3 April 2024].

Pratt, J., Gordon, P. and Plamping, D. (1999) *Working Whole Systems: Putting Theory into Practice in Organizations*. London: The King's Fund.

Pryce, A. and Chambers, N. (2011) Board brilliance revealed, *Health Service Journal*, 30 June [https://www.hsj.co.uk/board-brilliance-revealed-study-into-top-performing-boards-finds-19-top-organisations/5030841.article; accessed 2 April 2024].

Refsum, C. and Britnell, M. (2023) The missing millions: leadership and the global workforce crisis in healthcare, in N. Chambers (ed.) *Research Handbook on Leadership in Health-care*, Cheltenham: Edward Elgar Publishing.

Savage, M., Savage, C., Brommels, M., et al. (2020) Medical leadership: boon or barrier to organisational performance? A thematic synthesis of the literature, *BMJ Open*, 10: e035542. doi: 10.1136/bmjopen-2019-035542; accessed 1 April 2024.

Sheaff, R., Charles, N., Mahon, A., Chambers, N., Morando, V., Byng, R., et al. (2015) NHS commissioning practice and health system governance: a mixed-methods realistic evaluation, *Health Services and Delivery Research*, 3 (10).

Simonet, D. (2023) Agencification, policy reversal and the reforms of the French health care system, *Public Administration and Policy: An Asia-Pacific Journal*, 26 (3): 272–281 [https://www.emerald.com/insight/publication/issn/2517-679X; accessed 24 March 2024].

Simsek, Z. (2007) CEO tenure and organization performance: an intervening model, *Strategic Management Journal*, 28 (6) 653–662.

Smith, P.C., Anell, A., Busse, R., Crivelli, L., Healy, J., Lindahl, A.K., et al. (2012) Leadership and governance in seven developed health systems, *Health Policy*, 106 (1): 37–49.

Storey, J., Holti, R., Winchester, N., Green, R., Salaman, G. and Bate, P. (2010) *The Intended and Unintended Outcomes of New Governance Arrangements within the NHS*. London: National Institute for Health Research.

Tuohy, C.J. (2003) Agency, contract and governance: shifting shapes of accountability in the health care arena. *Journal of Health Politics Policy and Law*, 28 (2/3): 195–215.

Vainieri, M., Ferre, F., Giacomelli, G. and Nuti, S. (2019) Explaining performance in health care: how and when top management competencies make the difference, *Health Care Management Review*, 2019 Oct/Dec; 44 (4): 306–317 doi: 10.1097/hmr.0000000000000164. PMID: 28448307; PMCID: PMC6749958.

Veronesi, G., Kirkpatrick, I. and Vallascas, F. (2014) Does clinical management improve efficiency? Evidence from the English National Health Service, *Public Money & Management*, 34 (1): 35–42 doi: 10.1080/09540962.2014.865932.

Walshe, K. and Chambers, N. (2010) Healthcare reform and leadership, in S. Brookes and K. Grint (eds) *The New Public Leadership Challenge*. Basingstoke: Palgrave Macmillan.

Walshe, K. and Shortell, S.M. (2004) When things go wrong: how health care organizations deal with major failures. *Health Affairs*, 23 (3): 103–111.

Waring, J., Bishop, S., Clarke, J., Exworthy, M., Fulop, N.J., Hartley, J., et al. (2022) Healthcare Leadership with Political Astuteness and its role in the implementation of major system change: the HeLPA qualitative study, *Health and Social Care Delivery Research*, 10 (11). https://doi.org/10.3310/FFCI3260.

West, M. and Bailey, S. (2023) Healthcare leadership: cultures, climates and compassion, in Chambers, N. (ed.) *Research Handbook in Leadership in Healthcare*. Cheltenham UK: Edward Elgar Publishing.

WHO (World Health Organization) (2023) Monitoring universal health coverage. *2023 Global Monitoring Report* [https://www.who.int/data/monitoring-universal-health-coverage; accessed 4 January 2024].

Chapter

3

Quality improvement in healthcare

Joy Furnival

Introduction

Quality is a term widely used not only within healthcare but throughout society, with numerous references to the quality of care; commissioning; access to care; quality and payment systems; patient safety; the regulation of quality of care; and service user expectations of quality in this book alone. However, the study and development of quality are often hampered by lack of clarity of definition (Endeshaw, 2020).

There are many different definitions of quality in healthcare (see Table 3.1). Due to this, there are also many different approaches to both measuring and then improving quality (Busse et al., 2019). These different perspectives are often associated with a particular lens of quality, or with a particular professional group, or associated with sub-components of quality, such as patient safety, resilience or equity. This has increasingly led to a developing multi-disciplinary perspective of quality and quality improvement (Swinglehurst et al., 2015).

This chapter focuses on what is often termed 'quality improvement' (QI). It considers the development of QI, by reflecting on the different approaches that can be taken for improving quality and safety, both external to organizations, such as regulation (Talbot, 2010; Busse et al., 2019) and from within healthcare organizations, before outlining the underlying principles of the approaches to improvement. An example (the Virginia Mason Production System, drawing on the Lean approach) is provided later in this chapter to demonstrate how QI is used in practice in healthcare and to consider whether QI works. The chapter concludes with a discussion of the challenges and limitations of QI.

Why improve quality in healthcare?

Continued unexplained and unwarranted variations in healthcare system, organizational and clinical performance continue to challenge researchers, clinicians and managers alike (Busse, et al., 2019; Wiig and O'Hara, 2021). Variations across different domains and perspectives of

Table 3.1 Definitions of healthcare quality

Donabedian (1987)	Maxwell (1984)	Langley et al. (1996/2009)	Institute of Medicine and Committee on Quality Health Care in America (2001)	Darzi (2008)
• Manner of practitioner – patient interaction • Patient's own contribution to care • Care setting amenities • Facility in access to care • Social distribution of access • Social distribution of health improvements attributable to care	• Access to services • Relevance to need • Effectiveness • Equity • Social acceptability • Efficiency and economy	• Performance • Features • Time • Reliability • Durability • Uniformity • Consistency • Serviceability • Aesthetics • Personal interaction • Flexibility • Harmlessness • Perceived quality • Usability	• Safety • Effectiveness • Patient-centredness • Timeliness • Efficiency • Equity	• Patient Safety • Patient Experience • Care Effectiveness

quality continue to be described as excessive and receive ongoing attention (Murray et al., 2017; Bates and Singh, 2018). The sentinel book *To Err is Human: Building a Safer Health System* by the Institute of Medicine (2000) controversially suggested that, in contrast to saving lives, the excessive variation in healthcare safety performance might account for the third highest cause of death in the world. More recently, studies have shown that errors related to medical misdiagnosis are substantial (Marang-van de Mheen et al., 2023; Newman-Toker et al., 2023). Given this urgent need for improved quality, there is growing public concern, and it is argued that for those leading and practising medicine there are moral, ethical and personal motivations for quality improvement in healthcare (Bohmer, 2016; 2009).

The many ways of improving quality in healthcare

Due to the differing perspectives of quality in healthcare, there are also differing perspectives as to the most effective way of improving quality in care. Efforts to improve have sometimes been hampered by competing beliefs about *how* improvements are best achieved (Ham et al., 2016). Talbot (2010) outlines four categories for improving quality and performance. These are: managerial/contractual interventions; market/systemic change; user choice and voice; and capability-led interventions (see Table 3.2). The first three of these (managerial, market, and user voice) can all be described as 'externally led' ways of improving often with a third party, such as a commissioner or regulator, via a governmental body or through the development of patient/service user rights. Lillis and Lane (2007) outline how 'outside-in' perspectives for improvement have dominated literature and practice and that an increased focus on improving from within – capability-led approaches – is required.

Table 3.2 Categories of performance improvement

Managerial/ contractual interventions	Direct and top-down management control, contractual levers, minimum standards, use of performance reporting and management, typically using 'Red/Amber/Green' colour coding ratings. Direct, and potentially punitive, consequences where targets and standards are not met. Delegation of enforcement of minimum standards by regulatory agencies.
Market/systemic change	Systemic reforms to stimulate competition between organizations, use of transparency systems, such as benchmarking, explicit ratings and league tables, to stimulate competition. Potential subsidies to new entrants to markets to encourage competition. Requires independently produced data about performance and quality.
User choice and voice	Empowers users of services and products through formal rights and specific entitlements, including choice of service/product provider.
Capability-led interventions	Supports organizations through direct action and resource management approaches, including specific improvement approaches, such as Lean, IHI-QI, agile and other developmental and re-engineering interventions, to enhance leadership and management.

Source: Adapted from Talbot (2010).

Improving from within: quality improvement in healthcare

Just as the term 'quality' has a variety of meanings, there is a confusion of terminology for quality improvement, including for example Total Quality Management (TQM) (Henrique and Filho, 2018) continuous quality improvement (CQI) (Loper et al., 2022), and improvement science (Health Foundation, 2011). Terms have continued to proliferate, although such terms often appear to be interchangeable in practice (Jones et al., 2019).

New developments from differing professional fields have also influenced the terminology and practice of quality improvement in healthcare. Over the last two decades in parallel with the rise in quality improvement, there has been a rise in new approaches for patient safety, healthcare regulation and evidence-based care within healthcare, often because of, and in response to, significant failures in safe healthcare provision. Such approaches draw heavily on the same foundations as QI and often utilize the same improvement methodologies sometimes with unintended consequences, such as poor fidelity in practice and superficial application. This can lead to little improvement and in some cases worse performance than prior to their application (Peerally et al., 2016; Reed and Card, 2016; Staines et al., 2020).

Healthcare-specific improvement developments have arisen possibly because some people have thought that externally developed systematic approaches for improvement from other sectors, such as automotive and telecoms, may not be appropriate or have relevance in care settings due to the significant contextual differences. Care-specific improvement approaches have developed within healthcare to account for a service-orientated context where the person receiving care receives both the 'output' and the 'outcome' of the service.

In addition, within healthcare settings, the person receiving care is inherently part of the process of service delivery and experiences the process throughout care receipt (Subramooney and Pugh, 2015; Anderson and Ròvik, 2015). There are several prominent healthcare-specific improvement approaches and strategies (Busse et al., 2019). These include clinical governance (Adduci et al., 2024), clinical guidelines and pathways, the Institute for Healthcare Improvement (IHI) approach (IHI-QI) (2003; 2024), patient safety culture, and clinical audit (Stewart et al., 2016).

Some common approaches for QI that have originated outside of healthcare, each within different contexts, include Lean (Womack and Jones, 1996); the Theory of Constraints (TOC) (Goldratt and Cox, 2004; Bacelar-Silva et al., 2024), Six Sigma (Pyzdek and Keller, 2003) and Agile (Highsmith, 2010). More information on these can be found in Table 3.3.

Some selected prominent approaches for improvement are described in the following section.

Clinical governance

Clinical governance can be defined as 'a framework through which organisations are accountable for continuously improving the quality of services and safeguarding high standards of care by creating an environment in which clinical care will flourish' (Gottwald and Lansdown, 2014: 2). Clinical governance was developed as an overall approach as part of policy on quality, including safety, in the NHS in England (Scally and Donaldson, 1998; Wood et al., 2022) and spread quickly to other healthcare systems around the world. This led to the establishment of formal clinical audit programmes, increased focus on clinical effectiveness and risk management, among other things. Clinical governance can be viewed as an overall QI process, but one that focuses specifically on clinical issues while still highlighting the importance of organizational culture, individual behaviour and interaction.

IHI-QI

The Institute for Healthcare Improvement (IHI) was established in 1991 and has grown from a 'collection of grant-supported programs to a self-sustaining organization with worldwide influence' (IHI, 2024). Its mission is to 'improve health and care worldwide' (IHI, 2024). The IHI quality improvement approach (IHI-QI) is informed by the work of Shewhart (1931) and Deming (1984) as in common with most other improvement approaches (Scoville and Little, 2014). The key elements of its approach are the 'Model for Improvement' (Langley et al., 2009; Associates in Process Improvement, 2024), which aims to understand the goal of the improvement work, the tasks and adjustments to deliver care improvements and the measures that will provide evidence that the goal is being met. The Model for Improvement is typically used with a collaborative approach (IHI, 2003; 2024). Following these questions, as in common with other QI approaches, a series of Plan-Do-Study-Act (PDSA) learning cycles follows (Deming, 1984; Reed and Card, 2016).

The IHI-QI approach is one of the more commonly utilized approaches for QI in healthcare due to its simplicity and generalizability for many different priorities for improvement,

Table 3.3 Quality improvement approaches

Approach	Description	Key reference	Healthcare example	Origin
Agile	Use of an updated 'new' approach drawing from Lean but contextualized for software development operational challenges, to tackle new and urgent issues and swiftly leverage benefits	Highsmith (2010)	United Arab Emirates Public Hospital (Holden et al., 2021)	Silicon Valley
IHI – Quality Improvement (QI)	Based extensively on Plan-Do-Study Act (PDSA) (see later in this table) and built on the Model for Improvement. IHI-QI draws a fundamental distinction between the system to be improved and the techniques and methods used to improve it	Institute for Healthcare Improvement (2003; 2024)	East London NHS Foundation Trust and IHI (O'Sullivan et al., 2021)	Automotive and electronics adapted for healthcare
Lean	Focus on elimination of waste through identification of customer value and respect for people and society	*Lean Thinking* Womack and Jones (1996)	NHS 5 Trusts and Virginia Mason (Burgess et al., 2022; 2023)	Automotive
Plan-Do-Study-Act (PDSA) (also known as Plan-Do-Check-Act, (PDCA)).	An iterative four-step management method provided for the control and continuous improvement of processes and products. It is also known as the Deming or Shewhart circle/cycle/wheel, or plan–do–study–act (PDSA)	*The Improvement Guide* (Langley et al., 1996/2009)	Taylor et al. (2013)	Various
Six Sigma	The term 'six sigma' refers to a process that has at least six standard deviations (6s) between the process mean and the nearest specification limit	*The Six Sigma Handbook* (Pyzdek and Keller, 2003)	Irish Healthcare, (Teeling et al., 2023)	Electronics manufacturing
TOC	Every system has at least one constraint – anything that limits the system from achieving higher performance. The existence of constraints represents opportunities for improvement – they are not viewed as negative	*The Goal* Goldratt and Cox (1984)	Brazilian Healthcare, Bacelar-Silva et al., (2024)	Manufacturing

making it easy to teach/learn and scale, meaning that many different staff members from across teams, clinical pathways and organizations are more likely to be familiar with a model, and in particular the use of 'quality improvement collaboratives' as an improvement delivery mechanism for large-scale change (Perla et al., 2013). However, the IHI-QI approach can be criticized for being too project orientated and therefore non-continuous (Dixon-Woods and Martin, 2016). The collaborative approach has also been criticized for limitations in research design and for potential publication bias (Wells et al., 2018) meaning that efforts that show successful project results are more likely to be submitted and accepted for publication coupled with a potential underreporting of unanticipated results or failures, although these critiques are not unique to the IHI-QI approach.

Patient safety

Patient safety is an ongoing area of study and practice that has developed at least in part from QI (Dekker-van Doorn et al., 2020). Like quality improvement, the study of patient safety draws on a range of disciplines, including psychology, sociology, clinical epidemiology and informatics. Preventing things going wrong is as important as being able to analyse them when they go well, although prevention is often given less attention compared to analysis, perhaps because it often raises challenging and complex issues that cannot be easily addressed. While good progress in addressing patient safety has been made, pervasive challenges and causes of safety problems and harms remain across, for example, infection rates, diagnostics, medical and surgical errors, IT failures and clinical handovers despite these efforts (Bates and Singh, 2018; Zegers et al., 2020). Many of the key issues raised in the study of patient safety (Bates and Singh, 2018) are like the issues raised in the study of QI.

Learning activity 3.1

What QI approaches are in use within your organization? How have they been chosen? How can you get more involved in your organization's approach to QI?

Discuss these questions in your team or department and raise your responses with your organizational leads for QI.

Does it matter which QI approach is used?

Given the wide array of different approaches for improving quality, from both within and external to an organization in healthcare, it may be wise to consider which approach might be the most effective and easy to apply and in what circumstances. Differing approaches have different emphasis, and jargon, and in practice these approaches are often context or sector specific. For example, corporate digital and software teams often use an Agile

(Highsmith, 2010) approach incorporating multiple 'project' development cycles – rather like the QI project cycles used in IHI-QI. Localized clinical teams may often use an IHI-QI (Langley et al., 2009) approach, using a combination of projects with iterative PDSA improvement cycles. Large organizations working with external partners in the wider healthcare system may take a proprietary approach, such as that of Virginia Mason (Burgess et al., 2022; Burgess, 2023) who draw on Lean and other large-scale approaches for continuous improvement (Womack and Jones, 1996; Slack et al., 2022); (Table 3.3). But there is little evidence that any of the approaches are necessarily any better than another (Walshe, 2009; Health Foundation, 2021) and what might work for one team and one organization may not work for another, even if they work within the same clinical specialty or geography.

The use of QI approaches in practice is complex and many studies outline the challenges of sustaining improvements on an ongoing basis (Flynn et al., 2018; Lennox et al., 2018; Woodnutt, 2018; Braithwaite et al., 2020). In addition, the QI approaches that may be used are not mutually exclusive, as the approaches have much in common (Walshe, 2009; Ham, 2016). QI approaches are systematic interventions that require long-term consistency in application across an organization (Alderwick et al., 2017).

QI commonalities

There are some fundamental commonalities that underpin QI, whatever the approach chosen (Table 3.3), although the emphasis on them varies.

A process view

The QI approaches described in this chapter are based on the process view of organizations (Slack et al., 2022). Process management is defined as entailing three practices: mapping processes, improving processes and adhering to systems of improved processes (Holweg et al., 2018). It is argued that taking a process view is one of the key characteristics of organizations that are successful in QI along with adopting evidence-based practice, measurement for improvement, learning collaboratively and being ready and able to change (Turner et al., 2020). The process view has also been the basis for the development of systems thinking (Holweg et al., 2018), which is based on the following principles:

- A system needs a purpose to aid people in managing interdependencies.
- The structure of a system determines its performance.
- Changes in system structure have the potential for generating unintended consequences.
- The structure of a system dictates the benefits for people working in the system.
- The size and scope of a system influences the potential for improvement.
- The need for cooperation is a logical extension of interdependencies within systems.
- Systems must be managed and led.

The process view examines and improves the interaction between elements of the organization, including the individuals who work within them. It can also be seen in the clinical emphasis on pathways, the use of clinical guidelines and process mapping that can lead to clinical and resource utilization improvements (Trebble et al., 2010).

Flow

Managing the flow of patients through a healthcare process draws on approaches widely developed in manufacturing, as well as healthcare (Holweg at al., 2018; Johnson et al., 2020). Understanding and evaluating flow requires a more detailed understanding of demand and capacity, calling for whole system alignment of goals and objectives. A focus on flow to the customer and alignment are key elements of Agile and Lean approaches (Table 3.3).

Variation

Variation within a process is inherent and it is long argued that understanding and analysing the variation are keys to success in improvement (Shewhart, 1931). Patient variability is 'random' and cannot be eliminated or reduced but must be managed, whereas non-random variability should be reduced or eliminated. The measurement and reduction of variation is a key element of the Six Sigma approach to improvement and that of Lean through a focus on reducing unevenness (Table 3.3).

The role of the 'customer'

QI approaches developed from external to healthcare require the identification of the customer, who may be internal or external to the organization, and subsequently their needs. The purpose of the process must be clear before improvement can take place; however, the role of the customer varies depending on the approach used (Boaden et al., 2008; Turner et al., 2020):

- In Six Sigma, what is 'critical to quality' as far as the customer is concerned defines the measures identified to determine the 'defects' to be reduced.
- In Lean, the customer's conception of value (which might be thought of as the ratio of benefits to costs) defines which elements of processes are useful (value-adding), the rest being non-value adding, or 'waste'.
- Six Sigma, Agile and Lean are predicated on the principle that the system should seek to provide more quality to the customer and/or at lower cost.
- IHI-QI has less emphasis on the customer as a key driver of improvement.

The role of people

Many QI approaches are not explicit about the role of people (particularly staff) and assume that people will automatically be motivated to improve quality. The IHI-QI approach emphasizes the role of individuals in improvement, and the involvement of people is explicit in Lean (see Table 3.3). In addition, increasingly QI approaches take a co-design approach to improve in partnership with the people receiving care and the wider public (Bate and Robert, 2007). Attention is required for the roles and behaviours of all staff, and most especially leaders in developing a culture for improvement.

Learning activity 3.2

What problems are being tackled with the QI approach you have identified in use in your organization? What measurement and evaluation of the improvement work is being employed? How do feel about the QI work that is taking place?

As with Learning activity 3.1, discuss these questions in your team or department and raise your responses with your organizational leads for QI.

Lean at Virginia Mason Medical Center (VMMC)

Background

In 1998, VMMC, a 300-bedded, not-for-profit hospital and integrated care system with approximately 450 physicians made a financial loss for the first time in its history, which continued in 1999 (Blackmore et al., 2011). Following the appointment of a new CEO, the leadership team and external management consultants (previously from Boeing) worked together to develop a new strategy to ensure the highest level of safety, improved care delivery and the elimination of waste: the Virginia Mason Production System (VMPS), (Bohmer and Ferlins, 2005). This focused on delivering patient satisfaction and productivity through a zero-defect approach (Kaplan and Patterson, 2008) and required staff to constantly seek ways to deliver the highest quality and safest patient care on an ongoing basis. This was based on the Lean approach (see Box 3.1).

Box 3.1   Lean healthcare

The Lean approach has been developed in healthcare through the implementation of the Toyota Production System (Kaplan and Rona, 2004). There are numerous reports of the application of Lean in healthcare (for example, Boaden et al., 2008; Lindsay et al., 2020). Lean appears to be applied in the public sector without a full understanding of the underlying principles, so that it is considered to be a set of tools rather than a fundamental shift in culture (Radnor and Osborne, 2013). Critics suggest Lean is a 'management fad' and question the appropriateness of whole-scale adoption of 'production line' Lean within professionally dominated healthcare (Waring and Bishop, 2010; McCann et al., 2015). Nevertheless, Lean continues to develop within healthcare with large-scale and publicly funded programmes across large conurbations (Bhat et al., 2020; Burgess et al., 2022; Marsillo et al., 2022; Teeling et al., 2023).

An example of the Lean approach in practice: The Virginia Mason Production System (VMPS)

Staff visited Toyota in Japan to study the problem-solving approaches as part of the Toyota Production System and developed the VMPS, which included agreed definitions of quality, summarized as 'better, faster and more affordable' (Blackmore et al., 2011), to ensure there was clear agreement on goals and what high quality looked like. Rapid Process Improvement Workshops (RPIWs), (also known as Rapid Improvement Events, (RIEs)) were used; staff were excused from their day role to work in a problem-solving team, redesigning and standardizing processes, to eliminate error and ensure flow.

The physician compact

The VMMC leadership worked closely with the staff within the organization to make explicit the agreements between staff and the organization, particularly doctors, about what was expected from them in terms of improvement and in return what they could expect from the organization. This 'compact' for implementing VMPS was not without challenges, and some staff left the organization, but overall it helped to reduce misalignment between staff and the organization (Bohmer and Ferlins, 2005; Kenney, 2010; Kenny, 2015).

Impact

Results from over 10 years of operation include 91 per cent patient satisfaction and 95 per cent same day appointments (Blackmore et al., 2011). Pham et al., (2007) describe numerous cost savings achieved through pathway redesign: for example, savings of $750,000 annually through the substitution of stress echocardiograms for nuclear perfusion imaging. The Leapfrog Group ranked VMMC in the top 1 per cent of hospitals in the US (and also designated VMMC as 'Hospital of the Decade').

Many organizations are trying to emulate the success of VMMC, often on a larger scale; for example, the NHS in the North East of England (Erskine et al., 2009; Hunter et al., 2014; Hunter et al., 2015). More recently, the Virginia Mason Institute worked with five English Trusts over a five-year period in partnership with NHS England to spread the improvement approach further (Burgess et al., 2022).

The Virginia Mason Partnership with NHS England and five NHS Trusts

From 2015 onwards the NHS in England partnered with the Virginia Mason Institute (VMI), a body set up to spread learning about the VMPS beyond Seattle. Five NHS Trusts, who had not been successful at meeting national quality standards allowing them to become more autonomous 'Foundation Trusts', were selected via a competitive process to receive free support via the national bodies and regulators, NHS England and NHS Improvement. The partnership aimed to develop improvement capability within the organizations and derive learning for the wider NHS community. The partnership formally concluded in 2021, and an evaluation of the programme was conducted alongside by academics at Warwick Business School, funded independently by a national charity, the Health Foundation. Several structured approaches to generating and sharing learning continued beyond the life of the programme including the application of the 'compact' (Burgess et al., 2019; Burgess et al., 2022; Burgess, 2023).

The 'compact' (Burgess et al., 2019) for this national programme drew on learning from the Virgina Mason compact and set out the reciprocal commitments of the national body, NHS Improvement and the partner NHS Trusts. The commitments for all included behaving in a respectful way, at all levels, with transparency. At a national level integrity and candidness in feedback were cited and within NHS Trusts, prioritizing the use of the approach when under pressure and with the wider NHS system were requirements.

The evaluation (Burgess et al., 2022) developed six key lessons for leaders in healthcare to support the fostering of a culture of continuous improvement (Burgess, 2022; Vora, 2022).

These are:

1   **Build cultural readiness as a foundation for better quality improvement outcomes**. The study found that organizations who had built an agreed set of shared values prior to commencing the programme built a stronger foundation through this cultural work to enable their quality improvement efforts; this meant that those organizations got better outcomes overall from their quality improvement efforts.

2   **Embed quality improvement routines and practices into everyday practice.** The study found that when expectations were set so that everyone had a role in practising quality improvement as part of their daily work, every day, it meant that there was regular and routinized learning in real situations and in real time. This allowed quality improvement capability to be built across the organizations rapidly.

3   **Have leaders show the way and light the path for others.** The study found that it is important that leaders role model the importance of quality improvement and recognize that their behaviour signals the value of improvement and enables people to lead improvement from where they are at, including from the point of care. The study also found that leadership behaviour is a system issue, and that the use of quality improvement can help healthcare organizations move away from 'command and control' models to improvement at every level of the system.

4   **Relationships aren't a priority; they are a pre-requisite.** The study found that building improvement efforts can be expedited where attention is paid to both the technical and the social aspects of improvement. Using social network analysis, the study was able to evidence that systematic improvement methods work best where there are strong inter-connected relationships, based on trust and shared values.

5   **Hold each other to account for behaviours not just outcomes.** The study found that organizations needed to role model the behaviours expected for quality improvement, and this included the need to embed space for reflection and learning in formal meetings and leadership routines.

6   **The rule of the golden thread: not all improvement matters in the same way.** The study found that improvement is more likely to succeed as intended when improvement priorities and objectives are more closely aligned with the most significant organizational priorities and objectives, as this makes it easier to demonstrate outcomes from quality improvement endeavours in ways that matter to staff, patients and stakeholders.

Overall, this evaluation supports other work (for example: Zoutman and Ford, 2017) signalling that QI is a 'people-process', and that the 'role of people' is foundational in developing and creating the conditions in which quality improvement can thrive in the longer term.

Does quality improvement 'work'?

There have been a range of reviews of quality improvement research; all challenged by the same issues, which make it difficult to decide which approaches 'work'. Many of the papers are descriptive case studies based on a single site, rather than analytical reviews of the application of improvement approaches with few empirical or theoretical studies, although these are growing (see, for example, Burgess et al., 2022; Williams et al., 2022).

In addition, QI measurement mechanisms can be missing or inadequate with poor data quality, missing data sets and lacking reliability and may require more subjective assessment, which can be resource intensive (Parand et al., 2014). Further, due to the differing conceptualizations of what constitutes 'quality' and 'quality improvement', it can be challenging to set out the key aspects for measurement (Khalifa and Househ, 2021). Many dimensions of quality can lead to the establishment of multiple different metrics, adding to measurement burden and, due to unintended and unanticipated consequences of QI work, key areas may not be measured at all (Li and Evans, 2022). These challenges can hinder QI practice and its assessment, with a need to strengthen indicators to track improved quality (Iqbal et al., 2019).

Methodologically, many papers are relatively small-scale before-and-after studies, making it difficult to determine whether any reported changes are directly attributable to the QI intervention or not. In addition, many studies lack programme theory or theories of change, which would enable stronger evaluation by outlining the rationale and assumptions about mechanisms that are intended to link the improvement intervention with the intended outcomes (Davidoff et al., 2015; Ko and Dixon-Woods, 2023).

There is debate about the relevance (or otherwise) of randomized controlled trial methods to investigate the effectiveness of quality improvement approaches. Some argue that QI is a complex social intervention, for which methods designed to 'control out' the influence of context on the implementation of the intervention are not relevant. Trials may not be sensitive to the things that influence the success of change: the 'array of influences: leadership, changing environments, details of implementation, organisational history, and much more' (Berwick, 2008: 1183) and varying designs have been proposed to develop and evaluate complex interventions (BMJ, 2021).

There are few large-scale, rigorously conducted trials that provide conclusive evidence to support the assertion that implementing quality improvement programmes and methods leads to improved processes and outcomes of care (Dixon-Woods and Martin, 2016; Akmal et al., 2021; Ko et al., 2022). Very few studies contain any analysis of the economic implications (Crump, 2023; Evans et al., 2023; Øvretveit, 2009) or the impact of QI on cost. However, many authors argue for a more pluralistic approach to improvement with the choice of approach contingent on the problem at hand (Grol et al., 2008; Health Foundation, 2021).

The aim is not to find out 'whether quality improvement works', as the answer to that question is almost always 'yes, sometimes'. The purpose is to establish when, how and why the intervention works, to unpick the complex relationship between context, content, application and outcomes.

(Walshe, 2007: 58)

Table 3.4 Core challenges to organizing for quality

Challenge	Lack of this can lead to ...
Structural – organizing, planning and coordinating quality efforts	Fragmentation and lack of synergy between different parts of the organization doing quality improvement
Political – addressing and dealing with the politics of change surrounding any quality improvement effort	Disillusionment and inertia because quality improvement is not happening on the ground, and certain groups or individuals are resisting change
Cultural – giving quality a shared, collective meaning within an organization	Evaporation because the change has not been properly anchored in everyday thinking and routines
Educational – creating a learning process that supports improvement	Amnesia and frustration as lessons are forgotten or fail to accumulate, and improvement capabilities fail to keep abreast of growing aspirations
Emotional – engaging and motivating people by linking quality improvement efforts to inner sentiments and beliefs	Loss of interest and fade-out as the change effort runs out of momentum due to a failure to engage front-line staff
Physical and technological – the designing of physical systems and infrastructure that supports quality efforts	Exhaustion as people try to make change happen informally, without systematic routines for necessary everyday activities

Source: Bate et al. (2008).

There is little evaluative research regarding QI. The aforementioned evaluation of the Virginia Mason Partnership with NHS England and five trusts by the Health Foundation with Warwick Business School concluded that:

> our key findings ... signal the importance of developing continuous improvement capability across the NHS and illustrate the role of continuous improvement in shaping sustainable health care.
>
> (Burgess et al., 2022)

One durable attempt to distil common challenges in QI through a review of case studies of healthcare organizations provides a useful overview of the organizing challenges (Bate et al., 2008), (see Table 3.4).

Learning activity 3.3

In your organization and network how are you planning to evaluate your improvement activity? What challenges do you face and how can they be overcome? What is your role in that?

Create an action plan with your team using SMART principles to provide clarity on what improvement activity is coming up in the next year.

Conclusion

While over the last quarter of a century the focus has been on building the infrastructure to measure quality and safety, and to build skills to improve it, the next decade will need to leverage on these foundations at scale, demystifying improvement and democratising the knowledge around it. Given the variety of perspectives on quality improvement, especially those from a system perspective and those developed by professionals, there are challenges for all:

- The need to **build improvement capability** across whole organizations and health systems (Martin et al., 2023). The tendency for each new quality improvement approach to proclaim itself a magic bullet (Dixon-Woods and Martin, 2016) and to pseudo-innovate its own jargon, brand and esoteric knowledge must be resisted (Walshe, 2009). Concurrently, efforts are needed to strengthen fidelity in the use and execution of improvement approaches, regardless of brand and jargon (Akmal et al., 2021; Ko et al., 2022; Vaz and Araujo 2022).
- Healthcare professionals and leaders need to recognize their **roles, behaviours and responsibilities** to the wider system, with a need to balance clinical professional autonomy with transparent accountability, to support the ongoing improvement of clinical work and services (Martin et al., 2017; Burgess et al., 2022).
- **Data and insight** are necessary but insufficient by themselves to achieve high-quality care. The emergence of many dashboards, benchmarks, clinical audits and safety indices have all helped to understand where there is good and poor care, and to support the evaluation of quality improvement activities. However, a primary focus on collecting data is insufficient, and at worst collecting more data can divert energy and effort from the hard work of using existing data for the improvement and transformation of care (Bohmer, 2016; Ko et al., 2022; Wagstaff et al., 2022).

In the continually changing world of healthcare, quality is always going to be important, and the differing perspectives, local contexts and multidisciplinary approaches must be considered to improve quality.

Box 3.2   Summary

- Quality is a widely used term with a variety of meanings attributed to it.
- Approaches to quality improvement may have a focus on changing organizations, professionals and interactions between participants in the system. Externally led approaches for improvement, such as regulation and user choice and voice run alongside QI approaches.
- The principles common to all approaches to quality improvement are a focus on processes, consideration of flow and variation, an explicit role for the 'customer' and the role of 'people'.

- Clinically developed approaches to improvement include clinical audit, clinical governance and some approaches to patient safety. These approaches have much in common with approaches developed outside of healthcare including Lean, Six Sigma, Agile and the Theory of Constraints (see Table 4.3).
- Healthcare is different from other sectors in terms of quality improvement primarily because of the professional autonomy of many of its staff, but improvement is a challenge for all parties who need to simplify concepts, recognize their responsibilities and the limits of their authority.

Acknowledgements

This chapter author acknowledges previous authors and co-authors of this chapter from previous editions, which has been drawn upon in developing this updated version, particularly Ruth Boaden.

Learning resources

British Medical Journal (BMJ) Quality and Safety: BMJ Quality & Safety is an international peer reviewed journal focused on the quality and safety of health care and improvement science [http://qualitysafety.bmj.com/].

Institute for Healthcare Improvement: The IHI website includes resources about improvement science and healthcare case studies [www.ihi.org].

The Health Foundation: This website includes many health and care improvement resources particularly linked to patient safety and patient experience [http://www.health.org.uk/].

The Q Community: This sub-site also hosted by the Health Foundation, the Q Community hosts member generated improvement content accessible for members across the UK and Ireland [https://q.health.org.uk].

The Lean Enterprise Institute: The global Lean network website, with improvement case studies, resources and blogs for healthcare and non-healthcare sectors [http://www.planet-lean.com/].

References

Adduci, A., Perilli, A., Durante, F., De Mattia, E., Cicchetti, A., Ricciardi, W. et al. (2023) Clinical governance: an in-depth scientometric analysis, *International Journal of Healthcare Management*, 1–15. doi: 10.1080/20479700.2023.2214963.

Akmal, A., Podgorodnichenko, N., Foote, J., Greatbanks, R., Stokes, T. and Gauld, R. (2021) Why is quality improvement so challenging? A viable systems model perspective to understand the frustrations of healthcare quality improvement managers, *Health Policy*, 125 (5): 658–664.

Alderwick, H., Charles, A., Jones, B. and Warburton, W. (2017) *Making the Case for Quality Improvement: Lessons for NHS Boards and Leaders.* London: Kings Fund.

Anderson, H. and Ròvik, K.A. (2015) Lost in translation: a case-study of the travel of lean thinking in a hospital, *BMC Health Services Research*, 15 (401).

Associates in Process Improvement (2024) Model for Improvement. API Associates in Process Improvement (API) home page. [https://www.apiweb.org; accessed 7 May 2024].

Bacelar-Silva, G.M., Cox, J.F. and Rodriques, P. (2024) Achieving rapid and significant results in healthcare services by using the theory of constraints, *Health Systems*, 12 (1): 48–61.

Bate, P. and Robert, G. (2007) *Bringing User Experience to Healthcare Improvement: The Concepts, Methods and Practices of Experience-based Design.* Abingdon: Radcliffe Publishing Ltd.

Bate, P., Mendel, P. and Robert, G. (2008) *Organising for Quality: The Improvement Journey of Leading Hospitals in Europe and the United States.* Abingdon: Radcliffe Publishing.

Bates, D.W. and Singh, H. (2018) Two decades since 'To Err is Human': an assessment of progress and emerging priorities in patient safety, *Health Affairs*, 37 (11): 1736–1743.

Berwick, D.M. (2008) The science of improvement, *Journal of the American Medical Association*, 299: 1182–1184.

Bhat, S., Antony, J., Gijo, E.V. and Cudnew, E.A. (2020) Lean Six Sigma for the healthcare sector: a multiple case study analysis from the Indian context, *International Journal of Quality and Reliabilty Management*, 37 (1): 90–111.

Blackmore, C.C., Mecklenburg, R.S. and Kaplan, G.S. (2011) At Virginia Mason, collaboration among providers, employers, and health plans to transform care cut costs and improved quality, *Health Affairs*, 30: 1680–1687.

BMJ (2021) A new framework for developing and devaluating complex interventions: update of Medical Research Council guidance, *British Medical Journal*, 374:n2061.

Boaden, R., Harvey, G., Moxham, C. and Proudlove, N. (2008) *Quality Improvement: Theory and Practice in Healthcare*, Warwick, UK: NHS Institute for Innovation and Improvement.

Bohmer, R. (2009) *Designing Care: Aligning the Nature and Management of Healthcare.* Boston: Harvard Business Press.

Bohmer, R. (2016) The hard work of health care transformation, *New England Journal of Medicine*, 375 (8): 709–711.

Bohmer, R. and Ferlins, E.M. (2005) Virginia Mason Medical Center. *Harvard Business School*, 3: 1–28.

Braithwaite, J., Ludlow, K., Testa, L., Herkes, J., Augustsson, G.L., McPherson, E. and Zurynski, Y. (2020) Built to last? The sustainability of healthcare system improvements, programmes and interventions: a systematic integrative review, *BMJ Open*, 10 (6).

Burgess, N. (2022) Six key lessons from the NHS and the Virginia Mason Partnership. Warwick Business School [https://www.wbs.ac.uk/news/six-key-lessons-from-the-nhs-and-the-virginia-mason-institute-partnership/; accessed 28 May 2024].

Burgess, N. (2023) Partnership for improvement: how a leadership compact fostered relational change between five hospital chief executives and their regulator, in N. Burgess and G. Currie (eds) *Shaping High Quality, Affordable and Equitable Healthcare through Meaningful Innovation and System Transformation (Organisational Behaviour in Healthcare)*. Cham: Palgrave Macmillan. https://doi.org/10.1007/978-3-031-24212-0_3.

Burgess, N., Currie, G., Crump, B. and Dawson A. (2022) *Leading Change across a Healthcare System: How to Build Improvement Capability and Foster a Culture of Continuous Improvement. Summary Report of the Evaluation of the NHS-VMI Partnership*. Warwick Business School.

Burgess, N., Currie, G., Crump, B., Richmond, J. and Johnson, M. (2019) Improving together: collaboration needs to start with regulators, *British Medical Journal*, 367.

Busse, R., Klazinga, N., Panteli, D. and Quentin, W. (2019) *Improving Healthcare Quality in Europe: Characteristics, Effectiveness and Implementation of Different Strategies*. Copenhagen: Organisation for Economic Co-operation and Development (OECD).

Crump, B. (2023) Quantifying financial impact of quality improvement programmes: lessons and limitations, in *Shaping High Quality, Affordable and Equitable Healthcare: Meaningful Innovation and System Transformation*. Cham: Springer International Publishing.

Darzi, A. (2008) *High Quality Care For All – NHS Next Stage Review Final Report* in Department of Health (ed.), London: Crown.

Davidoff, F., Dixon-Woods, M., Leviton, L. and Michie, S. (2015) Demystifying theory and its use in improvement, *BMJ Quality and Safety in Healthcare*, 24: 228–238.

Dekker-van Doorn, C., Wauben, L., van Wijngaarden, J., et al. (2020) Adaptive design: adaptation and adoption of patient safety practices in daily routines, a multi-site study. *BMC Health Services Research*, 20: 426. https://doi.org/10.1186/s12913-020-05306-2.

Deming, W.E. (1984) *Out of the Crisis*. Cambridge, MA: MIT Press.

Dixon-Woods, M. and Martin, G.P. (2016) Does quality improvement improve quality? *Future Hospital Journal*, 3 (3): 191.

Donabedian, A. (1987) Commentary on some studies of the quality of care, *Health Care Financing Review*, Annual Supplement, 75–86.

Endeshaw, B. (2020) Healthcare service quality measurement models: a review, *Journal of Health Research*, 35 (2): 106–117.

Erskine, J., Hunter, D.J., Hicks, C., Mcgovern, T., Scott, E., Lugsden, E., et al. (2009) New development: first steps towards an evaluation of the North East Transformation System. *Public Money & Management*, 29: 273–276.

Evans, J., Leggatt, S.G. and Samson, D. (2023) A systematic review of the evidence of how hospitals capture financial benefits of process improvement and the impact on hospital financial performance, *BMC Health Services Research*, 23 (237): 1–3.

Flynn, R., Newton, A.S., Rotter, T., Hartfield, D., Walton, S., Fiander, M., et al. (2018) The sustainability of Lean in pediatric healthcare: a realist review, *Systematic Reviews*, 7: 137.

Goldratt, E.M. and Cox, J. (2004) *The Goal: A Process of Ongoing Improvement – 20th Anniversary Edition* (3rd edn.). USA: North River Press.

Gottwald, M. and Lansdown, G.E. (2014) *Clinical Governance: Improving the Quality of Healthcare for Patients and Service Users*. Maidenhead: Open University Press.

Grol, R., Berwick, D. and Wensing, M. (2008) On the trail of quality and safety in health care, *British Medical Journal*, 336: 74–76.

Ham, C., Berwick, D.J. and Dixon, J. (2016) *Improving Quality in the English NHS*. London: The Kings Fund.

Health Foundation (2011) *Improvement Science*. London: Health Foundation.

Health Foundation (2021) *Quality Improvement Made Simple* (3rd edn.). London: Health Foundation.

Henrique, D.B. and Filho, M.G. (2018) A systematic literature review of empirical research in Lean and Six Sigma in healthcare, *Total Quality Management and Business Excellence* 31 (3–4): 429–449.

Highsmith, J. (2010) *Agile Project Management: Creating Innovative Products* (2nd edn.). London: Pearson.

Holden, R.J., Boustani, M.A. and Azar, J. (2021) Agile Innovation to transform healthcare: innovating in complex adaptive systems is an everyday process, not a light bulb event, *BMJ Innovations*, 2: 22–32.

Holweg, M., Davies, J., De Mayer, A. and Lawson, B. (2018) *Process Theory: The Principles of Operations Management*. Oxford: Oxford University Press.

Hunter, D.J., Erskine, J., Hicks, C., Mcgovern, T., Small, A., Lugsden, E., et al. (2014) A mixed-methods evaluation of transformational change in NHS North East, *Health Service Delivery Research*, 2.

Hunter, D.J., Erskine, J., Small, A., Mcgovern, T., Hicks, C., Whitty, P., et al. (2015) Doing transformational change in the English NHS in the context of "big bang" redisorganisation, *Journal of Health Organization and Management*, 29: 10–24.

Institute for Healthcare Improvement (2003) *The Breakthrough Series: IHI's Collaborative Model for Achieving Breakthrough Improvement*. IHI Innovation Series White Paper. Boston, MA: Institute for Healthcare Improvement.

Institute for Healthcare Improvement (2024) Vison, Mission and Values, Boston, USA. [https://www.ihi.org/about/vision-mission-values; accessed 13 May 2024].

Institute of Medicine and Committee on Quality Health Care in America (2001) *Crossing the Quality Chasm*. Washington DC: Institute of Medicine.

Iqbal, U., Humayun, A. and Li, Y. (2019) Healthcare quality-improvement and measurement strategies and its challenges ahead, *International Journal for Quality in Health Care*, 31 (1): 1. https://doi.org/10.1093/intqhc/mzz009.

Johnson, M., Burgess, N. and Sethi, S. (2020) Temporal pacing of outcomes for improving patient flow: design science research in a National Health Service hospital, *Journal of Operations Management*, 66 (1–2): 35–53.

Jones, E., Furnival, J., and Carter, W. (2019) Identifying and resolving the frustrations of reviewing the improvement literature: the experiences of two improvement researchers, *BMJ Open Quality*, 8(3): e000701.

Kaplan, G.S. and Patterson, S.H. (2008) Seeking perfection in healthcare. *Healthcare Executive*, 23: 16–21.

Kaplan, G.S. and Rona, J.M. (2004) Seeking zero defects: applying the Toyota production system to healthcare. *16th National Forum on Quality Improvement in Healthcare*. Orlando, Florida.

Kenney, C. (2010) *Transforming Health Care: Virginia Mason Medical Center's Pursuit of the Perfect Patient Experience*. New York: Productivity Press.

Kenney, C. (2015) *A Leadership Journey in Health Care: Virginia Mason's story*. Boca Raton: CRC Press.

Khalifa, M. and Househ, M. (2021) Utilizing health analytics in improving the performance of hospitals and healthcare services: promises and challenges, in M. Househ, E. Borycki, and A. Kushniruk (eds) *Multiple Perspectives on Artificial Intelligence in Healthcare. Lecture Notes in Bioengineering*. Cham: Springer. https://doi.org/10.1007/978-3-030-67303-1_3.

Ko, C.Y. and Dixon-Woods, M. (2023) What is programme theory and why is it important to perioperative quality improvement?, in C.J. Peden, L.A. Fleisher and M. Englesbe (eds) *Perioperative Quality Improvement*.

Ko, C.Y., Martin, G. and Dixon-Woods, M. (2022) Three observations from improving efforts in surgical quality improvement, *JAMA Surgery*, 157 (12): 1073–1074.

Langley, G.J., Moen, R.D., Nolan, K.M., Nolan, T.W., Norman, C.L. and Provost, L.P. (1996/2009) *The Improvement Guide. A Practical Approach to Enhancing Organisational Performance*. San Francisco, CA: Jossey-Bass.

Lennox, L., Maher, L. and Reed, J. (2018) Navigating the sustainability landscape: a systematic review of sustainability approaches in healthcare, *Implementation Science*, 13 (1): 1–15.

Li, X. and Evans, J.M. (2022) Incentivizing performance in health care: a rapid review, typology and qualitative study of unintended consequences, *BMC Health Services Research*, 22: 690. https://doi.org/10.1186/s12913-022-08032-z.

Lillis, B. and Lane, R. (2007) Auditing the strategic role of operations, *International Journal of Management Reviews*, 9 (3): 191–210.

Lindsay, C.F., Kumar, M. and Juleff, L. (2020) Operationalising lean in healthcare: the impact of professionalism, *Production Planning & Control*, 31 (8): 629–643.

Loper, A.C., Jensen, T.M., Farley, A.B., Morgan, J.D., and Metz, A.J. (2022) A systematic review of approaches for continuous quality improvement capacity-building. *Journal of Public Health Management and Practice*, 28(2): E354–E361.

Marang-van de Mheen, P.J., Thomas E.J. and Graber, M.L. (2023) How safe is the diagnostic process in healthcare? *BMJ Quality and Safety*. First published online: 4 October 2023. doi: 10.1136/bmjqs-2023-016496.

Marsillo, M., Pissara, M., Rubio, K. and Shortell, S. (2022) Lean adoption, implementation and outcomes in public hospitals: benchmarking the US and Italy health systems, *BMC Health Services Research*, 22 (1): 122.

Martin, G., Stanford, S., and Dixon-Woods, M. (2023) A decade after Francis: Is the NHS safer and more open? *British Medical Journal*, 380: 513 [doi:10.1136/bmj.p513].

Martin, G.P., Kocman, D., Stephens, T., Peden, C.J. and Pearse, R.M. (2017) Pathways to professionalism? Quality improvement, care pathways and the interplay of standardisation and clinical autonomy, *Sociology and Health and Illness*, 39 (8): 1314–1329.

Maxwell, R.J. (1984) Quality assessment in health, *British Medical Journal*, 288: 1470–1472.

McCann, L., Hassard, J.S., Granter, E. and Hyde, P.J. (2015) Casting the lean spell: the promotion, dilution and erosion of lean management in the NHS, *Human Relations*, 68 (10): 1557–1577.

Murray, R., Jabbal, J., Thompson, J., Baird, B. and Maguire, D. (2017) The Kings Fund Quarterly Monitoring Report, 23. London: The Kings Fund.

Newman-Toker, D.E., Nassery, N., Schaffer, A.C., Yu-Moe, C.W., Clemens, G.D., Wang, Z., Zhu, Y., et al. (2023) Burden of serious harms from diagnostic error in the USA, *BMJ Quality and Safety*, First published online: 17 July 2023. doi: 10.1136/bmjqs-2021-014130.

O'Sullivan, O.P., Chang, N.H., Baker, P. and Shah, A. (2021) Quality improvement at East London NHS Foundation Trust: the pathway to embedding lasting change, *International Journal of Health Governance*, 26 (1): 65–72.

Øvretveit, J. (2009) *Does Improving Quality Save Money?* London: The Health Foundation.

Parand, A., Dopson, S., Renz, A. and Vincent, C. (2014) The role of hospital managers in quality and patient safety: a systematic review, *BMJ Open* 4: e005055. doi: 10.1136/bmjopen-2014-005055.

Peerally, M.F., Carr, S. and Waring, J. (2016) The problem with root cause analysis. *BMJ Quality and Safety*, 0: 1–6.

Perla, R.J., Bradbury, E. and Gunther-Murthy C. (2013) Large-scale improvement initiatives in healthcare: a scan of the literature, *The Journal for Healthcare Quality*, 35 (1): 30–40.

Pham, H.H., Ginsburg, P.B., Mckenzie, K. and Milstein, A. (2007) Redesigning care delivery in response to a high-performance network: The Virginia Mason Medical Center, *Health Affairs*, 26: w532–w544.

Pyzdek, T. and Keller, P.A. (2003) *The Six Sigma Handbook: A Complete Guide for Green Belts, Black Belts, and Managers at all Levels.* New York: McGraw-Hill.

Radnor, Z. and Osborne, S.P., (2013) Lean: a failed theory for public services? *Public Management Review*, 15 (2): 265–287.

Reed, J. and Card, A. (2016) The problem with plan-do-study-act cycles, *BMJ Quality and Safety*, 25: 147–152.

Scally, G. and Donaldson, L.J. (1998) Clinical governance and the drive for quality improvement in the new NHS in England, *British Medical Journal*, 317: 61–65.

Scoville, R. and Little, K. (2014) Comparing lean and quality improvemen. *Institute for Healthcare Improvement White Paper.* Cambridge, MA: Institute for Healthcare Improvement.

Shewhart, W.A. (1931) *Economic Control of Quality of Manufactured Product.* New York: Van Nostrand.

Slack, N., Brandon-Jones, A. and Burgess, N. (2022) *Operations Management.* London: Pearson Education Limited.

Staines, A., Amalberti, R., Berwick, D.M., Braithwaite, J., Lachman, P. and Vincent, C.A. (2020) COVID-19: patient safety and quality improvement skills to deploy during the surge, *International Journal for Quality in Health Care*, 33 (1), 2021, mzaa050. https://doi.org/10.1093/intqhc/mzaa050.

Stewart, K., Bray, B. and Buckingham, R. (2016) Improving quality of care through national clinical audit, *Future Hospital Journal*, 3 (3): 203.

Subramooney, M. and Pugh, S.D. (2015) Services management research: review, integration and future directions. *Journal of Management*, 41 (1): 349–373.

Swinglehurst, D., Emmerich, N., Maybin, J., Park, S. and Quilligan, S. (2015) Confronting the quality paradox: towards new characterisations of 'quality' in contemporary healthcare, *BMC Health Services Research*, 15: 240.

Talbot, C. (2010) *Theories of Performance: Organisational and Service Improvement in Public Domain.* Oxford: Oxford University Press.

Taylor, M.J., Mcnicholas, C., Nicolay, C.R., Darzi, A., Bell, D. and Reed, J.E. (2013) Systematic review of the application of the plan–do–study–act method to improve quality in healthcare, *BMJ Quality & Safety*.

Teeling, S.P., McGuirk, M., McNamara, M., McGroarty, M. and Igoe, A. (2023) The utilisation of lean six sigma methodologies in enhancing surgical pathways and surgical rehabilitation, *Applied Sciences*, 13 (12): 6920.

Trebble, T.M., Hansi, N., Hydes, T., Smith, M.A. and Baker, M. (2010) Process mapping the patient journey: an introduction, *British Medical Journal*, 341.

Turner, J.R., Thurlow, N. and Rivera, B. (2020) *The Flow System: Practitioner Tools for Navigating Complexity. In Cases on Performance Improvement Innovation.* IGI Global.

Vaz, N. and Araujo, C. (2022) Failure factors in quality improvement programmes: reviewing two decades of the scientific field, *International Journal of Quality and Service Sciences*, 14 (2): 291–310.

Vora, T. (2022) How to foster a culture of continous improvement [sketchnote], in Burgess (2022) *Six Key Lessons from the NHS and the Virginia Mason Partnership.* Warwick Business School [https://www.wbs.ac.uk/news/six-key-lessons-from-the-nhs-and-the-virginia-mason-institute-partnership/; accessed 28 May 2024].

Walshe, K. (2007) Understanding what works—and why—in quality improvement: the need for theory-driven evaluation, *International Journal for Quality in Health Care*, 19: 57–59.

Walshe, K. (2009) Pseudoinnovation in the development and dissemination of healthcare quality improvement methodologoies, *International Journal of Quality in Healthcare*, 21 (3): 153–159.

Wagstaff, D., Warmakulasuriya, S., Singleton, G., Moonesinghe, S.R., Fulop, N. and Vindrola-Padros, C. (2022) A scoping review of local quality improvement using data from UK perioperative National Clinical Audits, *Perioperative Medicine* 11 (43) online.

Waring, J.J. and Bishop, S. (2010) Lean healthcare: rhetoric, ritual and resistance, *Social Science & Medicine*, 71: 1332–1340.

Wells, S., Tamir, O., Gray, J., Naidoo, D., Bekhit, M. and Goldmann, D. (2018) Are quality improvement collaboratives effective? A systematic review, *BMJ Quality and Safety*, 27: 226–240.

Wiig, S. and O'Hara, J.K. (2021) Resilient and responsive healthcare services and systems: challenges and opportunities in a changing world, *BMC Health Services Research*, 21: 1037. https://doi.org/10.1186/s12913-021-07087-8.

Williams, S.J., Caley, L., Davies, M., Bird, D., Hopkins, S., and Willson, A. (2022) Evaluating a quality improvement collaborative: a hybrid approach, *Journal Of Healthcare Organisation and Management*, 36 (8): 987–1008.

Womack, J. and Jones, D. (1996) *Lean Thinking: Banish Waste and Create Wealth in Your Corporation.* New York: Simon and Schuster.

Wood, D.P., Robinson, C.A., Nathan, R. and McPhillips, R. (2022) A study of the implementation of patient safety policies in the NHS in England since 2000: what can we learn? *Journal of Health Organisation and Management*, 36 (5): 650–665.

Woodnutt, S. (2018) Is Lean sustainabile in today's NHS Hospitals? A systematic literature review using the meta-narrative and integrative methods, *International Journal for Quality in Health Care*, 30 (8): 578–586.

Zegers, M., Hanskamp-Sebregts, M. Wollersheim, H. and Vincent, C.A. (2020) Patient safety strategies, in M. Wensing, R. Grol and J. Grimshaw (eds) in *Improving Patient Care: Strategies for Change* (3rd edn.). Wiley Online Books.

Zoutman, D.E. and Ford, B.D. (2017) Quality improvement in hospitals: barriers and facilitators, *International Journal of Health Care Quality Assurance*, 30 (1): 16–24. https://doi.org/10.1108/IJHCQA-12-2015-0144.

Public health and global inequalities

Peymané Adab

Introduction

Global health inequalities contribute significantly to poor health outcomes across the world. Despite improvements in global life expectancy, substantial disparities persist. For example, life expectancies in some Sub-Saharan African countries remain below 60 years, compared to over 80 years in many European countries and Japan (The World Bank, 2022). Furthermore, while the gap in health service coverage between rich and poor has nearly halved in low- and middle-income countries over the last few decades, mortality in the under-fives remains significant, with wealth-related inequalities accounting for an estimated 1.8 million excess child deaths (World Health Organization, 2023). Approximately 4.5 billion people worldwide lack access to essential health services (WHO and World Bank, 2023), highlighting a major global health inequity. These inequalities are not just confined to low-income countries; most high-income nations also exhibit disparities in access to healthcare, quality of care and health outcomes across different population groups (MacKinnon et al., 2023). Addressing these global health inequalities requires a multifaceted approach, including targeted policies, improved data collection, and a commitment to universal health coverage to ensure that no one is left behind.

Healthcare managers stand at the forefront of change within healthcare organizations, guiding practice towards a future where health equity is not just an ideal, but a tangible reality. As a manager, it is important to understand that social determinants of health disproportionately affect segments of the population and therefore there is a role for proactively taking steps to mitigate these disparities.

This chapter focuses on global inequalities within a public health context, setting out what we mean by health inequalities, how they arise, and describing the pivotal role that management plays in addressing these challenges. The aim is to provide you with tools to critically analyse your practice, identify areas where inequalities may arise and implement solutions that promote inclusivity and accessibility.

Definitions

There are many kinds of health inequality, and many ways in which the term is used. When analysing inequalities, it is important to distinguish between differences that arise from biological factors, or pathogens, from those that are more amenable to change. The latter include inequalities that are a function of socioeconomic or political factors, or those that stem from differences in service provision. When inequalities result from vulnerability due to these external factors (termed as inequities), interventions may require unequal provision of services to compensate and avoid perpetuation of inequities (World Health Organization, 2021). Box 4.1 includes some important definitions to set the context for the remaining sections.

Box 4.1   Some definitions of public health and inequalities

Public health or 'population health' programmes generally refer to interventions or policies that impact on the health of the public (or a specific population) rather than individual treatments for people with established disease. Public health interventions target the root causes of ill health and seek to improve population well-being through influencing people's lifestyles and behaviours (e.g. to promote physical activity, reduce harms from alcohol, etc.), aspects of the environment and the wider economy that impact on people's health as well as maximizing the effectiveness, efficiency and equitability of our health services. Hence, public health includes activities that are under the control of local and national government, such as the quality of our air, children's schooling, the amount of disposable income people have (through taxation) or the amount of green space available for the public. Preventive activity (see below) is also a large and important subset of public health, including the control (prevention and management) of communicable diseases.

Prevention strategies target the various stages of a disease process (Kisling and Das, 2024) and include:

- *primordial prevention* – targeting underlying social and environmental conditions that promote disease, usually through laws and policies;

- *primary prevention* – targeting susceptible, but healthy individuals and populations to prevent disease onset, such as smoking prevention or immunization;
- *secondary prevention* – targeting early disease detection in apparently healthy individuals, usually through health screening;
- *tertiary prevention* – targeting those with a disease, with the aim of reducing the severity, often through rehabilitation programmes.

Inequality in public health refers to the uneven distribution of health or health resources (Williams et al., 2022). This can arise from factors related to biology or genetics, our geography and environment, or ability and resources to access health-promoting commodities and healthcare. It is a broad term that encompasses any measurable difference in health outcomes among individuals or groups.

Inequity is a subset of inequality defined as unfair, avoidable and systematic differences in health across the population, and between different groups within society (Braveman and Gruskin, 2003). Inequity arises from modifiable causes that can be prevented through changes in policy or practice. Although the term inequity and inequality are often used interchangeably, inequity implies a failure to act on preventable inequalities.

When we talk about health inequality, it is useful to be clear which measure is unequally distributed, and between which people (Williams, et al., 2022). The measures that are commonly used to look at differences between groups include those related to health status (e.g. disease prevalence, premature mortality rates, life expectancy), behaviours that impact health (e.g. unhealthy diet, smoking prevalence), access to care (e.g. through availability of services, financial means to access) and quality and experience of care (e.g. satisfaction with services). In addition, differences in the wider determinants of health, such as level of education or quality of housing and differential uptake of public health interventions, are important measures.

Types of inequalities and implications for practice

Health inequalities are not uniform and affect various groups of people differently. As healthcare managers, understanding these disparities is essential for informed decision-making and targeted interventions, as well as enabling advocacy for equitable policies and strategic allocation of healthcare resources.

The main factors that determine groupings of health inequalities include socioeconomic factors (e.g. income, education, occupation), certain characteristics including those protected in law (e.g. age, sex, ethnicity, disability), geography (e.g. regional divides, rurality, coastal areas) and being part of marginalized groups (e.g. homeless, traveller or prison populations). Some examples of how these factors are associated with measures of inequality and the implications for practice are summarized in Table 4.1 and these are explored in more detail in the rest of the chapter.

Table 4.1 Examples of groups affected by health inequalities, how they are affected and implications for health managers

Some factors affecting inequality	Health status measures	Potential mechanisms leading to inequalities	Role of health managers
Social class and socioeconomic factors	Individuals from lower compared with higher socioeconomic groups tend to have shorter life expectancies, higher rates of chronic diseases and increased mortality risk.	Financial constraints may impact health behaviours (e.g. poor diet), access to healthcare, quality of care received and adherence to treatments.	Understanding reasons for poor access to healthcare/poor adherence and implementing interventions to improve this.
Sex and gender	Women tend to have longer life expectancy compared to men, but a higher rate of chronic disease. LGBTQ+ people have disproportionately worse health outcomes compared to those who are heterosexual.	Men are more likely to engage in unhealthy behaviours (e.g. smoking). Women face some barriers in health seeking and quality of care. Discrimination and stigma against LGBTQ+ people negatively affect health seeking, access and quality of services.	Ensure services are gender equitable. Train staff regarding LGBTQ+ health issues and culturally competent care. Visible leadership (visibly support gender inclusivity).
Disability and ability	People with disabilities tend to have higher than expected rates of depression, asthma, diabetes, obesity and poor oral health.	Physical barriers, lack of accessible information and discriminatory attitudes impact healthcare access. Poorer access to education, lower employment and poverty exacerbate this.	Tailored care plans can accommodate diverse abilities. Accessible preventive health services to suit those of all abilities.
Geography	People living in rural and coastal communities tend in many countries to have higher rates of chronic disease.	Geographical isolation and shortage of health infrastructure impact access. Economic constraints and lower average incomes also contribute.	Targeted organization of healthcare services and innovative approaches for improving access (e.g. telemedicine).
Housing quality	Poor housing (e.g. overcrowding, inadequate heating, dampness) leads to higher rates of infections, respiratory, cardiovascular and mental health problems.	The relationship between poor housing and health is cyclical, self-perpetuating and linked to poverty. Additional to the physical effects, those living in unfit housing tend to have poorer access to employment, education, services and healthy food.	Ensure equitable healthcare services that are responsive to the needs of those living in poor housing. Support access to services and adequate community health programmes. Advocate for policies that address the root causes of poor housing.
Migrants and refugees as marginalized groups	These populations have higher rates of communicable diseases, mental health issues and chronic conditions.	Mix of factors including language and cultural differences, limited health service access and institutional discrimination all contribute.	Implement culturally sensitive healthcare policies (e.g. language support, culturally appropriate health education). Improve healthcare service access. Foster inclusive practices (e.g. training of healthcare providers).

Learning activity 4.1

For each of the following examples, consider whether there are inequities (unjust, avoidable differences), or whether the inequality is unavoidable. For those you consider as inequities, what are the root causes of the disparity (consider societal, economic, educational, service level, political and other factors)?

Example 1: The mean age of death for men experiencing homelessness in the UK is 45 years, compared to the life expectancy of 80 years for the general population.

Example 2: The prevalence of colon cancer in people aged <50 years is 13 per cent, compared to a prevalence of 56 per cent in those aged 65 years or more.

Example 3: A 2019 UK national dental survey shows that among 5-year-old children, 34 per cent of those living in the 10 per cent most deprived areas of the country and 14 per cent living in the 10 per cent least deprived areas had experienced dental caries.

Example 4: There were around 49,000 cases of malaria reported worldwide in 2022. Of these, 27 per cent were reported in Nigeria and 0 per cent in the UK.

Example 5: A study that examined the risk of malaria in children in Uganda found that the risk was 33–43 per cent lower in those living in higher income households (better housing and less food insecurity) and in those whose primary caregiver had a higher level of education.

You may want to revisit this activity at the end of the chapter to further reflect on strategies that could address the issue and what health managers can contribute to create equitable solutions (consider resource allocation and the needs of vulnerable populations).

Structural inequalities and intersectionality

While reflecting on the root causes of inequalities and the different factors that are associated with health inequities, you may have recognized that many of these are inter-related. Disadvantages tend to be concentrated in particular parts of the population. For example, people from less affluent backgrounds tend to have a higher prevalence of higher-risk health behaviours, worse access to care and less opportunity to lead healthy lives than those who are more affluent (McCartney et al., 2013; Goddard and Smith, 2001). Furthermore, these factors can reinforce each other to compound and magnify the health risks and challenges that disadvantaged groups face. There is a complex interaction between personal characteristics, the accessibility and quality of health and care services, individual behaviours and the wider determinants of health. This concept, known as 'intersectionality', can provide a framework through which service providers can better understand how different factors work together in disadvantaging population groups and creating inequalities (Holman et al., 2021; Williams et al., 2022).

When applying an intersectional lens, we need to recognize that each person is shaped by their simultaneous inclusion of multiple interconnected social categories (e.g. age, race, gender identity, social class) that interact within a context of connected power systems (e.g. oppression and discrimination) and structures (e.g. laws, policies), which then result in structural inequalities. By using an intersectional framework, the multiplicity of factors that affect an individual's or a group's health, their access to care and quality of treatment can be better understood. As health managers, this understanding can inform targeted interventions enabling the creation of more equitable health policies and practices.

Learning activity 4.2

Let us apply an intersectional lens to understand barriers that may face different people with diabetes who are registered with a local community health clinic, and how they can be addressed.

To better understand intersectionality and health, watch the video available on the For Equity website: [https://forequity.uk/general-resources/].

1   Consider the following questions around social categories:
  - How might ethnicity, age, occupation, disability and socioeconomic status intersect to influence access to healthy food options and contribute to diabetes risk?
  - How could language barriers and cultural or religious beliefs about health impact a patient's understanding of diabetes management?
  - Are there any gender-based factors that might influence diabetes risk or healthcare access in this community?
2   Now consider what discriminatory power systems may be operating within the clinic (staff and structures). Think about racism, sexism, homophobia, ableism, ageism, classism – among others. How might these impact accessibility and use of the diabetes service?
3   Finally consider wider structures within your country – including the legal, political, immigration, economic and educational systems, social and historical forces. How might they interact with social identities and contribute to health inequalities related to diabetes in your clinic's patient population?
4   Write down what strategies you could develop to address some of these inequalities. How can you utilize your understanding of intersectionality to:
  - improve access to culturally appropriate diabetes education materials and support groups?
  - reduce language barriers faced by patients through interpretation services or translated materials?
  - partner with community organizations to address social determinants of health, like food insecurity, that contribute to diabetes risk?
  - What are some of the challenges you might face in implementing intersectional approaches in your healthcare setting?

Causes of inequalities

Inequalities arise because of the different conditions in which we are born, live, work and age and are affected by the factors that determine how easy or difficult it is for people to access healthy choices equally. The mechanisms through which health inequalities emerge are diverse and interrelated, and the interplay between biological, social, economic and environmental contributors extend far beyond individual control (Dahlgren and Whitehead, 2006). A comprehensive understanding of the root causes of health disparities is essential for healthcare managers to implement policies and interventions that are informed by and designed to address the systemic factors that perpetuate inequalities.

Health inequalities are consistently observed within almost all countries where they have been studied (Braveman and Tarimo, 2002; Mackenbach et al., 2008) and are also apparent between countries across different social, economic and demographic groups.

Explanatory theories

Several theories have been proposed to explain the existence and persistence of health inequalities. Distinguishing between the underlying causes and mechanisms leading to inequalities is essential for informing action. There is general agreement that contrasting socioeconomic circumstances best explain how health inequalities arise. Some of the main theories (McCartney et al., 2013), summarized below, attempt to explain how variation in socioeconomic factors is shaped and influenced by wider systems and structures:

- *Social Causation, or Determinants Theory (Department of Health and Social Security, 1980; Canning and Bowser, 2010)*: This theory argues that the social conditions in which people live and work, such as poverty, unemployment, limited education, poor housing and limited access to healthy food all lead to increased stress. Reduced access to healthcare and less healthy lifestyles leads to poorer health.
- *Health Selection Theory, or the Drift Hypothesis (Blane et al., 1993)*: This theory suggests that people with better health tend to gravitate towards higher socioeconomic positions, while those with poor health have reduced earning potential and drift towards lower socioeconomic groups. This leads to an association between social class and health. (This theory is limited as it does not explain why disadvantaged groups have worse health across generations.)
- *Behavioural/Cultural Theories (Dean, 1989; Gruer et al., 2009)*: These theories claim that poor health outcomes are a result of unhealthy lifestyle choices made by individuals, such as smoking, poor diet and lack of exercise, which are more prevalent among certain social groups. (This theory is criticized as victim-blaming as it doesn't address the root causes of these behaviours.)
- *Structural/Materialist Theories (Department of Health and Social Security, 1980; Acheson, 1998; Marmot et al., 2020)*: These argue that social structures influencing the distribution of power, wealth and resources and systems, such as discrimination, systematically disadvantage certain groups. This can lead to unequal access to healthcare, education, housing and opportunities for healthy living.

The concept of intersectionality complements these theories and allows us to understand how inequalities may arise. Another concept, 'the inverse care law', formulated by Julian Tudor Hart (Tudor Hart, 1971), describes a paradox in healthcare; people who need the most care are often the ones who receive the least. It describes the cycle of disadvantage whereby individuals and communities facing greater health challenges often have the least access to quality healthcare services, resources and preventative measures, thus further amplifying health inequalities.

In summary, no single theory is sufficient in explaining how inequalities arise, but all are rooted in some supportive evidence and provide insights into mechanisms. Health inequalities can therefore arise throughout the life course through a complex interplay of differences in social contexts that lead to stress, limited access to structural resources or variations in health behaviours, which themselves may be rooted in historic, neighbourhood or social contexts. Institutional factors, such as the healthcare, educational and governmental systems, as well as political and economic policies, can further exacerbate or perpetuate inequalities through unequal access to services or lack of investment in public health infrastructure. Geographical factors also influence both physical and social structures and global influences, such as trade policies or global pandemics, can further exacerbate inequalities.

The theories and concepts discussed in this section will help to explain the patterns of inequalities discussed in the following section and form the basis for the section on interventions for tackling inequalities and the role of health managers within this.

Global and national inequalities in health

In this section we will explore in more detail some data on health inequalities, including how to evaluate such data. Gathering and analyzing data in this way allows us to identify where inequalities lie, who is affected and therefore what interventions are needed. Through this knowledge, health services can be tailored and adapted to meet the needs of diverse groups, as well as empowering managers to allocate resources more effectively to ensure that those who are most in need receive appropriate care. Later in the chapter we will discover why such actions, beyond being an imperative for social justice, contribute to overall public health improvement. In addition to informing interventions to improve services, understanding health inequalities can help healthcare managers to anticipate and respond to emerging health trends and challenges. For example, if certain conditions are more prevalent in specific communities, preventive measures can be focused in those areas. Within a globalized world, awareness of international health trends can also help us better prepare services to meet emerging health challenges.

Health inequalities at the global level

Globally, there is an abundance of evidence of inequalities between countries, with higher disease burden and premature mortality in low- and middle-income countries, compared to high income regions. Widening inequalities, closely linked to higher rates of poverty and lower levels of education, is associated with these poorer health outcomes (Marmot, 2015; Leonard, 2024). For example, data from 2021 show that life expectancy at birth for a child born in Nigeria was 52.7 years, compared to 84.8 years for one born in Japan (Dattani et al., 2023). Life expectancy is a measure that is determined by a combination of factors including socioeconomic status, access to healthcare, diet, lifestyle and the environment (Raleigh, 2024). Around 70 per cent of all maternal deaths globally (number of women who die of pregnancy related causes while pregnant or within a short time after pregnancy) in 2020 were recorded in sub-Saharan Africa (Taylor, 2023). Such deaths are an indicator of wider societal health, including child health, and are largely preventable. Mortality rates from chronic diseases, including cardiovascular disease, are also increasing more rapidly in the developing Global South compared with the highly developed Global North (Stuckler, 2008; Li et al., 2022). There are several sources of data that allow us to examine data on global variations in health measures. Monitoring trends and types of inequalities facilitates both the evaluation and development of evidence-informed, equity-oriented policymaking (Hosseinpoor et al., 2023).

Learning activity 4.3

For this activity, think about the country where you are living or working, and what may be the main priorities for the health system in that country to address inequalities. We will do this by exploring the WHO Health Inequality Data Repository: [https://www.who.int/data/inequality-monitor/data].

You can start with downloading the Life expectancy and mortality dataset: [https://www.who.int/data/sets/health-inequality-monitor-dataset#gho].

Try looking at the data on healthy life expectancy at age 60 years (should take you to this webpage: [https://www.who.int/data/gho/data/indicators/indicator-details/GHO/gho-ghe-hale-healthy-life-expectancy-at-age-60]). How does the data from your country compare with that from other countries? Explore this within the WHO region, as well as globally.

Explore the data further, looking at both the datasets and visuals, examining how the measure has changed over time and varies for males compared to females. You will notice that for most countries, the measure has increased over time and is higher in women compared to men. However, there are exceptions to this. What are the patterns you see for your country and how does this compare to the regional and global trends? What do you think may explain any differences you observe and what role do you think healthcare managers can play in addressing any inequalities you observe?

Now start to explore other tables, selecting inequality indicators that may be more relevant to your country and work setting. Again, consider how the patterns you observe can help healthcare managers prioritize actions within the health system that you are familiar with.

Health inequalities at regional and country level

Inequalities are not confined to between countries. There are also regional inequalities and disparities within countries. You can explore some of the regional differences within the activity above, using the WHO inequality dataset. For example, the probability of dying from cardiovascular disease, cancer, diabetes or chronic respiratory disease for adults aged 30–70 years within Europe in 2019 ranged from 28.3 per cent in Tajikistan to 7.9 per cent in Switzerland (with a European average of 16.3 per cent). Monitoring and exploring data in this way allows us to consider the reasons behind these variations. For instance, differences in economic status, healthcare infrastructure, public health policies and lifestyle choices are likely to contribute to these disparities.

Furthermore, inequalities are also seen within countries and are not confined to low-income settings. Some of the gaps in life expectancy seen between affluent and disadvantaged communities within a single country can be similar to the average life-expectancy gap seen between high- and low-income settings (Marmot, 2017). Some examples are summarized in Box 4.2.

Box 4.2 Examples of within-country inequalities

- In the WHO inequality dataset above on chronic disease mortality risk for Europe, in both Tajikistan and Switzerland, the probability of premature death was slightly higher in men compared with women (31.8 per cent and 9.6 per cent respectively). However, in other countries, such as Turkey, the probability of death from these chronic diseases was almost double in men (21.0 per cent) compared to women 10.8 per cent). The sex differences may be explained by gender-related behaviours and social norms (for example, higher rates of smoking and alcohol consumption in men in certain cultures) or different occupational exposures and hazards. Moreover, men may be less likely to seek medical help or adhere to prescribed treatment, potentially due to cultural perceptions of masculinity and self-reliance.
- Within Scotland (UK) in 2018–20, the gap in life expectancy between men and women from the most affluent, compared to the most deprived areas, was 13.5 and 10.2 years respectively (Miall, 2022).
- On average, a 60-year-old woman in the poorest area of England has a diagnosed illness equivalent to that of a 76-year-old woman in the wealthiest area (Watt et al., 2022).
- Qualitative studies suggest that women from ethnic minority backgrounds in the UK experience 'stereotyping, disrespect, discrimination and cultural insensitivity' when using maternal and neonatal healthcare services (Kapadia et al., 2022).
- In the USA, there is widening gap in life expectancy, with the wealthiest Americans living 10–15 years longer than the poorest (Dickman et al., 2017). Contributing factors include healthcare system financing, which requires a

larger share of household income going towards health services in poor and middle-class families, compared to those who are more affluent. Additionally, highly racially rooted wealth inequalities dating from historical structures, some of which persist, mean the median family wealth for the white population is almost ten times that of African Americans and around five times that of Hispanics (Kochhar and Mosliami, 2023).

- In India, factors such as gender, caste, wealth, education and geography contribute to within-country health inequalities, such as under-five mortality rates being higher in children whose mothers have no education compared to those with mothers having secondary or higher education (106 and 49 per 1000 births, respectively) (Balarajan et al., 2011).

Effective healthcare management involves the collection and analysis of health data to allow surveillance, identify at-risk populations and monitor the impact of health interventions. Such data also informs the development of strategies that improve access to care, promote health education and encourage preventive measures, targeting groups that have the greatest need. This includes advocating for policies that address the root causes of health disparities, such as poverty and education, and tailoring healthcare services to meet the specific needs of different population groups.

Impact of inequalities

So far, we have described health inequalities and explored some of the causes and mechanisms. Before moving on to examine how to address these, it is worth reflecting on the reasons why inequalities matter and different motivations to take action.

Moral and justice considerations

By definition, inequities represent unfair and reversible disparities and therefore there are moral and justice imperatives for us to act to tackle health inequities. Modifiable inequalities violate the principles of equity and justice and equitable access to healthcare is a fundamental human right. Some examples of modifiable inequalities in health service provision include:

- high cost of services, making them unaffordable to those with low incomes
- inequitable access to treatments and interventions due to affordability or supply issues
- low accessibility of services due to limited provision for those who work long hours, live in rural areas
- poor access due to language or communication barriers or disabilities.

The right to health was first articulated in the World Health Organization (WHO) constitution in 1946 (Binagwaho and Mathewos, 2023). It is further enshrined in several international treaties, and is a legal obligation in many countries. It includes access to timely, acceptable and affordable healthcare of appropriate quality, as well as the underlying determinants of health, such as safe and potable water, sanitation, food, housing, health-related information and education, and gender equality.

Social considerations

Furthermore, from a social perspective, poor health leads to a cycle of disadvantage through its adverse impacts on educational and employment opportunities, leading to further generational poverty and ill health. An increasing body of literature, including work by the epidemiologist Richard Wilkinson, provides evidence of the detrimental effects of health inequalities on society. A divided society with extremes of wealth and poverty, associated with thriving and deteriorating health, leads to instability and an overall decline in well-being. Wilkinson argues that it's not just absolute poverty that harms health, but the gap between the rich and the poor in a society (Wilkinson and Pickett, 2009). This and similar work (Lago et al., 2018) demonstrate that interventions that aim to create a more equitable society in terms of income distribution can improve well-being, and overall health for everyone, not just those who are more deprived.

Learning activity 4.4

Listen to Richard Wilkinson's TED Talk: [https://m.youtube.com/watch?v=Ndh58GGCTQo].

- What health problems are highlighted to be linked with income inequality?
- What explanations are offered for these associations?
- What interventions could a health manager in your country implement to try to address some of these inequalities?

Although a lot of the focus of research has been on socioeconomic and income disparities, there is evidence that health benefits extend to other forms of equity as well. For example, a study examining the association between gender inequality and life expectancy using panel data from OECD countries during the period 1990–2017, showed a linear association between greater gender equity and higher life expectancy (Veas et al., 2021). A similar direction of effect was reported in a systematic review of studies that examined the association between gender equity in different countries and different health outcomes (Milner et al., 2021).

Economic considerations

Beyond these considerations, health inequities have economic impacts, resulting from productivity loss and increased healthcare burden. In the UK, the Marmot Review (Marmot et al., 2010) estimated the annual societal cost of health inequalities to be around £31 billion (2010 prices), while US studies estimate the annual cost from racial and ethnic health disparities at $451 billion (2018 prices) (LaVeist et al., 2023). The additional hospitalization costs associated with the higher disease burden associated with deprivation was estimated to be £4.8 billion per year in the UK (2011 prices) (Asaria et al., 2016). Overall, there is accumulating evidence globally that investing in health equity would lead to considerable returns on investment (Yerramilli et al., 2024).

Other considerations

These include the importance of health as a key component within the UN Sustainable Development Goals, and tackling health inequities will significantly support the achievement of these broader goals. Finally, particularly considering the experiences of the COVID-19 pandemic, addressing health inequalities would contribute to a more stable and resilient society, with lower risk of community transmission in the face of pandemics.

In summary, tackling health inequalities is not just a moral obligation, but also a pertinent social and economic investment. Reducing inequity, including within healthcare delivery services, leads to a fairer society with better productivity and improved health for everyone.

Interventions to tackle inequalities

Policy reviews and reports

Internationally, several prominent reports have attempted to analyse and describe health inequalities, the determinants of inequities and recommend actions to address them. In the UK, one of the first was the Black Report (Department of Health and Social Security, 1980; Gray, 1982), a pioneering UK study highlighting stark differences in health outcomes across social classes and attributing these to a range of social determinants, such as income, education and employment conditions. The report recommended comprehensive policy measures, including strengthening of community health and primary care, as well as broader social policies, such as improvements in child benefits, housing and minimum working conditions as potential solutions. Following this, the Acheson Report (Acheson, 1988) further investigated health disparities in the UK, emphasizing the need for health impact assessments for all policies and advocating for a cross-sectoral approach to health that included partnerships between health and local government to tackle education, housing and income distribution.

More recently, the updated Marmot Review (Marmot et al., 2020) revisited a previously commissioned UK government report on addressing health inequalities. This highlighted a widening health gap between the rich and poor and a slowdown in life expectancy, with a notable decline among the poorest women. The report suggested that austerity policies, cuts to public services and funding for education were key drivers of these declines. The importance of the social determinants of health and addressing these through policies and strengthening of the public health infrastructure were emphasized.

In the US, a key report by the Institute of Medicine (Smedley et al., 2003) exposed racial and ethnic disparities in healthcare access and quality, highlighting significant disadvantage, discrimination and care for minority ethnic groups compared to white populations, resulting in poorer health outcomes for these groups. The report recommended reforms in healthcare financing, workforce diversity and cultural competency training.

At an international level, The World Health Organization's Commission on the Social Determinants of Health landmark report (World Health Organization, 2003) highlighted the profound impact of social factors, like income, education and housing, on health outcomes. It called for a global approach to addressing these determinants to achieve health equity. More recently the World Health Organization and Lancet Commission on Ending Childhood Obesity report (Nishtar et al., 2016) drew attention to the global rise of childhood obesity and its unequal distribution across socioeconomic groups. It advocated for multisectoral interventions addressing factors like poverty, unhealthy food environments and marketing practices.

Further reports such as the OECD's 'Health at a Glance' series (OECD, 2023), and reports on health inequalities from the World Bank, including Inequalities in Health in Developing Countries (Wagstaff, 2002) provide comparative data on health inequalities and suggest solutions for developed and developing countries respectively. The World Bank studies shed light on the challenges faced by low-income countries, including limited access to healthcare services and the impact of infectious diseases on marginalized populations. These reports often emphasize the role of international aid and the need for strengthening health systems to achieve equity in health.

Common themes emerging from reviews and international studies on health inequities

Overall, the many policy reports and reviews from across the world highlight several recurring themes for tackling health inequities:

- A recognition that health inequalities are not merely a result of individual lifestyle choices but are deeply rooted in structural and social factors.
- The need to implement multifaceted approaches that address the broader determinants of health, in particular, highlighting the importance of upstream, low-agency interventions that address the root causes of inequalities. This includes interventions to tackle poverty and discrimination through social policies and community development initiatives.
- Recommendations to improve access to healthcare. This may be through expanding health insurance coverage, reducing geographic barriers to care or ensuring culturally competent services.
- Emphasis on public health initiatives that promote healthy behaviours, healthy food environments and early childhood development programmes.
- The importance of data collection and analysis to monitor social determinants and health outcomes disaggregated by social identity and allow evaluation of interventions.

- The value of holding policymakers accountable for reducing health disparities and advocacy for policies that promote equity and social justice in health.
- A recognition that implementing recommendations requires political will, intersectoral collaboration and sustained investment in public health infrastructure and social services.

By understanding these reports and their recommendations in their national and international contexts, healthcare managers can gain valuable insights into the complex causes of health inequalities and identify local strategies (and as appropriate contribute at a national level) to create a more just and equitable system of healthcare.

Examples of specific interventions

Although most countries still grapple with how to reduce health inequalities and move towards equity, there are several examples of successful interventions at different levels. Below we explore some of these in more detail.

Social interventions

There is increasing evidence that schooling and education has beneficial effects on health outcomes, including reducing mortality (Balaj et al., 2024). In particular, education of women and girls reduces gender health inequalities (Ross et al., 2012), with outcomes hypothesized to be realized through a combination of economic, social and educational mechanisms (Braveman and Gottlieb, 2014). Healthcare providers and managers can support initiatives that promote women's education through partnering with local organizations like schools and community centres to offer health education and address social determinants of health. Furthermore, managers have a critical role in promoting gender equity through supporting women towards leadership roles within healthcare (Mousa et al., 2021).

Economic measures

Fiscal and economic strategies, such as implementation of tax systems to change demand for products that could influence health, are examples of upstream, low-agency initiatives that can contribute to reducing health inequalities. For example, there is high-quality evidence that the intervention with the greatest potential to reduce socioeconomic inequalities in smoking is to increase tobacco price via taxation (Sarah et al., 2014). An example of healthcare managers supporting such initiatives was in the US, where they launched a campaign with citizens to support Proposition 56, a ballot initiative to increase the cigarette tax by $2 per pack called *Proposition 56: A New Era in State Funded Healthcare and Research in California* (Tobacco-Related Disease Research Program (TRDRP), 2016; Purushothaman et al., 2023). This was done through public education campaigns, lobbying and formation of community partnerships.

Another example of a successful economic strategy comes from Scandinavian countries. Norway and Sweden's progressive tax system results in redistribution of wealth and reduced income inequality, which in turn is associated with better health outcomes. Among other policies, this has meant that Norway has a sustained plan for addressing the social determinants of health (Fosse, 2022). Modelling studies from Scotland also demonstrate that income-based policies have the potential to reduce health inequalities and mortality (Richardson et al., 2020). Although such strategies require government action, healthcare leaders have a role in partnering with government agencies and lobbying for change.

Health service action

There is an abundance of past and ongoing research on interventions to reduce health inequalities within the health sector, focusing on increasing access, acceptability and targeting services to those in most need. Rather than describing these in detail, it is worth highlighting available resources and summary reviews. Some of these are summarized in Box 4.3.

Box 4.3   Some resources that summarize tools and interventions for addressing health inequalities for health managers

Resources:

Living evidence maps of published research on *'What Works'* to address health inequalities in primary care. https://www.heec.co.uk/component-library/evidence-maps/

List of resources and guidance through the CLEAR collaboration on actions that healthcare professionals can use to address health inequalities in their practice (Andermann, 2016)

A framework of overarching principles to guide primary care facilities and reduce health inequalities, based on a review of the literature (Gkiouleka et al., 2023).

An umbrella review of interventions to address health inequalities within the health sector Garzón-Orjuela et al., 2020), that concludes interventions should be intersectoral and multidisciplinary.

Key themes:

- Focusing on people's individual behaviours and how to change those are largely ineffective (Vilhelmsson and Östergren, 2018).
- It is important to shift the focus to systems processes and practices. This includes making services flexible, inclusive and community centred.
- Benefits of universal access to healthcare services
- Coordinating services across the system to make them more connected improves accessibility
- Using an intersectionality lens allows us to identify and address institutional structures and practices that create barriers to meaningful engagement with those who are marginalized
- Action is needed at multiple levels and requires partnership and intersectoral working
- Importance of monitoring and measurement of inequalities, as a tool for improving outcomes and for evaluation of interventions

---

Learning activity 4.5

Go back to activity 4.3, where you used the WHO Health Inequality Data Repository.

This resource has an associated health equity assessment tool, HEAT, which is available from: https://whoequity.shinyapps.io/heat/#

Using this resource, explore some of the datasets to examine trends in inequalities by different dimensions (e.g. age, sex, socioeconomic group) for your country of interest.

Also look at how data from your country compares with other countries and draft a summary note of the key inequalities challenges facing your nation and its health system.

In summary, addressing inequalities requires a multifaceted approach that moves beyond interventions focused solely on individual behaviour. Healthcare managers must understand these factors to effectively address and reduce health disparities.

Role of healthcare managers

Throughout the chapter, the role of healthcare managers in tackling public health inequalities has been discussed. Here, these are summarized and include some additional suggestions where management can play a key role.

Awareness, training and continuous professional development

Through this chapter, you will have learnt about the nature and importance of the social determinants of health. You will have discovered that health outcomes are not equally distributed, explored some of the social groups that are more vulnerable, and measures used to assess health inequalities, as well as some of the reasons behind these. In each section, the type of actions that managers can take both within and outside of the health system have been highlighted. As health managers it is essential to keep up to date with emerging findings on how to address health inequalities, for example, through continuing professional development (CPD) activities or being part of learning networks, such as the Health Anchors Learning Network [https://haln.org.uk/], which provides opportunities for health professionals and managers to share learning and to use case studies to inform their practice. You might also take up opportunities to develop relevant skills for addressing health inequalities as part of wider health management, such as communication, partnership working and advocacy.

Monitoring and evaluation

The importance of data collection, analysis and communication was emphasized in earlier parts of the chapter. Data is important for prioritizing action, monitoring evaluation and as a lever for change. It is important to ensure data covers both the categories of characteristics that determine groups of interest (such as age, sex, ethnicity, socioeconomic group), as well as the measures or outcomes that indicate inequalities (e.g. mortality, service access, satisfaction). Involving communities and service users is important in determining what measures to include that are meaningful to those we serve.

Workforce diversity, health and well-being

Health managers have a critical role in overseeing the health and well-being of their workforce, and to ensure that health inequities among their employed staff are also tackled (Ross et al., 2020; Hemmings et al., 2021). Health services are often large employers and have a responsibility as a workforce and role model to others. Increasing staff diversity is not just about fairness, but also improves productivity, creativity and understanding, and, as we explored earlier in the chapter, the well-being of the entire workforce. Managers should ensure all their staff are provided with good quality work (i.e. work that is free of health-adverse effects, while being beneficial to the worker) (Public Health England, 2020) and that the workforce culture supports health equity. As large employers, healthcare organizations can also use their purchasing power, in both employment and commissioning, to benefit their local population, improving their health and reducing inequalities.

Partnership working

In previous sections, the importance of partnership working was emphasized as an essential tool for effective action for reducing inequalities. Partnerships across the health sector, integrating and co-ordinating care, are important in order to improve access and provide more flexibility, which in turn are all likely to reduce inequalities. However, multisectoral partnerships and working with other agencies are also necessary. As we have seen, many of the root causes of health inequalities lie in social and economic conditions, and interventions and strategies to address these often lie outside of the health service. Therefore, working with schools, housing, local and regional government, police, fire services and others to tackle the social determinants of health is essential. Partnerships should also be with charities and third-sector organizations and private companies to ensure that the needs of the wider population are considered and diverse community groups are included. Such partnerships often develop organically in local settings, but increasingly case studies and overviews describe the elements and principles of successful partnerships. For example, a US group have developed principles to guide the design of cross-sector partnerships to address childhood adversity, considering how to integrate healthcare with food support, legal, housing and financial services (Liu et al., 2022). Further consideration of partnership working, in the context of integrated care, is made in Chapter 15 (Integrated care).

Advocacy

Healthcare managers can act as powerful advocates for individuals, communities, the health workforce and the general population. In order to improve health and reduce inequalities, many strategies involve actions from other organizations. Health managers are experts and trusted professionals, often linked with professional and national membership organizations that have power to lobby and advocate for change. Legislative, fiscal and economic measures that are effective in reducing health inequalities require government action. Health managers can use their knowledge, provide data to influence decision-makers to ensure policies consider health equity and thus contribute to the development of fairer health systems. For example, the Royal College of Physicians in England has convened a coalition of over 140 organizations to campaign for a cross-government strategy to reduce inequalities (https://www.rcplondon.ac.uk/projects/inequalities-health-alliance). In many other countries, including the US (Counts et al., 2021) and Canada (Andermann, 2016), health professionals and organizations also play an active role in lobbying and advocacy to address the upstream social determinants of health.

Conclusion

This chapter has described global health inequalities, including some of the patterns of inequity, the measures used and explored the root causes and theories of why some groups of the population have poorer health. We have also examined some of the interventions that have been shown to effectively address some inequalities and the role of healthcare managers. To be effective, strategies should tackle systems and structures and require collaborative, multisectoral collaboration.

Understanding health inequalities is fundamental for healthcare managers to fulfil their role effectively. It enables them to provide targeted, equitable care, improve resource allocation, respond to health trends, and advocate for systemic change. By doing so, they not only meet the immediate needs of patients and communities but also contribute to the long-term goal of achieving health equity.

Learning resources

World Health Organization: WHO is the United Nations agency that connects nations, partners and people to promote health. It is responsible for providing leadership on global health matters, shaping the health research agenda, setting norms and standards, articulating evidence-based policy options, providing technical support to countries and monitoring and assessing health trends. Extensive data on a range of health topics for WHO member states is accessible on their website [http://www.who.int/], some of which has been referred to throughout the chapter. Particularly relevant links include:

WHO Health Inequality Data Repository: [https://www.who.int/news/item/20-04-2023-who-releases-the-largest-global-collection-of-health-inequality-data], which is the most comprehensive global collection of publicly available disaggregated data and evidence on population health and its determinants.

WHO Health Inequality Monitor: [https://www.who.int/data/inequality-monitor], which provides evidence, tools, resources, and training on health inequality monitoring.

Institute for Health Metrics and Evaluation (IHME): This is an independent population health research organization based at the University of Washington School of Medicine. The Institute works with collaborators around the world to develop timely, relevant and scientifically valid evidence, aiming to inform health policy and practice. It provides data and articles and reviews on some of the world's most important health problems and discusses strategies to address these, including topic-related health inequalities [https://www.healthdata.org/].

The King's Fund: The King's Fund is an independent charitable organization focusing on health and care in England. Within their Insight and Analysis section, there are several articles that discuss and review aspects of health inequalities, some of which are referenced in the chapter [https://www.kingsfund.org.uk/].

Public Health Scotland Learning Zone: This includes a range of learning resources on public health and health inequalities for people working in the health sector. Although the focus is on Scotland, there is valuable transferrable information that is applicable to other health systems. The resources are highly accessible and include videos and reflective activities [https://learning.publichealthscotland.scot/course/view.php?id=580].

US Centre for Disease Control and Prevention (CDC), Social Determinants of Health section: The CDC is a science-based, data-driven, service organization in the US aimed at protecting the public's health. As the social determinants of health are an important health policy priority in the US, the CDC offers a range of resources on how these affect health and health inequalities and how to address them [https://www.cdc.gov/about/priorities/why-is-addressing-sdoh-important.html].

References

Acheson, D. (1988) Report of the Committee of Inquiry into the future development of the public health function. London: HMSO.

Andermann, A. (2016) Taking action on the social determinants of health in clinical practice: a framework for health professionals, *Canadian Medical Association Journal*, 188(17–18): E474-e483. http://dx.doi.org/10.1503/cmaj.160177.

Asaria, M., Doran, T. and Cookson, R. (2016) The costs of inequality: whole-population modelling study of lifetime inpatient hospital costs in the English National Health Service by level of neighbourhood deprivation, *Journal of Epidemiology and Community Health*, 70(10): 990–6. http://dx.doi.org/10.1136/jech-2016-207447.

Balaj, M., Henson, C.A., Aronsson, A., Aravkin, A., Beck, K., Degail, C. et al. (2024) Effects of education on adult mortality: a global systematic review and meta-analysis, *The Lancet Public Health*, 9(3): e155–e165. http://dx.doi.org/10.1016/S2468-2667(23)00306-7.

Balarajan, Y., Selvaraj, S. and Subramanian, S.V. (2011) Health care and equity in India, *The Lancet*, 377(9764): 505–15. http://dx.doi.org/10.1016/s0140-6736(10)61894-6).

Binagwaho, A. and Mathewos, K. (2023) The right to health: looking beyond health facilities, *Health and Human Rights*, 25(1): 133–135.

Blane, D., Smith, G.D. and Bartley, M. (1993) Social selection: what does it contribute to social class differences in health?, *Sociology of Health and Illness*, 15(1): 1–15 [https://doi.org/10.1111/j.1467-9566.1993.tb00328.x.

Braveman, P. and Gottlieb, L. (2014) The social determinants of health: it's time to consider the causes of the causes, *Public Health Reports*, 129 Suppl 2(Suppl 2), 19–31. http://dx.doi.org/10.1177/00333549141291s206.

Braveman, P. and Gruskin, S. (2003) Defining equity in health, *Journal of Epidemiology and Community Health*, 57(4), 254–8 (http://dx.doi.org/10.1136/jech.57.4.254).

Braveman, P. and Tarimo, E. (2002) Social inequalities in health within countries: not only an issue for affluent nations, *Social Science & Medicine*, 54(11): 1621–35. http://dx.doi.org/10.1016/s0277-9536(01)00331-8.

Canning, D. and Bowser, D. (2010) Investing in health to improve the wellbeing of the disadvantaged: reversing the argument of Fair Society, Healthy Lives (the Marmot Review), *Social Science & Medicine*, 71(7): 1223–1226. http://dx.doi.org/10.1016/j.socscimed.2010.07.009.

Counts, N.Z., Taylor, L.A., Willison, C.E. and Galea, S. (2021) Healthcare lobbying on upstream social determinants of health in the US, *Preventive Medicine*, 153, 106751. https://doi.org/10.1016/j.ypmed.2021.106751.

Dahlgren, G. and Whitehead, M. (2006) European Strategies for Tackling Social Inequities in Health: Levelling up Part 2. World Health Organization Regional Office for Europe. (https://dssbr.ensp.fiocruz.br/wp-content/uploads/2020/10/European-strategies-for-tackling-social-inequities-1.pdf; accessed 18 December 2024).

Dattani, S., Rodes-Guirao, G.L., Ritchie, H., Ortiz-Ospina, E. and Roser, M. (2023) Life Expectancy [https://ourworldindata.org/life-expectancy?utm_source=substack&utm_medium=email; accessed 18 December 2024].

Dean, M. (1989) Christmas, the poor, and the development of a UK underclass, *The Lancet*, 334(8678): 1536–1537. http://dx.doi.org/10.1016/S0140-6736(89)92989-9.

Department of Health and Social Security (1980) Inequalities in Health: Report of a Research Working Group (The Black Report). London: DHSS, 1980.

Dickman, S.L., Himmelstein, D.U. and Woolhandler, S. (2017) Inequality and the health-care system in the USA, *The Lancet*, 389(10077). 1431–1441. http://dx.doi.org/https://doi.org/10.1016/S0140-6736(17)30398-7.

Fosse, E. (2022) Norwegian policies to reduce social inequalities in health: developments from 1987 to 2021, *Scandinavian Journal of Public Health*, 50(7): 882–886. http://dx.doi.org/10.1177/14034948221129685.

Garzón-Orjuela, N., Samacá-Samacá, D.F., Luque Angulo, S.C., Mendes Abdala, C.V., Reveiz, L. and Eslava-Schmalbach, J. (2020) An overview of reviews on strategies to reduce health inequalities, *International Journal for Equity in Health*, 19(1): 192. http://dx.doi.org/10.1186/s12939-020-01299-w.

Gkiouleka, A., Wong, G., Sowden, S., Bambra, C., Siersbaek, R., Manji, S., et al. (2023) Reducing health inequalities through general practice, *The Lancet Public Health*, 8(6): e463–e472. http://dx.doi.org/10.1016/S2468-2667(23)00093-2.

Goddard, M. and Smith, P. (2001) Equity of access to health care services: theory and evidence from the UK, *Social Science & Medicine*, 53(9): 1149–62. http://dx.doi.org/10.1016/s0277-9536(00)00415-9.

Gray, A.M. (1982) Inequalities in health. The Black Report: a summary and comment, *International Journal of Health Services*, 12(3): 349–80. http://dx.doi.org/10.2190/xxmm-jmqu-2a7y-hx1e.

Gruer, L., Hart, C.L., Gordon, D.S. and Watt, G.C.M. (2009) Effect of tobacco smoking on survival of men and women by social position: a 28 year cohort study, *British Medical Journal*, 338, b480. http://dx.doi.org/10.1136/bmj.b480.

Hemmings, N.B., Buckingham, H., Oung, C. and Palmer, W. (2021) Attracting, supporting and retaining a diverse NHS workforce. London: Nuffield Trust.

Holman, D., Salway, S., Bell, A., Beach, B., Adebajo, A., Ali, N., et al. (2021) Can intersectionality help with understanding and tackling health inequalities? Perspectives of professional stakeholders, *Health Research Policy and Systems*, 19(1): 97. http://dx.doi.org/10.1186/s12961-021-00742-w.

Hosseinpoor, A.R., Bergen, N., Kirkby, K. and Schlotheuber, A. (2023) Strengthening and expanding health inequality monitoring for the advancement of health equity: a review of WHO resources and contributions, *International Journal for Equity in Health*, 22(1): 49. http://dx.doi.org/10.1186/s12939-022-01811-4.

Kapadia, D., Zhang, J., Salway, S., Nazroo, J., Booth, A., Villarroel-Williams, N., et al. (2022) Ethnic inequalities in healthcare: a rapid review, NHS Race & Health Observatory.

Kisling, L.A. and Das, J.M. (2024) Prevention Strategies in StatPearls. Treasure Island (FL): StatPearls Publishing.

Kochhar, R.M. and Moslimani, M. (2023) Wealth surged in the pandemic, but debt endures for poorer Black and Hispanic families. Pew Research Center [www.pewresearch.org/wp-content/uploads/sites/20/2023/12/RE_2023.12.04_Race-Wealth_Report.pdf; accessed 13 June 2024].

Lago, S., Cantarero, D., Rivera, B., Pascual, M., Blázquez-Fernández, C., Casal, B., et al. (2018) Socioeconomic status, health inequalities and non-communicable diseases: a systematic review, *Z Gesundh Wiss*, 26(1): 1–14. http://dx.doi.org/10.1007/s10389-017-0850-z.

LaVeist, T.A., Pérez-Stable, E.J., Richard, P., Anderson, A., Isaac, L.A., et al. (2023) The economic burden of racial, ethnic, and educational health inequities in the US, *Journal of the American Medical Association*, 329(19): 1682–1692. http://dx.doi.org/10.1001/jama.2023.5965.

Leonard, C. (2024) The sociology of global health: inequality, disease-related stigma, and the rise of nongovernmental organizations, *Sociology Compass*, 18(2): e13176. http://dx.doi.org/https://doi.org/10.1111/soc4.13176.

Li, Y., Cao, G.-y., Jing, W.-z., Liu, J. and Liu, M. (2022) Global trends and regional differences in incidence and mortality of cardiovascular disease, 1990–2019: findings from 2019 global burden of disease study, *European Journal of Preventive Cardiology*, 30(3): 276–286. http://dx.doi.org/10.1093/eurjpc/zwac285.

Liu, P.Y., Beck, A.F., Lindau, S.T., Holguin, M., Kahn, R.S., Fleegler, E., et al. (2022) A framework for cross-sector partnerships to address childhood adversity and improve life course health, *Pediatrics*, 149 (Supplement 5). http://dx.doi.org/10.1542/peds.2021-053509O.

Mackenbach, J.P., Stirbu, I., Roskam, A.J.R., Schaap, M.M., Menvielle, G., Leinsalu, M., et al. (2008) Socioeconomic inequalities in health in 22 European countries, *New England Journal of Medicine*, 358(23): 2468–2481. http://dx.doi.org/10.1056/NEJMsa0707519.

MacKinnon, N.J., Emery, V., Waller, J., Ange, B., Ambade, P., Gunja, M., et al. (2023) Mapping health disparities in 11 high-income nations, *JAMA Network Open*, 6(7): e2322310. http://dx.doi.org/10.1001/jamanetworkopen.2023.22310].

Marmot, M. (2015) The health gap: the challenge of an unequal world, *The Lancet*, 386(10011), 2442–2444 [http://dx.doi.org/10.1016/S0140-6736(15)00150-6.

Marmot, M. (2017) The health gap: the challenge of an unequal world: the argument, *International Journal of Epidemiology*, 46(4): 1312–1318. http://dx.doi.org/10.1093/ije/dyx163.

Marmot, M., Allen, J., Boyce, T., Goldblatt. P. and Morrison, J. (2020) Health Equity in England: The Marmot Review 10 years on, Institute of Health Equity [health.org.uk/publications/reports/the-marmot-review-10-years-on; accessed 18 December 2024].

Marmot, M., Allen., T., Bell, J., Black, C., Broadfoot, P., Cumberlege, J., et al. (2010) Fair Society, Healthy Lives. The Marmot Review [https://www.instituteofhealthequity.org/resources-reports/fair-society-healthy-lives-the-marmot-review; accessed 18 December 2024].

McCartney, G., Collins, C. and Mackenzie, M. (2013) What (or who) causes health inequalities: theories, evidence and implications?, *Health Policy*, 113(3): 221–227. http://dx.doi.org/https://doi.org/10.1016/j.healthpol.2013.05.021.

Miall, N., Fergie, G. and Pearce, A. (2022) Health Inequalities in Scotland: Trends in Deaths, Health and Wellbeing, Health Behaviours, and Health Services since 2000. Scotland: MRC/CSO Social and Public Health Sciences Unit, University of Glasgow.

Milner, A., Kavanagh, A., Scovelle, A.J., O'Neil, A., Kalb, G., Hewitt, B., et al. (2021) Gender equality and health in high-income countries: a systematic review of within-country indicators of gender equality in relation to health outcomes, *Women's Health Reports* (New Rochelle), 2(1): 113–123. http://dx.doi.org/10.1089/whr.2020.0114.

Mousa, M., Boyle, J., Skouteris, H., Mullins, A.K., Currie, G., Riach, K., et al. (2021) Advancing women in healthcare leadership: a systematic review and meta-synthesis of multi-sector evidence on organisational interventions, *EClinicalMedicine*, 39, 101084. http://dx.doi.org/10.1016/j.eclinm.2021.101084.

Nishtar, S., Gluckman, P. and Armstrong, T. (2016) Ending childhood obesity: a time for action, *The Lancet*, 387(10021): 825–827. http://dx.doi.org/10.1016/S0140-6736(16)00140-9.

OECD (2023) Health at a Glance 2023: OECD Indicators. Paris: OECD Publishing. (https://doi.org/10.1787/7a7afb35-en.

Public Health England (2020) *Local action on health inequalities: Promoting good quality jobs to reduce health inequalities*. London: Public Health England. [https://www.instituteofhealthequity.org/resources-reports/local-action-on-health-inequalities-promoting-good-quality-jobs-to-reduce-health-inequalities-/local-action-on-health-inequalities-promoting-good-quality-jobs-to-reduce-health-inequalities-full-report.pdf].

Purushothaman, V., Cuomo, R.E., Li, J. and Mackey, T.K. (2023) Examining the association between California tobacco licensed retail density and public support or opposition to state anti-tobacco legislation, *Tobacco Prevention & Cessation*, 9, 2. http://dx.doi.org/10.18332/tpc/156460.

Raleigh, V. (2024) What is happening to life expectancy in England?, The Kings Fund [https://www.kingsfund.org.uk/insight-and-analysis/long-reads/whats-happening-life-expectancy-england; accessed 20 May 2024].

Richardson, E., Fenton, L., Parkinson, J., Pulford, A., Taulbut, M., McCartney, G., et al. (2020) The effect of income-based policies on mortality inequalities in Scotland: a modelling study, *The Lancet Public Health*, 5(3): e150–e156. http://dx.doi.org/10.1016/S2468-2667(20)30011-6.

Ross, C.E., Masters, R.K. and Hummer, R.A. (2012) Education and the gender gaps in health and mortality, *Demography*, 49(4): 1157–83. http://dx.doi.org/10.1007/s13524-012-0130-z.

Ross, S., Jabbal, J., Chauhan, K., Maguire, D., Randhawa, M. and Dahir, S. (2020) Workforce race inequalities and inclusion in NHS providers, United Kingdom: The King's Fund https://policycommons.net/artifacts/1715931/workforce-race-inequalities-and-inlcusion-in-nhs-providers/ accessed 18 December 2024].

Sarah, H., Amanda, A., David, C. and Stephen, P. (2014) Impact of tobacco control interventions on socioeconomic inequalities in smoking: review of the evidence, *Tobacco Control*, 23(e2): e89. http://dx.doi.org/10.1136/tobaccocontrol-2013-051110.

Smedley, B.D., Stith, A.Y. and Nelson, A.R. (eds) (2003) Unequal Treatment: Confronting Racial and Ethnic Disparities in Health Care. Institute of Medicine (US) Committee on Understanding and Eliminating Racial and Ethnic Disparities in Health Care. Washington, DC: National Academies Press. DOI: 10.17226/12875.

Stuckler, D. (2008) Population causes and consequences of leading chronic diseases: a comparative analysis of prevailing explanations, *Milbank Quarterly*, 86(2): 273–326. http://dx.doi.org/10.1111/j.1468-0009.2008.00522.x.

Taylor, L. (2023) Maternal health is now deteriorating in much of the world, UN report shows, *British Medical Journal*, 380, 454. http://dx.doi.org/10.1136/bmj.p454.

Tobacco-Related Disease Research Program (TRDRP) (2016) Proposition 56: A New Era in State Funded Healthcare and Research in California (https://trdrp.org/news/prop-56-state-funded-medical-research-healthcare%20.html; accessed 12 June 2024].

Tudor Hart, J. (1971) The inverse care law, *The Lancet*, 297(7696): 405–412. http://dx.doi.org/10.1016/S0140-6736(71)92410-X.

Veas, C., Crispi, F. and Cuadrado, C. (2021) Association between gender inequality and population-level health outcomes: panel data analysis of organization for Economic Co-operation and Development (OECD) countries, *eClinicalMedicine*, 39. http://dx.doi.org/10.1016/j.eclinm.2021.101051.

Vilhelmsson, A. and Östergren, P.O. (2018) Reducing health inequalities with interventions targeting behavioral factors among individuals with low levels of education: a rapid review, *PLOS One*, 13(4): e0195774. http://dx.doi.org/10.1371/journal.pone.0195774.

Wagstaff, A. (2002) Inequalities in Health in Developing Countries: Swimming against the Tide?, Policy Research Working Paper 2795. The World Bank Development Research Group Public Services and Human Development Network Health, Nutrition, and Population Team.

Watt, T., Raymond, A. and Rachet-Jacquet, L. (2022) Quantifying health inequalities in England: the Health Foundation [https://www.health.org.uk/news-and-comment/charts-and-infographics/quantifying-health-inequalities; accessed 18 December 2024].

WHO and World Bank (2023) Tracking Universal Health Coverage: 2023 Global monitoring report, Geneva [https://iris.who.int/bitstream/handle/10665/374059/9789240080379-eng.pdf?sequence=1; accessed 18 December 2024].

Wilkinson, R.D. and Pickett, K. (2009) *The Spirit Level: Why More Equal Societies Almost Always Do Better.* New York, NY: Bloomsbury Publishing.

Williams, E., Buck, D., Babalola, G., Maguire, D. (2022) What are health inequalities? The King's Fund [https://www.kingsfund.org.uk/insight-and-analysis/long-reads/what-are-health-inequalities; accessed 20 May 2024].

World Bank (2022) Life expectancy at birth, World development indicators.

World Health Organization (2003) The world health report 2003: shaping the future, World Health Organization.

World Health Organization (2021) State of inequality: HIV, tuberculosis and malaria. Geneva: World Health Organization.

World Health Organization (2023) Health Inequality Data Repository [https://www.who.int/data/inequality-monitor/health-inequality-data-repository; accessed 1 March 2024].

Yerramilli, P., Chopra, M. and Rasanathan, K. (2024) The cost of inaction on health equity and its social determinants, *BMJ Global Health*, 9 (Suppl 1). http://dx.doi.org/10.1136/bmjgh-2023-012690.

Equality, diversity and inclusion

Dr Sandie Dunne

Introduction

It is without doubt that one of the most pertinent issues in health policy in the twenty-first century is that of equality, diversity and inclusion (EDI). This is seen in policy and strategy documents from major nations across the globe (Government of Canada, 2017; Australian Government Department of Health and Aged Care, 2023; NHS England, 2023a; New Zealand Government Ministry of Health / Manatū Hauora, 2023).

This chapter sets out to explore key concepts in relation to EDI to help readers understand the thinking and development of key ideas behind these terms and to raise healthcare managers' awareness of current debates related to healthcare, with reference to equity and social justice. In doing so, it will provide examples from international health systems and explore key issues in terms of policy and practice for managers at work. By the end of this chapter, health and care managers will be able to develop skills in building more inclusive teams and organizational cultures that promote social justice, equality, diversity and inclusion within their workplaces.

Theorizing equality, diversity and inclusion – understanding key EDI concepts in relation to social justice and equity

While the acronym EDI has become commonplace in western democracies, such as the UK, it is perhaps wiser to start a discussion of equality, diversity and inclusion by referring to the US acronym of DEI – diversity, equity and inclusion. This is because to achieve equality (and equity) one must recognize a starting point that all individuals are unique or different. It is from this that equality (and equity) can be promoted, advanced towards and both practised and managed, through being inclusive.

However, before advancing any of these definitions further, it is important to acknowledge that, like most academic definitions, these terms are contested, differing across context, time and disciplines, due, in large parts, to the very nature of uniqueness and difference. This means their application in, for example, education, with respect to gender, in terms of the environment of health, requires circumspection and consideration that such terminology can be interpreted differently by different people in different contexts.

To begin, this section will consider social justice, before outlining definitions of diversity, inclusion, equality and equity.

Social justice

Justice is the concept of fairness. Social justice is fairness as it manifests in society. That includes fairness in healthcare, employment, housing, education and more. The concept of social justice came to prominence in the eighteenth century (Zajda et al., 2006) and in Rawls' (1971: 4) definition of the principles of social justice as providing '...a way of assigning rights and duties in the basic institutions of society; [they] define the appropriate distribution of benefits and burdens of social co-operation'. Social justice depends on four essential goals: human rights, access, participation and equity. We often connect the social determinants of health (Dahlgreen and Whitehead, 1991; 2021), that is, the factors that contribute to our health and well-being to the conditions of social justice.

For many, social justice is associated with a quid pro quo of 'give and take', in which individuals fulfil their role in society (some might call this 'responsibilities' or 'cooperation') and receive in return recognition from society in the form of 'rights (Banai et al., 2011); that is to say, benefits and burdens of being a member of society' (Rawls, 1971): taxation, public health, education, public services, employment rights, the regulation of markets, to ensure a fair distribution of wealth and equal opportunity (Bejan, 2021; Hayvon, 2024).

More recently, the emphasis has moved to breaking down of barriers related to social mobility, the creation of safety nets and economic as well as distributive justice, in a context of opportunities and deprivations (Rhodes et al., 2012: 2), recognizing that inequalities are likely to be 'baked in' to society through the passage of time (Khan, 2018), caused by different ideologies, modes and models of government and governance that have led to unfairness and injustice (Rodriguez-Bailon et al., 2017).

Diversity

Diversity is about understanding that every person is unique or different. At the heart of promoting diversity is a willingness to embrace people's differences with respect to their beliefs, abilities, preferences, backgrounds, values and identities (Roberson and Perry, 2021). Within organizations, diversity could be considered as the composition of groups or workforces (Roberson, 2004). These could be demographic differences among members (McGrath et al., 1995) or resulting from potential behavioural differences among cultural groups (Larkey, 1996).

These may be due to observable and non-observable characteristics (Milliken and Martins, 1996), such as gender, race, ethnicity and age, which are legally protected from discrimination, particularly in the United States and United Kingdom (Roberson, 2004; see also Box 5.1: UK Equality Act, 2010) and also include cultural, cognitive and technical differences (Kochan et al., 2003). Thompson (2020: 6) furthers this by stating that '… these are not only dimensions of diversity in a sociological sense, they are also dimensions of experience in a psychological sense', part of lived experience.

Box 5.1   UK Equality Act (2010) (UK legislation)

This Act of UK Parliament offers legal protection from discrimination in the workplace and society. This legislation brought previous anti-discrimination laws under a single Act, strengthening protections and making the law easier to understand – clearly setting out the ways in which it is unlawful to treat someone. It is against the law to discriminate against anyone based on any of these protected characteristics:

- age
- disability
- gender reassignment
- marriage and civil partnership
- pregnancy and maternity
- race
- religion or belief
- sex
- sexual orientation

The Australian Government Department of Health and Aged Care (2023) has set out its diversity and inclusion strategy through a series of workplace initiatives, actions plans, staff networks and associations with breastfeeding, disability, cultural and linguistic, carer, LGBTI+ and indigenous (Aboriginal and Torres Strait Islander) organizations. Its belief is that diversity supports innovation, develops good policy, better understands and serves clients and attracts a wider range of talented staff.

Inclusion

To recognize and promote diversity, inclusion could be considered the practice of actively managing diversity, through 'targeted recruitment initiatives, education and training, career development and mentoring programs to increase and retain workforce heterogeneity in organizations' (Cox, 1993; Morrison, 1992, as cited by Roberson, 2004: 4). Some organizations rely on broader programmes and initiatives that remove barriers to diversity, such as employee participation, communication strategies and community relations (Ramonetti and Pilato, 2019; Griffin, 2020; Scott and Kline, 2022) to allow the full range of employee skills and competencies to be demonstrated in organizations (Harvey, 1999).

Equality and equity

While equality is about offering the same rights and opportunities to all people regardless of their characteristics, and income, equity recognizes that individuals start at different points so giving them the same rights and opportunities will not close any gaps in terms of wealth, assets, capital or status and will result in continuing inequality. The World Health Organization (2024a) defines health equity as 'the absence of unfair, avoidable or remediable differences among groups of people, whether those groups are defined socially, economically, demographically, or geographically or by other dimensions of inequality (e.g. sex, gender, ethnicity, disability, or sexual orientation)'.

Employing the metaphor of a 100-metre sprint, equity acknowledges that some people will start at the start line, whereas others have a structural advantage due to their characteristics (e.g. wealth, status, education) and therefore will start 50 metres closer to the finish line. That is to say, equity means offering rights and opportunities fairly, acknowledging people's differences so there is fair access to those opportunities. To achieve equity requires action to be taken by providing various levels of support depending on the specific needs or abilities of those individuals. Figure 5.1 demonstrates the differences between equality and equity.

The difference between equality, equity and justice is significant. Although they all promote fairness, equality achieves this through treating everyone the same regardless of need, while equity achieves this through treating people differently dependent on need, and justice seeks to remove the barriers that create the need in the first place. This difference impacts the strategies developed to address inequality and to remove discriminatory barriers.

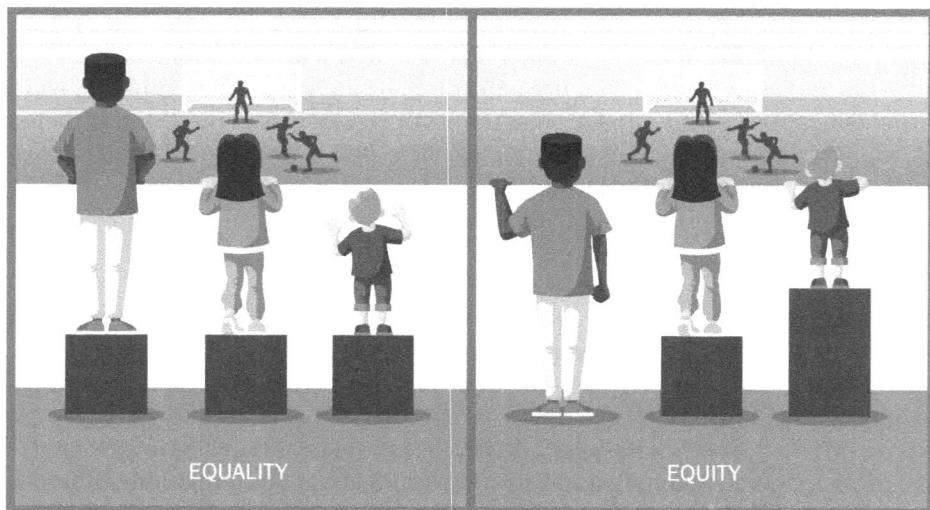

Figure 5.1 Equality vs equity

Power and privilege in healthcare

This section focuses on power and privilege and introduces some key concepts that build knowledge about social justice, equity, diversity and inclusion.

Central to the idea of inequality is the idea that one group has power over another, and this power imbalance leads to inequality, discrimination and exclusion (McCartney et al., 2020). There are many expressions of power described in Box 5.2.

Box 5.2 Key points to note regarding power and privilege

Power and privilege

- Power and privilege are often invisible to those with privilege.
- Those with privilege do not necessarily feel or experience privilege.
- If you have privilege (white, male, heterosexual, non-disabled), your life may not be easy, it is just that your privilege (white, male, heterosexual, non-disabled) is not one of the things that make it hard.
- Those without privilege see the privilege of others.

If we think about how society may favour individuals of white heritage, we may refer to this as white supremacy or white privilege (see Box 5.3). This is a construction of power that does not attach the intention to be a white supremacist to a particular individual. It may encourage white people think about how their behaviours may contribute to the system that favours them and also encourage thinking about changing behaviours to change the impact of white dominance. It may prompt changes in the way we organize. For example, we may change our recruitment policies and practices to be more equitable, which changes hierarchical representation. The NHS have produced EDI toolkits, a set of resources to support teams, to explore and discuss EDI issues. An example is Imperial College Healthcare NHS Trust's 'How to guide' for EDI toolkits: https://www.imperial.nhs.uk/-/media/website/about-us/how-we-work/equality-and-diversity/how-to-guide-toolkits.pdf.

Box 5.3 White privilege

White privilege is a term coined by Peggy McIntosh (1988; 2003) where she describes white privilege as 'like an invisible weightless knapsack of special provisions, maps, passports, codebooks, visas, clothes, tools, and blank checks… As a white person, I realized I had been taught about racism as something that puts others at a disadvantage, but had been taught not to see one of its corollary aspects, white privilege, which puts me at an advantage… I have come to see white privilege as an invisible package of unearned assets that I can count on cashing in each day, but about which I was "meant" to remain oblivious' (McIntosh, 1988: 2).

Invisible backpack of privilege

What's in your backpack?

McIntosh's work on race has been further developed to explore gender and sexuality, using the following privilege statements as a way of exploring power and difference.

- I can arrange to protect my children most of the time from people who might not like them.
- I do not have to educate my children to be aware of systemic racism for their own daily physical protection.
- I can speak in public to a powerful male group without putting my race on trial.
- I can do well in a challenging situation without being called a credit to my race.
- I am never asked to speak for all the people of my racial group.
- I can be pretty sure that if I ask to talk to the "person in charge", I will be facing a person of my race.
- I can easily buy posters, post-cards, picture books, greeting cards, dolls, toys, and children's magazines featuring people of my race.
- I can go home from most meetings of organizations I belong to feeling somewhat tied in, rather than isolated, out-of-place, outnumbered, unheard, held at a distance or feared.

Other and othering

'Othering' is the process of casting a group, an individual or an object into the role of 'the Other' and establishing one's own identity through opposition to and, frequently, vilification or abuse of this Other. In this way white people 'other' Black Indigenous People of Colour (BIPOC), LGBTQIA+ and so on. Othering comes from a form of power over the Other. As Akbulut and Razum (2022: 4) describe, 'othering can affect health in different ways as it occurs in multiple dimensions and forms that vary according to marginalized groups and institutional as well as social contexts'.

A common microaggression and way of othering is asking the question, 'Where are you from?' In this way racism compromises cultural affiliation and the sense of home, where people of colour all have examples of this 'not belonging' feeling (Kinouani, 2021). As Nobel Laureate, Toni Morrison (2017: 3) put it:

> Our tendency to separate and judge those not in our clan as the enemy, as the vulnerable and deficient needing control, has a long history … Race has been a constant arbiter of difference, as have wealth, class and gender – each of which is about power and the necessity to control.

Othering is based on the idea that identities are socially constructed (see Box 5.4) and are created in the context of history and power, whereby certain groups are socially constructed as different by other groups who have power, in this way we say people are 'Othered' in a process of racialization that shapes societal norms as dominant for one group over another (AbdulMagied, 2020).

Box 5.4   Social construction

Understanding how society is organized through relations of power (often referred to as 'socially constructed') is important for understanding structural inequalities and raising our awareness of the unequal impact of difference. Organizations mirror or reflect the way power works in society. For example, most hierarchies remain white and male at the top/senior levels. Understanding the construction of that power helps us think about how to change things to bring greater equity and justice to our organization's ways of working and to wider society.

This process of othering has a history in relation to different identities; for example, slavery is the process that othered black people in order to justify exploiting slaves as free labour and racism continues historically to justify unequal treatment of black people by white people who hold economic power; the gender and black pay gap are recent examples of unequal treatment in the workforce. As the writer Chimamanda Ngozi Adichie (2009) once said:

> Power is the ability not just to tell the story of another person, but to make it the definitive story of that person. Show a people as one thing, only one thing, over and over again, and that is what they become.

When we talk about 'Power Over', we can also use the terms hegemony or hegemonic power to describe the dominance of one group over another; for example, we may refer to male hegemonic power describing the dominance of men over women (see Box 5.5).

Box 5.5   Power (Batliwala, 2010; Veneklasen and Miller, 2002)

Expressions of power vary:

- Power To: Ability to take action, innate ability or power acquired through skill, knowledge, training or other forms of personal development
- Power Over: Overt ability to use relational or positional power to shape events, frequently viewed as negative, but arguably sometimes of positive use
- Power With: Collective power through relationships and acts of solidarity
- Power Within: The power which can be acquired through acts of working on self; requires deep personal learning and reflection
- Power Under: Positive or negative power which results from experiences of hardship, oppression. The strength of which originates from struggle.

Sources of Power (French and Raven, 1959)

- Formal (positional) power – a role, title, or job description granted by the organization.
- Resource power – control of (or access to) desirable resources.
- Status power – esteem or respect due to perceived social ranking.
- Charismatic power – personality, vision, enthusiasm and/or charm.
- Convening power – ability to assemble diverse, even isolated, individuals & groups.
- Expert (technical) power – advantageous knowledge, skills, or technical capabilities
- Informational power – possession or access to valued information.
- Reward power – provide personal, political, or economic rewards.
- Coercive power – provide personal, political, or economic penalties or punishments.
- Social power – connections to critical individuals and networks.
- Reverent power – commanding admiration and respect

How we exercise and experience power can be subtle and is often described as micro-aggressions (see Box 5.6).

As has been shown, power and privilege play a key role in extending inequalities and promoting social injustice across society. While there are many areas of inequality, the next two sections will focus on race and gender.

Learning activity 5.1

Consider the following questions to explore privilege and power you have as a health-care manager.

1 What privilege(s) do I hold and how has this influenced my role as a manager?
2 How does privilege operate in my team and organization – who benefits and who does not?
3 How can I use my power and privilege as a manager to create more inclusive teams and cultures?

Create a short learning activity to explore and discuss issues related to power and privilege and how that impacts on EDI in your team, department or organization.

Race, racism and ethnicity in healthcare

Racism describes the system of racial inequality, based on the belief that some groups are innately superior to other groups (Rattansi, 2020). Racism rests on the prejudices (attitudes), symbols (such as language), actions and policies (discrimination) that reproduce the false ideology that other groups are inferior to white people (Devakumar et al., 2022). It also relies on power structures, such as historical and cultural relations established through colonialism and our social institutions; for example, government, law, education, media and science (Devakumar et al., 2022).

Both the term and the idea are relatively modern and were developed in the context of colonization and slavery and the division of human beings along racial lines in order to justify the slave trade. In order to justify slavery, theories of racial categories were developed and underlie the modern foundations of racial division (Linnean Society, 2024).

If we think in terms of social construction (see Box 5.4 earlier), we may think differently about terms such as 'minorities'. For example, in terms of numbers, Black Indigenous People of Colour (BIPOC) are not a minority of people in the world and in fact are the global majority, and women are not a minority in gender terms; instead, it is useful to think about power relations that lead to both BIPOC and women being 'minoritized', i.e., subordinated in status and excluded. Moreover, such thinking was evident throughout history to justify domination by white people. Apartheid in South Africa is one example of this process of categorization and domination by white supremacists. 'BAME' may also be considered a categorization of people by colour designed for ethnic monitoring of those minoritized by systems of power (Bunglawala, 2019; Fakim and Macaulay, 2020; DaCosta et al., 2021).

When we talk about 'race' we know that we are using a social construct that divides humans by colour and it is difficult to separate out the idea that race is socially constructed through relations of power and not a real division; race only exists where there is racism or racist supremacy, but that racism itself and its impact are very real. These terms are used interchangeably but need to be thought about separately if we are to deconstruct and understand how racism occurs (see Box 5.6).

Box 5.6   Key terms associated with race and racism

Racial trauma

Broadly speaking, trauma describes responses to frightening events. It refers to a long-lasting sense of overwhelm, unsafeness and distress that follows exposure. Racial trauma is therefore a framework to describe the physical and emotional responses that can follow exposure to racism at an individual and group level, it is the collective harm that racism can inflict (Kinouani, 2021).

Anti-racism

- Anti-racist: a person who opposes racism and promotes racial justice,
- Anti-racism: the policy or practice of opposing racism and promoting racial tolerance (Kendi, 2019).

Colonialism

Racial categories have their origins in slavery and colonialism; the historical and political processes by which groups and nation states enrich themselves through economic and social control of other countries and sub-groups. Colonial forces used violence and ideology to legitimize the idea that white people were superior to other groups, thus creating white supremacy. (Andrews, 2021).

Microaggressions

'Microaggression' is a term that refers to commonplace, everyday or casual and commonplace daily acts of racism (but equally applies to sexism) that may be verbal, behavioural or environmental indignities, which communicate hostile, derogatory, or negative attitudes toward stigmatized or culturally marginalized groups (Skinner-Dorkenoo et al., 2021). These microaggressions are still aggressions and are experienced as microaggressions whether they are intentional or unintentional and are sometimes referred to as 'everyday racism' (or 'everyday sexism') (Sue et al., 2007).

In the UK, the COVID-19 pandemic not only replicated existing health inequalities but, in some cases, increased or exacerbated them, with a disproportionate impact on certain population groups, including older people, disabled people, Black and People of Colour, and geography. including disparities in local communities (Lawrence, 2020).

> In the early weeks of the Covid pandemic, as mounting evidence began to show that Black, Asian and minority ethnic communities were dying at a disproportionate rate... It was immediately apparent that the impact on people's health was inseparable from economic prospects and experiences of discrimination... It is often said, but perhaps not fully appreciated, that behind each statistic is a human story. For me, amplifying the voices of those who are all too often invisible has been the driving force behind my many years of campaigning.
>
> (Lawrence, 2020: 4).

There are many ways in which racism manifests itself at work. We need to be comfortable about being uncomfortable and learn to talk about race and racism in our roles as a manager and with our teams. A recent survey (Kline and Warmington, 2024) found that managers and staff find it difficult to talk about race and racism in the NHS (see Learning resources: Race).

Gender, sexuality and identity

In the UK, the Gender Recognition Act (2004) covers the legislation in relation to gender. Gender self-identification is developing in many countries; for example, New Zealand introduced a self-identification process in 2023 (New Zealand Government Ministry of Justice, 2023).

This section covers some of the key terms used in this area of social justice, equity, diversity and inclusion but there are also more commonly used terms such as 'cisgender', shortened to 'cis' (cis woman/cis man), that also describe ways of being and thinking about gender (see Box 5.7). Our understanding about gender identity is evolving and debates continue to be the subject of ideological and social development in a more gender fluid approach to thinking.

Box 5.7   Key terms related to sex and gender

Affirmed gender identity: The gender that a person identifies with (Hidalgo et al., 2013).

Assigned sex: The sex given to a person at birth, usually based on the genitalia they have (Clarke, 2022).

Cisgender: Denoting or relating to a person whose sense of personal identity and gender corresponds with their birth sex (Lindqvist et al., 2020). A cisgender person (sometimes cissexual, informally abbreviated cis) is one whose gender identity matches their sex assigned at birth. For example, someone who identifies as a woman and was identified as female at birth is a cisgender woman. The word cisgender is the antonym or opposite of transgender.

Gender: Often expressed in terms of masculinity and femininity, gender is largely culturally determined and is assumed from the sex assigned at birth (Lindqvist et al., 2020).

Gender affirmation surgery/gender reassignment surgery: Refers to surgical alteration, often referring to lower or top surgery, but can refer to any surgery (Akhavan et al., 2021).

Gender binary: The (inaccurate) idea that there are only two genders – male and female (and that everyone will fit into this) (Lindqvist et al., 2020).

Gender dysphoria: Used to describe when a person experiences discomfort or distress because there is a mismatch between their sex assigned at birth and their gender identity. This is also used as the clinical diagnosis for someone who does not feel comfortable with the sex they were assigned at birth (Cooper et al., 2020).

Gender identity: A person's innate sense of their own gender, whether male, female, or something else (see non-binary below), which may or may not correspond to the sex assigned at birth (Wood and Eagly, 2013).

Identity politics: A term that describes a political approach wherein people of a particular gender, religion, social background, class, or other identifying factors, develop political agendas that are based upon theoretical interlocking systems of oppression that may affect their lives and come from their various identities. Contemporary applications of identity politics describe people of specific race, ethnicity, sex, gender identity, age, economic class, disability status, education, religion, language, and geographic location (Das, 2020). These identity labels are not mutually exclusive but are in many cases compounded or intersect (Cerezo et al., 2020).

Non-binary: A person who feels the gender binary of man or woman does not fit their gender identity (Schudson and Morgenroth, 2022). The gender pronouns that a person identifies with should be used. There are many terms for someone who identifies like this, and it is down to personal preference. For example, genderfluid, bi-gender, polygender, etc.

Pronoun: Words we use to refer to people's gender in conversation–for example, 'he' or 'she'. Some people may prefer others to refer to them in gender neutral language and use pronouns such as they/theirs/them (Johnson et al., 2021).

University of California Davis (2023) has developed a LGBTQIA+ Resource Center glossary. Its purpose is to develop a shared understanding of the language commonly used in conversations about social justice, equity, diversity and inclusion in relation to LGBTQIA+ people. This is not an exhaustive set of concepts to frame our thinking or terms used (Stonewall, 2023), nor does it reflect the entirety of the discriminatory issues, or the harmful impact lived experiences have on individuals and groups of people (see Box 5.8).

Box 5.8   LGBTQIA+ What do the acronyms mean? (Cherry, 2023)

L (Lesbian): A lesbian is a woman/woman-aligned person who is attracted to only people of the same/similar gender.

G (Gay): Gay is usually a term used to refer to men/men-aligned individuals who are only attracted to people of the same/similar gender. However, lesbians can also be referred to as gay.

B (Bisexual): Bisexual indicates an attraction to all genders. The recognition of bisexual individuals is important since there have been periods when people who identify as bisexual (or bi for short) have been misunderstood as being gay. Bisexuality has included transgender, binary and non-binary individuals since the release of the 'Bisexual Manifesto' in 1990.

T (Transgender): Transgender is a term that indicates that a person's gender identity is different from the gender associated with the sex they were assigned at birth. 'Trans' is an umbrella term to describe people whose gender is not the same as, or does not sit comfortably with, the sex they were assigned at birth. Trans people may describe themselves using one or more of a wide variety of terms, including (but not limited to) transgender or non-binary.

Queer or questioning: The process of exploring your own sexual orientation and/or gender identity.

Intersex: Where sexual anatomy or chromosomes are different from traditional markers of male and female.

Asexual: Describes individuals who generally do not feel sexual desire or attraction to any group of people but can have romantic feelings towards someone.

+ (Plus): The 'plus' is used to signify all of the gender identities and sexual orientations that are not specifically covered by the other initials in the acronym; for example, pansexual, not limited in sexual choice with regard to biological sex, gender or gender identify.

Women's rights: Feminism and waves of feminism – black feminism

Feminism is broadly the advocacy of women's rights based on the equality of the sexes, and is related to the theory of the political, economic and social equality of the sexes (Krolòkke and Sòrensen, 2006). Feminism, or the women's movement, is often described as happening in 'waves'. Generally speaking, the first wave was about women's right to vote and the second wave the women's liberation movement from the 1960s. Both of these waves are largely seen as representing white and middle-class women (hooks, 2000), with the third wave including black feminists who see women's lives as intersectional, demonstrating how race, ethnicity, class, religion, gender and nationality are all significant factors when discussing feminism.

Patriarchy

Patriarchy describes a system or culture of male dominating forms of power over women (Ortner, 2022). Patriarchy is a system of society or government in which the father or eldest male is head of the family and descent is through the male line (Cremer, 2021). More broadly, patriarchy is a system of society or government in which men hold the power and women are largely excluded from it (Brännmark, 2021). This concept of patriarchy underpins much of feminist thought (Tong and Botts, 2024). The gender pay gap is an example of patriarchal dominance in the workforce (Griffiths, 2023) (see Box 5.9).

> ### Box 5.9 Case Study – the UK gender pay gap in the NHS (NHS England, 2023b)
>
> The gender pay gap report is based on the government's methodology for calculating difference in pay between female and male employees, considering full-pay relevant employees of NHS England and NHS Improvement.
>
> 'Equal pay' means being paid equally for the same/similar work. 'Pay gap' is the difference in the average pay between two groups.
>
> As of 31 March 2022, NHS England and NHS Improvement's 11,449 employees comprised 68.7 per cent women and 31.3 per cent men. This was an increase of 0.9 per cent more women in the organization as a whole, compared to the previous year.
>
> The gender pay gap trend for NHS England and NHS Improvement is positive, with improvements made from the previous year. The mean gender pay gap was 14.7 per cent in March 2022, representing a reduction in the gap of 1.5 per cent percentage points. The median gender pay gap has remained at 14 per cent in March 2022, equating to no change in percentage points since March 2021.

Intersectionality

Intersectionality describes the ways in which a person's social and political identities (gender, race, class, sexuality, disability) combine to create unique modes of privilege and discrimination. Intersectionality is seen as a more meaningful description of the multiple impacts of discrimination, where an individual's identities overlap with a number of 'minority' or protected characteristics including race, ethnicity, gender identity, class, language, religion, diverse-ability, sexuality, mental health, age, education, body size and many more (Collins and Bilge, 2020; Duckworth, 2020).

Crenshaw (1989) coined the term to explain a feminist perspective to the view that women experience oppression in varying configurations and in varying degrees of intensity. Accordingly cultural patterns of oppression are not only interrelated but are bound together and influenced by the intersectional systems in society including race, gender, class, sexuality and diverse-ability (a term used by NHS England Senior Influencers Group for disability; some disabled people identify as diversely abled and reject other terms to describe their identity). Critical to Crenshaw's approach is to challenge white feminist notions that all women are the same. She argues inequality does not impact all women in the same way and questions who gets to speak and whose voices are heard (Crenshaw, 2014).

Inequality in healthcare

By now it is probably evident that issues related to race and gender (not to mention disability, class, age and so on) have a major impact on health and well-being. This section will draw together issues related to inequality and inequity in healthcare, beginning with the social determinants of health.

Social determinants of health

The social determinants of health (SDH) are the non-medical factors that influence health outcomes. They are the conditions in which people are born, grow, work, live and age, and the wider set of forces and systems shaping the conditions of daily life. These forces and systems include economic policies and systems, development agendas, social norms, social policies and political systems (World Health Organization, 2024b).

Understanding the connection between social determinants of health and health outcomes helps us to provide a structure for how national health care systems can assess and influence these determinants, as anchor institutions as well as care providers (see Figure 5.2).

Health inequalities are systematic, avoidable and unjust differences in health and wellbeing between different groups of people (Whitehead and Dahlgren, 2006; Hutler, 2022). There is clear evidence that reducing health inequalities improves life expectancy and reduces disability across the social gradient (Marmot, 1986; Gutin and Hummer, 2021). Tackling health inequalities is therefore a core part of improving access to services, quality of services and health outcomes for the whole population. Health inequalities include socioeconomic position, occupation, housing, geographic deprivation and membership of a vulnerable group

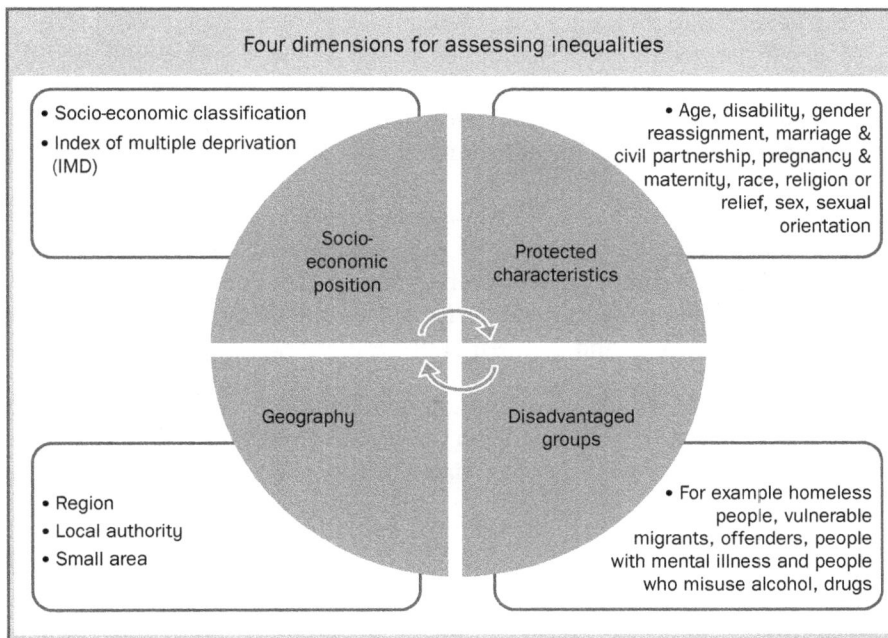

Figure 5.2 Four dimensions for assessing inequalities
Source: PHE (2018).

and these dimensions overlap and intersect (Whitehead and Dahlgren, 2006; Otu et al., 2020). In Australia, New Zealand and Canada there are specific strategies for indigenous populations (see Box 5.10).

Box 5.10 Indigenous health strategies to tackle inequality in Australia, New Zealand and Canada

In Australia, with regard to Aboriginal and Torres Strait Islander health, the government's approach, through its Closing the Gap strategy (Coalition of Peaks, 2020) has been to focus on priority areas of reform, to work inclusively on:

- shared decision-making;
- building a community controlled provider sector;
- the transformation of mainstream institutions that identify and eliminate racism and are culturally safe and responsible to this specific population's needs; and
- the use of locally relevant data.

In neighbouring Aotearoa New Zealand, one of its government's key strategies is around Māori health (along with whole system, Pacific Islander, disabled, rural and women's health). Four key tenets underpin the *Whakamaua: Māori Health Action Plan 2020–2025* (New Zealand Government Ministry of Health / Manatū Hauora, 2020):

1 Māori exercising their authority to improve their health and well-being
2 ensuring the health and disability system is fair and sustainable and delivers more equitable outcomes for Māori
3 addressing racism and discrimination in all its forms
4 protecting mātauranga Māori throughout the health and disability system.

In Canada, the government has set out goals in relations to First Nations, Inuit and Métis (indigenous populations) health under the principle of being a funding and governance, rather than a designing and delivery, partner (Government of Canada, 2023a). This means that these indigenous populations will assume responsibility for the design, administration, management and delivery of programmes, in order to:

- increase First Nations' control in their own health services;
- enable improved coordination with provincial/territorial health systems; and
- create the conditions needed to address health inequities faced by First Nations people.

Key to the delivery of this new approach is the co-development of new distinctions-based Indigenous health legislation to improve access to high-quality, culturally relevant health services (Government of Canada, 2023b).

Learning activity 5.2: Health inequalities

- With your team or departmental colleagues, consider how you understand different types of health inequality in your areas.
- What data do you rely on to understand health inequalities and how do you use this data to drive improvement?
- Create a short action plan to focus on your top three priorities.

Words matter: language in social justice, equality, equity, diversity and inclusion

The language and terminology used in social justice, equity, diversity and inclusion is always evolving; this is because language is a product of our thinking, and it is important because what we say also indicates what we think (Aspinall, 2020). Language changes as our knowledge and understanding of the issues also change; new ways of thinking and describing the issues change the language we use and the importance we attach to naming these issues (Aspinall, 2020).

In social justice, equity, diversity and inclusion the context of the language we use is therefore important and often relates to the history and development of the words or terms over time, so what may have been appropriate or useful at one point in history may not be adequate in another (Aspinall, 2020). For example, since the early Gay Liberation Movement the terms lesbian, gay or bisexual have been expanded to meet the changes in thinking about gender and identity (Mavhandu-Mudzusi et al., 2023). We now use LGBTQIA+ with the plus, leaving room for other ways of identifying (see Box 5.7). Including plus in the acronym is more inclusive of those who may not feel represented by the other terms. The purpose of the acronym is to represent the tremendous diversity of how people choose to identify (Blakemore, 2021).

The language we use in social justice, equality, equity, diversity and inclusion may also suggest a view or a position often described as an ideology; that is a system of ideas or theory (Ross et al., 2020). We often use terms that also imply that a view or ideology is contentious or likely to cause an argument; for example, 'political correctness' or 'PC', or 'woke'. In social justice, equality, equity, diversity and inclusion we believe that what we are called and what we call others is really important because it conveys understanding of another person's identity and lived experience (Baker-Bell, 2020). Doing so shows respect and acknowledgement for our differences, and it implies acceptance of those differences (Noels et al., 2020).

Changing the conversation: generating deeper understanding and meaning by exploring assumptions and bias

Changing the conversations we have about social justice, equality, equity, diversity and inclusion will help us explore our differences so that we can work together more effectively (Winters, 2020). If we work together constructively to understand the issues associated with social justice, equity, diversity and inclusion we can work to improve everyone's lived experience (Winters, 2020).

This means we need to develop a common language and understanding of how our differences are constructed. One of the most significant claims that something is socially constructed is that it could be constructed differently (Gergen, 2022). So, it is possible for us to think differently about power in healthcare systems, and this would contribute to making the constructions that depend on this thinking change (Ross et al., 2020). This idea is central to the task of developing change; opening up possibilities for us all not just to think differently but also to act differently, calling us all to make an active choice in relation to what is being constructed (Ross et al., 2020).

Assumptions may be unconscious and lead to 'unconscious bias': the tendency to think and act more positively towards others who are like you and to think and act more negatively towards those who are perceived as different to you (Suveren, 2022).

Learning activity 5.3: Language and bias: a common example in healthcare settings

You are in a team meeting and the Chair invites team members to suggest ways to improve team working. A woman on the team makes a suggestion but the Chair does not respond; a male colleague then makes the same suggestion and the Chair responds to say the suggestion is great and will be implemented.

- Consider what feedback you would give to the Chair.
- Consider what assumptions you may be making about the gender of the Chair in this example.
- Think of an assumption or bias you may hold that you can share with your team and ask your team to explore their biases or assumptions with you.
- Explore with colleagues why you may hold this bias or assumption.

The questions we ask ourselves can lead to very different conversations and have the potential to be transformational. When we use terms like 'heteronormative' we are referring to the idea that a society is organized in favour of heterosexual people. In this case heterosexual people will benefit from heteronormative privilege and also the impact of exclusion of LGBTQIA+ people. Regardless of their own view, this benefit will still be conferred on straight people, just by being heterosexual (Toorn et al., 2020).

If we are talking about how society favours men, using terms like patriarchy and sexism, this does not mean all men are sexist or that all men agree with patriarchy (hooks, 2000). But in a society that favours men the impact will be felt by everyone. Similarly, when we think about gender, we may also think about disparities in pay, i.e. the gender pay gap (Box 5.9 earlier).

When we think or talk about the 'ableist' way that the environment privileges those considered 'non-disabled' and consider how the social and environmental factors exclude disabled people it raises our awareness (Kattari, 2020). Having these conversations and thinking differently leads us to be more open to creating social, cultural and environmental access for all (Lazarus et al., 2020).

'But what can I do?': constructive conversations support and challenge

Sometimes the language we use around social justice, equality, equity, diversity and inclusion is used to disparage others; it is a way of belittling or reducing the importance of someone or of something that person represents. This is a way to use language, terms or words negatively to blame or put down others. In trying to develop our understanding of each other and the issues of inequality this is not helpful and does not encourage an environment where we can have meaningful conversations that lead to real change and transformation: conversations that change the way we work and live in a more equal way (Charity Hudley et al., 2024).

By using language and exploring ideas constructively, we can help each other develop our understanding, compassion and empathy, help make sense of our lived experience and issues of inequality, and make meaningful change happen (Charity Hudley et al., 2024).

Lived experience: links to social determinants of health

Increasingly listening to the voices of lived experience helps us make sense of the ways in which discrimination impacts our health and well-being, as well as determining our social, economic and educational life chances.

Studies by David Williams (McKenna and Williams, 2019), Michael Marmot (Marmot et al., 2020) and more recently Doreen Lawrence (2020) use lived experience to understand the social determinants of health and the impact of discrimination on our patients, users and communities.

Conclusions: implications for healthcare managers

This chapter has outlined the key definitions, aspects and some of the contentions regarding equality, diversity and inclusion, as well as equity and social justice, within society and more specifically within healthcare systems. It has linked these to the core concepts of social justice and equity.

Issues of power, privilege, race and gender all contribute to health inequalities and this chapter has set out how managers will be able to lead, manage and practise more inclusively. By doing so, it builds on work elsewhere in this volume on compassionate and inclusive leadership (Chapter 2), the evidence-based practice and the research to practice gap (Chapter 6) and the importance of inclusive leadership behaviours in engaging with staff and service users (Chapter 21).

It provides a call-to-action for healthcare managers in terms of anti-discriminatory practice, challenging discrimination and oppression in healthcare and ensuring that all workers in healthcare, along with all patients, service users and clients, are treated inclusively and valued for their contributions. This is mirrored in the UK Messenger Review into Healthcare Leadership (see Box 5.11).

Box 5.11   EDI implications for healthcare managers (Kline, 2022): The UK Messenger Review into Healthcare Leadership (Messenger and Pollard, 2022)

Kline's assessment of The Messenger Review emphasizes the central importance of equality, diversity and inclusion in improving patient care and safety accepting that: 'although by no means everywhere, acceptance of discrimination, bullying, blame cultures and responsibility avoidance has almost become normalised in certain parts of the system'.

How an organization performs and behaves in relation to EDI is a clear indicator of its maturity and openness and is a clear determinant of how an organization fares in a rapidly changing social and work context.

EDI is about respectful relationships and underpins a wider culture of respect, but is currently partial, inconsistent and elective and in some places tokenistic.

One of the core messages of The Messenger Review is that the system must:

> ...embed inclusive leadership practice as the responsibility of all leaders... educate leaders to ensure they understand their role in demonstrating and improving inclusive leadership. This must include a more central role for EDI in leadership training and development which, in turn, requires greater skills and understanding of the topic from those delivering the training.

Embedding inclusion means:

- applicants to management posts, especially senior posts, are required to demonstrate what they have personally done to promote equity
- managers and especially senior leaders taking time to reflect on their own roles and practices, placing themselves in the shoes of those disadvantaged by discrimination and being relentlessly proactive in changing behaviours and practices contributing to discrimination, including within career progression

- leaders who understand that embedding inclusion requires it to be seen as a core part of improvement work, underpinned by accountability
- they must be prepared to have uncomfortable discussions, in particular about racism.

To truly improve health and care services, managers must embrace all the talents available, for moral, ethical, creative and productive reasons. To achieve this, it is vital that healthcare managers promote equality, diversity and inclusion in their work and ensure positive action is taken to eliminate discrimination in all healthcare practice every day (see Box 5.12).

Box 5.12   Positive action and positive discrimination

Positive action

This is the deliberate introduction of measures to eliminate or reduce discrimination or its 'effects'. It is about encouraging people from demonstrably under-represented groups in the workplace. Positive action describes a range of measures allowed under the Equality Act 2010. These can be lawfully taken to encourage and train people from under-represented groups to support them.

Positive discrimination

Positive discrimination favours one group over another. For example, by increasing the numbers from a minority group because they have protected characteristics in that group or giving preferential treatment to that individual or group because of their protected characteristics rather than their suitability: this is unlawful.

The key difference between positive action and positive discrimination is that positive action is lawful under the Equality Act 2010, whereas positive discrimination is unlawful.

Learning resources

Diversity

Atcheson, S. (2018) *Allyship – The Key To Unlocking The Power Of Diversity*. [https://www.forbes.com/sites/shereeatcheson/2018/11/30/allyship-the-key-to-unlocking-the-power-of-diversity/#5515d0bb49c6].

Continued

Learning resources   *Continued*

Gender and sexuality

Ellis Ross, T. (2018) A woman's fury holds lifetimes of wisdom. TED Talk. [https://www.youtube.com/watch?v=JoUZ929qoLk].

Imkaan is a UK-based, black feminist organization dedicated to addressing violence against women and girls. Produced by Purple Drum and The End Violence Against Women (EVAM) Coalition, who are the UK's largest coalition of organizations working to eradicate violence against women and girls, this short film *I'd just like to be free* (2016) details young women speaking out about sexual harassment. [https://www.youtube.com/watch?v=lJ-qpvibpdU].

Things Not to Say to Gay People:
[https://www.youtube.com/watch?v=ujxl5WZJHL4].

Things Not to Say to a Non-Binary Person:
[https://www.youtube.com/watch?v=8b4MZjMVgdk].

Things Not to Say to a Bisexual Person:
[https://www.youtube.com/watch?v=7oHkF8YnJG0].

Health inequality

American Public Health Association (2018) Interview with Professor David Williams (Harvard University) on health inequality, 12 November.
[https://www.youtube.com/watch?v=iyJy3p7_kHs].

Race

Akala (2015) Black History: The Lost Pages of Human History. Oxford Union.
[https://www.youtube.com/watch?v=WUtAxUQjwB4&feature=youtu.be].

Allyship Toolkit – https://thetoolkit.wixsite.com/toolkit/beyond-allyship
[http://whitepriv.blogspot.com/2010/02/10-ways-to-be-and-ally.html].

Andrews, K. (2020) Oxford Union Society Debates: British Education Does Perpetuate Racism [https://www.youtube.com/watch?v=DLjisEPSus0].

Andrews, K. (2021) *The New Age of Empire: How Racism and Colonialism Still Rule the World.* London: Penguin.

brap is a UK charity transforming the way to think and do equality. They support organizations, communities and cities with meaningful approaches to learning, change, research and engagement. Their latest report *Too Hot To Handle* (2024) written by Roger Kline and Joy Warmington brings together key learning from tribunal cases and survey responses from over 1,300 English NHS staff to explore how healthcare organizations respond to allegations of racism [https://www.brap.org.uk/post/toohottohandle].

DiAngelo, R. (2018) *White Fragility: Why It's So Hard for White People to Talk About Racism* [https://youtu.be/45ey4jgoxeU].

Guardian News (2020) *Coronavirus: why black, Asian and minorities may be more at risk* [https://www.youtube.com/watch?v=XPF35H9RLNE&feature=youtu.be].

Hirsch, A. (2020) *After coronavirus, black and brown people must be at the heart of Britain's story* [https://www.theguardian.com/commentisfree/2020/may/07/coronavirus-black-brown-people-britain-ethnic-minorities].

Malik, N. (2020) Otegha Uwagba: 'I've spent my entire life treading around white people's feelings' [https://www.theguardian.com/books/2020/nov/14/otegha-uwagba-ive-spent-my-entire-life-treading-around-white-peoples-feelings].

NHS England Workforce Race and Equality Standard (2020) *Professor David Williams: Seminar on 'race and health – the global overview'* [https://www.youtube.com/watch?v=i1xHs3DxfLE&feature=youtu].

The Runnymede Trust is a British race equality and civil rights think tank. They generate research to challenge structural racism in Britain. Their report *Broken Ladders* (2022) focuses on the myth of meritocracy for women of colour in the UK workplace. [https://www.runnymedetrust.org/publications/broken-ladders].

Unconscious Bias

Asana.19 unconscious biases to overcome and help promote inclusivity [https://asana.com/resources/unconscious-bias-examples].

References

AbdulMagied, S. (2020) Othering, identity, and recognition: the social exclusion of the constructed 'Other', Faculty of Humanities, Psychology, and Theology: Åbo Akademi University, 2020 [https://www.doria.fi/handle/10024/177835; accessed 14 July 2024].

Adichie, C.N. (2009) The danger of a single story. TED Talk [https://www.ted.com/talks/chimamanda_ngozi_adichie_the_danger_of_a_single_story?language=en; accessed 14 July 2024].

Akbulut, N. and Razum, O. (2022) Why Othering should be considered in research on health inequalities: theoretical perspectives and research needs, *SSM - Population Health*, Nov 5; 20:101286. doi: 10.1016/j.ssmph.2022.101286. PMID: 36406107; PMCID: PMC9672483.

Akhavan, A.A., Sandhu, S., Ndem, I. and Ogunleye, A.A. (2021) A review of gender affirmation surgery: what we know, and what we need to know, *Surgery*, Jul; 170 (1): 336–340. doi: 10.1016/j.surg.2021.02.013. Epub 2021 Mar 16. PMID: 33741180.

Andrews, K. (2021) *The New Age of Empire: How Racism and Colonialism Still Rule the World*. London: Penguin.

Aspinall, P.J. (2020) Ethnic/racial terminology as a form of representation: a critical review of the lexicon of collective and specific terms in use in Britain, *Genealogy*, 4 (3): 87. doi: 10.3390/genealogy4030087.

Australian Government Department of Health and Aged Care (2023) Diversity and inclusion [https://www.health.gov.au/about-us/work-with-us/what-we-offer/diversity-and-inclusion; accessed 14 July 2024].

Baker-Bell, A. (2020) *Linguistic Justice: Black Language, Literacy, Identity, and Pedagogy*. New York: Routledge.

Banai, A., Ronzoni, M. and Schemmel, C. (2011) *Social Justice, Global Dynamics: Theoretical and Empirical Perspectives*. Florence: Taylor and Francis.

Batliwala, S. (2010) Feminist Leadership for Social Transformation: Clearing the Conceptual Cloud. Creating Resources for Empowerment in Action (CREA) [https://creaworld.org/wp-content/uploads/2020/11/feminist-leadership-clearing-conceptual-cloud-srilatha-batliwala.pdf; accessed 14 July 2024].

Bejan, T.M. (2021) Rawls's Teaching and the Tradition of Political Philosophy, *Modern Intellectual History*, 18 (4): 1058–1079.

Blakemore, E. (2021) From LGBT to LGBTQIA+: the evolving recognition of identity, *National Geographic*, October [https://www.nationalgeographic.com/history/article/from-lgbt-to-lgbtqia-the-evolving-recognition-of-identity; accessed 14 July 2024].

Brännmark, J. (2021) Patriarchy as institutional, *Journal of Social Ontology*, 7 (2): 233–254. https://doi.org/10.1515/jso-2021-0033.

Bunglawala, Z. (2019) Please, don't call me BAME or BME! GOV.UK [https://civilservice.blog.gov.uk/2019/07/08/please-dont-call-me-bame-or-bme/; accessed 14 July 2024].

Cerezo, A., Cummings, M., Holmes, M. and Williams, C. (2020) Identity as resistance: identity formation at the intersection of race, gender identity, and sexual orientation, *Psychology of Women Quarterly*, 44 (1): 67–83. doi: 10.1177/0361684319875977.

Charity Hudley, A.H., Mallinson C. and Bucholtz, M. (2024) *Inclusion in Linguistics*. Oxford: Oxford University Press.

Cherry, K. (2023) What Does LGBTQIA+ Mean? Understand why the acronym is used and what it stands for [https://www.verywellmind.com/what-does-lgbtq-mean-5069804; accessed 14 July 2024].

Clarke, J.A. (2022) Sex assigned at birth, *Columbia Law Review*, 122 (7): 1821–1898. https://www.jstor.org/stable/27178460.

Coalition of Peaks (2020) National Agreement on Closing the Gap: Coalition of Peaks [https://www.coalitionofpeaks.org.au/national-agreement-on-closing-the-gap; accessed 14 July 2024].

Collins, P.H. and Bilge, S. (2020) *Intersectionality*. Medford, MA: Polity Press.

Cooper, K., Russell, A., Mandy, W. and Butler, C. (2020) The phenomenology of gender dysphoria in adults: a systematic review and meta-synthesis, *Clinical Psychology Review*, 80. doi: 10.1016/j.cpr.2020.101875.

Cox, T.H., Jr. (1993) *Cultural Diversity in Organizations: Theory, Research and Practice*. San Francisco, CA: Berrett-Koehler.

Cremer, D.J. (2021) Patriarchy, religion, and society, in J. Marques (ed.) *Exploring Gender at Work: Multiple Perspectives*. Cham: Palgrave Macmillan.

Crenshaw, K. (1989) Demarginalizing the intersection of race and sex: a Black feminist critique of antidiscrimination doctrine, feminist theory and antiracist politics, *University of Chicago Legal Forum*, 1989: 8. [https://chicagounbound.uchicago.edu/uclf/vol1989/iss1/8; accessed 21 July 2024].

Crenshaw, K. (2014) Justice Rising: moving intersectionally in the age of post-everything, LSE Public Lecture, 26 March [https://www.lse.ac.uk/lse-player?id=10ad7291-17e2-43d5-823a-973b18ba3117; accessed 14 July 2024].

DaCosta, C., Dixon-Smith, S. and Singh, G. (2021) Beyond BAME: rethinking the politics, construction, application, and efficacy of ethnic categorisation. Stimulus Paper, April [https://pureportal.coventry.ac.uk/files/41898015/Beyond_BAME_final_report.pdf; accessed 14 July 2024].

Dahlgreen, G. and Whitehead, M. (1991) *Policies and Strategies to Promote Social Equity in Health*. Stockholm: Institute for Future Studies.

Dahlgren, G. and Whitehead, M. (2021) The Dahlgren-Whitehead model of health determinants: 30 years on and still chasing rainbows, *Public Health*, 199: 20–24. doi: 10.1016/j.puhe.2021.08.009. Epub 2021 Sep 14. PMID: 34534885.

Das, R. (2020) Identity politics: a Marxist view, *Class, Race and Corporate Power*, 8 (1): 5. doi: 10.25148/CRCP.8.1.008921.

Devakumar, D., Selvarajah, S., Abubakar, I., Kim, S-S., McKee, M., Sabharwal, N.S., et al. (2022) Racism, xenophobia, discrimination, and the determination of health, *The Lancet*, 400 (10368): 2097–2108.

Duckworth, S. (2020, Aug 19) Intersectionality [Infographic]. Flickr [https://flic.kr/p/2jy46K4; accessed 14 July 2024].

Equality Act (2010) c39. United Kingdom of Great Britain and Northern Ireland. London: HMSO [https://www.legislation.gov.uk/ukpga/2010/15/contents; accessed 22 July 2022].

Fakim, N. and Macaulay, C. (2020) 'Don't call me BAME': Why some people are rejecting the term. BBC News [https://www.bbc.co.uk/news/uk-53194376; accessed 14 July 2024].

French, J.R.P., Jr. and Raven, B.H. (1959) The bases of social power, in D. Cartwright (ed.), *Studies in Social Power* (pp. 150–167). Ann Arbor, MI: Institute for Social Research.

Gender Recognition Act (2004) United Kingdom of Great Britain and Northern Ireland [https://www.legislation.gov.uk/ukpga/2004/7/contents; accessed 14 July 2024].

Gergen, K.J. (2022) *An Invitation to Social Construction: Co-Creating the Future*. London: SAGE Publications [http://digital.casalini.it/9781529784633 online; accessed 14 July 2024].

Government of Canada (2017) Employment Equity, Diversity and Inclusion at Health Canada and the Public Health Agency of Canada [https://www.canada.ca/en/health-canada/campaigns/jobs-health-canada-public-health-agency-canada/employment-equity-diversity-inclusion.html; accessed 21 July 2024].

Government of Canada (2023a) Indigenous Health Care in Canada [https://www.sac-isc.gc.ca/eng/1626810177053/1626810219482; accessed 21 July 2024].

Government of Canada (2023b) Co-developing Distinctions-based Indigenous Health Legislation [https://www.sac-isc.gc.ca/eng/1611843547229/1611844047055; accessed 21 July 2024].

Griffin, K.A. (2020). Institutional Barriers, Strategies, and Benefits to Increasing the Representation of Women and Men of Color in the Professoriate, in L. Perna (eds) *Higher Education: Handbook of Theory and Research*, 35, Cham: Springer, https://doi.org/10.1007/978-3-030-11743-6_4-1.

Griffiths, E. (2023) The Intractable nature of the gender pay gap: a comparative perspective – conclusions and reflections and Reflections, in F. Hamilton and E. Griffiths (eds) *The Evolution of the Gender Pay Gap: A Comparative Perspective*. London: Routledge.

Gutin, I. and Hummer, R. (2021) Social inequality and the future of US life expectancy, *Annual Review of Sociology*, 47: 501–520. https://doi.org/10.1146/annurev-soc-072320-100249.

Harvey, B.H. (1999) Technology, diversity and work culture – key trends in the next millennium, *HR Magazine*, 44: 58–59.

Hayvon, J.C. (2024) Action against inequalities: a synthesis of social justice & equity, diversity, inclusion frameworks, *International Journal for Equity in Health*, 23: 106. https://doi.org/10.1186/s12939-024-02141-3.

Hidalgo, M.A., Ehrensaft, D., Tishelman, A.C., Clark, L.F., Garofalo, R., Rosenthal, S.M., Spack, N.P. and Olson, J. (2013) The gender affirmative model: what we know and what we aim to learn, *Human Development*, 1 October; 56 (5): 285–290. https://doi.org/10.1159/000355235.

Hooks, b. (2000) *Feminism is for Everybody*. London: Pluto Press.

Hutler, B. (2022) Causation and injustice: locating the injustice of racial and ethnic health disparities, *Bioethics*, 36: 260–266. https://doi.org/10.1111/bioe.12994.

Johnson, I.R., Pietri, E.S., Buck, D.M. and Daas, R. (2021) What's in a pronoun: exploring gender pronouns as an organizational identity-safety cue among sexual and gender minorities, *Journal of Experimental Social Psychology*, 97: 104194. https://doi.org/10.1016/j.jesp.2021.104194.

Kattari, S.K. (2020) Ableist microaggressions and the mental health of disabled adults, *Community Mental Health Journal*, 56: 1170–1179. https://doi.org/10.1007/s10597-020-00615-6.

Kendi, I.X. (2019) *How to be an Antiracist*. London: Bodley Head.

Khan, O. (2018) Economic inequality and racial inequalities in the UK: Current evidence and the possible effects of systemic economic change. London: Runnymede Trust [https://friendsprovidentfoundation.org/wp-content/uploads/2024/01/Runnymede-report.pdf; accessed 21 July 2024].

Kinouani, G. (2021) *Living While Black: The Essential Guide to Overcoming Racial Trauma*. London: Ebury Press.

Kline, R. (2022) Don't Shoot the Messenger, LinkedIn. 13th June [https://www.linkedin.com/pulse/dont-shoot-messenger-roger-kline/; accessed July 2023].

Kline, R. and Warmington, J. (2024) Too Hot to Handle: Why Concerns About Racism Are Not Heard …Or Acted Upon. January, brap [https://27aa994b-a128-4a85-b7e6-634fb830ed15.usrfiles.com/ugd/27aa99_9a9468c5e4da43288da375a17092d685.pdf; accessed 21 July 2024].

Kochan, T., Bezrukova, K., Ely, R., Jackson, S., Joshi, A., Jehn, K., et al. (2003) The effects of diversity on business performance: report of the diversity research network, *Human Resource Management*, 42, 3–21.

Krolökke, C. and Sörensen, A.S. (2006) *Gender Communication Theories & Analyses: From Silence to Performance.* SAGE Publications, Inc.

Larkey, L.K. (1996) The development and validation of the workforce diversity questionnaire, *Management Communication Quarterly*, 9: 296–337.

Lawrence, D. (2020) An Avoidable Crisis: The disproportionate impact of Covid-19 on Black, Asian and minority ethnic communities [https://uploads-ssl.webflow.com/5f5bdc0f30fe 4b120448a029/5f973b076be4cadc5045fad3_An%20Avoidable%20Crisis.pdf; accessed 10 December 2024].

Lazarus, J.V., Baker, L., Cascio, M., Onyango, D., Schatz, E., Smith, A.C, et al. (2020) Novel health systems service design checklist to improve healthcare access for marginalised, under-served communities in Europe, *BMJ Open*, 10: e035621. doi: 10.1136/bmjopen-2019-035621.

Lindqvist, A., Sendén, M.G. and Renström, E.A. (2020) What is gender, anyway: a review of the options for operationalising gender, *Psychology & Sexuality*, 12 (4): 332–344. https://doi.org/10.1080/19419899.2020.1729844.

Linnean Society (2024) Linnaeus and Race [https://www.linnean.org/learning/who-was-linnaeus/linnaeus-and-race; accessed 14 July 2024].

Marmot, M., Allen, J., Boyce, T., Goldblatt, P. and Morrison, J. (2020) Health Equity in England: The Marmot Review 10 Years On. February [https://www.health.org.uk/publications/reports/the-marmot-review-10-years-on; accessed 14 July 2024].

Marmot, M.G. (1986) Social inequalities in mortality: the social environment, in R.G. Wilkinson (ed.) *Class and Health: Research and Longitudinal Data.* London: Routledge.

Mavhandu-Mudzusi, A.H., Ndou, A., Mamabolo, L., Netshapapame, T., Ngwenya, T., Marebane, T., et al. (2023) Terms which LGBTQI+ individuals prefer or hate to be called by, *Heliyon*, 9 (4): e14990, April. https://doi.org/10.1016/j.heliyon.2023.e14990.

McCartney, G., Dickie, E., Escobar, O. and Collins, C. (2020) Health inequalities, fundamental causes and power: towards the practice of good theory, *Sociology of Health & Illness*, 43 (1): 20–39. https://doi.org/10.1111/1467-9566.13181.

McGrath, J.E., Berdahl, J.L. and Arrow, H. (1995) Traits, expectations, culture and clout: the dynamics of diversity in work groups, in S.E. Jackson and M.N. Ruderman (eds), *Diversity in Work Teams.* Washington, DC: American Psychological Association.

McIntosh, P. (1988) White Privilege: Unpacking the Invisible Knapsack. Working Paper 189. White Privilege and Male Privilege: A Personal Account of Coming to See Correspondences through Work in Women's Studies, Wellesley College Center for Research on Women [https://www.wcwonline.org/images/pdf/White_Privilege_and_Male_Privilege_Personal_Account-Peggy_McIntosh.pdf; accessed 20 July 2024].

McIntosh, P. (2003) White privilege: unpacking the invisible knapsack, in S. Plous (ed.), *Understanding Prejudice and Discrimination.* London: McGraw-Hill.

McKenna, H. and Williams, D. (2019) Professor David Williams on racism, discrimination and the impact they have on health. London: King's Fund [https://www.kingsfund.org.uk/audio-video/podcast/david-williams-racism-discrimination-health; accessed 14 July 2024].

Messenger, G. and Pollard, L. (2022) Health and Social Care Review: Leadership for a collaborative and inclusive future. GOV.UK, 8 June [https://www.gov.uk/government/publications/health-and-social-care-review-leadership-for-a-collaborative-and-inclusive-future; accessed 14 July 2024].

Milliken, F. and Martins, L. (1996) Searching for common threads: understanding the multiple effects of diversity in organizational groups, *Academy of Management Review*, 21: 402–433.

Morrison, A.M. (1992) *The New Leaders: Guidelines on Leadership Diversity in America*. San Francisco, CA: Jossey-Bass.

Morrison, T. (2017) *The Origin of Others*. Cambridge, MA / London: Harvard University Press.

New Zealand Government Ministry of Health / Manatū Hauora (2020) Whakamaua: Māori Health Action Plan 2020-2025 [https://www.health.govt.nz/our-work/populations/maori-health/whakamaua-maori-health-action-plan-2020-2025; accessed 21 July 2024].

New Zealand Government Ministry of Health / Manatū Hauora (2023) Achieving equity [https://www.health.govt.nz/about-ministry/what-we-do/achieving-equity; accessed 21 July 2024].

New Zealand Government Ministry of Justice (2023) Change the sex/gender on a birth certificate [https://www.justice.govt.nz/family/change-the-sexgender-on-a-birth-certificate/; accessed 21 July 2024].

NHS England (2023a) NHS equality, diversity, and inclusion improvement plan [https://www.england.nhs.uk/long-read/nhs-equality-diversity-and-inclusion-improvement-plan/; accessed 21 July 2024].

NHS England (2023b) Gender Pay Gap Report [https://www.england.nhs.uk/publication/gender-pay-gap-report/; accessed 14 July 2024].

Noels, K.A., Yashima, T. and Zhang, R. (2020) Language, identity, and intercultural communication, in J. Jackson (ed.). *The Routledge Handbook of Language and Intercultural Communication* (2nd edn). Oxon: Routledge.

Ortner, S.B. (2022) Patriarchy, *Feminist Anthropology*, 3: 307–314. https://doi.org/10.1002/fea2.12081.

Otu, A., Ahinkorah, B.O., Ameyaw, E.K., Seidu, A.A. and Yaya S. (2020) One country, two crises: what Covid-19 reveals about health inequalities among BAME communities in the United Kingdom and the sustainability of its health system? *International Journal for Equity in Health*, Oct 27; 19 (1): 189. doi: 10.1186/s12939-020-01307-z. PMID: 33109197; PMCID: PMC7590239.

Public Health England (2018) Local action on health inequalities: Understanding and reducing ethnic inequalities in health. *PHE publications*. OGL 3.0 [https://assets.publishing.service.gov.uk/media/5b607232e5274a5f6ab8603f/local_action_on_health_inequalities.pdf; accessed 29 November 2024].

Ramonetti, M. and Pilato, V. (2019) Keeping the equity, inclusion, and diversity conversations going, *Urban Library Journal*, 25 (1).

Rattansi, A. (2020) *Racism: A Very Short Introduction*. Oxford: Oxford University Press.

Rawls, J. (1971) *A Theory of Justice*. Cambridge, MA: Harvard University Press, Belknap Press.

Rhodes, R., Battin, M. and Silvers, A. (2012) (eds) *Medicine and Social Justice: Essays on the Distribution of Health Care* (2nd edn). Oxford: Oxford University Press https://doi.org/10.1093/acprof:osobl/9780199744206.001.0001.

Roberson, Q.M. (2004) Disentangling the Meanings of Diversity & Inclusion. Working Paper 04-05, Cornell Center for Advanced Human Resource Studies [https://ecommons.cornell.edu/server/api/core/bitstreams/d4c6f6d3-5615-42ac-b8ee-55c1809bcf7f/content; accessed 14 July 2024].

Roberson, Q. and Perry, J.L. (2021) *Inclusive Leadership in Thought and Action: A Thematic Analysis*. London: Group & Organization Management (GOM).

Rodriguez-Bailon, R., Bratanova, B., Willis G.B., Lopez-Rodriguez, L., Sturrock, A. and Loughnan, S. (2017) Social class and ideologies of inequality: how they uphold unequal societies, *Journal of Social Issues*, 73 (1): 99–116. [https://spssi.onlinelibrary.wiley.com/doi/abs/10.1111/josi.12206; accessed 21 July 2024].

Ross, S., Jabbal, J., Chauhan, K., Maguire, D., Randhawa, M. and Dahir, S. (2020) Workforce Race Inequalities and Inclusion In NHS Providers. July, London: King's Fund [https://assets.kingsfund.org.uk/f/256914/x/eeb3fa7cd3/workforce_race_inequalities_inclusion_nhs_providers_2020.pdf; accessed 27 July 2024].

Scott, C.L. and Klein L.B. (2022) Advancing traditional leadership theories by incorporating multicultural and workforce diversity leadership traits, behaviors, and supporting practices: implications for organizational leaders, *Journal of Leadership, Accountability and Ethics*, 19 (3). https://doi.org/10.33423/jlae.v19i3.5320.

Schudson, Z.C. and Morgenroth, T. (2022) Non-binary gender/sex identities, *Current Opinion in Psychology*, 48: 101499. https://doi.org/10.1016/j.copsyc.2022.101499.

Skinner-Dorkenoo, A.L., Sarmal, A., André, C.J., and Rogbeer, K.G. (2021) How Microaggressions Reinforce and Perpetuate Systemic Racism in the United States, *Perspectives on Psychological Science*, 16 (5): 903–925. https://doi.org/10.1177/17456916211002543.

Stonewall (2023) List of LGBTQ+ terms [https://www.stonewall.org.uk/list-lgbtq-terms; accessed 14 July 2024].

Sue, D.W., Capodilupo, C.M., Torino, G.C., Bucceri, J.M., Holder, A.M.B., Nadal, K.L., et al. (2007) Racial microaggressions in everyday life: implications for clinical practice, *American Psychologist*, 62 (4), 271–286. https://doi.org/10.1037/0003-066X.62.4.271.

Suveren, Y. (2022) Unconscious bias: definition and significance, *Current Approaches in Psychiatry*, 14 (1): 414–426. DOI: 10.18863/pgy.1026607.

Thompson, N. (2020) *Anti-Discriminatory Practice: Equality, Diversity and Social Justice* 9th edn.). London: Bloomsbury Publications, Red Globe Press.

Tong, R. and Botts, T.F. (2024) *Feminist Thought: A More Comprehensive Introduction*. Oxon, UK; New York: Taylor & Francis.

Toorn, J., Pliskin, R. and Morgenroth, T. (2020) Not quite over the rainbow: the unrelenting and insidious nature of heteronormative ideology, *Current Opinion in Behavioral Sciences*, 34. https://doi.org/10.1016/j.cobeha.2020.03.001.

University of California Davis (2023) LGBTQIA Resource Center Glossary. July 21st [https://lgbtqia.ucdavis.edu/educated/glossary; accessed 14 July 2024].

VeneKlasen, L. and Miller, V. (2002) Power and empowerment, PLA Notes, 43: 39–41 [https://www.iied.org/sites/default/files/pdfs/migrate/G01985.pdf; accessed 27 July 2024].

Whitehead, M. and Dahlgren, G. (2006) Concepts and principles for tackling social inequities in health: Levelling up Part 1. World Health Organization [https://www.enothe.eu/cop/docs/concepts_and_principles.pdf; accessed 28 July 2024].

Winters, M-F. (2020) *Inclusive Conversations: Fostering Equity, Empathy, and Belonging across Differences*. Oaklands, CA: Berrett-Koehler Publishers.

Wood, W. and Eagly, A. (2013) Gender identity, in M.R. Leary and R.H. Hoyle (eds) *Handbook of Individual Differences in Social Behavior*. New York: Guilford Publications.

World Health Organization (2024a) Health equity [https://www.who.int/health-topics/health-equity#tab=tab_1; accessed 14 July 2024].

World Health Organization (2024b) Social determinants of health [https://www.who.int/health-topics/social-determinants-of-health#tab=tab_1; accessed 14 July 2024].

Zajda, J., Majhanovich, S. and Rust, V. (2006) *Education and Social Justice.* Springer [https://link.springer.com/book/10.1007/1-4020-4722-3; accessed 28 July 2024].

Research and evaluation

Tara Lamont and Gareth Hooper

Introduction

Why do managers need research? Those leading and shaping services may not need to carry out research themselves, but they need to be able to draw on existing evidence and understand in broad terms the quality and weight of that research to make decisions. Managers also need to know when and how to get others to evaluate service changes (Lamont et al., 2016). This is important to assess whether planned changes have had the desired impact on people and services. There may also be unintended effects on other parts of the system. Without research and evaluation, we do not know which changes are working well for which people or how services might be optimized to deliver better care.

Healthcare is dynamic and complex, with increasing pressures on services and changes to how that care is delivered. In the last decade, more complex care, from diagnostics to dialysis and chemotherapy, is now delivered at home or in the community (Corbett et al., 2015). Hospitals themselves have changed beyond recognition, with a greater volume of day cases and minimally invasive surgery. At the same time, patients are living longer with multiple and complex long-term conditions that require inter-agency collaboration and input from a number of professionals. There have been considerable changes in role scope and practice, with increasing numbers of non-medical prescribing and enhanced skills in a range of healthcare staff (Evans et al., 2021).

But changes have not always been evaluated, and it is difficult at times to understand the real gains of service changes and innovations. Managers need to be able to engage confidently in dialogue with clinicians about costs and benefits of therapeutic advances. This might include challenges to well-held views, for instance, recent evidence showing little or no added benefit of recently approved cancer drugs (Brinkhuis et al., 2024). There can be a degree of 'techno-optimism' – for instance, in the actual benefits of assistive technology in keeping older people out of hospital (Howard et al., 2021) – which does not take into account evidence of challenges in implementing and maintaining technical solutions to optimal effect. Other areas where research evidence indicates new care models falling somewhat short of intended goals include evaluation of different forms of integrated care pilots introduced in the UK (Lewis et al., 2021) showing limited impact on emergency hospital admissions.

In other areas, evidence may show under-use of potentially beneficial aspects – such as an early study showing effectiveness of advanced nurse practitioners (Htay and White-head, 2021) or conditions for effective use of paramedics in primary care settings (Eaton et al., 2021). Research can also sometimes confound long-established truths – analysis of English NHS data suggested that smaller hospitals are not generally associated with lower quality of care (Gaughan et al., 2020). Research can provide necessary caution when extrapolating likely savings or impact from new changes in light of what we know from robust evaluations. It can also point to new areas of practice with potential to make a difference that could be worth adopting or considering.

Why else do managers need to know about research? Healthcare managers need to understand the benefits of research in their organizations – not least as there is good evidence that research-active hospitals tend to have better patient outcomes (Boaz et al., 2015). During the pandemic, having a networked research-ready set of hospitals able to carry out platform trials at pace enabled the UK to break new ground in establishing low-cost, effective treatments for people with COVID-19 (RECOVERY Collaborative Group, 2021). Research activity is an important part of what healthcare organizations do and the financial support they receive, both commercial and through large programmatic funding from major research funding bodies. Your organization may be involved as a study site or sponsor of research with specific responsibilities and activity, involving staff in costing contracts, financial and project management, oversight of research governance, data management and more. You may not need to get closely involved with research that is done, but understanding and supporting research activity in your organization is critical for the modern manager.

In this chapter, we will look at examples of managers **using evidence to support decisions** at individual and organizational level and **planning evaluations** of different kinds to assess impact of changes. This is an exciting time for health services research, with expanding investment in real-world applied research in areas from workforce to evaluation of large-scale service transformation. Managers need to know enough about available resources and activities to harness research and research evidence to strengthen decisions about care.

Using evidence to support decisions

Why managers should look to evidence

Managers and service leaders increasingly want answers to pressing and practical questions. What will help me most in retaining ward staff in a busy hospital – from team-based self-rostering to structured onboarding? Will expanding virtual wards reduce emergency admission of frail older people in my organization? What model of same-day emergency care services works best? Which kinds of childhood obesity prevention or immunization programmes get most uptake from high-risk groups? How should we staff a new cross-agency homeless health and well-being pathway?

Learning activity 6.1

Take one of the five example problems mentioned that is relevant to your organization or a similar current issue or concern in your organization and try to find one or two research studies that seem relevant. Discuss the results with someone leading work on this area in your organization. How helpful are the findings to them? Did you find it easy to access research or know where to look (general internet or resources like Google Scholar)? Did you find the answer to your question in a single source? How far back would you need to look? Would research from different countries be useful – and if not, why? Was there mention of value for money or only clinical outcomes?

A quick search on the internet will bring you information but it may not be reliable or high quality. More information on how to search and what to look for when interpreting findings is given in the next section.

Box 6.1   Case study – early evaluation of telehealth and telecare

It is important that managers know enough about evidence to ask questions and have reasonable scepticism about claims that seem too good to be true. This is particularly necessary where political or commercial interests are in play – or just a natural optimism and belief by clinical or other champions introducing a new technology or service.

A good example of research with highly positive findings was the Whole System Demonstrator evaluation of telehealth and telecare. This was a complex programme of work involving over 6000 patients with conditions like COPD, diabetes and heart failure in 238 practices across three sites in Newham, Kent and Cornwall in the UK. This was the largest trial of telehealth and telecare ever conducted, which involved expertise and input from six different academic teams.

In advance of the publication of results in academic journals, headline findings were published on the government website at the end of 2011 (Department of Health, 2011). These showed startlingly positive results – 'when used correctly, telehealth can deliver a 15% reduction in A&E visits, a 20% reduction in emergency admissions, a 14% reduction in elective admissions, a 14% reduction in bed days and an 8% reduction in tariff costs. More strikingly they also demonstrate a 45% reduction in mortality rates'.

The same announcement identified at least three million people with long-term conditions or social care needs who could benefit from using telehealth and telecare. This was great news for industry and other stakeholders.

But published results over the next two years told a rather different story. Using routine data, the main trial of telehealth showed lower mortality and emergency admission rates for those using telehealth, but the latter could be linked to an unexplained increase in emergency admissions for patients in the control arm (Steventon et al., 2012). The authors presented headline findings carefully in the original paper, as follows:

What this study adds:

- Among people with chronic obstructive pulmonary disease, heart failure, or diabetes, a broad class of telehealth technologies could be associated with reduced rates of mortality and emergency hospital admission

- This effect, however, could be linked to short term increases in hospital use observed in the control group that may have been affected by recruitment processes during the trial

- The estimated scale of hospital cost savings for commissioners of care is modest, and the cost of the telehealth intervention should also be taken into account

Further analysis (Steventon, 2015) suggested that these findings about lower emergency admissions could not be generalized to routine practice. The nested economic analysis showed that telehealth was not cost-effective in addition to usual care (Henderson et al., 2013). A linked study showed no benefit of telecare on quality of life or well-being (Cartwright et al., 2013). And organizational analysis showed that system-level integration to support telecare and telehealth was not evident in the study sites (Hendy et al., 2012).

So, the headline findings promoted by policymakers accurately reported data from the trial, but this did not tell the whole story. This example shows that it is easy to cherry-pick results to support a decision. But the cautious and balanced view of experienced researchers is important to understand the weight of evidence and what it means for large investment or decisions. And despite the flaws of academic scientific publishing and peer review, the system of checks and balances in high-quality journals does help to eliminate bias and report findings accurately. This makes it more likely that correct inferences are drawn and the right interpretations made to support important decisions. Managers need to employ scepticism and enlist the help of others to understand what research means.

It is a paradox that as more research-based (and other) information becomes available, it may be increasingly difficult for managers to interpret and assess. Over two million biomedical articles a year are indexed in the PubMed database every year, landing at a rate of around two papers a minute (Landhuis, 2016). An estimate in 2014 that scientific output doubles every nine years (Van Noorden, 2014) is probably conservative, given accelerated increase in volume of research studies around COVID-19 and the rise of open access journals and modes of publishing. Given increasing awareness of the flawed nature of much published research, addressing the wrong questions or with weak study design or delivery (Glasziou and Chalmers, 2018), it is no wonder that managers may find it difficult to know where to start in finding 'good enough' evidence.

But it is important to persist. There is a proud history in the UK of developing robust approaches to testing and synthesizing evidence, particularly randomized trials looking at the comparative effectiveness of treatments, to standardize best clinical practice. The evidence-based medicine movement, seen as disruptive and radical in the 1970s, has now become embedded as mainstream health practice, with most NHS organizations now engaged in trials and effectiveness studies and national standards enshrined through the work of the National Institute of Health and Care Excellence (NICE). There is an interesting debate around evidence-based management. It is now well understood that the paradigm of evidence-based medicine cannot be imported wholesale to the management of services. As noted in a key paper (Walshe and Rundall, 2001), managers may struggle to access a dispersed social science literature without clear hierarchy of evidence or easy synthesis of findings on complex problems.

There are real differences between the paradigms of clinical and managerial knowledge and no easy solutions, but there is growing recognition by many management and business schools of the limitations of a complacent, evidence-free culture in which the anecdote or business case study triumphs over systematic knowledge. Proponents of evidence-based management decry the poor uptake of known effective management practices, such as goal setting and performance feedback or poor use of academic management information by general managers (Rousseau, 2006).

How managers might find useful evidence

Let us return to health and how you might go about finding best evidence on problems or innovations from e-rostering to community diagnostic hubs. If you are wanting to carry out a reasonably thorough scan, short of a formal evidence review, you will probably need to enlist the help of people with skills, like library staff and information analysts. Many health organizations employ library staff or research teams as well as institutions to provide learning and management support. National healthcare thinktanks and foundations such as the Health Foundation, Nuffield Trust and Kings Fund in the UK also have useful libraries and resources, including accessible overviews of evidence for service-facing audiences.

Thinking carefully about the scope of your search is important. Would learning from international literature be relevant on recruiting general practitioners in rural areas? Are family doctors or generalists equivalent? How recent does this need to be – would research from before 2010 be relevant and is there a logical cut-off in terms of service or policy change?

Formal published research can be accessed through different databases, with broad coverage on health issues in repositories, such as Medline and more healthcare-oriented resources, such as CINAHL (nursing and allied health literature) or HMIC (health management and policy) or broader social research such as SSCI (Social Sciences Citation Index). But you may also want to access 'grey literature', i.e. information that is not from peer reviewed academic journals, such as UK-based service evaluations, local audits or good practice summaries published on websites such as NICE (which includes evidence-based quality standards on questions, such as best discharge from inpatient mental health settings).

You can also extend your search by using one core paper that is particularly helpful and following references 'back' that are identified in that paper and looking 'forward' to more recent publications citing the core paper. This is known as forward and backward citation tracing – or more loosely as 'snowballing'. The key is to identify core papers that might yield the highest value and relevant papers.

Once you have a list or database of possibly useful papers you can read the title and abstract to get a sense of whether it fits your search question. You will probably only want to read the full text of a few and may need further help to access these from a university or healthcare library – or even a local library. There is a bigger debate about how those outside universities can access research findings, with many funders now requiring researchers to publish in open access form. To know what is available, start with the Directory of Open Access Journals (DOAJ) [https://doaj.org/]. In the meantime, you can often find full text versions of articles in Google Scholar search results or contact authors directly if you have identified an article of interest by email or through academic social media-style sites, such as ResearchGate [https://www.researchgate.net/] and Acaemia.edu [https://www.academia.edu/].

How managers might make sense of evidence

In terms of making sense of the papers and assessing the quality, this will depend on your question. If you want to find out whether a new form of community nursing reduces emergency admissions, a small descriptive study of a frailty team in one locality without any measurement of impact or comparator will be of limited use as results may not translate to another setting. If you wanted to know about the experience of call-handlers in triaging patients, a quantitative study analysing routine data would not be so relevant as these research approaches would not give insights or information about what matters to staff and why. Quality of papers will partly be about the scale of study, explicit research design and how well the paper explains existing evidence and the gap that this research fills.

Complex organizational questions are different from well-defined clinical treatments or interventions. Assessing services and parts of systems will usually require a mixture of quantitative and qualitative data collection. Certain kinds of observational data, from cross-sectional surveys to large routine datasets like Hospital Episode Statistics in the UK or Organisation for Economic Co-operation and Development (OECD) health data (see: https://www.oecd.org/health/) can be analysed using statistical techniques to identify patterns and factors associated with certain outcomes. However, these kinds of studies may not provide evidence of causal relations that enable definitive statements about the impact of certain changes. Reviewing published evidence on a particular service problem will therefore need a level of judgement in assessing what can be reasonably asserted about impact and a range of studies may be needed to establish the state of knowledge.

As a busy manager, it is a good idea to look for reliable and high-quality evidence reviews that synthesize research in a systematic way, adjusting for the weight or quality of different sources. These tend to be more reliable than single studies and can present evidence showing mixed results. Reliable sources for high-quality reviews related to service delivery and organization, as well as critical appraisal tools, are given in the Learning resources section at the end of this chapter.

Box 6.2   Case study – evidence on twelve-hour nursing shifts

There is increasing use of 12- rather than 8-hour nursing shifts in the UK, Europe, the US and elsewhere. In this country, there is no central data on nurse shift patterns by organization but a study in 2014 (Griffiths et al., 2014) found around a third of day shifts on acute hours were 12 hours. The proportion is likely to be greater now, but most organizations appear to operate a mixed economy of shift patterns.

A recent narrative overview by leading workforce experts provides a helpful place to consider what the evidence tells us (Dall'Ora et al., 2022). The authors concluded that there was limited robust evidence to support claims that 12-hour shifts are more cost-effective or generate greater satisfaction and well-being for staff. Unusually for an area of workforce research, there is reasonably good research on nurse activity and outcomes due to a series of large-scale, cross-sectional observational studies surveying more than 30,000 nurses in 12 European countries. This provides a robust level of evidence to interrogate some of the key stated claims for longer shifts, although authors noted that the literature base also included many studies with small samples and weak design, for instance, simple before–after studies without controls or comparators.

The central proposition is that longer shifts lead to more productive care, addressing nurse shortages, by reducing overlaps between shifts with fewer nurse hours to be rostered each day. Also, there is anecdotal evidence that staff prefer it, and this will support retention and well-being. Counter to this is the suggestion that nurses working 12-hour shifts may be more fatigued, leading to errors and harm to patients and not all staff prefer this working mode.

Taking each stated benefit in turn, the review noted there was very little evidence to support reduced costs or greater productivity with 12-hour shifts. Direct evidence showed no reduction in nursing hours worked per day, as assumed, and higher sickness absence in places with greater proportions of 12-hour shifts. In addition, removing overlap and handover between shifts appeared to result in missed information about patients who may be deteriorating or need attention or for staff education and development.

There was less reliable information on fatigue and error (often self-reported by nurses in research studies) and so it was difficult to assess the impact of longer shifts on quality of care.

The proposition that longer shifts would improve recruitment and retention was not supported by existing evidence. But there is research showing nurses value choice and flexibility around shift patterns and reports that longer shifts provide better work–life balance, which can contribute to nurse well-being and could plausibly impact on decisions to stay or leave.

This review helpfully assesses existing evidence around central claims made about the value of nurse shift patterns. While propositions of reduced costs and greater productivity might not be supported by existing evidence and impact on quality of care remains uncertain, there are benefits for some if not many of better work–life balance in fewer longer shifts.

What can managers do with this information? Given known risks of fatigue, poor handover or communication of risk, potential harms and mixed satisfaction, managers may want to try mitigating these effects while maximizing benefits that could lead to better well-being and improved recruitment and retention. Enabling a mixed economy of shifts according to preference may be optimal and requires organizational flexibility. Evidence often provides complex answers to complex questions, but it is helpful to know the signals from best available research that has been sifted and interpreted by those with content and research knowledge of a field.

Evidence-informed organizations

So far, we have focused on how individuals might best gather and make sense of evidence for specific problems, but it is also worth considering how you as a manager can support the everyday use of evidence in an organization.

Some research evidence can help us with what works and does not work in embedding a research-using culture in health organizations (Swan et al., 2017), drawing on findings from Swan and others, which suggest:

- Managers of all backgrounds find it hard to make sense of and apply evidence in their everyday work.
- Managers tend to make less use of formal research. They value examples and experience of others, as well as local information and intelligence.
- Evidence does not speak for itself. Organizations need skills, not just technical around critical appraisal capacity, but also to engage experts and frame research for different audiences.
- Having skilled individuals, like public health staff, on the spot to contextualize and interpret evidence helps managers use evidence when making decisions.

A recent study of how health and care boards use research evidence showed that this did not happen systematically (Parkinson et al., 2021). Individual board members would rarely seek published evidence themselves but would rely on clinical leads and others to package up and synthesize relevant research. Examples where organizations made explicit use of research evidence include decisions about new services like telehealth (particularly in relation to pandemic pressures and service shifts), new treatment, such as those for opiate misuse, and organizational research topics, such as workforce stability. But it was still rare for organizations to actively seek or expect to use evidence as part of routine decision-making, and often hard for decision-makers to find evidence that was relevant and timely for particular decisions they were making.

In terms of practical actions, there are a number of steps which organizations can take as noted in recent national strategies to embed research in the everyday work of healthcare. This might include identifying a named director or board member in an organization to take a lead on research. Having a research champion can improve general research literacy and awareness at different levels, but it is also everybody's business to ask if there might be relevant evidence to support decisions, from local evaluations in neighbouring systems to reviews and evaluations in published literature or reliable overviews from intermediary bodies. It should also be a broader goal to foster a culture in which asking the right questions is encouraged and valued. These might include:

- Could we look to other forms of intelligence here? Who or where might hold relevant evidence including lived experience of staff and relevant patient groups?
- Have others adopted services like these and what impact did it have?
- Is there evidence to support this particular model of care in relation to existing alternative services?
- What might good enough evidence be to support this decision?

Other initiatives that may be helpful to stimulate interest and confidence in using research include mechanisms like journal clubs, well established in medical and nursing professional development that could be extended to other staff. Having meetings or workshops to celebrate local research activity or to hear from a leading expert giving overview of what is known on a hot topic from weekend working to use of AI in diagnostics can also stimulate interest and engagement. There are many different ways in which organizations can help staff to think about how they could use research more in everyday work and decisions.

Research to make you think...

In this chapter we have concentrated on the instrumental value of research to support best decisions, but there is also the benefit of research in stimulating new ways of thinking about problems or viewing the world. Some research can help us to change the conversation. For instance, research has helped us to understand that clinicians' 'resistance to technology' may be founded on cultural and system blocks that are avoidable (Greenhalgh et al., 2014). Similarly, Dixon-Woods theory of 'candidacy' helps us think differently about poor uptake of services, playing on staff assumptions and structural barriers that may inhibit care for minoritized populations (Dixon-Woods et al., 2006). Some of these research terms permeate into mainstream management thought. It is not unusual at general staff training sessions to include notions of contrasting 'work as imagined' or idealized views of a managed environment versus 'work as done' or the reality of messy, complex daily work practices, concepts drawn originally from the academic literature around resilience and patient safety (Hollnagel, 2015). What many of these thought-changing research studies share is a grounding in qualitative and observational research, where staff and services are closely monitored in ethnographic research. There is value in qualitative research to understand staff and patient experience, interactions and how systems work in practice, as well as other kinds of quantitative analysis in research on services and care.

Learning activity 6.2

Take a table of contents from a recent journal like *Sociology of Health and Illness* or *BMJ Quality and Safety* and pick a title that intrigues you. Or perhaps choose a couple of titles from different journals on the same topic. Get hold of the articles – which may involve trying a few avenues, as suggested earlier. Try to write a five-sentence summary and a social media post that describes the nature of the topic and why it is interesting or gives new insights into an existing health or healthcare problem. Or how the study is disappointing as it does not tell you what you need to know. Discuss with a few colleagues and get them to bring an article that interests them next time. You will have started your own journal club!

Planning evaluations of new or changing services

Spectrum of evaluation effort

Complex multi-method evaluations may take many years to complete. Typical funded national evaluations from experienced teams combining expertise in qualitative research, routine data analysis and health economics, with full data governance and ethical approvals, may take 3 to 5 years to complete. These substantive studies are needed in order to advance knowledge and provide robust evidence, but services are dynamic and change rapidly. Completed evaluations may come too late to inform funding or commissioning decisions, and services and contexts may have changed in the meantime.

Over the past 5 to 10 years, we have seen growth in rapid evaluation capacity and capability in the UK. Some of the largest applied health funders have invested in multiple centres to provide 6- to 9-month mixed methods evaluations of new service changes, from home pulse oximetry (Fulop et al., 2023) to mental health support teams in schools (Ellins et al., 2023).

The methods have also advanced to enable rapid appraisal, ethnography and real-time evaluation designs, with a marked increase in the number of recent publications setting out approaches to evaluation in shorter time frames (Vindrola-Padros et al., 2021). At times, the evaluation itself is compressed, but there has also been a trend towards longer evaluations with multiple feedback loops to share interim findings with decision-makers and assessments planned in cyclical stages. Even shorter projects require intense engagement with decision-makers and patient groups from the start and thorough early scoping at the start pays dividends (Smith et al., 2023). There are of course trade-offs between the quality of evidence – for instance, it is often difficult to get robust summative (definitive) impact assessment in less than six months – and the timeliness of research.

The first step when planning an evaluation is to think about the aims of the improvement and how the intended changes might work to achieve that effect. A useful tool for illustrating how the expected outcomes will be achieved from the available resources is a logic model. Also known as a theory of change or programme theory, this requires a structured and sequenced approach to show why the intervention is expected to work.

A logic model is a visual plan, based on an underlying theory, of how the resources and activities of a health programme will achieve the intended outcomes (Kaplan and Garrett, 2005). Logic models often share the same features:

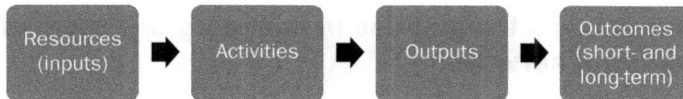

Figure 6.1 General logic model

An example of a logic model to reduce falls in older people might be written as:

Table 6.1 Example logic model to reduce falls

Resources (inputs)	Activities	Outputs	Outcomes
Community physiotherapists	Delivering physical exercises to older people in the community	Fewer falls in the older population	Improved quality of life and reduced demand for healthcare services

The starting point for a service change is the problem that needs to be solved. In this example, it might be that there is a higher-than-expected number of emergency admissions for hip fractures following falls in the community and associated delayed discharge in hospital. Tackling this problem is important as it leads to a reduction in quality of life for patients and greater demand on the healthcare system. It then must follow that some falls are preventable and could reduce the demand on healthcare services. Only if this logical assumption is satisfied does the logic model work. It follows that the theory of change could be written as:

To improve the quality of life of older people and reduce their demand for healthcare services we should reduce the number of falls in the population.

This statement can be verified by a local audit to determine how many falls there are per year in the target population and how much healthcare resources are consumed by treating patients. An assumption within the logic model is that (some) falls are preventable and could reduce the demand on healthcare services. Only if this logical assumption is satisfied does the logic model work. In the logic model, one reason falls can be prevented is by patients becoming stronger through physical training. The activity can be framed as an If-Then statement: *If* older people are physically stronger, *then* they will have fewer falls. A systematic review has been carried out and does conclude that physical training of older people does reduce the risk of a fall (Sherrington et al., 2019). The logic model has validity due to existing evidence.

Within the logic model you will have to consider allocation of resources and what you would have to do to move the resources from treatment to prevention. Making the economic case for reallocation of resources can be challenging, especially if the expected gains do not offset any costs for change. Building business cases for change are often a synthesis of local data and findings from published research: together, they can be used to estimate the effects of changing the service and quantify the costs and benefits gained.

Box 6.3   Case study – inequalities in mortality and morbidity in UK maternity services

The UK, like other high-income countries, routinely collects data relating to outcomes in healthcare. Routinely collected data at the patient level can demonstrate where outcomes are not satisfactory, either across a population or at an individual patient level. Health inequities are where population sub-groups experience poorer outcomes associated with a characteristic such as sex, age or ethnicity. The National Perinatal Epidemiology Unit at Oxford University conduct research in several areas of maternity care. One area is the Mothers and Babies: Reducing Risk through Audits and Confidential Enquiries across the UK (Knight et al., 2023) to monitor the health outcomes of maternity care. Their report shows that women and babies from Black, Asian and minority ethnic backgrounds are at greater risk of dying than women with a white background.

As a healthcare manager you could be asked to determine how your hospital should address the findings of the MBRRACE-UK report. To do this you will need evidence of the problem at your hospital and a theory of change to reduce disparities in mortality.

Quantifying the mortality at your hospital

The MBRRACE-UK report contains national data, but you will need an estimation of the disparities at your hospital. Working with an analyst using local data, you could estimate how many women in maternity services are at increased risk of mortality. This estimation will be the baseline data that you can compare with future changes made to the service to determine the impact of the change.

Evidence-based changes

Making changes to maternity services must be based on evidence. If not, the likelihood of success is low, and scarce resources will be wasted. The evidence to support the changes could include published research and clinical expertise, as well as patient perspectives. A qualitative evidence synthesis (MacLellan et al., 2022) found several organizational failings that directly affected women from Black, Asian and minority ethnic backgrounds when receiving care from maternity services in the UK that may have contributed (and continue to contribute) to inequitable outcomes. The synthesis suggested technocratic systems, poor communications, mistreatment and failure of women-centred care contributed to excess mortality. Using clinical and patient expertise on how changes could be made could form a theory of change and used within a logic model to plan for improvements in care.

Reducing disparities in maternity outcomes can be achieved through implementation of evidence-based interventions. Midwife-led continuity of care demonstrates reduced risk of preterm babies and lower risk of losing babies (Sandall et al., 2016), but like many areas of healthcare, single interventions must be looked at in the wider context of activities that improve safety, such as culture and teamwork (Liberati et al., 2019).

Using research to inform a theory of change

Using the data from MBRRACE-UK and the evidence synthesis from MacLellan et al., along with local data, and the interventions suggested by Sandall et al. and Liberati et al., a theory of change can be developed to reduce disparities between ethnic groups. An alongside quantitative evaluation will verify whether the intervention has been successful.

The design of the evaluation, the data collected and the methods used for analysis will depend on the level of investment in a new service or change and the importance of the question. For a small local decision, you may not need to do much more than collect some before and after data, but for national service changes, it will be important to develop robust designs that can not only demonstrate effect but attribute it to that particular intervention rather than other trends happening across all services. This can help to counteract various forms of bias that could lead to false interpretations of data. These include common challenges, such as confounding or regression to the mean.

Confounding is where a positive response to treatment or service change is observed (Jager et al., 2008). But many other changes may be happening that contribute to changes in service activity, such as new policy directives or tariff alterations. Some study designs are better than others at being able to attribute the effect to the change alone. Similarly, *regression to the mean* alludes to the fact that data showing much higher or lower activity tends to be much closer to average when measured the second time (Barnett et al., 2005). We know that data varies naturally above and below a long-term average, but it is easy to see a positive reading and forget this. In sport, footballers may go through periods of scoring goals regularly or not scoring at all. After a period of not scoring any goals, the player may change something: their training, their diet or which sock they put on first! If they then go on to score lots of goals, they may attribute it to the changes they made rather than just the natural variation in data in the short-term. Similar situations occur in healthcare, where a new service might seem to reduce emergency admissions but a return to the long-term average without the intervention could also happen.

While you may not be commissioning one of these robust evaluations yourself, you may be involved as one of several sites undergoing changes that are being evaluated by an independent research team. It is helpful to understand at a high level different kinds of study design for evaluation and what they can tell you (Clarke et al., 2019; see Table 6.2).

Many complex service changes will need mixed-methods approaches, foregrounding the importance of qualitative research in understanding how new models of care are implemented or affect ways of working for staff and patients. Qualitative research might range from interviews and focus groups to forms of observational activities to see how staff and patients interact. Good examples of current mixed-methods studies in the UK evaluating national service changes include assessing the impact of surgical hubs or optimized alcohol

Table 6.2 Quantitative study designs for evaluation

	Description	*Strengths*	*Weaknesses*
EXPERIMENTAL			
Randomized controlled trial	Randomly assign patients to treatment or control	Standardize context so only difference is effect of treatment – can make causal claims	Requires time, money, expertise Services more complex than drug therapies, leading to outcomes that lack context and may not reflect the real-world setting
QUASI-EXPERIMENTAL			
Stepped wedge trial	Clusters of services introduced to new changes over time, in steps, with remainder acting as controls	More pragmatic than classic trial as follows service changes as they happen Some strengths of randomized trials	Requires time, money, expertise Complex and policy changes may make staged introduction of change difficult
Interrupted time series	Data collected at a number of time points before and after introduction of new service	Multiple timepoints allow for more sophisticated assessment of impact	May be difficult to identify exact start of new service model Reliance on routine data
Difference in difference	Similar to interrupted time series but with matched control group	More possible to attribute effect to intervention	As above
SIMPLE			
Before-after (without control)	Repeat activity data before and after introducing service change	Easy to do	Subject to bias and difficult to attribute to change alone

care teams. These studies use a range of qualitative methods including observational work, as well as careful quantitative activity with interrupted time series using routine data and modelling longer-term impact.

You are unlikely to commission a stepped wedge trial or interrupted time series study of a local change, but it is important that you do what you can to be sure you know whether the intended changes are having an effect returning to the original logic model. This might mean asking yourself what a good enough comparator might be, for instance, using data from a neighbouring locality if not national reference data on current activity or outcomes. It is also worth asking which staff groups or services, adjacent or connected, could be affected by the planned change. How could you best reach them and find out any unintended consequences in other parts of the system? Without replicating a high-cost national evaluation study, there are important questions you can ask and think about possible data sources or proxy means of understanding impact on the ground.

Conclusions

What is 'good enough' evidence scanning and evaluation?

We hope that in this chapter we have given you a greater sense of how research can be used by managers and organizations in different ways. This includes the need to understand enough about what to look for in research papers around a problem or decision and how to interpret findings, without needing a full grasp of all technical details of a non-inferiority trial or a meta-ethnography. You can strengthen your critical intelligence muscles by asking whether headline findings on the impact of a single service change is likely to be true or what more information we need to be sure. This includes knowing where to go for sound overviews and 'packages' of relevant information, as well as who to ask to help you if you want to carry out a simple search yourself. Some examples have been given of real problems, from investment in remote monitoring for chronic conditions or changes to nurse shift patterns, and how to make sense of conflicting or mixed evidence.

We have also given some examples of service changes where you might want to carry out a simple evaluation yourself or get others to help. In any situation, you need some structured approaches to understand what effect is intended and the likely mechanisms to achieve them and how you can measure change in a way that is reasonably robust. We have also signposted useful resources and support for carrying out or commissioning evaluations.

While this chapter has focused on the actions of individual managers in using research evidence or evaluating services, we also touch on the responsibility of organizations to promote evidence use. We know that healthcare organizations that take part in research and use research are likely to be high-performing organizations. We hope too that we have given a flavour of the rich and vibrant state of health and health services research at the moment. There has never been a better time to dip into the world of applied research to address the real problems facing managers today, from staffing shortages to increasing demands on general practice, outpatients and hospital care. Research has helped us to scale up innovations, from day case surgery to early supported discharge in stroke and make better decisions about where and how services are best provided. Managers need to know enough to ask the right questions to support decisions to improve patient care.

Learning resources

Useful research sources

NIHR Journals Library: In the UK, the National Institutes for Health and Care Research (NIHR) is the largest funder of applied health and healthcare research. The Journals Library provides an open access repository of completed studies that are peer reviewed and protocols for live projects with useful background sections. This is a great resource to browse and search for useful topics, as many have been commissioned to address the most important uncertainties facing service and clinical leaders. The findings from the Health and Social Care Delivery Research programme are particularly relevant to managers, including rapid evidence syntheses and rapid evaluations on service delivery questions. Recently published studies range from evaluation of new psychiatric decision units to impact of special measures on challenged organizations [https://www.journalslibrary.nihr.ac.uk/].

Healthcare thinktanks: Intermediary organizations or thinktanks provide accessible and good overviews of topical areas in management and healthcare, often with scoping reviews that may be more rapid than formal evidence syntheses, case studies and large-scale analytics. Recent outputs from the Health Foundation include reports on sustainable healthcare and staff retention [https://www.health.org.uk/]; from the Nuffield Trust on supply of clinical staff and the state of NHS dentistry [https://www.nuffieldtrust.org.uk/]; and The Kings Fund on hospital discharge and inequalities in waiting lists. The Kings Fund also has experienced librarians and resources for managers [https://www.kingsfund.org.uk/].

Other organizations like the Institute of Fiscal Studies have generated useful evidence on workforce and retention issues, as well as condition-specific organizations and charities from Diabetes UK to MIND on particular services and care groups.

Cochrane Collaboration: The Cochrane Collaboration provides high-quality systematic reviews, focusing particularly on synthesizing comparative effective evidence (largely trials) on clinical treatment and interventions. There is also a group on Effective Practice and Organisation of Care (EPOC) which includes more service delivery topics, from staff substitution to hospital at home schemes [http://www.cochrane.org/].

Campbell Collaboration: The Campbell Collaboration carries out high-quality reviews on the effects of interventions in social, behavioural and educational contexts. Coordinating groups are centred on topics, such as disability and ageing, with a wide range of individual reviews [http://www.campbellcollaboration.org/].

Evidence for Policy & Practice Information (EPPI) Centre: UK-based review centre at University College London that includes focus on health, education, welfare and public policy. Recent publications range from reviews on volunteering during the pandemic to public health services of community pharmacies [https://eppi.ioe.ac.uk/cms/].

Appraising evidence

Critical appraisal tools: If you want to get into the nitty-gritty of assessing individual studies, there are checklists and worksheets to help you (but you may not need this level of detail). These include resources at the Centre for Evidence-based medicine (CEBM), at the University of Oxford with critical appraisal worksheets focused largely on clinical evidence. [https://www.cebm.ox.ac.uk/resources/ebm-tools/critical-appraisal-tools].

Similarly, the Joanna Briggs Institute in Australia has developed well-rated critical appraisal tools, originally directed at nursing literature but covering a wide range of healthcare-related study types, including economic studies and qualitative research as well as trials and other research [https://jbi.global/critical-appraisal-tools].

Evaluation tools

The Magenta Book: The Magenta Book is written and published by the UK government as a guide to evaluation for both commercial and non-commercial evaluation. Written to guide evaluations that will be used by governments in decision making, it is a comprehensive guide that is applicable to evaluations across many settings including healthcare [https://www.gov.uk/government/publications/the-magenta-book].

The Strategy Unit: Focused on evaluation in healthcare, this guide includes quantitative, qualitative, economic and mixed-methods evaluation design, process and impact and ethical considerations when carrying out service evaluation [https://www.strategyunitwm.nhs.uk/sites/default/files/2022-01/MDSN-Interactive-Evaluation-Guide.pdf].

References

Barnett, A.G., Van der pols, J.C. and Dobson, A.J. (2005) Regression to the mean: what it is and how to deal with it, *International Journal of Epidemiology*, 34: 215–220.

Boaz, A., Hanney, S., Jones, T. and Soper, B. (2015) Does the engagement of clinicians and organisations in research improve healthcare performance: a three-stage review, *BMJ Open*, 5(12): e009415.

Brinkhuis, F., Goettsch, W.G., Mantel-Teeuwisse, A.K. and Bloem, L.T. (2024) Added benefit and revenues of oncology drugs approved by the European Medicines Agency between 1995 and 2020: retrospective cohort study, *British Medical Journal*, 384: e077391.

Cartwright, M., Hirani, S.P., Rixon, L., Beynon, M., Doll, H., Bower, P., et al. (2013) Effect of telehealth on quality of life and psychological outcomes over 12 months (Whole Systems Demonstrator telehealth questionnaire study): nested study of patient reported outcomes in a pragmatic, cluster randomised controlled trial, *British Medical Journal*, 346.

Clarke, G.M., Conti, S., Wolters, A.T. and Steventon, A. (2019) Evaluating the impact of healthcare interventions using routine data, *British Medical Journal*, 365.

Corbett, M., Heirs, M., Rose, M., Smith, A., Stirk, L., Richardson, G., et al. (2015) The delivery of chemotherapy at home: an evidence synthesis, *Health and Social Care Delivery Research*, 2015; 3(14). https://doi.org/10.3310/hsdr03140.

Dall'Ora, C., Ejebu, O.-Z. and Griffiths, P. (2022) Because they're worth it? A discussion paper on the value of 12-h shifts for hospital nursing, *Human Resources for Health*, 20: 1–7.

Department of Health (2011) Whole System Demonstrator Headline Findings [Online] [https://www.gov.uk/government/publications/whole-system-demonstrator-programme-headline-findings-december-2011; accessed 29 February 2024].

Dixon-Woods, M., Cavers, D., Agarwal, S., Annandale, E., Arthur, A., Harvey, J., et al. (2006) Conducting a critical interpretive synthesis of the literature on access to healthcare by vulnerable groups, *BMC Medical Research Methodology*, 6: 1–13.

Eaton, G., Wong, G., Tierney, S., Roberts, N., Williams, V. and Mahtani, K.R. (2021) Understanding the role of the paramedic in primary care: a realist review, *BMC Medicine*, 19, 145.

Ellins, J., Hocking, L., Al-Haboubi, M., Newbould, J., Fenton, S.-J., Daniel, K., et al. (2023) Early evaluation of the Children and Young People's Mental Health Trailblazer programme: a rapid mixed-methods study, *Health and Social Care Delivery Research* 11, 08.

Evans, C., Poku, B., Pearce, R., Eldridge, J., Hendrick, P., Knaggs, R., et al. (2021) Characterising the outcomes, impacts and implementation challenges of advanced clinical practice roles in the UK: a scoping review, *BMJ Open*, 11, e048171.

Fulop, N.J., Walton, H., Crellin, N., Georghiou, T., Herlitz, L., Litchfield, I., et al. (2023) The impact of COVID-19 Oximetry @home on mortality and the use of hospital inpatient services. A rapid mixed-methods evaluation of remote home monitoring models during the COVID-19 pandemic in England, *Health and Social Care Delivery Research*, 11(13).

Gaughan, J., Siciliani, L., Gravelle, H. and Moscelli, G. (2020) Do small hospitals have lower quality? Evidence from the English NHS, *Social Science & Medicine*, 265: 113500.

Glasziou, P. and Chalmers, I. (2018) Research waste is still a scandal—an essay by Paul Glasziou and Iain Chalmers, *British Medical Journal*, 363.

Greenhalgh, T., Stones, R. and Swinglehurst, D. (2014) Choose and book: a sociological analysis of 'resistance' to an expert system, *Social Science & Medicine*, 104, 210–219.

Griffiths, P., Dall'Ora, C., Simon, M., Ball, J., Lindqvist, R., Rafferty, A.-M., et al. (2014) Nurses' shift length and overtime working in 12 European countries: the association with perceived quality of care and patient safety, *Medical Care*, 52: 975–981.

Henderson, C., Knapp, M., Fernández, J.-L., Beecham, J., Hirani, S.P., Cartwright, M., et al. (2013) Cost effectiveness of telehealth for patients with long term conditions (Whole Systems Demonstrator telehealth questionnaire study): nested economic evaluation in a pragmatic, cluster randomised controlled trial, *British Medical Journal*, 346.

Hendy, J., Chrysanthaki, T., Barlow, J., Knapp, M., Rogers, A., Sanders, C., et al. (2012) An organisational analysis of the implementation of telecare and telehealth: the whole systems demonstrator, *BMC Health Services Research*, 12: 1–10.

Hollnagel, E. (2015) Why is work-as-imagined different from work-as-done? in R.L. Wears, E. Hollnagel and J. Braithwaite (eds) *Resilient Health Care: The resilience of everyday clinical work*. vol. 2, Ashgate Studies in Resilience Engineering. Farnham: Ashgate. [http://www.ashgate.com/isbn/9781472437822].

Howard, R., Gathercole, R., Bradley, R., Harper, E. and Davis, L. (2021) The effectiveness and cost-effectiveness of assistive technology and telecare for independent living in dementia: a randomised controlled trial, *Age and Ageing*, 50: 882–890.

Htay, M. and Whitehead, D. (2021) The effectiveness of the role of advanced nurse practitioners compared to physician-led or usual care: a systematic review, *International Journal of Nursing Studies Advances*, 3: 100034.

Jager, K., Zoccali, C., Macleod, A. and Dekker, F. (2008) Confounding: what it is and how to deal with it, *Kidney International*, 73: 256–260.

Kaplan, S. A. and Garrett, K. E. (2005) The use of logic models by community-based initiatives, *Evaluation and Program Planning*, 28(2): 167–172. https://doi.org/10.1016/j.evalprogplan.2004.09.002.

Lamont, T., Barber, N., De Pury, J., Fulop, N., Garfield-Birkbeck, S., Lilford, R., et al. (2016) New approaches to evaluating complex health and care systems, *British Medical Journal*, 352.

Landhuis, E. (2016) Scientific literature: information overload, *Nature*, 535: 457–458.

Lewis, R.Q., Checkland, K., Durand, M.A., Ling, T., Mays, N., Roland, M., et al. (2021) Integrated care in England–what can we learn from a decade of national pilot programmes? *International Journal of Integrated Care*, 21.

Liberati, E.G., Tarrant, C., Willars, J., Draycott, T., Winter, C., Chew, S., et al. (2019) How to be a very safe maternity unit: an ethnographic study, *Social Science & Medicine*, 223: 64–72.

MacLellan, J., Collins, S., Myatt, M., Pope, C., Knighton, W. and Rai, T. (2022) Black, Asian and minority ethnic women's experiences of maternity services in the UK: a qualitative evidence synthesis, *Journal of Advanced Nursing*, 78: 2175–2190.

Knight, M., Bunch, K., Felker, A., Patel, R., Kotnis, R., Kenyon, S., et al. (eds.) on behalf of MBRRACE-UK (2023) Saving Lives, Improving Mothers' Care Core Report - Lessons learned to inform maternity care from the UK and Ireland Confidential Enquiries into Maternal Deaths and Morbidity 2019–2021. Oxford: National Perinatal Epidemiology Unit, University of Oxford.

Parkinson, S., Bousfield, J., Millar, R., George, J. and Marjanovic, S. (2021) *Communicating Research Evidence to Boards in Health and Care Organisations: A Scoping Study*. RAND Corporation. https://doi.org/10.7249/RRA1267-1.

RECOVERY Collaborative Group (2021) Dexamethasone in hospitalized patients with Covid-19, *New England Journal of Medicine*, 384: 693–704.

Rousseau, D.M. (2006) Is there such a thing as 'evidence-based management'? *Academy of Management Review*, 31: 256–269.

Sandall, J., Soltani, H., Gates, S., Shennan, A. and Devane, D. (2016) Midwife-led continuity models versus other models of care for childbearing women, *Cochrane Database of Systematic Reviews*, 4(4). https://doi.org/10.1002/14651858.CD004667.pub5.

Sherrington, C., Fairhall, N.J., Wallbank, G.K., Tiedemann, A., Michaleff, Z.A., Howard, K., et al. (2019) Exercise for preventing falls in older people living in the community, *Cochrane Database of Systematic Reviews*, 1(1), Cd012424. https://doi.org/10.1002/14651858.CD012424.pub2.

Smith, J., Ellins, J., Sherlaw-Johnson, C., Vindrola-Padros, C., Appleby, J., Morris, S., et al. (2023) Rapid evaluation of service innovations in health and social care: key considerations, *Health and Social Care Delivery Research*, 11.

Steventon, A. (2015) Rapid Response: Why did the Whole Systems Demonstrator report reductions in emergency hospital admissions? Insights from new analyses, *British Medical Journal*. [www.bmj.com/content/344/bmj.e3874/rr; accessed 18 February 2025].

Steventon, A., Bardsley, M., Billings, J. and Dixon, J. (2012) Effect of telehealth on use of secondary care and mortality: findings from the Whole System Demonstrator cluster randomised trial, *British Medical Journal*, 344.

Swan, J., Gkeredakis, E., Manning, R.M., Nicolini, D., Sharp, D. and Powell, J. (2017) Improving the capabilities of NHS organisations to use evidence: a qualitative study of redesign projects in Clinical Commissioning Groups, *Health and Social Care Delivery Research*, 5(18). https://doi.org/10.3310/hsdr05180.

Van Noorden, R. (2014) Global scientific output doubles every nine years. Nature news blog. [https://blogs.nature.com/news/2014/05/global-scientific-output-doubles-every-nine-years.html; accessed 29 November 2024].

Vindrola-Padros, C., Brage, E. and Johnson, G.A. (2021) Rapid, responsive, and relevant? A systematic review of rapid evaluations in health care, *American Journal of Evaluation*, 42: 13–27.

Walshe, K. and Rundall, T.G. (2001) Evidence-based management: from theory to practice in health care, *The Milbank Quarterly*, 79: 429–457.

The politics of healthcare and the health policy process

Ruth Thorlby and Mark Exworthy

Introduction

'Politics' concerns the exercise of power and the resolution of conflicts over resources (Moran, 1999; Freeman, 2000; Marmor, 2013). It is most conventionally thought of in relation to the activities of governments within nation states, the process by which certain groups, parties or individuals assume the authority to raise taxes and set and enforce the rules within which the activities of states take place, from law and order, to defence, education and healthcare. Hence, it is essential to the conduct and delivery of healthcare in any health system.

In all high-income countries, the resources expended on healthcare are large and growing, and the scope of conflicts over these resources is broad, involving a range of interest groups, ideas and institutions (the most central of which is the state) (see also Shearer et al., 2016). Even in health systems where the bulk of healthcare is provided and purchased privately, the state remains a powerful player, for example, paying for healthcare for older or poorer people, and in setting the rules by which healthcare providers function and how doctors are licensed.

The politics of healthcare or the politics of health?

The politics of 'health' is potentially a much broader field than the politics of 'healthcare' (see Box 7.1). A person's health is shaped by a multitude of factors, such as their genetic inheritance, family, communities, work, income, housing, food and physical environment, all of which are influenced by the activities of multiple players, including government and multinational companies (see Chapter 4, Public health and global inequalities).

Box 7.1   The politics of health or healthcare?

Some have argued that establishing the scope of politics is in itself a political act in relation to health and healthcare (Bambra et al., 2005). Critics of those who have confined the analysis of politics to healthcare rather than health argue that it runs in the face of over four decades of evidence that health is shaped much more by social, economic and cultural factors than by access to medical treatments and services. Viewed from this perspective, a fully rounded study of the politics of health in relation to the acts of government and the state should combine analysis of all the different interests and influences on government policy, including employment, the food industry, transport policy and welfare policy more broadly. Bambra and colleagues argue that the exclusion of wider health from the politics of healthcare also derives from the dominance of political science by those who use behaviouralist, institutional and rational choice theories, particularly in the United States.

This chapter will focus on the politics of healthcare rather than health. The primary unit of analysis is the nation state and the interaction of different groups within it. However, the politics played out at a national level pervades individual healthcare providers: the politics of, and within, a large hospital, for example, are highly complex. This might be called the small 'p' politics within organizations (Clarke et al., 2021).

Why is an understanding of politics important for healthcare managers?

Why should a chapter on the politics of healthcare and the health policy process be included in a textbook about healthcare management? A healthcare manager with a good grasp of the politics of healthcare is more able to understand the way the healthcare system in their country operates, the policies which might be possible (or not), the behaviour of the different political actors, from a national level through to the teams around them in their own institutions, and the forces that might shape the future.

The structure of this chapter

This chapter starts with a brief description of the scope of the resources in a healthcare system (see also Chapters 9, 10 and 11) that generate political challenges and describes the common challenges faced by all countries in terms of medical technology and changing population need (Conflict over what?). It then sets out the main players that influence the way those resources are distributed in most high-income countries: on the supply side, the professional and other interest groups (doctors, hospital associations, insurers), on the demand side (patients, patient groups, the public as voters and payers of taxes or insurance premiums), and in the middle, in a mediating role, the state or government (The main players). The size and configuration of these players varies between countries: the chapter then explores the main groupings of health system politics (Types of healthcare politics).

Next, we consider the dynamics of change and healthcare policymaking, by describing some of the theories put forward by political scientists and sociologists to explain how policymaking happens within the healthcare politics of individual countries, why some policies succeed and others fail (The politics of policymaking – politics in action). Finally, the chapter looks ahead to the main drivers of change facing healthcare politics in the future (Healthcare politics: what does the future hold?)

This chapter attempts to take an international perspective on the politics of health. It draws primarily on examples from high-income countries, as health systems have been established for longer. But it is hoped that these insights will be applicable to other countries, particularly as the burden of non-communicable, chronic illness is now becoming more prominent in many regions of the globe (Murray, 2015) (see Chapter 4). And the experience of health system design, both positive and negative, holds lessons for lower- and middle-income countries as they develop and reform their own health systems (Gabani et al., 2023).

Conflict over what?

The 'triple aim' is a concept that helps to explain the competing objectives of all healthcare systems. It comprises: access, cost and quality. (They might also be described as population health, efficiency and outcomes; Berwick et al., 2008). While it is not possible to maximize all three, healthcare systems (as political systems) need to find ways to reconcile them according to the society's preferences, available resources and clinical/technological capabilities. Politics lies at the heart of the triple aim; it is not to be avoided but rather calls for more/better involvement by all parties, especially those who are traditionally neglected or excluded, such as patients (Alford, 1975).

Note that the triple aim has evolved to the 'quadruple aim', noting the centrality of workforce (from recruitment and retention to morale and job satisfaction) (Bodenheimer and Sinsky, 2014).

Costs of healthcare

The story of the latter half of the twentieth century is of increasingly large sums of money spent both publicly and privately on 'healthcare'. The different drivers of this increase are more fully explored in Chapter 10, but it is the striking upward trend since 1960 in the proportions of national wealth spent on healthcare (gross domestic product or GDP) in all high-income nations that is important here.

As economies have grown, these percentages translate into huge sums in cash terms. Take the example of Germany; the total spend on healthcare in 2021 (public and private) was 474 billion euros (Destatis, 2023), or 12.9 per cent of GDP (OECD/European Observatory, 2023). In 2018, 5.7 million people were employed in the healthcare sector (12.3 per cent of all people employed in Germany). The number of people working in the healthcare sector increased by 41 per cent between 2000 and 2018 (Blümel et al., 2020).

The demands on how these resources should be used has increased substantially in recent years, beyond the delivery of treatment and care. These include preparedness for another pandemic (OECD, 2023), and climate change; see, for example, the English NHS (NHS England, 2022). Digital technology (including AI) is also rapidly expanding the range and scope of possible healthcare (World Health Organization, 2021). New sets of actors (from global tech firms to small start-ups) are entering the healthcare field, shifting the political dynamics therein.

The scale of activity in modern healthcare is, historically speaking, a relatively recent phenomenon. Doctors and hospitals were places to be avoided until the end of the nineteenth century, when innovations in surgery and medical technology transformed hospitals from places that were 'receptacle[s] for the sick poor, and a dangerous source of disease', into institutions that were 'central to the practice of new scientific medicine' (Moran, 2000). Medicine and healthcare, particularly the care delivered in hospitals, have become highly valued attributes of modern societies. As Moran puts it: '[h]ealthcare facilities in modern industrial societies are great concentrations of economic resources – and because of that they are also the subject of political struggle' (Moran, 1999: 1).

The reason that this political struggle is so profound in healthcare is partly because of its interaction with the other crucial legacy of the late nineteenth and first half of the twentieth century: the near-universal adoption of the idea of healthcare as a 'special' good, a service which should not depend on a person's income, and which governments – as representatives of the collective will of societies – have a responsibility to organize. By the middle of the twentieth century, most high-income countries had established universal access to healthcare, funded collectively, either by general taxation or social insurance.

Rising healthcare expenditure can be seen as a moral good. As societies become wealthier, it is a political expression of their values that they can and do spend more on healthcare (as populations age, costs rise and technologies provide more opportunities). However, such rising expenditure can be seen as inimical if it crowds out other spending (such as education), whether by government or the individual.

Conflict between whom? The main players

In his 'structural interest theory', Alford (1975) sought to describe and explain the paralysis of reform in the New York city health system. He argued that reform was a political struggle between 'dominant' and 'challenging' interests. The (medical) profession represented the former while an array of state, corporate and organizational groups represented the latter. Beyond these was a 'repressed' interests, namely patients, citizens and taxpayers whose views were overlooked, neglected or ignored. These interest groups vie for power, which lies at the heart of the politics of healthcare. Alford's theory has enduring quality as much of the political conflict in health systems remains as he described nearly 50 years ago. We adopted his basic structure below: the state, the profession and users (e.g. Checkland et al., 2009; Peckham et al., 2024).

The state

The central player at the heart of the political struggle is the state. The sums of money spent on healthcare by high-income countries are vast and even in countries where private providers and insurers have a large role – for example the United States – the government is still a major player in funding safety net healthcare for vulnerable groups, regulating the market, licensing healthcare providers and professionals, and setting the rules within which competition in the market takes place (Rice et al., 2020).

The central role of the state in healthcare is a recent development in Europe: until the eighteenth century, states raised taxes primarily for the purposes of defence against external enemies and law enforcement at home:

> By 1980 almost all European states had guaranteed access [to healthcare] to almost all of their citizens. In 1880, none of them did
>
> (Freeman, 2000: 14)

A central role for states in ensuring affordable access to healthcare is a global goal. In 2015, the UN's Sustainable Development Goals included an aim for universal health coverage by 2030. Although progress is slow (World Health Organization, 2023), proponents of universal health coverage see an active role for the state in ensuring public funding for healthcare (UHC 2030, 2023).

Stewardship and governance

Traditional approaches to describe the role of the state in healthcare have distinguished between countries with a 'hierarchical' – or command and control type of government – and more market-based approaches to financing and providing healthcare (Exworthy et al., 1999). The former implied a state that defined the rules, allocated resources and directly purchased or provided healthcare; the latter, a state that aimed to regulate and incentivize private purchasers and providers. Since most countries use a mix of approaches, an alternative way of thinking about the activities of the state has been developed by the World Health Organization (WHO), as part of a framework to understand how well health systems are performing. Originally conceptualized as 'stewardship' ('the careful and responsible management of the well-being of the population', World Health Organization, 2000), a more recent iteration identifies the key functions of governance (generally performed by governments) in relation to the health system (Papanicolas et al., 2022; see Box 7.2).

Box 7.2   Functions of governance

- Setting a strategic vision for the health system, contained in a set of policies, guidelines and laws for which the government can be held accountable.
- Ensuring that a range of stakeholders, including academia, professional and provider organizations, civil society organizations, representatives of marginalized communities and the public are able to contribute to policymaking decisions.

- Enabling the collection and use of intelligence, data and information to assess the performance of the health system.
- The capacity to use legislation and regulation to achieve health system goals and ensure compliance with legislation.

Source: Papanicolas et al. (2022).

The professions

A countervailing force to the power of the state has been the organized power of the medical 'profession'. By the middle of the twentieth century, doctors as a profession were considered to be the most important players in European health systems (Freeman, 2000), enjoying both affluence and authority on a personal level but also collectively. Their professional organizations had negotiated both autonomy for individual clinicians to practise with a minimum level of interference and control over the market in terms of who could be called a doctor.

The power of the medical profession has been challenged in the last few decades of the twentieth century and beginning of the twenty first, with the increasing pressure on health spending forcing encroachment into the clinical autonomy of doctors, with the state enforcing prices, setting fees for reimbursement and scrutinizing, (and often specifying) the amount of medical care to be given in each individual clinical encounter, via clinical guidelines or other evidence-based recommendations of best practice (Exworthy, 2015). Stemming from the challenge from the state has been the challenge from managerialism, often called New Public Management (NPM) (Ferlie et al., 2007). NPM challenged professional dominance by making their professional practice and knowledge more explicit, measurable and manageable. NPM was initially resisted by the medical professions but is now more accepted as the norm, in healthcare and more widely (Exworthy and Halford, 1999; Hyndman and Lapsley, 2016).

Role of professional organizations

Relationships between the organized medical profession and the state in many countries can typically be characterized as oppositional. Often, the creation of universal healthcare was met by hostility and resistance from doctors, who felt their autonomy to practise (and charge) freely for their services was under threat.

In Canada doctors in several provinces resisted the gradual nationalization of healthcare, culminating in an ultimately unsuccessful 23-day doctors' strike in Saskatchewan in 1962 after the province became the first to introduce a single-payer system (Marchildon and Schrijvers, 2011) (see also Tuohy, 1999, Chapter 7). In New Zealand, similar resistance was partially successful – as universal healthcare was introduced in the late 1930s, primary care doctors mobilized to preserve their autonomy and still retain the right to charge their patients individually (Cumming et al., 2014). Germany, one of the first countries to introduce a form of compulsory insurance in 1883, saw the medical profession unite to try to limit the power of social health insurance funds after the fact, in the early years of the twentieth century (Busse and Blümel, 2014).

Despite these episodes of opposition, most political scientists describe the relationship between these two players as deeply intertwined and mutually dependent (Moran, 1999; Harrison and McDonald, 2008), or the politics of the 'double bed' as Klein (1990) colourfully described it. States need the (medical) profession to deliver electorally popular health services and the profession needs the state to provide financial resources and effective regulation to safeguard their autonomy.

Box 7.3   The role of professional organizations in the United Kingdom

The professional organization of doctors substantially predates the emergence of the modern state. In the UK, the College of Physicians (later to become the Royal College of Physicians) was founded in 1518 (Harrison and McDonald, 2008). It was created to license practitioners of medicine, and in 1563 it laid down a set of professional requirements, including undertaking training and examinations, refraining from criticizing other members, and not working with unlicensed physicians. A second College was formed in 1540 for surgeons (later to become the Royal College of Surgeons) and Apothecaries gained their Royal Charter in 1617.

Three important features are visible from the early history of these professional groups. First, they all demonstrate the hallmarks of 'self-regulation' (i.e. retaining the right to decide who is to be called a 'doctor' or 'surgeon'). Self-regulation has been eroded in recent decades following high-profile medical scandals and evidence of performance variations (Dixon-Woods et al., 2011). Second, the source of this authority is the state (at this point the monarchy). Third, there is already evidence of a hierarchy between the professional groups. Formal state licensing did not arrive in the UK until the nineteenth century, with the creation of the General Medical Council in 1858, which maintained a register of 'registered medical practitioners', and specified the content of medical training (Harrison and McDonald, 2008).

A fourth feature of medical professional power also emerged in the nineteenth century, reflecting the lobbying or union function of representing doctors' interests (Eckstein, 1960). In the UK this took the form of the Provincial Medical and Surgical Society, later to become the British Medical Association (BMA) in 1855.

International experience

Most countries have physician organizations that perform the functions of licensing practitioners on the one hand and representing doctors' interests on the other. There are variations in how concentrated the power of these professional bodies is, or whether they are split along specialty lines, or regionally. Table 7.1 below, which draws on Freeman (2000) and the

Table 7.1 Medical organizations in five countries

Country	Professional licensing	Union representation
France	Ordre des Médecins: national, regional and departmental. Registers physicians, oversees guidelines, and board of peers for disciplinary and ethical matters.	Multiple unions for self-employed doctors, fragmented along geographic and occupational lines. Separate Union of Hospital Physicians (Syndicat National des Praticiens Hospitaliers) for doctors employed by public hospitals. Learned societies also play a lobbying role.
Germany	Licensing, ethics, discipline and continuing education handled at regional state level by physician's chambers (Arztekammer). Doctors are legally obliged to become members. To treat patients under statutory sickness insurance funds, doctors must also be members of Association of Sickness Fund Doctors regionally.	Hartmannbund represents doctors in independent local practice, acting as an interest group in the policymaking process, Marburger Bund represents hospital doctors with a direct trade union function, as hospital doctors are salaried employees. Many other specialist groups exist and have a lobbying role.
Italy	Doctors must be licensed both nationally by the Ministry of Health, and at a provincial level by one of over 100 medical associations (Ordini dei Medici), which are semi-public and carry out disciplinary actions. National umbrella organization (FNOM) based in Rome establishes ethics code.	Doctors' interests have traditionally been represented via political parties (especially Christian Democrats) rather than medical professional organizations.
Sweden	National Board of Health and Welfare licenses doctors. Disciplinary measures, including withdrawal of the right to practise, are handled by separate Medical Responsibility Board.	Swedish Medical Association (Sveriges Läkarförbund) represents majority of doctors of all disciplines, with over 90% membership rate.
UK	Doctors are licensed by the General Medical Council (GMC). The GMC also licenses medical schools and conducts disciplinary hearings. Specialist medical qualifications are approved by the respective Royal Colleges.	The British Medical Association represents all doctors in contract and pay negotiations with government, with a membership of over two thirds of practising doctors.

Source: Freeman, 2000; Rand Europe, 2009; Chevreul et al., 2010; European Observatory, 2012; Busse and Blümel 2014.

Health Systems in Transition series, summarizes the attributes of medical organizations in five countries.

As is evident from Table 7.1, there are differences between countries in how their doctors' interests are represented, which has consequences for how policy emerges (discussed below). All countries have some form of body that licenses and protects doctors' interests: the drive for doctors to pursue their collective self-interest through self-regulation seems universal.

There is considerable debate among political scientists and sociologists about how unique doctors are in this respect compared with other professions. Theorists such as Freidson have argued that the most important variable of 'professionalism' is the extent to which its dominance can gain control over their own work without interference from outside and win the trust of governments and consumers in the process (Freidson, 1994). Others have argued that erosion of professional power has come from increasingly educated patients (Haug, 1976) or from the increasingly corporate organization of medical provision (Navarro, 1988). Doctors who combine medical practice with managerial roles, increasingly common in some health systems, have also been described as creating a distinct professional identity (McGivern et al., 2015).

Doctors have a unique standing with society and health systems because of their connection to science and technology and their contact with individual patients (Moran, 1999). For several decades in the last century, doctors were able to function in most countries with minimal interference from the state. But, as pressures on healthcare spending have increased, the state has grown in its capacity to 'see into' the work of the professions, as data on their activity, costs and quality of doctors' work has grown (Moran, 1999). This was the heart of the NPM project from the 1980s onwards. Despite evidence of variations in practice and multiple scandals, doctors continue to retain high levels of public trust (Ipsos, 2022).

Learning activity 7.1

Identify the professional organizations in your country:

- (i) Who sets the standards (of performance), (ii) who monitors those standards, and (iii) Who disciplines doctors (if necessary)?
- Who licenses doctors?
- Are these membership organizations? Who pays for them? How many doctors and what kinds of doctors are members?
- Do they have the power to strike?

Having identified these organizations, make an assessment of their influence on the policy and direction of the healthcare system in your country. Do you detect any change in this influence over the past decade?

Other interest groups

While the presence of doctors' professional associations is common to all health systems, the political force of other entities, such as hospitals, or insurance companies varies according to the anatomy of the health system in question. In countries dominated by private providers, hospital groups (corporate) and hospital associations (representative) wield considerable lobbying power. For example, the American Hospital Association (AHA) represents over 5,000 hospitals in the US and declared revenue of over $130 million in 2022 (AHA, 2022).

All countries represent potential markets for pharmaceutical products and medical equipment, and the large pharmaceutical companies in particular act as powerful interest groups at national and regional levels. Determining the scale and nature of their influencing activity depends on whether countries require disclosure of lobbying of policymakers. In the US, which requires disclosure of money spent on influencing policymakers, $225 million was spent on campaign contributions in 2018 by the pharmaceuticals and health products industry, and $421 million on lobbying (Open Secrets, 2018). In the European Union (EU), by contrast, disclosure is voluntary: €36 million was declared by pharmaceutical companies on activities to influence decision making in the EU in 2021, but campaign groups believe the actual figure may be higher (Corporate Europe Observatory, 2021).

Think tanks have increasingly become important stakeholders in health politics. They play a key role in framing the nature of the 'problem' to be addressed as well as the solutions that they recommend. While some are independent, some are explicitly political, being aligned to certain economic ideologies, for example, the Adam Smith Institute or the Institute of Economic Affairs (Stone, 2001). Also, there are others who are less transparent in their funding, analysis and political influence, features compounded by off-the-record policy discussions and limited involvement of the wider public (Shaw et al., 2014).

Management consultancies also play an often-unseen role in health politics. Their ability to 'sell' their ideas to health ministries and healthcare organizations reflects their growing power and influence (Saint-Martin, 1998; Penno and Gauld, 2017; Begley and Sheard, 2021).

The role of patients and citizens in the politics of healthcare is complex and evolving and is discussed in more detail in Chapter 22. Most political scientists draw a distinction between the role played by individuals as patients and their broader role as voters and payers of taxes, social or private insurance contributions that fund health services. Furthermore, engaged citizens in social democratic systems represent a collective entity with distinct (though overlapping) interests.

The relationship between individual patients and their physicians has traditionally been characterized as hierarchical and paternalistic, with most of the power being in the hands of the physician. This has shifted over time, as patients have become better educated and informed, and non-medical alternatives, such as self-help movements, have increased. In the UK, patient-led organizations began to emerge in the 1960s, against a wider societal movement that questioned the 'power and authority of professions-including medicine' (Mold, 2010). A recent overview of patient groups in 10 European countries found considerable variation in how these groups function and are funded. In some countries, such as the UK, Sweden and Finland, health consumer and patient groups were 'politically mature' and heavily engaged with policymakers, while at the other end of the spectrum, in Austria for example, organizations were primarily focused on self-help and giving assistance (Baggott and Forster, 2008). A more recent systematic review of studies on patient and public involvement (PPI) across Europe (in both healthcare and research) found a similarly uneven picture, with PPI most embedded and formalized in the UK, Scandinavian countries and the Netherlands (Biddle et al., 2021). Overall, there is limited evidence of the impact of patient and public involvement on policymaking, partly due to the multiple techniques used to engage (ranging from surveys to citizen's juries) and absence of systematic evaluation (Baumann et al., 2022).

The collective voice of citizens is most obviously exercised through democratic processes, but how directly this impacts on healthcare and health policymaking varies considerably according to individual health systems. In centralized national health systems, such as the English NHS, health is often a dominant issue in general election campaigns, although manifestos rarely contain much policy detail. Equally, with a health system funded by general taxation, the transparency between taxes and service provision is rather opaque. Direct democratic influence may be stronger where health systems are devolved, for example, in the case of Sweden. The funding and provision of healthcare services are the responsibility of 21 regions, while care for older people and disabled people is organized by 290 municipalities. Elections for national, regional and municipal governments are held on the same day every 4 years. Although turnout for elections is high (over 85 per cent), a survey in 2022 found that 41 per cent of people thought that the funding and provision of healthcare was the responsibility of the national government, suggesting that democratic accountability for healthcare might not be as strong as it could be (Janlöv, 2023).

A third strand of user influence has been fostered by policymakers in the past two decades, with the evolution of reform policies that actively encourage patients to make choices and act more like consumers in other markets, for example, in Denmark and England (Dent and Pahor, 2015). Patients in Denmark have had a choice of hospital since 1993: while patients are satisfied with having a right to choose, evaluations suggest that in practice very few choose to travel further for their care (Vrangbaek, 2015). Patient choice in England was a strong policy theme in the 1990s but in practice it was an 'over-simplification of reality' (Victoor et al, 2012), not least because patients are not always willing or able to travel to providers with capacity and/or short waiting times (Exworthy and Peckham, 2006). Moreover, the policy has faded somewhat as financial crises mean less (spare) capacity to which patients could 'move' (Iacobucci, 2023).

Varieties/types of health care systems – the consequences of politics?

What we have set out above is a description of the range of possible political actors in healthcare systems. Although many countries face very similar challenges (such as rising costs, longer living populations and more chronic disease), the actual form of their healthcare systems is very different, the product of historical circumstance and political choices.

Political scientists have classified welfare states according to archetypes, for example, laissez-faire liberalism (e.g. United States) or Bismarckian insurance states (e.g. Germany). Esping-Anderson (1990) built on this by grouping nations into three different welfare 'clusters'. In the liberal cluster are states with a strong work ethic and welfare systems characterized by means-testing and strict entitlement rules (e.g. the US and Australia). A second cluster, exemplified by Germany, France and Italy, consists of conservative, corporatist welfare states, with a broader set of state-organized entitlements than the first cluster, but preserving traditional family structures through the exclusion of non-working women from insurance coverage and under-developed childcare. The third cluster, 'social democratic' has universal entitlement at its heart, and is underpinned by equality of rights rather than equality of minimum standards (Esping-Anderson, 1990).

Moran (2000) and Wendt et al. (2009) among others have attempted to refine these basic welfare state categories in order to better reflect the complexity of the politics of the healthcare state. Unlike simple cash transfers, delivering healthcare requires a huge organizational, professional and economic infrastructure between the funder and recipient. Power struggles and the exercise of political control also occur within this system, not just at its entry point. Wendt (2009) defines three different dimensions of control over healthcare systems:

1 **Financing**. Is it the state, private individuals or insurers, or non-governmental social organizations that obtain and provide the money for healthcare?
2 **Health service provision**. Is it state bodies, private firms or professionals, or non-governmental social organizations that actually deliver and own the means of delivering healthcare?
3 **Regulation or governance**. Is it the state, private individuals or insurers, or non-governmental social organizations that determine how the system is run, set targets and priorities and govern relations with professionals, technology policy and contracts?

Moran also draws attention to the question of who governs 'consumption' by determining who can access healthcare, and how costs are controlled. His classification and Wendt's both suggest as reference points 'ideal types', where all three dimensions are controlled by the same element of the system (Burau and Blank, 2006). For instance, England is generally seen as an ideal type of the state system. Its National Health Service is funded almost entirely from central taxation and the state either directly controls, or owns at arm's length, the NHS trusts that provide most hospital care and other secondary care. Note that primary care doctors are independent contractors (see Chapter 14). Other frequently cited examples are the United States as an ideal type of the private system, and Germany as an ideal example of social insurance. Of course, these healthcare systems do not always match the ideal types in every detail; they are approximations. To account for this reality, the Wendt (2009) typology allows for 'mixed systems', where the three dimensions of control are divided between two or all three of the private, state and social groups. This gives a potential total of 27 different health system types. A classification of three real countries in the present day, giving examples of different mixes of control, is shown in Table 7.2.

In practice, most health systems tend to have either private or state provision (or a mix of them), and to have predominantly state regulation (Wendt, 2009). Wendt (2009) argues that this categorization is a useful way to gauge the depths of reforms, based on whether they move systems across the category boundaries. Only truly historic reforms will shift multiple dimensions, so that an ideal mostly private-based system becomes mostly public. The 1938 creation of a national health system in New Zealand is an example of such major and profound reform: primary care doctors opted out and remained in the private sector, (but more recently have participated in more integrated provision via primary care organizations; see Chapter 14).

Table 7.2 Examples of countries' mix of control of their health system

	Regulation	*Financing*	*Provision*
United States	Private/state. Market competition is relied on generally to drive quality and determine financial viability. Voluntary and state boards also accredit providers. Insurance is now federally regulated and mandated.	Private/state. With most healthcare paid for by tax-subsidized private insurance, the USA is the archetypally privately funded system. However, the role of state funding has grown over decades, covering primarily poorer and older people.	Private/social. Hospitals are mostly either charitable or for-profit, with the proportion of each varying by state. Primary care is provided by private clinics or not-for-profit community centres.
New Zealand	State. Overall strategy, targets for improvement, and standards for providers are set by the government.	State. The government pays the majority of costs from general taxation, although patients also pay some out-of-pocket charges.	State/private. Public sector bodies provide most hospital and community care, with some private clinics. Primary care is provided through privately owned practices.
Japan	State/private. Patients have a wide choice of provider but not of insurer, which is usually determined by employment. Insurers are regulated by central government. Providers are regulated for basic standards of safety by central government. Local government regulates other aspects.	Social. The central government, municipal governments, and voluntary organizations linked to different professions and corporations all provide health insurance for different groups. Patients also contribute co-payments at the point of use, at up to 30% of total cost.	Mixed. The majority of Japanese hospitals, which dominate the health system, are run on a not-for-profit basis. However, local government and the private sector also run significant numbers.

Source: Adapted from Tatara and Okamoto, 2009; Saltman et al., 2013; Cumming et al., 2014

More modest or gradual reforms might be understood as a shift within one dimension. In 2006, the Netherlands introduced a system of 'managed competition' between both insurers and providers, following a long-term and incremental process of reform (Kroneman et al., 2016). However, treating this as a full shift in regulation from state to private would be an oversimplification: government bodies now had a new role regulating a complex market-based yet publicly funded health system.

Learning activity 7.2

Using the classification of state, social and private control, think about which institutions in your country's heath system exert most influence on:

1   financing of healthcare
2   provision of healthcare
3   regulation of healthcare

What recent or ongoing struggles have there been about changing who controls these elements of your country's healthcare system?

What single change to each of the three dimensions above would you propose for your country's health system and why?

Health politics in action: policymaking

This section addresses the question of what drives health reforms, and what factors determine whether policies succeed in some countries at certain points in time, and why they fail at others.

Understanding the role of political institutions on policymaking

One perspective on understanding the role of political institutions on health policymaking and interest-group bargaining has been set out by Ellen Immergut, in a study of Sweden, France and Switzerland (Immergut, 1992). In comparing the process of legislating for universal health insurance in the three countries, she argues that it is important to understand the design of each country's unique political systems, and in particular the 'veto points' available for those – including interest groups – to block or modify proposed legislative changes.

In Sweden's parliamentary democracy, the first chamber of parliament represents an important veto point, but in practice, stable parliamentary majorities underpinned by stable voting patterns meant that there was no real veto point for opponents of national health insurance, and the government was able to enact strong reforms, including regulating doctors' fees, and restricting the rights of doctors to practise privately. The absence of a powerful veto point shaped the behaviour of Sweden's Medical Association, which tended to take a cooperative stance, channelled through 'participation in expert commissions and written responses to government proposals' (Immergut, 1992: 223) while minimizing the likelihood of a rival doctors' professional association breaking away as it would have had even less access to the executive.

In France, reforms to create a universal national insurance scheme resulted in many of the features of the Swedish system – including regulation of doctors' fees – but the process took far longer as it was shaped by a different democratic reality. The power of the executive government was dependent on the support of parliamentary coalition partners, who behaved opportunistically and vetoed legislation in Parliament. Doctors' professional interests could be pursued on a wider front than in Sweden, with doctors active as politicians and able to influence directly the leadership of some of the parties.

In Switzerland, the evolution of health policy was shaped by referendum politics, which represented the most important veto point, allowing direct electoral influence over the actions of the executive. However, referendum verdicts could often run counter to the parliamentary election results. Interest groups could call for referenda, giving minorities powerful influence over policymaking, and Immergut argues that the resulting shape of Switzerland's health system – government-subsidized health insurance but with a much more regressive distribution of coverage than in Sweden – is the product of this political system that enabled the professional doctors' groups to resist state interference.

Path dependency

One of the frameworks used by political scientists to explain why radical policy change does or does not happen is the concept of 'path dependency'. This theory, originally derived from the economic history literature, suggests that policy decisions made at a particular time shape the likelihood of subsequent decisions (Greener, 2005). As time goes by, these decisions shape the path into the future, increasing the probability of continuing on the same path and decreasing the probability of deviation. Radical reform is never impossible but becomes increasingly unlikely (Wilsford, 1994). The primary situation where this has been applied by political scientists is the failure of the United States to deliver universal access to healthcare for its citizens for so many decades, in contrast to many other high-income countries. The defeat in Congress of President Clinton's reforms in 1993 – to expand healthcare coverage – has been seen as a prime example of the power of US political institutions that are 'not designed to accommodate large-scale reform; in fact, they are designed to actively thwart it' (Wilsford 1994: 271).

Less than two decades later, the same political institution – Congress – passed the Affordable Care Act (ACA), in 2010. President Obama allowed Congress to lead the drafting of the Act (in contrast to Clinton), which allowed powerful interest groups (including the insurance industry) to influence the Congressional leaders as they developed the legislation, albeit watering it down in the process (Rocco and Waddan, 2024). Republican opposition to 'Obamacare' has continued, with opposition played out at state-level (several states opted out). The logic of path dependency reasserted itself again, when a Republican controlled government failed to overturn the legislation in 2017, with opposition from interest groups who had, by then, 'accommodated themselves' to the ACA (Rocco and Waddan, 2024).

The Canadian political scientist Carolyn Tuohy has refined the path dependency framework further, by focusing attention on the 'windows of opportunity' that open up to politicians and policymakers, their interaction with the 'logic' of previous reforms and their impact on structures and institutions within healthcare politics (Tuohy, 1999). She argues that when the 'relatively rare conditions' opened a window of opportunity in the early 1990s for the UK Prime Minister to take action, the internal 'logic' of the NHS system both facilitated and tempered the impact of the reform. On the one hand, the hierarchical character of the NHS facilitated the top-down implementation of these apparently radical reforms – ushering in a market-inspired split between purchasers and providers – through the traditional mechanisms of guidance and directives from the centre. On the other hand, the traditionally collegial nature of relationships within the local NHS and the relatively primitive level of data on clinical outcomes and cost meant that many of the contracts between the new purchasers and providers looked very like the old 'block contracts' and agreements that they were meant to replace.

The 'logic' of these reforms endured. The Labour party went on to adopt market-inspired policies of competition between providers and patient choice, and competition also underpinned the 2012 reforms introduced by the Coalition government. Tuohy has characterized these various policy iterations as examples of different forms of policy change (Tuohy, 2018). The 1990s reforms were an example of 'big bang' change, whereas Labour's were incremental in nature, introduced piecemeal and therefore avoiding major political confrontation. The 2012 reforms are an example of 'mosaic' policy change in which radical ideas were subject to extensive consultation and revision (as with the ACA in the US).

Learning activity 7.3

Think of a change (policy reform) that you would like to be made to your country's healthcare system.

What would most likely prevent it from happening? What would encourage reform taking place? Who would be the key stakeholders involved?

In which circumstances might it become possible for it to happen?

Map out a path of dependency for a previous change that has taken place in your healthcare system, using the approach suggested by either Wilsford or Tuohy.

The small 'p' of healthcare politics

So far, this chapter has primarily addressed politics as it applies to national governments, party politics and major policy reforms. However, it can also be contrasted with the politics within and between organizations, stakeholder groups and even individuals. Organizations are thus the arena for political struggles between competing interests. Indeed, such small 'p' politics (or micro-politics) are perhaps the more common experiences of people working in health and care services. This is because any change is a political process, involving 'winners' and 'losers'. Most theories of change rely on the engagement (or 'buy-in') of key groups (such as clinical staff) (Best et al., 2012); this is the essence of micro-politics. Ferris et al. (2007) defines political skill as the 'ability to effectively understand others at work and use such knowledge to influence others to act in ways that enhances one's personal and/or organisational objectives'.

It is increasingly recognized that practitioners (especially those in leadership positions) need to acquire and develop a set of skills to navigate the process of micro-politics within organizations and in wider health systems (Hartley and Benington, 2011).

Health and care practitioners need skills to navigate the politics of organizations at the interpersonal, inter-professional and inter-organizational levels (Waring et al., 2023). Such political skills can be developed and exercised within and between organizations. At an inter-personal level, such skills include persuasion and influence for dealing with 'difficult' people. Inter-professionally, these skills relate to understanding the political climate. Inter-organizationally, political skills are needed to build legitimacy and support through coalitions of actors, especially those over whom no direct authority can be exercised.

The acquisition and use of these skills of political astuteness should be recognized as a means to an end (not the end in itself). A central purpose of such astuteness is the creation of a 'receptive context' for implementing change (Pettigrew et al., 1992). However, an individual alone is rarely sufficient to precipitate or sustain organizational change. Waring et al. (2022) discuss the basis of micro-politics as comprising the 'interplay between skills (capabilities), strategies (plans) and actions (doings)'. Politics must thus be seen as a collective action, the skills for which are unevenly distributed.

Conclusion: the future of healthcare politics

Theodore Marmor neatly summarized the politics of healthcare as the process of 'resolving – or at least attenuating – conflicts about resources, rights and values' (Marmor, 2013: 407). These conflicts are likely to grow in the future, resulting in healthcare remaining as one of the most dynamic arenas for politics to play out in countries.

The scope for the diagnosis and treatment of diseases will increase, particularly as genomic medicine develops (see Chapter 19). These new technologies for fighting illness (chronic and acute) will result in longer lifespans and longer periods in a person's life in which disease can be detected and treated. But this raises its own challenges, as research is beginning to reveal the scale of multi-morbidity especially in older populations (Barnett et al., 2012; Watt et al., 2023) and exposing the limitations of services and clinical guidelines based on single disease models (Guthrie et al., 2012). The care of frailer, older patients may enhance the need for the discretionary autonomy of clinicians, particularly generalists, but it will also require access to better non-medical social care, which has been considered beyond the scope of universal healthcare services in many countries to date (see Chapter 17).

These trends will increase the possibilities of what clinicians are able to offer patients, but at the same time will intensify the search by governments (and all those paying for care) to understand value, monitor outcomes and set reasonable limits, especially if healthcare remains in the wider public's mind as something that should be available to all with minimal financial barriers.

Recently, existing health system challenges have been augmented by a series of new ones. These include pandemic preparedness, climate change and digital technology. In parallel, the huge growth of data collected on the incidence of disease and the use of services, coupled with better IT systems, will increase the ability of those managing healthcare to assess the volume and quality of healthcare. However, accountability based on such availability of data and outcomes has so far been limited; i.e. there are large amounts of data but the (political) will to use and act on it appears to often be lacking. On the other hand, it also opens debates about public expectations of healthcare systems, including 'responsible' use of health services by patients.

From the perspective of healthcare managers, an awareness of the institutions, values and interests that underlie healthcare politics is invaluable as a means of shedding light on the day-to-day tasks of managing and improving healthcare. At any one time, myriad decisions about resources are being made by each clinician as they treat their patients. Efforts to contain costs and improve quality will often encroach on clinical autonomy, and patients will want access to treatments that will prolong life and improve the quality of life. An ability to think through and act upon the broader politics of healthcare management will help disentangle the sort of approaches that might work to improve care, the level at which problems need to be solved (for example, what is in the control of local managers to change, and what will require regional and national action), and the most effective ways to work with, rather than against, the grain of society's values.

Learning activity 7.4

Take an example of a recent major new health policy introduced into your country.

- Given what you know of the politics of your country, what seems to have worked with this new policy and why? Did the policy improve clinical outcomes, or cost-effectiveness, or increase patient satisfaction?
- What seems not to have worked? How did this policy overcome 'path dependency' of the previous approach?
- If you were giving advice to policymakers, what would you suggest that they do differently if starting again with the introduction of this health policy?

Learning resources

World Health Organization European Observatory on Health Systems and Policies: The Observatory produced reports on individual health systems, and also comparative research on policy developments and reform initiatives across Europe.

Reports are updated on a regular basis, and many are available in another official language as well as English. [https://eurohealthobservatory.who.int/].

OECD Health Policies and Data: This offers extensive background data about health spending, policies and systems, as well as information about wider social policy, such as family support, pensions and migration. [http://www.oecd.org/els/health-systems/].

OECD Health Systems Characteristics Survey: Latest survey results from 2023, available through an interactive website, which allows comparisons of the funding and service delivery models between 32 countries. [https://data-explorer.oecd.org/?pg=0& fc=Topic].

Ian Greener's 'game': [https://t1ber1us.itch.io/the-health-policy-game-beta].

The *New England Journal of Medicine Politics of Health Reform* section: This US-based academic journal regularly publishes papers exploring single country and international comparative health policy. [http://www.nejm.org/medical-research/politics-of-health-care-reform].

The Milbank Quarterly: This US-based academic journal publishes many analytical and comparative studies of health policy and politics. [http://www.milbank.org/the-milbank-quarterly].

References

Alford, R. (1975) *Health Care Politics*. Chicago: University of Chicago Press.

American Hospital Association (2022) AHA 2022 IRS form 990. [https://www.aha.org/legal-documents/2022-11-18-american-hospital-association-2021-irs-form-990; accessed 7 December 2024].

Baggott, R. and Forster, R. (2008) Health consumer and patients' organizations in Europe: towards a comparative analysis, *Health Expectations*, 11: 85–94.

Bambra, C., Fox, D. and Scott Samuel, A. (2005) Towards a politics of health, *Health Promotion International*, 20(2): 187–193.

Barnett, K., Mercer, S., Norbury, M., Watt, G., Wyke, S. and Guthrie, B. (2012) Epidemiology of multimorbidity and implications for healthcare, research, and medical education: a cross sectional study, *The Lancet*, 380: 37–43 [www.thelancet.com/journals/lancet/article/PIIS0140-6736(12)60240-2/fulltext; accessed on 25 February 2025].

Baumann, L. Reinhold, K. and Brütt, A. (2022) Public and patient involvement in health policy decision-making on the health system level – A scoping review, *Health Policy*, 126(10): 1023–1038. https://doi.org/10.1016/j.healthpol.2022.07.007.

Begley, P. and Sheard, S. (2021) From 'honeymoon period' to 'stable marriage': the rise of management consultants in British health policymaking, *Bulletin of the History of Medicine*, 95(2): 227–255.

Berwick, M., Nolan, T. and Whittington, J. (2008) The triple aim: care, health, and cost, *Health Affairs*, 27(3): 759–769. https://doi.org/10.1377/hlthaff.27.3.759.

Best, A., Greenhalgh, T., Lewis, S., Saul, J.E., Carroll, S. and Bitz, J. (2012) Large-system transformation in health care: a realist review, *The Milbank Quarterly*, 90: 421–456. https://doi.org/10.1111/j.1468-0009.2012.00670.x.

Biddle, M., Gibson, A. and Evans, D. (2021) Attitudes and approaches to patient and public involvement across Europe: a systematic review, *Health and Social Care in the Community*, Jan; 29(1): 18–27. doi: 10.1111/hsc.13111. Epub 2020 Jul 23. PMID: 32705752.

Blümel, M., Spranger, A., Achstetter, K., Maresso, A. and Busse, R. (2020) Germany: health system review. Health Systems in Transition, *European Observatory on Health Systems and Health Policies*, 22(6): i–273. [https://iris.who.int/bitstream/handle/10665/341674/HiT-22-6-2020-eng.pdf?sequence=1; accessed 24 February 2025].

Bodenheimer, T. and Sinsky, C. (2014) From triple to quadruple aim: care of the patient requires care of the provider, *The Annals of Family Medicine*, Nov 2014, 12(6): 573–576; doi: 10.1370/afm.1713.

Burau, V. and Blank, R. (2006) Comparing health policy: an assessment of typologies of health systems, *Journal of Comparative Policy Analysis, Research and Practice*, 8(1): 63–67.

Busse, R. and Blümel, M. (2014) Germany: health system review. Health Systems in Transition, *European Observatory on Health Systems and Health Policies*, 16(2).

Checkland, K., Harrison, S. and Coleman, A. (2009) 'Structural interests' in health care: evidence from the contemporary national health service, *Journal of Social Policy*, 38(4): 607–625. doi:10.1017/S0047279409003262.

Chevreul, K., Durande-Zaleski, I., Bahrami, S., Hernandez-Quevedo, C. and Mladovsky, P. (2010) France Health Systems Review, *European Observatory Health Systems in Transition*, 12(6).

Clarke, J.M., Waring, J., Bishop, S., Hartley, J., Exworthy, M., Fulop, N.J., et al. (2021) The contribution of political skill to the implementation of health services change: a systematic review and narrative synthesis, *BMC Health Services Research*, 21: 260. https://doi.org/10.1186/s12913-021-06272-z.

Corporate Europe Observatory (2021) Big Pharma's lobbying firepower in Brussels: at least €36 million a year (and likely far more). May 2021 [online] [https://corporateeurope.org/en/2021/05/big-pharmas-lobbying-firepower-brussels-least-eu36-million-year-and-likely-far-more; accessed 7 December 2024].

Cumming, J., McDonald, J., Barr, C., Martin, G., Gerring, Z. and Daube, J. (2014) New Zealand health system review, *Asia Pacific Health Systems in Transition*, 4(2).

Dent, M. and Pahor, M. (2015) Patient involvement in Europe – a comparative framework, *Journal of Health Organization and Management*, 29(5): 546–55.

Destatis, Federal Statistical Office of Germany (2023) Press release, no. 136 Health expenditure exceeded 474 billion euros in 2021 [https://www.destatis.de/EN/Press/2023/04/PE23_136_236.html; accessed 7 December 2024].

Dixon-Woods, M., Yeung, K. and Bosk, C.L. (2011) Why is U.K. medicine no longer a self-regulating profession? The role of scandals involving 'bad apple' doctors, *Social Science and Medicine*, Nov; 73(10):1452–1459. doi: 10.1016/j.socscimed.2011.08.031. Epub 2011 Sep 21. PMID: 21975027.

Eckstein, H. (1960) *Pressure Group Politics: The Case of the British Medical Association*. Stanford, CA: Stanford University Press.

Esping-Anderson, G. (1990) *The Three Worlds of Welfare Capitalism*. Princeton, NJ: Princeton University Press.

European Observatory on Health Systems and Policies (2012) Sweden: Health System Review, *Health Systems in Transition*, 14(5).

Exworthy, M. (2015) The Iron Cage and the gaze: interpreting medical control in the English health system, *Professions and Professionalism*, 5(1). doi: 10.7577/pp.944.

Exworthy, M. and Halford, S. (eds) (1999) *Professionals and the New Managerialism in the Public Sector*. Philadelphia, PA: Open University Press.

Exworthy, M. and Peckham, S. (2006) Access, choice and travel: implications for health policy, *Social Policy & Administration*, 40: 267–287. https://doi.org/10.1111/j.1467-9515.2006.00489.x.

Exworthy, M., Powell, M. and Mohan, J. (1999) Markets, bureaucracy and public management: the NHS: quasi-market, quasi-hierarchy and quasi-network?, *Public Money & Management*, 19(4): 15–22. doi: 10.1111/1467-9302.00184.

Ferlie, E., Lynn L. and Pollitt, C. (eds) (2007) *The Oxford Handbook of Public Management* (online edn, Oxford Academic, 2 Sept. 2009) https://doi.org/10.1093/oxfordhb/9780199226443.001.0001.

Ferris, G.R., Treadway, D.C., Perrewé, P.L., Brouer, R.L., Douglas, C. and Lux, S. (2007) Political skill in organizations, *Journal of Management*, 33: 290–320. https://doi.org/10.1177/0149206307300813.

Freeman, R. (2000) *The Politics of Health in Europe*. Manchester: Manchester University Press.

Freidson, E. (1994) *Professionalism Reborn: Theory, Prophecy, And Policy*. Cambridge: Polity Press.

Gabani, J., Mazumdar, S. and Suhrcke, M. (2023) The effect of health financing systems on health system outcomes: a cross-country panel analysis, *Health Economics*, 32(3): 574–619. https://doi.org/10.1002/hec.4635.

Greener, I. (2005) The potential of path dependence in political studies, *Politics*, 25(1): 62–72. https://doi.org/10.1111/j.1467-9256.2005.00230.x

Guthrie, B., Payne, K., Alderson, P., McMurdo, M. and Mercer, S. (2012) Adapting clinical guidelines to take account of multimorbidity, *BMJ*, 12(3): 345.

Harrison, S. and McDonald, R. (2008) *The Politics of Healthcare in Britain*. London: Sage.

Hartley, J. and Benington, J. (2011) Political leadership, in A. Bryman, D. Collinson, B. Jackson, K. Grint and M. Uhl-Bien (eds) *Sage Handbook of Leadership*. London: Sage.

Haug, M.R. (1976) The erosion of professional authority: a cross-cultural inquiry in the case of the physician, *The Milbank Memorial Fund Quarterly. Health and Society*, 54(1): 83–106. https://doi.org/10.2307/3349670.

Hyndman, N. and Lapsley, I. (2016) New public management: the story continues, *Financial Accountability & Management*, 32(4): 385–408. https://doi.org/10.1111/faam.12100.

Iacobucci, G. (2023) New push for patient choice will not automatically cut waiting times, leaders warn, *BMJ*, 381: 1209. doi:10.1136/bmj.p1209.

Immergut, E. (1992) *Health Politics. Interests and Institutions in Western Europe*. New York: Cambridge University Press.

Ipsos (2022) Doctors and scientists are seen as the world's most trustworthy professions, The 2022 Ipsos Global Trustworthiness Index. [https://www.ipsos.com/sites/default/files/ct/news/documents/2022-07/Global%20trustworthiness%202022%20Report.pdf; accessed 24 February 2025].

Janlöv, N., Blume, S., Glenngård, A.H., Hanspers, K., Anell, A. and Merkur, S. (2023) Sweden: Health system review. European Observatory on Health Systems and Policies, *Health Systems in Transition*; 25(4): i–198 [https://iris.who.int/bitstream/handle/10665/372708/9789289059473-eng.pdf?sequence=8; accessed 24 February 2025].

Klein, R. (1990) The state and the profession: the politics of the double bed, *BMJ*, Oct 3; 301(6754):700–2. doi: 10.1136/bmj.301.6754.700. PMID: 2224241; PMCID: PMC1664062.

Kroneman, M., Boerma, W., van den Berg, M., Groenewegen, P., de Jong, J., van Ginneken, E. (2016) The Netherlands: health system review, *Health Systems in Transition*, 2016; 18(2): 1–239.

Marchildon, G. and Schrijvers, K. (2011) Physician resistance and the forging of public healthcare: a comparative analysis of the doctors' strikes in Canada and Belgium in the 1960s, *Medical History*, 55(2): 203–222.

Marmor, T. (2013) Healthcare politics and policy. The business of medicine: a course for physician leaders, *Yale Journal of Biology and Medicine*, 86: 407–411.

McGivern, G., Currie, G., Ferlie, E., Fitzgerald, L. and Waring, J. (2015) Hybrid manager–professionals' identity work: the maintenance and hybridization of medical professionalism in managerial contexts, *Public Administration*, 93: 412–432. https://doi.org/10.1111/padm.12119.

Mold, A. (2010) Patient groups and the construction of the patient-consumer in Britain: an historical overview, *Journal of Social Policy*, Oct; 39(4): 505–521. doi: 10.1017/S0047279410000231. PMID: 20798768; PMCID: PMC2925204.

Moran, M. (1999) *Governing the Health Care State. A Comparative Study of the United Kingdom, the United States and Germany*. Manchester: Manchester University Press.

Moran, M. (2000) Understanding the welfare state: the case of health care, *British Journal of Politics and International Relations*, 2(2): 135–160.

Murray, C. (2015) Global, regional, and national age–sex specific all-cause and cause-specific mortality for 240 causes of death, 1990–2013: a systematic analysis for the Global Burden of Disease Study 2013, *The Lancet*, 385(9963): 117–171.

Navarro, V. (1988) Professional Dominance or proletarianization?: Neither, *The Milbank Quarterly*, 66: 57–75. https://doi.org/10.2307/3349915.

NHS England (2022) Delivering a 'Net Zero' National Health Service. [https://www.england.nhs.uk/greenernhs/wp-content/uploads/sites/51/2022/07/B1728-delivering-a-net-zero-nhs-july-2022.pdf; accessed 7 December 2024].

OECD (2023) Ready for the Next Crisis? Investing in Health System Resilience, OECD Health Policy Studies, OECD Publishing, Paris. https://doi.org/10.1787/1e53cf80-en.

OECD/European Observatory on Health Systems and Policies (2023) Germany: Country Health Profile 2023, State of Health in the EU, OECD Publishing, Paris/European Observatory on Health Systems and Policies, Brussels. [https://eurohealthobservatory.who.int/publications/m/germany-country-health-profile-2023; accessed 7 December 2024].

Open Secrets (2018) Health sector summary. [https://www.opensecrets.org/industries/indus?cycle=2024&ind=H; accessed 7 December 2024].

Papanicolas, I., Rajan, D., Karanikolos, M., Soucat, A. and Figueras, J. (eds) (2022) Health system performance assessment: a framework for policy analysis, Geneva: World

Health Organization; (Health Policy Series, No. 57). [https://iris.who.int/bitstream/han dle/10665/352686/9789240042476-eng.pdf?sequence=1; accessed 7 December 2024].

Peckham, S., Bailey, S. and Huggins, D. (2024) Chapter 7: Institutions, interests and ideas: framing and explaining entrepreneurial policy change in the UK health system, in *Research Handbook on Health Care Policy*. Cheltenham: Edward Elgar Publishing. https://doi.org/10.4337/9781800887565.00011.

Penno, E. and Gauld, R. (2017) The role, costs and value for money of external consultancies in the health sector: a study of New Zealand's District Health Boards, *Health Policy*, April; 121(4): 458–467. doi: 10.1016/j.healthpol.2017.02.005. Epub 2017 Feb 21. PMID: 28259501.

Pettigrew, A., Ferlie, E. and McKee, L. (1992) Shaping strategic change - The case of the NHS in the 1980s, *Public Money & Management*, 12(3): 27–31. doi: 10.1080/09540969209387719.

RAND Europe (2009) International Comparison of Ten Medical Regulatory Systems. RAND Corporation [https://www.rand.org/pubs/technical_reports/TR691.html; accessed 7 December 2024].

Rice, T., Rosenau, P., Unruh, L.Y., Barnes, A.J. and van Ginneken, E. (2020) United States of America: health system review, *Health Systems in Transition*, 22(4): i–441.

Rocco, P. and Waddan, A. (2024) Chapter 21: The pathologies of the United States health care regime, in *Research Handbook on Health Care Policy*, Cheltenham: Edward Elgar Publishing. doi: 10.4337/9781800887565.00025.

Saint-Martin, D. (1998) Management consultants, the State, and the politics of administrative reform in Britain and Canada, *Administration & Society*, 30(5): 533–568.

Saltman, R. and van Ginneken, E., Rice, T., Rosenau, P., Unruh, L. and Barnes, A. (2013) United States of America health system review, *European Observatory on Health Systems and Policies*, 15(3): 1–431.

Shaw, S.E., Russell, J., Greenhalgh, T. and Korica, M. (2014) Thinking about think tanks in health care: a call for a new research agenda, *Sociology of Health and Illness*, 36: 447–461.

Shearer J., Abelson J., Kouyaté B., Lavis, J.N., and Walt, G. (2016) Why do policies change? Institutions, interests, ideas and networks in three cases of policy reform, *Health Policy and Planning*, November; 31(9): 1200–1211. https://doi.org/10.1093/heapol/czw052.

Stone, D. (2001) Think tanks, global lesson-drawing and networking social policy ideas, *Global Social Policy*, 1(3): 338–360.

Tatara, K. and Okamoto, E. (2009) Japan health system review, *European Observatory on Health Systems and Policies*, 11(5).

Tuohy, C. (1999) *Accidental Logics: The Dynamics of Change in the Health Care Arena in the United States, Britain and Canada*. Oxford: Oxford University Press.

Tuohy, C. (2018) *Remaking Policy: Scale, Pace, and Political Strategy in Health Care Reform*. Toronto: University of Toronto Press.

UHC2030 (2023) From commitment to action. Action agenda on universal health coverage from the UHC movement. [https://www.uhc2030.org/fileadmin/uploads/uhc2030/Documents/UN_HLM_2023/Action_Agenda_2023/UHC_Action_Agenda_long_2023.pdf; accessed 24 February 2025].

Victoor, A., Delnoij, D.M., Friele, R.D. and Rademakers, J.J.D.J.M. (2012) Determinants of patient choice of healthcare providers: a scoping review, *BMC Health Services Research*, 12, article 272. https://doi.org/10.1186/1472-6963-12-272.

Vrangbaek, K. (2015) Patient involvement in Danish health care, *Journal of Health Organization and Management*, 2015, 29(5): 611–662.

Waring, J., Bishop, S., Clarke, J., Exworthy, M. and Hartley, J. (2023) Chapter 7: Healthcare leadership with political astuteness, in *Research Handbook on Leadership in Healthcare*, Cheltenham, UK: Edward Elgar Publishing. https://doi.org/10.4337/9781800886254.00014.

Waring, J., Bishop, S., Clarke, J., Exworthy, M., Fulop, N.J. and Hartley, J. (2022) Healthcare Leadership with Political Astuteness and its role in the implementation of major system change: the HeLPA qualitative study, *Health and Social Care Delivery Research*, 10(11).

Watt, T., Raymond, A., Rachet-Jacquet, L., Head, A., Kypridemos, C., Kelly, E., et al. (2023) Health in 2040: projected patterns of illness in England, *The Health Foundation* [https://www.health.org.uk/reports-and-analysis/reports/health-in-2040-projected-patterns-of-illness-in-england; accessed 7 December 2024].

Wendt, C., Frisina, L. and Rothgang, H. (2009) Healthcare system types: a conceptual framework for comparison, *Social Policy & Administration*, Oxford: 43(1).

Wilsford, D. (1994) Path dependency, or why history makes it difficult but not impossible to reform healthcare systems in a big way, *Journal of Public Policy*, 14(3): 251–283.

World Health Organization (2000) World health report 2000. Geneva: WHO. [https://www.who.int/publications/i/item/924156198X; accessed 7 December 2024].

World Health Organization (2021) Global Strategy on Digital Health. [https://www.who.int/docs/default-source/documents/gs4dhdaa2a9f352b0445bafbc79ca799dce4d.pdf; accessed 7 December 2024].

World Health Organization (2023) Tracking universal health coverage: 2023 global monitoring report. Geneva: World Health Organization and International Bank for Reconstruction and Development / The World Bank; 2023. [https://iris.who.int/bitstream/handle/10665/374059/9789240080379-eng.pdf?sequence=1; accessed 24 February 2025].

Global health: governance in a new geopolitical era

Scott L. Greer and Matthias Wismar

Introduction: what is global health?

Global health is hard to define. It is partly difficult to define for logical reasons: most things are in some way global, since we all share a planet; and most things affect health. It is also partly difficult to define for political reasons. Given that anything, everything and nothing is intrinsically global health, the actual meaning of 'global health' is a somewhat untidy set of problems, institutions, policies and budgets engaged in diverse activities, such as development assistance, infectious disease surveillance, research and humanitarian response. It is politically constructed, and the phrase is more spoken in the rich countries of the 'Global North' (See Box 8.1). It is also a field with many practitioners and commentators who are extremely sensitive to inequality and hypocrisy, and who can find a lot of it in the politics of health in an unequal world.

Box 8.1 What are countries?

In a world of almost 200 countries, it is hard to discuss global health without some categories. During the Cold War, there was talk of the First (Western, rich), Second (Communist) and Third (poor and/or non-aligned) worlds. Some used a distinction between 'advanced industrial democracies' and 'developing countries'. These have both fallen aside, since they contain judgements about both democracy and development that are hard to defend.

Now, it is common to speak of low- and middle-income countries (LMICs), to be distinguished from high-income countries (HICs) or broken down for more specificity into low-income (LIC) and middle-income (MIC) countries. MICs usually have their own resources, while LICs' health policies tend to depend on donors for financing and therefore must contend with donor pressures on their governments, as well as many donors' reluctance to partner with governments at all. These categories can be a bit questionable. For example, the World Bank categorizes Equatorial Guinea as an upper-middle-income country due to oil wealth, but as that wealth is monopolized by a tiny elite most of its people live in a very low-income environment. One solution is to use a country's Human Development Index (HDI) score, compiled by the United Nations Development Programme instead of simple gross domestic product (GDP) measures. The HDI score is based on the extent to which a country gives its citizens a 'a long and healthy life, being knowledgeable and having a decent standard of living' (UNDP, 2024). HDI scores above 0.8 out of 1 usually are taken as a sign of a country with very high human development (and Equatorial Guinea's stagnant 0.588 HDI score is below average for the middle tier of human development).

It is also common to speak of the Global North and the Global South, loosely distinguishing between the rich countries and the poor but adding an implicit sense of political mission and attention to global hierarchy, often at the expense of nuance. To assert that the Global South includes everything from world powers like China and India to the poorest countries on Earth raises the question of what the Global South might actually have in common.

Because it is political, definitions of global health have shifted (Table 8.1) (Brown et al., 2006). Over time, unsurprisingly, the term 'global health' has shifted more and more to refer to what might better be called international health, even if activities such as managing development assistance, are just what the original global health movement was trying to escape.

Reading through these different definitions, we can see that there are two ways to think about global health. One is about global health problems and defines the field as somehow being about shared health issues. The other is about governance, the set of political institutions, such as the World Health Organization (WHO) or leading governments, whose actions and pronouncements define some problems as global health.

Global health problems

Since everything is somehow global, and everything affects health, it is possible to define global health as essentially everything. In practice, there are a narrower range of issues that are discussed in global health circles and dealt with by governments and civil society as global health. The simplest guide would be the preoccupations and duties of the WHO.

One set of issues are the ones we might call international health – essentially, overseas development assistance and all that comes with it, from capacity building to subsidized loans. They did not go away or even become less important as a second set of more truly global

Table 8.1 Terminology in global health

Term	Meaning
Public health	The overarching field of study and practice concerned with improving population health and creating more equal health outcomes by a variety of evidence-based means, at any territorial scale.
Global health	Study and practice of issues that directly or indirectly affect health but transcend boundaries.
International health	Study and practice of health issues of countries other than one's own, with a focus on low- and middle- income countries, often in the context of development aid.
Comparative health	Study and practice of comparing different systems' and states' approaches to healthcare and public health.
Healthcare management and policy; health services research	Study and practice of the financing and delivery of healthcare services.

Source: Adapted by authors from Brown et al. (2006).

issues, ones that obviously affected the whole world, took a place on the stage. The most obviously health-related ones are the infectious disease outbreaks that, after HIV/AIDS, began to preoccupy policymakers. In some cases, as with COVID-19, they are truly novel and quickly afflict the globe; in others, such as Zika, they were 'neglected tropical diseases' when they affected poor and marginal populations (Hotez, 2021) but were promoted to global problems when they affected big cities in Brazil and, ultimately, Miami (Greer and Singer, 2017).

The broad term for policies to address such eruptions of risk is 'health security' and there are arguments that addressing threats to health security in any one country depends on addressing them in all countries (Lakoff and Collier, 2008; Fidler and Gostin, 2008). In practice, rich countries in particular are very good at insulating themselves from many circulating risks in a variety of ways, so it is not so clear that most elements of health security are *necessarily* global. Their advantages include better underlying health, healthcare systems that can quickly catch and treat sick people, sanitation, water and food systems that slow or block disease transmission, public health agencies that can track diseases and intervene to nip outbreaks in the bud. Thus, for example, tuberculosis control is almost invisible in rich countries because a relatively healthy, nonsmoking population is less likely to catch the disease, because there is effective and sometimes mandatory treatment for people with it, because there are public health agencies that try to identify and treat every person with the disease, and therefore because the overall population has a vanishingly low prevalence (which in turn makes it easier for public health agencies to focus on the populations at risk). Likewise, rich countries have been able to trace cases of Ebola, essentially confining outbreaks of the disease to West and Central Africa and were able to gain access to vaccines for COVID-19 and pandemic influenza quickly. The result is that while the most efficient and equitable way to control global health risks might be through global action, that might not be the easiest programme to sell in an unequal world. The public good of global health can often be turned into a club accessible to rich countries that can afford good healthcare, strong public administration, and effective surveillance – as well as expensive priority access to vaccines.

Then there are undeniably global issues of which health is a part. Climate change might be the single biggest one (see Naylor and Pinto, Chapter 12 in this volume). Not only does climate change have many effects on health, from spreading vector-borne diseases, such as malaria, as warm winters happen in more places, to heatstroke to lung problems from giant fires. The health sector is also a non-trivial contributor to climate change, whether through surgical gases, infrastructure, food purchasing or driving to hospitals (Holmes and Willison, 2024).

A second is the interface with ecosystems and animals. One Health is a WHO initiative with the agenda of uniting human, veterinary and ecosystem health. It grows from the fact that problems such as antimicrobial resistance (overuse of antibiotics and corresponding resistance among bacteria) span agriculture and human health, emerging infectious diseases are often associated with deforestation and damage to ecosystems, and food supply chains can contain public health threats (Lerner and Berg, 2015; Destoumieux-Garzón et al., 2018; Schmiege et al., 2020). Given the global nature of the issues involved, it is widely viewed as a global health issue. In both cases the problem is global even if many of the actions, such as 'greening' hospitals or ending deforestation, are very local. Here, the problem matches a global problem with any kind of global governance that could commit countries to actions, such as reducing deforestation or carbon emissions.

Finally, there are a set of problems created by global governance mechanisms themselves. These typically occur when a specific mechanism, such as trade and investment law, is too effective and distorts priorities. Thus, for example, the use of trade law challenges to tobacco control was a part of tobacco companies' war on public health regulation (Jarman, 2014), while pharmaceutical and other technology companies use intellectual property and other forms of global trade law to defend their interests (Shadlen et al., 2020; Ibata-Arens, 2021) (also see Box 8.2).

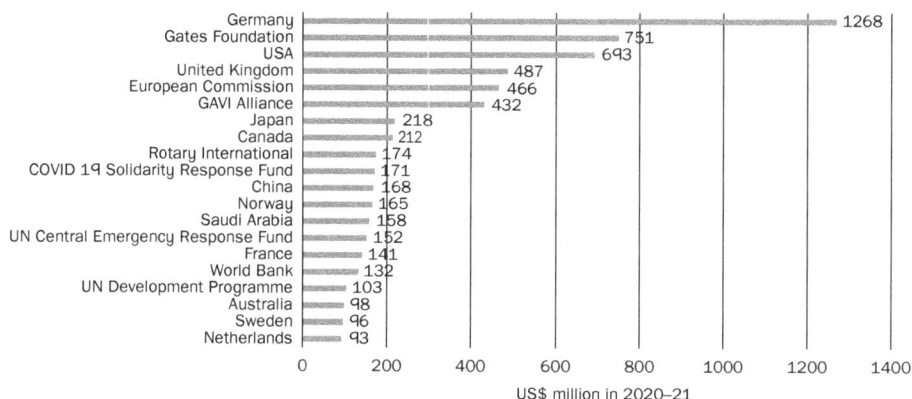

Figure 8.1 Top contributors to WHO
Data sourced from: https://www.who.int/about/funding/contributors

Global health governance in a geopolitical era

Global health governance is irrevocably part of global power politics, and the landscape of global health is shaped by power, war and inequality. This landscape contains a few key kinds of actors.

Multilateral organizations

Multilateral organizations are at the centre of global health governance. In particular, the World Health Organization, a part of the United Nations (UN), is at the core of the multilateral health world (Cueto et al., 2019). The WHO is headquartered in Geneva and its governing body is the World Health Assembly, which has one of the largest memberships of any multilateral body (194 members) and operates on a one-country-one-vote basis. One country, one vote gives smaller and poorer countries a great deal of power in the World Health Assembly relative to big and rich countries, and it leads to strong relationships between small countries and the WHO secretariat (Corbett et al., 2021). It elects an Executive Board, which provides more focused oversight.

The WHO's budget is based on a mixture of assessed and voluntary contributions; members are asked to provide funds in relation to their economic size, and donors of all kinds can donate to WHO activities. Not all countries provide their assessed funds at all or in a timely manner, and it is relatively easy for donors to use voluntary contributions to shape WHO agendas and activities (Chorev, 2012). Big and rich countries that are one vote among many in the World Health Assembly can exert their influence through the budget. In particular, Germany, the Bill and Melinda Gates Foundation, the United States, the UK, the European Commission and Gavi, The Vaccine Alliance are major contributors to the WHO budget (see Figure 8.1). To add further complexity, the WHO has very strong regional offices with elected leaders, one of which (the Pan-American Health Organization) existed for decades before the WHO was formed. There has never been consensus as to whether the regional offices are supposed to take directions from Headquarters in Geneva, and tensions have had to be managed (Cueto et al., 2019).

WHO, by design, delivers very few services, although it coordinates or participates in more administratively ambitious relief operations in which other agencies, governments and civil society actually deliver services. Its two greatest postwar triumphs, the eradication of smallpox and the near eradication of polio (the world is tantalizingly close), were both works of coordination, information and entrepreneurship (Stepan, 2011). In terms of coordination, the WHO is effectively the key part of any global health agreement or partnership. Even its critics agree that a global effort without WHO participation will be seen as partial.

The WHO also helps set and catalyze global health agendas. That includes particularly influential high-level agendas, such as Health for All ('"Health for all" means that health is to be brought within reach of everyone in a given country. And by "health" is meant a personal state of wellbeing, not just the availability of health services') (Mahler, 1981) or Universal Health Coverage ('Universal health coverage (UHC) means that all people have access to the full range of quality health services they need, when and where they need them, without financial hardship' (World Health Organization, n.d.).

WHO's work also includes many more technical outputs. This guidance might not always influence big, rich countries (although documents such as the International Classification of Diseases (ICD), which is in its tenth edition (ICD-10) and underpins payment systems around the world, or the WHO-FAO *Codex Alimentarius*, discussed shortly, certainly do). For smaller and poorer countries, seeking friendly and trustworthy advice on technical health topics, backed up by expert advice, can be vital. It also has reasonably good relations with a large number of problematic regimes, reserving judgement on a wide range of ethical questions in order to pursue health objectives and allowing it to influence policy in places where other organizations go unheard. If a small or poor country wants advice on technical health issues, WHO is often the first place it will go because, unlike every other form of advice, WHO advice is free, established through relatively clear globally credible processes, and more accountable to member states than to quirky donors. For governments that cannot afford strong government science and policy bureaucracies, WHO will do the work for them.

The WHO is also the secretariat servicing the Framework Convention on Tobacco Control (WHO FCTC) and the International Health Regulations (IHR); at the time of writing, it was coordinating negotiations on a prospective Pandemic Accord for which it would be the secretariat (see Box 8.2). Finally, WHO is a permanent institutional lobbyist for health in world politics (Lall, 2023).

Box 8.2   The pandemic treaty

COVID-19 showed some of the limitations of international public health law, in particular the International Health Regulations (IHR), in preventing pandemics or facilitating a response (Fidler, 2004). In December 2021, a special session of the World Health Assembly started negotiations on a new 'pandemic treaty' that would more comprehensively prepare the world to anticipate, prevent and respond to future pandemics. It would be different from the IHR in that the IHR are essentially focused on the rules for reporting outbreaks, reflecting their origins not in public health but in efforts to maintain international trade despite outbreaks. The pandemic treaty draft, therefore, contained a broad range of new duties and authorizations for member states relevant to more effective global responses.

Much of the treaty was relatively uncontested, though the populist far right in a number of countries spread disinformation about it (Taylor, 2024). Its provisions include commitments to comprehensive pandemic prevention plans, with components ranging from surveillance (which is also in the IHR) to wastewater, vaccination and veterinary health measures; strengthening and protecting healthcare workforces (see Box 8.5); building domestic healthcare and health information capacity; authorizing WHO to convene a network for making supply chains more resilient; and requesting more transparency in procurement and attention to the needs of other countries in procurement during a pandemic (e.g. setting aside a share of products acquired to share with less fortunate countries).

As one might expect, the core of the treaty – its potential value and the political conflict surrounding it – lies in intellectual property and data. As two observers wrote, 'Think of a pandemic treaty as a grand social bargain [with] two objectives: the open exchange of scientific information in real time, and the equitable allocation of medical countermeasures' (Gostin and Finch, 2024). This means two kinds of sharing, whose value to global health is inarguable but involves countries in very asymmetrical relationships. One creates an obligation to share technology in a pandemic so that every country can (at least try to) replicate technologies developed in the most technologically sophisticated countries. Richer countries with strong pharmaceutical and knowledge-based industries were naturally sceptical, preferring to control intellectual property and letting governments choose what to donate and companies what to transfer. This kind of transfer has long been contentious in global health. It will ask a country like Indonesia (often the home of new strains of influenza) to share data that is used to produce vaccines. Indonesia and other countries are then asked to buy those vaccines, while depriving them of the samples and data that gave them leverage (Gatter, 2014).

Much of the pandemic treaty commits governments to make better health policies and implement them well. Governments will often agree to such commitments with no intention or capability to follow through (LICs, however well intentioned, have a point when they point out that the commitments to building healthcare, health information and surveillance systems are expensive!). It is the parts that create legal obligations on sharing samples, data, technology and know-how that directly affect powerful actors and governments, which is why they were sticking points.

Learning activity 8.1

You are in charge of ensuring adequate personal protective equipment (PPE), medicines and vaccine availability for a large hospital in a medium-sized high-income country. Your hospital does not currently have the budget to stockpile and in some cases (e.g. vaccines, medicines with quick expiration) it is not feasible anyway. What do you ask your government to do and why?

WHO is not alone in the global health space. Even within the UN system, it has only about four per cent of the total staff (about 8,900 people) and budget. Within the UN system, other agencies with some kind of health mission include UNAIDS, which focuses on HIV/AIDS, and UNICEF, focused on children's health including vaccines. Other UN agencies with their own mandates and agendas are at work as well. Some have direct influence on health, as with the World Food Programme, United Nations Population Fund, and the United Nations High Commission for Refugees. Some are less obvious. The United Nations Office for Project Services

(UNOPS) provides infrastructure and project management for UN agencies. The Food and Agriculture Organization (FAO), among its other activities, produces a great deal of synthesis and guidance relevant to One Health issues and co-produces with WHO the Codex Alimentarius, the core global set of standards for food and feed hygiene. The Codex Alimentarius is a key set of standards and practices in addressing all sorts of problems, from antimicrobial resistance to toxins in food to overuse of pesticides.

The World Trade Organization (WTO), meanwhile, exists outside the UN. Its role is to codify and enforce global trade through its judicial system, which includes an appellate body similar to a court. WTO rules, along with other international legal instruments, have been used to challenge public health regulations in areas, such as tobacco control, pharmaceutical pricing and trade (Massard de Fonseca, 2013; Jarman, 2019).

Finally, among formal global multilateral institutions with a major effect on health policy and health, there are the IFIs: the international financial institutions. This term refers to the International Monetary Fund (IMF) and the World Bank (WB), which in turn refers to a family of linked development banks under the shared WB umbrella. If the WHO and its disease eradication campaigns led by doctors dominated the global health stage from World War Two until the 1980s, the IFIs became the dominant actors in global health policy in the 1980s and remained that way until recently, empowering economists at the expense of WHO and its doctors (Chorev, 2012). The IMF is essentially a bank of last resort for countries in deep economic trouble, normally meaning a currency crisis or inability to service their debt. It is traditionally headed by a European and the United States has a blocking minority of votes that allow it to veto decisions. Even though the IMF generally does not provide enough money to wholly end a crisis, its involvement and successful negotiations are taken by private markets that the country is, once more, safe for investment.

The IMF will extend emergency loans when private sources of capital will not, but at the price of policy reforms intended to rectify the country's fiscal situation (a process known as structural adjustment). On paper, it stands to reason that the IMF would combine immediate support with longer term reforms, but the record of structural adjustment lending at being implemented, having intended effects or producing economic growth and stability is poor. Its effect on health is better documented because decades of structural adjustment have often included huge cuts to health budgets, policies such as user fees and policies such as elimination of subsidies that affect health. It is hard to time health issues; babies do not get to choose when they are born, and few of us can choose when to get sick, so even if structural adjustment solves problems and produces better economies later, the damage done to people at the time can be hard to avoid or remedy. The result has been substantial documented damage to health and equity over the years (Kentikelenis and Stubbs, 2023), damage that the poor track record of structural adjustment on its own terms makes even harder to justify (Kentikelenis, 2017; Greer, 2014). User fees, for example, were often recommended. They deter care-seeking in unhelpful ways in rich countries and can lead to very dangerous results in poorer ones where fewer people can afford the fees (as with fees for HIV testing in Kenya) (Stein, 2008). In the Eurozone, the IMF along with the European Commission and European Central Bank was part of the 'troika' that imposed spending cuts and economic reforms on Greece, Ireland, Italy, Portugal and Spain; the result has been a lost decade of economic growth for most of them and health systems that were weakened when they had to confront COVID-19 (Peralta-Santos et al., 2021).

The World Bank, traditionally headed by a US citizen, exists to support development lending. In the immediate post-World War Two years, it often supported big infrastructure projects such as dams and railroads, but it shifted after the Cold War towards poverty reduction, which includes support for health projects and initiatives aimed at helping the poorest people in the poorest countries. This includes health expenditures, though there is a natural tension between health expenditures and loans. Health expenditures tend to work best when they are sustainable and most of the money goes on staff; this is an awkward fit with term loans, which are better suited to a defined project with an end point, such as building a hospital.

Outside this formal, treaty-bound world of UN agencies and their near partners, there is a set of partnerships developed as private philanthropies and collaborations. These organizations, such as Gavi, the Vaccine Alliance (in a partnership with WHO, UNICEF, the Gates Foundation and the World Bank, as previously mentioned) and ACT-A (see Box 8.4) are mechanisms that allow international organizations and philanthropies to team up for specific actions and programmes without the constraints (or accountability to every government) of the UN bodies. They gain some effectiveness from this and are a preferred vehicle for private sector and philanthropic actors, but their form also raises questions about accountability and priorities (though it is easy to overstate the democratic accountability of the alternative model, which are the UN organizations and IFIs). If the WHO was pushed aside in the 1980s by IFIs and their supporters in rich countries, giant philanthropies, notably the Bill and Melinda Gates Foundation, and their preference for management consultants, are again changing the locus of power and its chosen conceptual language. Thus, for example, IFIs are more likely to write recommendations addressed to governments – especially finance ministers – that suggest policy changes, such as alterations to the structure of healthcare financing or professional regulations and draw on analyses of market incentives, while the big charities are much more likely to focus on programmes and organizations, such as particular interventions to improve an area of health (e.g. maternal and child health or vaccinations) and take a detailed interest in how they are operated while often choosing to work with civil society organizations rather than governments. The politics of expertise in global health – who is determined an expert by whom – are important, reflect inequality within and between countries and are always contested (Kentikelenis et al., 2023).

This world is complex but has a certain logic and division of labour, even if parts of the system work at cross-purposes. It shows a combination of design and accident, with new organizations, such as UNAIDS and GAVI, responding to new actors and agendas and then becoming institutionalized; and also, power politics, with powerful countries and donors trying to act as effectively as possible, while less powerful countries try to maintain systems in which they have more voice.

One logic is that money talks. Big government donors such as the EU, Japan, UK and United States exert a great deal of influence. It is hard to overstate the power of the Bill and Melinda Gates Foundation in global health, since it is one of the largest, most agile and least politically constrained actors. It is also hard to overstate the centrality of HIV/AIDS in global health governance, not just because of its salient politics but because of the immense size of the United States' President's Emergency Plan for AIDS Relief (PEPFAR) programme for HIV/AIDS treatment. In both cases, a large funding source exercises a sort of gravitational pull. The sheer scale of PEPFAR helps to underpin the largest single sector of global health activity, with programmes, conferences, careers and often very successful policies built around what ultimately is a US budget line.

A corollary of the second logic is that governments will often ask international organizations to address wicked problems. World politics is full of problems that remain intractable for decades, ranging from frozen conflicts (e.g. Moldova, Cyprus), to hot wars (Gaza, Yemen, a steadily increasing share of the Maghreb), to tragic flows of refugees and internally displaced people (e.g. from Syria, Afghanistan and Haiti), to interstate disagreement on crucial issues (climate change) to reluctance to take the blame for problems (as with governments in debt). The real functions of international organizations are often to do governments' dirty work – to take unpopular actions and make the best of a situation when there is no good 'solution' visible. Success at doing dirty work looks to the outside world like a failure to achieve a mandate even when it is actually success at doing a key job for the organization.

International organizations are often called on to do such work for governments, as when the World Bank turns down unjustifiable projects, the IMF coordinates swingeing cuts in place of worse policies imposed by bond and currency market traders, WHO cooperates with regimes that show no respect for health or human rights, or UN peacekeepers contribute to freezing conflicts. Part of the job of multilateral organizations is precisely to take the blame for intractable problems that would be even worse without somebody doing the dirty work (O'Brien, 1985; Greer, 2016; Wenham and Davies, 2023). Part of the job of diplomacy in general is to find words and topics that keep people around the table, on the assumption that even hypocritical talk is better than war. Viewed through this lens, what might look like multilateral organizations failing their formal mandates is actually them doing their real job of serving governments in multiple ways that include taking the blame for failures.

Regional international organizations

Global institutions are not the whole of global health governance. There are hundreds of international organizations with a less than global ambition or membership, as diverse as the Association of Southeast Asian Nations (ASEAN), the Economic Community of West African States (ECOWAS), the Southern Common Market (known in Spanish as MERCOSUR), the Shanghai Cooperation Organisation (SCO), made up primarily of China's Western neighbours and Russia, and the African Union (AU). Many of them have only a limited formal engagement with health issues and fail to deliver on what little they promise. But they can also have indirect effects, as with trade or legal agreements that constrain and shape health systems and economies, as with the strong protection for intellectual property and exports of processed food in the North American free trade agreement, coordination in talks with donors in ASEAN, and the European Union's (EU) many economic rules that influence healthcare policy (Amaya et al., 2015; Greer et al., 2022). The EU is technically a regional international organization, but in global health it behaves much more like a great power, and its political authority is far broader and more established than that of the other regional bodies (Greer et al., 2022). Internally, it looks more like a federation than an international organization (Greer, 2020). (See Box 8.3 for more details on supra-national actors.)

Box 8.3 Comparative health data

Comparing health systems is difficult because countries have little incentive to invest much in system-level data, and still less to invest in making data more comparable when it might thereby become less useful to them. As a result, widely distributed numbers from excess mortality to counts of hospital beds to COVID-19 infection numbers are often literally unbelievable because of differences in the way numbers are gathered and reported. There are a few strong producers of comparative health system data and information:

Commonwealth Fund: a US-based charity known for survey-based research on the performance of health systems in selected countries, especially Australia, Canada, Germany, the Netherlands, New Zealand, the UK (sometimes with specific discussion of Scotland) and the US. It is a valuable source of their respective policy performance and complements other sources because of its use of surveys.

European Observatory on Health Systems and Policies: a partnership of governments, the EU and others that produces a variety of useful resources, including thematic studies of health policy issues, country health reports, ongoing policy monitoring and extensive book-length Health Systems in Transition reports that are often the best – and sometimes only – rigorous portrayal of all dimensions of a health system. Its model is being adopted elsewhere, notably by a Canada-based North American Observatory and an African Observatory. It has often differentiated between the UK's four health systems, which is not the norm in international comparisons that typically either report UK average data or just present English information.

EU: it has multiple agencies (such as the European Centre for Disease Control and Prevention), data sources (such as Eurostat), research projects and networks that work to make data on health issues comparable and useful for policy. This data is unfortunately scattered across the EU's websites, but the most comprehensive portal is the web page for the Directorate-General for Health.

Organization for Economic Cooperation and Development: born shortly after World War Two as an essentially transatlantic club of rich countries, but has been slowly expanding with new members, such as Chile, Colombia and Mexico. It is a club for finance ministers, and its huge programme of work on health and health policy reflects their preoccupation on quality and efficiency. It does tremendously important work on comparative health policy, underpinned by decades of work standardizing reporting so that there is some comparability in numbers such as hospital beds per capita. It has an unusually strong interest in the UK's four health systems and their different data and policies.

World Health Organization: including its diverse regional offices, it manages a range of databases but shifting politics within the organization led to it gathering, vetting and producing less data in recent years, a situation which a number of leaders in WHO are trying to remedy.

UN Agencies and IFIs such as the IMF, UNAIDS or UNICEF also collect and distribute more or less comparable data in their areas of expertise. The **United Nations Development Programme** collects data for and publishes the Human Development Index (HDI).

Great powers and geopolitics

Great powers do not work exclusively through formal multilateral governance, and what they do shapes global health. This section notes three, the EU, People's Republic of China and the United States, but other powers as diverse as the Gulf Monarchies, UK, Brazil, Japan, Russia and Australia also actively pursue strategic goals through global health policy. We saw this in particular with 'vaccine diplomacy' and 'vaccine nationalism' during the COVID-19 pandemic (Jarman et al., 2023; Greer et al., 2025). The purpose of this section is simply to show how global health is part of larger geopolitical games with very high stakes.

The EU is a major force in global health that has only recently started to develop an overall strategic approach (Greer, Rozenblum et al., 2024; Greer et al., 2025). Much of its power comes from its role as a huge and regulated market, which means that its stances on issues such as international trade law, intellectual property and regulatory standards have a global impact. It is also a major donor on a par with the United States and the Bill and Melinda Gates Foundation, and while many of its member states' foreign health aid budgets are exiguous, its contributions are very big. In 2023 the European Commission issued its first Global Health Strategy, which its member states governments then endorsed in 2024 European Council Conclusions. The institutional focus of the EU's approach is in the two units responsible for health and 'Institutional partnerships', which largely means development. Other areas of EU work that have major global ramifications, such as its trade, agricultural, and professional qualifications (i.e. workforce migration) policies, were left out (Greer, Rozenblum et al., 2024). The EU strategy and the Conclusions are particularly strong on a number of issues including support for reproductive freedom and human rights – and participation and support for the WHO. The UK, despite the convulsive politics of Brexit, has often aligned with the EU in its development priorities and support for multilateral organizations. It, like the EU member states, can perceive that multilateral organizations are relatively stable and hospitable environments for small and medium powers and therefore supports strengthening such forums.

This explicit EU focus on supporting global multilateralism stands out in contrast to the approaches taken by two other big powers, the US and China. Both of them chafe against multilateral forums that emphasize the equality of sovereign states. The United States, under Democratic presidents, such as Barack Obama and Joseph Biden, has had a tendency to combine support for multilateral institutions with efforts to build what amounted to parallel organizations of US allies and aid recipients, notably the Global Health Security Agenda under Obama. Under Republican President Donald Trump, longstanding conservative suspicion of the UN curdled into outright attacks on the WHO and an effort to leave it during the COVID-19 pandemic. The US would have to legislate to actually leave WHO, but as Trump showed a president can block its work, stop collaborating and stop sending its mandatory contributions fairly easily. The Biden Administration quickly re-established support for WHO, but also maintained the Obama administration's preference for dense bilateral relationships. The United States' April 2024 *Global Health Security Strategy*, which maps out plans for a second Biden term makes an interesting contrast to the EU's strategy, showing both a high level of awareness of the many ways the US exerts influence bilaterally, regionally and multilaterally across many policy areas – and also focusing not on 'global health' but on 'global health security' (The White House, 2024).

The Trump administration showed particular animosity towards WHO, but it was not supportive of multilateralism in general. For example, the US kept the WTO appellate body below quorum by refusing to make appointments, effectively paralyzing global trade law from 2019, including for the duration of Biden's first 4 years in office. In other words, the US is alternating between a political party that supports multilateral organizations, but it prefers to work with its allies on its own terms, and a party that is at a peak of hostility to multilateralism. Given the power of its president and the razor-edge closeness of its recent elections, this alternation raises questions about any US international commitment.

The People's Republic of China (PRC) is perhaps more consistent in its foreign policy, with nothing like the political swings of the US in recent years. Like the US it is frustrated by international organizations in which it has the same single vote as any less powerful country, and like the US (under Democrats) it has invested in influencing multilateral organizations, while also investing in influence over like-minded governments in organizations it leads. Its Belt and Road Initiative, a huge and evolving package of infrastructure projects and loans (Chinyong Liow et al., 2021), has financed a vast amount of infrastructure around the world. This initiative extends Chinese economic and political influence, giving poorer country governments more strategic and economic options, offering a model that emphasizes sovereignty and noninterference, enabling new investments and economic options and also creating huge debts to China for some countries (Economy, 2021). It remains to be seen how the PRC, a relative newcomer to international creditorship, will deal with debt crises and whether it will find itself converging or in conflict with the IFIs, OECD countries and private lenders. It is notable that Chinese policy focuses on infrastructure rather than health, and competition with the PRC might be pushing other official donors and lenders such as the EU towards a focus on infrastructure as they bid for the friendship of governments.

Learning activity 8.2

You are in the health ministry of a leading wealthy country in the OECD and are seeking additional staff resources in the ministry to work on global health governance. What topic or organization would you want to focus on and why would your superiors be persuaded to grant you the extra staff?

The politics of decoupling

Until around 2016 most conversations around global governance focused on the construction of rules for an integrating world. Debates in global health focused on the health impact of economic bodies, such as the IMF and WHO, and their rules, and ways that their actions could promote, or at least not undermine, health goals. The focus was on the construction and maintenance of a set of shared rules in an increasingly integrated world and the place of health in those systems.

Since 2016, global politics took a turn away from this model. Decoupling – the intentional separation of integrated economies – became a goal for governments ranging from Western countries decoupling from China and sanctioning Russia to Brexit to the multilateralism-sceptical Trump administration's actions. The COVID-19 pandemic and other shocks led to an interest in supply chains and production capacity, with a variety of countries realizing that while a fully global supply chain for vaccines or medical products might be technically efficient, it was vulnerable to political interference and disruption in times of crisis. As a result, governments began to put more effort into managing supply chains and locating key productive capacity within their borders, while actors as diverse as the United States under Trump and Russia under Putin explicitly undermined multilateral organizations and successfully paralyzed parts of the UN.

The result is a shift from a world of US-backed multilateral rules and complex international supply chains to a more contested landscape in which richer countries are trying to assure the resilience of their health product supply chain by reshoring production. Elements of the rules that preoccupied health researchers a decade ago now seem less important, while we must consider the international and equity effects of decoupling and its potential effects on, for example, international scientific collaboration.

From a health perspective, the effects of changing geopolitics can be quite direct, as when COVID-19 showed the complexity and fragility of cross-border supply chains for key products, such as protective equipment and vaccines. With COVID-19 vaccines, for example, the EU and UK blamed each other for supply interruptions in 2021, while India, 'the world's pharmacy', at one point suspended exports of vaccines to poorer countries in order to focus on vaccinating its own population. It is hard to fault the Indian government for this or imagine any other government would have done differently. The obvious solution is therefore to depend less on India or any other one producer even if that reduces overall efficiency. In particular, many countries have developed an interest in re-localizing production of key facilities such as vaccine plants in order to have important productive and research capacity under their control, in which case technology transfer becomes even more important (Massard da Fonseca and de Moraes Achcar, 2023; 2024). This has extended to international health policies that support creation of vaccine production capacity in Africa, a continent that was particularly poorly treated in global COVID-19 vaccination politics (see Box 8.4).

Box 8.4 COVID-19 vaccines and vaccine diplomacy

COVID-19 vaccination development was a triumph of science. The virus was identified and sequenced in January 2020, and within a year a variety of vaccines, made with different technologies, were available. Compared to any previous disease, this was remarkable. How did different countries, located in different parts of the world, engage (Jarman et al., 2023; Greer et al., 2025)?

The buyers

Rich countries' governments quickly acted to support vaccine development and place orders for themselves. While the details differed, the UK, US, EU and others fronted money to pharmaceutical companies and researchers with plausible plans while negotiating 'advance purchase' agreements to secure supplies and price. Betting on multiple companies with different production and administration spread risk, and some vaccines did indeed come faster or were more popular. Regulators sped review while maintaining their standards, conscious that an appearance of rushing or side effects could discredit vaccination. While many mostly remember waits, delays and polemics in December 2020 and early 2021, and it seems likely the EU negotiated much lower prices than the others, the result was that by the late spring of 2021 citizens of wealthy countries almost all had access to vaccinations.

The multilateralists

The multilateral organizations, led by GAVI and WHO, also moved quickly to try to address the virus as a global problem and shared a similar understanding of the structure of pharmaceutical industries (Perroud, 2025). They set up the ACT-A accelerator to speed vaccine development and production, and COVAX as a mechanism to purchase and distribute vaccines. Countries that joined COVAX would be able to use it as a purchasing club (buying at COVAX negotiated prices) or receive donated doses. The moral commitment was that no country should have enough doses for more than twenty per cent of its population until *every* country had enough doses for twenty per cent of its population. Rich countries and middle-income vaccine producers, such as India and Brazil, it seems, never had any intention of abiding by that rule. They, instead, used COVAX as a convenient mechanism for foreign aid, donating money and doses. The result was that COVAX became a mechanism of international health, converting donations from rich countries into charity for poor countries. Unsurprisingly, it never had anywhere near the resources that it would have taken to achieve universal vaccination by 2024.

The disruptors

Not every country's leadership saw its interests aligned with the rich countries or the multilateralists. One example is Russia, a disruptive global actor by any standard. It opted for a locally produced, quickly authorized vaccine and made it available before other vaccines were available. In some cases, it worked with other countries to enable local production, and it gave supplies to countries that otherwise waited a long time for inadequate supplies from COVAX or donors. In doing so the Russian government ignored every standard (WHO and other) of vaccine testing and production – but it was successful in using Sputnik-V as a tool of diplomacy.

The critics

Each of these three approaches relied on the basic model of publicly funded research converted, with additional public support, into the publicly regulated private property of pharmaceutical companies. The companies then produced the vaccines, which governments, multilateral organizations and private buyers then purchased. In other words, each model left the basic structure of the global pharmaceuticals sector intact. The critics who pointed this out were mostly marginal, in civil society and academia. No powerful stakeholder tried to use the moment to rethink the relationship between public and private.

Of course, this categorization is a bit too clean, and countries contain contradictions. For example, elements of the United States military during the Trump presidency tried to counter Chinese vaccine diplomacy in the Philippines by running campaigns on social media that tried to discredit Chinese vaccines and perhaps all vaccines (Bing and Schectman, 2024).

Box 8.5   Global health and the health workforce

Assuring a capable and sustainable health workforce might be the number one challenge for health managers around the world, but it has long been 'too hard' to address for governments. They would quickly tire of the cacophony of special interest demands from different professional groups that workforce policy involves (one analyst characterized workforce policy as 'piety, platitudes, and pork') (Fox, 1996). In richer countries, moreover, there is a simple solution to planning failures and shortages: the international health workforce market (Glinos, 2012). The result was a global, and poorly understood, 'brain drain' in which the healthcare workforce of richer countries often comes from poorer countries – as with Romanians working in Italy, Indians and Filipinos working in the US or the Gulf Monarchies, or Central Asians working in Russia, often in the less desirable places and jobs. Brain drain can be a disaster for LICs with very few local professionals, or an export sector for some countries that benefit from remittances such as the Philippine, (Kingma, 2006) – or both (Record and Mohiddin, 2006).

Workforce mobility also creates endless highly complex problems of credentialling, with multiple tensions: professional regulation, professional self-interest, shortages and real gaps between the content and standards of training in different countries. The EU has built up a body of law on the topic, which shows us how hard it is to create a stable legal framework for professional mobility across borders (notably, old federations such as Australia, Canada and the US have limited internal professional mobility and weak cross-border mutual recognition) (Matthijs et al., 2019). The EU's impressive achievement in creating cross-border professional mobility created extensive conversations about the definitions and roles of different professions, which in turn enabled reforms in some areas.

The NHS systems of the UK, for example, might be icons of national identities around the UK, famously and disingenuously instrumentalized on the 'Brexit bus' (Hervey et al., 2023), but they have always depended on recruiting labour from abroad (Seaton, 2023). UK governments have never chosen to train 'enough' healthcare workers, and NHS workforce plans are both rare and generally unstrategic. At first this dependency on foreign workers meant recruitment from the Empire and Commonwealth; later it came to mean recruitment from the EU, in part because successive UK governments explicitly tried to limit NHS recruitment from LICs with workforce shortages. After Brexit the UK became a major global magnet for health professionals from around the world, replacing its dependence on Europeans with dependence on citizens of LMICs (McCarey et al., 2022), and UK visa rules that required higher salaries than were paid in the care sector were one of the contributors to its crisis in long term and social care. The result is that the NHS, by far the largest employer in any country of the UK, does not just depend on international immigration but also, by virtue of its sheer size, affects the ethnic composition of many places around the UK.

Learning activity 8.3

- You are in charge of developing a sustainable healthcare workforce strategy for a set of hospitals in a rich country. It can include direct outreach to health systems, educators or providers in three countries. What criteria would you use to decide which countries you would approach, and why?
- You are in charge of developing the global side of a sustainable healthcare workforce strategy for a medium-sized rich country. What is the single biggest ethical problem you face and why?

Conclusions

Global health is a field full of contradictions: people with the best possible motivations exposed to the worst examples of hypocrisy and inequality; universal rights juxtaposed with geopolitical competition and ugly regimes; existential threats to the species in competition with the pettiest forms of selfishness. People working in global health are often particularly likely to be sensitive to the contradictions and compromises involved, which makes it an area particularly filled with critiques and passionate debates about principles.

Global health governance is also changing. For decades the phrase meant, essentially, the foreign trade, aid and debt policies of governments and non-governmental organizations of the rich democracies. Since around 2000, the rise and increasing geopolitical energy of powers, such as Brazil, Russia, India, China and South Africa (the BRICS), has meant that more and more of global health has become part of complex geopolitical contexts with policy tools, arguments and stakes that might have huge health effects but are conducted without much regard for health or human rights. For decades, the conversation about global health governance was about how to build rules and institutions to promote health in a global, capitalist system. More and more, it is about how to promote health and human rights in a world of geopolitical conflict and competition, with new actors and new options for everybody. Addressing global health problems, from climate change to healthcare supply chains, will become an increasingly complex and politically contested process. This changed world will be more complex and offer different options; whether it can be made good for human rights and health remains to be seen.

Learning resources

For statistical and comparative information sources, see Box 8.3. For further reading:

- On the general history of 'global health' as a field, (Packard, 2016)
- On the WHO and the way it developed, (Chorev, 2012; Cueto et al., 2019)
- On the IFIs and health, (Kentikelenis and Stubbs, 2023)
- On the EU Global Health Strategy (European Commission, 2022; European Council, 2024; Greer, Mauer et al., 2024)
- On the US Global Health Security Strategy of 2024, (The White House, 2024)
- On the Belt and Road Initiative as part of overall Chinese strategy, from two different perspectives, the PRC government at http://english.www.gov.cn/belt-AndRoad/ and (Economy, 2021)
- On the comparative politics of COVID-19 vaccine acquisition and vaccination, (Jarman et al., 2023; Greer et al., 2025)

The websites of organizations such as the WHO and EU can be vast and difficult to navigate, retaining huge amounts of information about programmes that are effectively defunct while also suffering from particularly bad cases of 'link rot' in which the pages remain but their URL is broken. In general, if you find anything important on a website, it is wise to save it offline for future reference.

References

Amaya, A.B., Rollet, V. and Kingah, S. (2015) What's in a word? The framing of health at the regional level: ASEAN, EU, SADC and UNASUR, *Global Social Policy*, 15(3): 229–260.

Bing, C. and Schectman, J. (2024) Pentagon ran secret anti-vax campaign to undermine China during pandemic, Reuters [https://www.reuters.com/investigates/special-report/usa-covid-propaganda/; accessed 30 November 2024].

Brown, T.M., Cueto, M. and Fee, E. (2006) The World Health Organization and the transition from 'international' to 'global' public health, *American Journal of Public Health*, 96(1): 62–72. doi:10.2105/AJPH.2004.050831.

Chinyong Liow, J., Liu, H. and Xue, G. (eds) (2021) *Research Handbook on the Belt and Road Initiative*. Cheltenham, UK & Northampton, MA, USA: Edward Elgar Publishing.

Chorev, N. (2012) *The World Health Organization between North and South*. Ithaca, NY: Cornell University Press.

Corbett, J., Xu, Y.-C. and Weller, P.M. (2021) *International Organizations and Small States: Participation, Legitimacy and Vulnerability*. Bristol: Bristol University Press.

Cueto, M., Brown, T.M. and Fee, E. (2019) *The World Health Organization: A History*. Cambridge: Cambridge University Press.

Destoumieux-Garzón, D., Mavingui, P., Boetsch, G., Boissier, J., Darriet, F., Duboz, P., et al. (2018) The One Health concept: 10 years old and a long road ahead, *Frontiers in Veterinary Science*, 5: 14.

Economy, E.C. (2021) *The World According to China*. Oxford: Polity.

European Commission (2022) EU Global Health Strategy: Better Health for All in a Changing World. [Available at: https://health.ec.europa.eu/document/download/25f21cf5-5776-477f-b08e-d290392fb48a_en?filename=international_ghs-report-2022_en.pdf; accessed on 22 February 2025].

European Council (2024) EU Global Health Strategy – Better Health for All in a Changing World – Council Conclusions. [Available at: https://data.consilium.europa.eu/doc/document/ST-5908-2024-INIT/en/pdf; accessed on 22 February 2025].

Fidler, D.P. and Gostin, L.O. (2008) *Biosecurity in the Global Age Biological Weapons, Public Health, and the Rule of Law*. Stanford: Stanford University Press.

Fidler, D.P. (2004) *SARS, Governance and the Globalization of Disease*. Basingstoke: Palgrave Macmillan.

Fox, D.M. (1996) From piety to platitudes to pork: the changing politics of health workforce policy, *Journal of Health Politics, Policy and Law*, 21(4): 825–844.

Gatter, R. (2014) The new global framework for pandemic influenza virus-and vaccine-sharing, in I.G. Cohen (ed.), *The Globalization of Health Care: Legal and Ethical Issues*. New York: Oxford University Press.

Glinos, I. (2012) Worrying about the wrong thing: patient mobility versus mobility of health care professionals, *Journal of Health Services Research & Policy*, 17(4): 254–256. doi:10.1258/jhsrp.2012.012018.

Gostin, L.O. and Finch, A. (2024) The World Desperately Needs a New Pandemic Treaty, Scientific American [https://www.scientificamerican.com/article/the-world-desperately-needs-a-new-pandemic-treaty/; accessed 30 November 2024].

Greer, S.L. (2014) Structural adjustment comes to Europe: lessons for the Eurozone from the conditionality debates, *Global Social Policy*, 14(1): 51–71.

Greer, S.L. (2016) Powering and puzzling in global public health, *European Journal of Public Health*, 26(3): 369–370.

Greer, S.L. (2020) Health, federalism and the European Union: lessons from comparative federalism about the European Union, *Health Economics, Policy and Law*, 1–14. doi:10.1017/S1744133120000055.

Greer, S.L. and Singer, P.M. (2017) Addressing Zika in the United States: polarization, fragmentation, and public health, *American Journal of Public Health*, 107(6), 861–862.

Greer, S.L., Amaya, A.B., Jarman, H., Legido-Quigley, H. and McKee, M. (2022) Regional international organizations and health: a framework for analysis, *Journal of Health Politics, Policy and Law*, 47(1): 63–92.

Greer, S.L., Massard da Fonseca, E., Jarman, H. and King, E.J. (2025) *Vaccination Politics: The Comparative Politics and Policy of COVID-19 Vaccinations*. Ann Arbor, MI: University of Michigan Press.

Greer, S.L., Mauer, N., Jarman, H., Rockwell, O., Falkenbach, M., Kickbusch, I., et al. (2024) *European Support for Improving Global Health Systems and Policies*. Brussels: European Observatory on Health Systems and Policies.

Greer, S.L., Rozenblum, S., Fahy, N., Panteli, D., Jarman, H., Brooks, E., et al. (2024) *Everything You Always Wanted to Know About European Union Health Policy but Were Afraid to Ask* (4th edn.). Brussels: European Observatory on Health Systems and Policies [https://eurohealthobservatory.who.int/publications/i/everything-you-always-wanted-to-know-about-european-union-health-policies-but-were-afraid-to-ask-fourth-revised; accessed 30 November 2024].

Hervey, T., Antova, I., Flear, M.L. and Wood, M. (2023) *Not What the Bus Promised: Health Governance After Brexit*. London: Bloomsbury Publishing.

Holmes, I.A. and Willison, C.E. (2024) SDG13, climate action: health systems as stakeholders and implementors in climate policy change, in S.L. Greer, M. Falkenbach, J. Figueras and M. Wismar (eds), *Health for All Policies: The Co-Benefits of Intersectoral Action*. Cambridge: Cambridge University Press.

Hotez, P.J. (2021) *Forgotten People, Forgotten Diseases: The Neglected Tropical Diseases and Their Impact on Global Health and Development*. New York: John Wiley & Sons.

Ibata-Arens, K.C. (2021) *Pandemic Medicine: Why the Global Innovation System Is Broken, and How We Can Fix It*. Boulder, CO: Lynne Rienner Publishers.

Jarman, H. (2014) *The Politics of Trade and Tobacco Control*. Basingstoke: Palgrave Macmillan.

Jarman, H. (2019) Normalizing tobacco? The politics of trade, investment, and tobacco control, *The Milbank Quarterly*, 97(2): 449–479. doi:10.1111/1468-0009.12393.

Jarman, H., Massard da Fonseca, E. and King, E.J. (2023) The political economy of vaccines during the COVID-19 pandemic, *Journal of Health Politics, Policy and Law*, 10910797. doi:10.1215/03616878-10910797.

Kentikelenis, A.E. (2017) Structural adjustment and health: a conceptual framework and evidence on pathways, *Social Science & Medicine*, 187: 296–305.

Kentikelenis, A. and Stubbs, T. (2023) *A Thousand Cuts: Social Protection in the Age of Austerity*. Oxford: Oxford University Press.

Kentikelenis, A., Seabrooke, L. and Sending, O.J. (2023) Global health expertise in the shadow of hegemony, *Studies in Comparative International Development*, 58(3): 347–368. doi:10.1007/s12116-023-09405-z.

Kingma, M. (2006) *Nurses on the Move: Migration and the Global Health Care Economy.* Ithaca, NY: Cornell University Press.

Lakoff, A. and Collier, S.J. (2008) *Biosecurity Interventions: Global Health and Security in Question.* New York: Columbia University Press.

Lall, R. (2023) *Making International Institutions Work: The Politics of Performance.* Cambridge: Cambridge University Press.

Lerner, H. and Berg, C. (2015) The concept of health in One Health and some practical implications for research and education: what is One Health? *Infection Ecology & Epidemiology,* 5(1): 25300. doi:10.3402/iee.v5.25300.

Mahler, H. (1981) The meaning of 'Health for All by the Year 2000', *American Journal of Public Health,* 106(1): 36–38.

Massard da Fonseca, E. (2013) Intellectual property enforcement in the European Union, in S.L. Greer and P. Kurzer (eds) *European Union Public Health Policies: Regional and Global Perspectives.* Abindgon: Routledge.

Massard da Fonseca, E., Shadlen, K.C. and de Moraes Achcar, H. (2023) Vaccine technology transfer in a global health crisis: actors, capabilities, and institutions, *Research Policy,* 52(4): 104739.

Massard da Fonseca, E. and de Moraes Achcar, H. (2024) SDG9, industry, innovation, and infrastructure: technology and knowledge transfer as means to generate co-benefits between health and industrial Sustainable Development Goals, in *Health for All Policies: The Co-Benefits of Intersectoral Action.* Cambridge: Cambridge University Press.

Matthijs, M., Parsons, C. and Toenshoff, C. (2019) Ever tighter union? Brexit, Grexit, and frustrated differentiation in the single market and Eurozone, *Comparative European Politics,* 17(2): 209–230. doi:10.1057/s41295-019-00165-6.

McCarey, M., Dayan, M., Jarman, H., Hervey, T., Fahy, N., Bristow, D., et al. (2022) *Health and Brexit: Six Years On.* London: Nuffield Trust.

O'Brien, C.C. (1985) U.N. Theater, *The New Republic,* 17–19.

Packard, R.M. (2016) *A History of Global Health: Interventions Into the Lives of Other Peoples.* Baltimore, MD: Johns Hopkins University Press.

Peralta-Santos, A., Saboga-Nunes, L. and Magalhães, P.C. (2021) A tale of two pandemics in three countries: Portugal, Spain, and Italy, in S.L. Greer, E.J. King, A. Peralta-Santos and E. Massard da Fonseca (eds) *Coronavirus Politics: The Comparative Politics and Policy of COVID-19.* Ann Arbor, MI: University of Michigan Press. [https://www.press.umich.edu/11927713/coronavirus_politics/?s=description; accessed 30 November 2024].

Perroud, J. (2025) Multilateral approaches to COVID-19 vaccines, in S.L. Greer, H. Jarman, E.J. King and E. Massard da Fonseca (eds), *Vaccination Politics: The Comparative Politics and Policy of COVID-19 Vaccination.* Ann Arbor, MI: University of Michigan Press.

Record, R. and Mohiddin, A. (2006) An economic perspective on Malawi's medical "brain drain", *Global Health,* 2, 12. doi:10.1186/1744-8603-2-12.

Seaton, A. (2023) *Our NHS: A History of Britain's Best Loved Institution.* New Haven, CT: Yale University Press.

Schmiege, D., Perez Arredondo, A.M., Ntajal, J., Minetto Gellert Paris, J., Savi, M.K., Patel, K., et al. (2020) One Health in the context of coronavirus outbreaks: a systematic literature review, *One Health,* 10: 100170. doi:10.1016/j.onehlt.2020.100170.

Shadlen, K.C., Sampat, B.N. and Kapczynski, A. (2020) Patents, trade and medicines: past, present and future, *Review of International Political Economy*, 27(1): 75–97.

Stein, H. (2008) *Beyond the World Bank Agenda: An Institutional Approach to Development.* Chicago: University of Chicago Press.

Stepan, N.L. (2011) *Eradication: Ridding the World of Diseases Forever?* Ithaca, NY: Cornell University Press.

Taylor, L. (2024) WHO pandemic treaty: 'Torrent of fake news' has put negotiations at risk, says WHO chief, *British Medical Journal*, 384, q243. doi:10.1136/bmj.q243.

The White House (2024) U.S. Government Global Health Security Strategy (GHSS) 2024. Washington, DC. [https://www.whitehouse.gov/wp-content/uploads/2024/04/Global-Health-Security-Strategy-2024-1.pdf; ; accessed 30 November 2024].

UNDP (2024) Human Development Reports, Human Development Index (HDI) [https://hdr.undp.org/data-center/human-development-index#/indicies/HDI; accessed 30 November 2024].

Wenham, C. and Davies, S.E. (2023) What's the ideal World Health Organization (WHO)? *Health Economics, Policy and Law*, 18(3): 329–340.

World Health Organization. (n.d.) Universal Health Coverage [https://www.who.int/health-topics/universal-health-coverage#tab=tab_1; accessed 30 November 2024].

Healthcare financing

Suzanne Robinson

Introduction

Healthcare funding more than doubled over the past two decades reaching around 9.8 per cent of global gross domestic product (GDP) and is usually the largest single industry (World Health Organization, 2021). Increased demand from an ageing population and technological advances mean that healthcare expenditure continues to grow, while on the supply side there is constant pressure because resources are scarce. People are living longer with more complex chronic health conditions that are costly to the system. Healthcare systems continually face pressure to curb spending as they compete for public funding (Holman, 2020; OECD, 2023a).

Over the last 20 years, health systems have been impacted by two major shocks: the economic downturn of 2008 and the impact of COVID-19 in 2020 (OECD, 2023a). Just as health spending and GDP had started to recover from the global crises the effects of the pandemic including lockdowns and other public health measures restricted economic activity, and additional funding spent on the pandemic saw health and public spending on non-COVID activities fall.

Increasing financial pressures make public sector borrowing a less attractive economic policy option in developed countries, where policymakers are increasingly looking towards the structure and organization of healthcare systems – including revenue collection (the demand side) and organization of service provision (the supply side) – as a means of managing ever-increasing pressures on health expenditure. As resources become scarce governments often look to funding reforms to support efficiency gains. When considering healthcare funding, governments and health managers alike need to consider several elements, including those of efficiency and equity, with their aim in resource allocation to provide efficient, effective and equitable health services for their populations (see Box 9.1 for definitions).

Box 9.1 Defining terms

Efficiency: 'Health system efficiency seeks to capture the extent to which the inputs to the health system, in the form of expenditures and other resources, are used to secure valued health system goals' (Cylus et al., 2017).

Equity: 'Providing care that does not vary in quality because of personal characteristics such as gender, ethnicity, geographic location, and socioeconomic status' (Institute of Medicine, 2001). Policymakers are faced with making sure resources are spent efficiently; they safeguard ethical principles around access and distribution of resource.

Gross domestic product (GDP): 'the standard measure of the value added created through the production of goods and services in a country during a certain period' (OECD, 2024a). GDP is the single most important indicator to capture these economic activities.

Given the importance of healthcare financing and its relationship to healthcare performance, it is paramount for health leaders and managers to understand healthcare funding systems. Having a clearer understanding helps decision-makers make informed decisions about budget allocation, policy development and planning, focusing on improving the overall efficiency, equity and effectiveness of healthcare systems, ultimately increasing health outcomes for their communities.

In this chapter, we look at healthcare funding, including an overview of revenue collection methods and mechanisms for the distribution of funds across the health system. It considers healthcare expenditure and focuses on funding pressures and their sources and the various health system responses. The chapter finalizes by considering how governments and health leaders can respond to funding pressures. Learning activities are used to illustrate and analyse the problems and practices of health funding in the developed world, attempting to draw out common themes and challenges facing policymakers and healthcare managers.

Healthcare funding: an analytical framework

Financing and provision of healthcare represent a transaction between providers who transfer resources to patients, and patients or third parties who transfer resources to providers; this has been described as the healthcare triangle, see Figure 9.1 (Mossialos et al., 2002).

While countries have different funding systems, the underlying logic is the same. The simplest transaction occurs when direct payments are made between patients and providers of healthcare services. Due to the uncertainty of ill health and the high cost of healthcare, most healthcare systems include a third-party element. This entity, whether public or private, collects resources from individuals and determines how to distribute them to providers. This third-party element offers financial protection against the risk of becoming ill and allows that

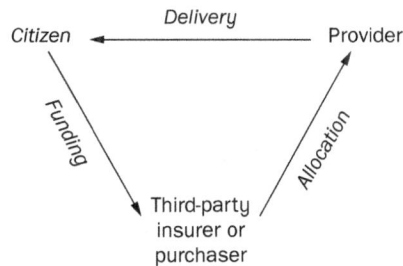

Figure 9.1 Healthcare triangle
Source: Mossialos et al. (2002).

risk to be shared among the protected population. Third-party provision may cover part or all of a country's population, once revenue has been collected it can then be used to reimburse either patients or providers of services. The funding system is therefore a way in which funds are collected, either via primary (patient) or secondary (third-party) sources, and then distributed to providers.

Functional components of healthcare financing are divided into three main categories:

1   **Revenue collection:** The way money is moved around the system and is concerned with sources of funding (examples include individuals or employers); mechanisms of funding (examples include direct or indirect taxes and voluntary insurance); and collection agents (examples include central or regional government). The main mechanisms of revenue collection are through taxation, social insurance contributions, voluntary insurance premiums and out-of-pocket payments (further discussion of these concepts later).
2   **Fund-pooling:** Occurs when a population's healthcare revenues are accumulated, with financial risk being shared between the population, rather than by each individual contributor. Fund-pooling incorporates both equity and efficiency considerations. Equity in-so-far as risk is shared among the pool or group, rather than it being assumed by individuals; and efficiency as pooling can lead to increases in population health and reduces uncertainty around healthcare expenditure (Smith and Witter, 2004: iii).
3   **Purchasing:** There are a wide range of purchasing activities in operation, some of which involve governments acting as both collection agent (raising revenue through general or local taxation), and purchaser of services from providers. Strategic issues around purchasing include decisions around what is to be purchased, such as the selection criteria for interventions. Other aspects include how to make a choice of providers and what mechanisms to use for purchasing.

Revenue generation

This section outlines the different methods of revenue generation and their associated effects on healthcare costs. Insurance-based methods – including private or public, compulsory or voluntary – are in operation across all healthcare systems. In addition, all countries have some form of direct payments by citizens made up of charges and/or co-payments for

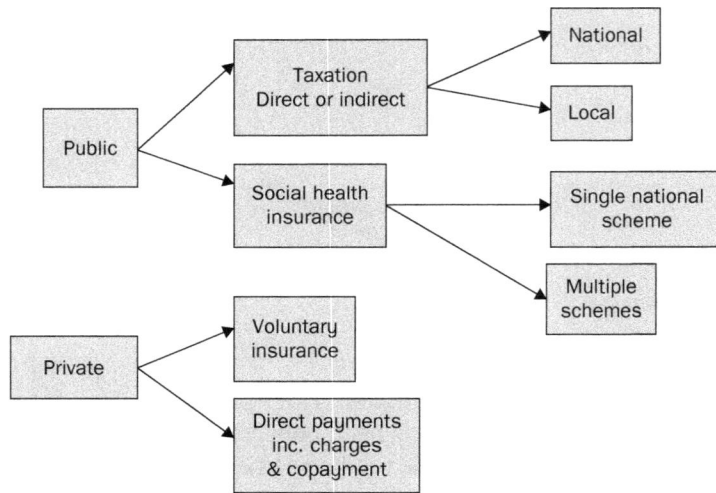

Figure 9.2 Different forms of revenue generation methods.

medications, medical appointments, pathology and diagnostic procedures at various levels. There are several different schemes in operation across countries including: charges to visit family doctors; charges or co-payments for treatment or services (i.e. hospital stays or dental care) (Thomson et al., 2010).

Figure 9.2 highlights the public and private revenue sources – methods that fall within the public sphere use financial mechanisms to achieve a set of social objectives, such as redistributing resources across the population. In contrast, private sources, such as voluntary insurance, focus on an individual's need and self-interest, rather than that of the wider population (Saltman and Dubois, 2004).

There are no 'pure models' but rather a blend of revenue generation methods in operation across OECD countries (Toth, 2021), with most countries having some form of compulsory insurance in operation (Joumard et al., 2010). While we see a mix of models there is often a predominant method strongly influenced by a society's underlying norms and values.

For some societies, healthcare is seen as a social and collective good, while for others it is perceived as a commodity that can be bought and sold (Chambers, 2020). However, even in countries that subscribe to the latter, there are usually funding mechanisms that allow redistribution of funds to those who cannot pay for healthcare.

Work by Joumard and colleagues (2010) group countries across six similar types of healthcare funding systems (see Table 9.1), ranging from those with higher market mechanisms around insurance and provision (Groups 1 and 2) to those that have high public insurance and regulation (see Joumard et al., 2010 and Anandaciva, 2023 for further discussion). Having an understanding of the predominant method is important because it allows for a greater understanding of what and how funding mechanisms drive the system and to make comparisons across and within systems. However, it is also important to understand the impact of the ancillary methods and how they interact with the predominant funding method (Toth, 2021).

Table 9.1 Countries grouped by similar funding systems

Group	Country	Funding system
Group 1	Germany, Netherlands, Slovak Republic, Switzerland	Market mechanisms regulating insurance coverage and service provision.
Group 2	Australia, Belgium, Canada, France	Basic public insurance coverage with private insurance beyond basic care. Extensive market regulating provision, with high gatekeeping and regulation.
Group 3	Austria, Czech Republic, Greece, Japan, Korea, Luxembourg	Basic public insurance coverage with limited private insurance. No gatekeeping function and extensive private supply.
Group 4	Iceland, Sweden, Turkey	High public insurance coverage limited private supply and high price regulation, limited gatekeeping.
Group 5	Denmark, Finland, Mexico, Portugal, Spain	High public insurance coverage, high level of gatekeeping and regulation, budget constraints limited.
Group 6	Hungary, Ireland, Italy, New Zealand, Norway, Poland United Kingdom	High public insurance, highly regulated with strict gatekeeping function, high budget constraint.

Source: Adapted from Joumard et al. (2010) and Anandaciva (2023).

General taxation

The UK has an example of a healthcare system that is funded predominantly through general (direct) taxation. The UK Treasury sets out what budget will be spent on healthcare, and once that is set, resources are distributed to the purchasers of care, with the majority of services being free to users at the point of provision. Other countries that primarily use a universal, tax-based funding mechanism include Denmark, Finland, New Zealand and Spain.

Funding healthcare through general taxation is seen as a progressive way of raising revenue. In most countries, tax is proportional to income, with those on higher incomes paying more tax than those on lower incomes, thus allowing for redistribution of resources from wealthy to poor, from healthy to sick, and from those of working age to the young and old. In addition, the financing of services is divorced from provision of services, which is important for equitable access, with resource being based on clinical need rather than ability to pay (Savedoff, 2004).

However, there is evidence to suggest that access to care is also affected by age, gender, education, wealth and race (for further discussion see Pickett and Wilkinson, 2010). Furthermore, while tax-based models are progressive, the degree to which the whole system of funding is progressive depends on what other funding mechanisms are being utilized. For example, even though general taxation is used to fund healthcare in Portugal the high share of out-of-pocket payments makes the overall system regressive (Wagstaff and van Doorslaer, 2000; Ping Yu et al., 2008). Evidence from Australia shows that out-of-pocket charges for GPs are impacting individuals' healthcare decisions and appear to be based on the ability to pay rather than the most effective care pathway (Fiebig et al., 2021).

Box 9.2 outlines the advantages and disadvantages of tax-based revenue generation.

Box 9.2   General taxation advantages and disadvantages

Advantages of tax-based revenue generation:

- Equitable progressive revenue raising – but dependent on wider system funding.
- Efficient administration, utilizing existing tax system and avoiding additional costs for the health sector.
- Strong incentives to control cost through government regulations, providers not easily able to increase revenue by raising prices or premiums, as in private insurance and social insurance (van der Zee and Kroneman, 2007; Kos, 2019).

Disadvantages of tax-based revenue collection:

- Dependency on economic conditions, health services linked to economy and government taxation policies. Economic downturns can lead to reductions in tax revenues, leading to tough choices around public spending.
- Health spending continues to rise; it may impact other public sector services, such as education and housing, which can have a negative impact on population health.
- The fact that taxes are not hypothecated in many countries means that the population is unable to judge the fiscal viability (i.e. affordability) of health services (Mckenna et al., 2017).

Local taxation

Denmark's healthcare is predominantly funded through general taxation, but unlike the UK, in Denmark the central government reallocates tax income to the local regions and municipalities, which finances around 77 per cent of the regional activity with a further 20 per cent of healthcare funding being generated through local taxes (Tikkanen et al., 2020a). Analysis has shown that local taxes are generally less progressive than national taxes (i.e. local taxes often take a larger proportion of tax from people whose income is low), as is demonstrated by the experience of Denmark and other countries, such as Finland, Sweden and Switzerland, who also have a high proportion of revenue generated by local taxation (McDaid, 2003; Health Policy Consensus Group, 2005; Ping Yu et al., 2008).

There are suggestions that local taxation could lead to inefficient resource allocation and priority setting (Abimbola et al., 2019; Rotulo et al., 2022). In the absence of a national system of redistribution, local taxation could create regional inequity. For example, if local tax rates vary by region this could lead to horizontal inequities (i.e. equal use of healthcare services for equal medical needs irrespective of any other characteristic, such as income, sex, race, etc.) (Pulok et al., 2020). Gundgaard (2006) suggests that the Danish system is generally equitable, however in sectors with a high degree of co-payments some horizontal inequity exists. Similarly, San Sebastián et al. (2017) identified horizontal equity in healthcare use in Sweden with higher use of GP services for those on higher incomes. Robust governance structures that focus on cost containment, efficiency and sustainability of health funding have been established by a number of central governments. For example, in Denmark the 'budget law' sets budgets for regions and sanctions are enforced if budgets are exceeded; similar laws apply in Sweden (Tikkanen et al., 2020a; Mossialos et al., 2015).

One of the advantages of local tax funding over national taxation is that decentralization can allow for greater transparency in terms of revenue raised and local spending (Abimbola et al., 2019). There is also greater direct political accountability for healthcare funding and expenditure, with local politicians being closer to their electorate than their national counterparts. Healthcare is separated from national priorities allowing for local needs to be more easily met (Abimbola et al., 2019).

Social insurance

Social health insurance tends to be a hypothecated tax – that is funds are specifically earmarked for health. There are large variations in the features of social health insurance systems across countries. Box 9.3 sets out some of the typical features of social health insurance systems. Social health insurance tends to be financed by mandatory earning contributions, with various arrangements for the unemployed (Wagstaff, 2010; Wickens and Brown, 2023).

Box 9.3 Typical features of social health insurance systems

- Insurance is compulsory for the majority or whole population.
- Insured individuals pay a regular, usually wage-based contribution, which may be a flat rate or variable.
- Employers may also pay a contribution.
- There may be one or more independent 'sickness funds' or social insurers.
- Individuals may or may not be able to choose which sickness fund they join.
- Transfers are made from general taxation to cover premiums of the unemployed, retired and other disadvantaged and vulnerable groups
- All allow for the pooling of revenue, typically insurance is not risk related.

Source: Adapted from McDaid (2003: 167).

Countries that operate a predominantly social health insurance system include Germany, France, Austria, Switzerland, Belgium, the Netherlands, Luxembourg and Japan. In addition, several central and eastern European countries have also adapted such models. Examples include Hungary, Lithuania, Czech Republic, Estonia and Poland (see European Observatory on Health Systems and Policies, 2024). Several countries have made substantial changes to their funding systems, due to ever-increasing financial pressures and a focus on having universal health coverage. Examples include in Germany, the reduction in sickness funds over a number of years have been intended to drive down costs and complexity (Blümel et al., 2020). In 2016 France implemented the Universal Health Protection Law aimed at providing systematic coverage to all French residents (Or et al., 2023).

Under social health insurance schemes, premiums tend to be collected directly by sickness funds (Austria, France, Switzerland) or distributed from a central state-run fund (Israel, Luxembourg) with Belgium using both methods. With the exception of France and Switzerland, sickness funds are private, not-for-profit organizations that are governed by an elected board. The rules under which sickness funds operate are usually led by national legislation (Saltman et al., 2004). The funds use revenues raised to fund contracts with providers who vary in terms of private not-for–profit, private for-profit and publicly operated. The number, size and structure of sickness funds varies between countries. Germany has around 110 funds covering around 88 per cent of the population (see Blümel et al., 2020 for further information), with Luxemburg merging multiple sickness funds into one single payer in 2009 (European Commission, 2016).

Funding using social health insurance tends to be more transparent than tax-based methods and traditionally this meant that health services were distanced from the political arena, with concerns tending to be around contribution rates rather than political matters.

The majority of social health insurance systems do require some level of subsidies from general and/or local taxation. For example, a large part of hospital care is paid for by general taxation in Austria and Switzerland. Van der Zee and Kroneman (2007) compared social insurance systems with general taxation-based systems and found that the latter seemed better at cost containment, while the former demonstrated greater population satisfaction with the system.

Private insurance

Private insurance can be classified into the following categories: substitutive, supplementary or complementary (Mossialos et al., 2002). Private healthcare insurance markets often develop around publicly funded systems, and, in many countries, private insurance plays a residual role in terms of healthcare funding. For example, in systems such as in the UK and Australia private insurance provides supplementary coverage to the public system and can enable faster access to certain services, such as elective hospital care (Buchmueller and Couffinhal, 2004: 4). In Australia there has been dissatisfaction with private insurance, and over the last 8 years there has been a decline in those taking out private insurance especially in younger age groups (Australian Medical Association, 2023). This is despite government subsidies and financial penalties. Duckett and colleagues suggest the current system is an 'unhappy mix' with private insurance offering additional services but also competing with the public sector by offering substitute services (see Duckett and Nemet, 2019).

There are mixed views on the role of private insurance; one argument is that it can relieve capacity and cost pressures from the public system, improving access and quality of care in the public sector. In contrast, there are concerns that an expanding private sector can divert resources from the public sector and increase issues of equity as those who are privately insured (usually on higher incomes) avoid public waiting lists and obtain faster access to care (Cheng, 2014). Analysis conducted by the OECD (2004) demonstrates that substitute private insurance can increase health expenditures and increase service usage, with limited efficiency gains. Private health insurance also tends to have a higher administrative burden than public or social insurance (Mueller et al., 2017).

Systems that rely heavily on private insurance are often criticized due to their inequitable nature; that is, these systems are based on a person's ability to pay for care rather than on clinical need (Wilper et al., 2009). Van Doorslaer et al. (2008: 97) demonstrate that 'unequal distribution of private health insurance coverage by income contributes to the phenomenon that the better-off and the less well-off do not receive the same mix of services.'

The country with one of the largest private health insurance components is the US, with private health insurance accounting for around 34 per cent of total expenditure in 2018. The introduction of the Patient Protection and Affordable Care Act (ACA) in the US was intended to provide affordable health insurance coverage for the majority of American citizens, improve access to primary care and reduce overall healthcare costs (Doherty, 2010). The ACA saw the establishment of 'shared responsibility' between government, employers and individuals for ensuring all Americans have access to affordable healthcare (Mossialos et al., 2015). Government figures for 2024 suggest that there has been a decline in the rate of uninsured Americans from 16 per cent in 2010 to 7.2 per cent in 2023 (The White House, 2024). While the reforms address one of the major barriers to care (insurance), the lack of primary care physicians limits access to primary care (Zhang et al., 2020).

Learning Activity 9.1 Exploring funding within your home country

The government of the day is looking to evaluate the country's healthcare funding revenue collection methods. You are part of an expert group that has been asked to identify and assess the major advantages and disadvantages in the current system and compare these with the experiences of other OECD countries.

Consider the following:

1. Examine the funding revenue collection methods in your country, focusing on how funds are sourced, allocated and managed within the system. What are the perceived advantages what are the perceived weakness?
2. Evaluate the implications of the identified disadvantages and advantages on healthcare management and delivery within your country. What does that mean for health professionals and patients?

Note: The Commonwealth Fund and European Observatory (see Resource list) provide country profiles and assess the impacts of funding models on health system performance.

Out-of-pocket payments and charges for healthcare

Out-of-pocket payments and charges involve individuals paying for all, or some, of their medical costs and make up a proportion of healthcare spending in all health systems. Out-of-pocket payments and charges are the main mechanisms that allow for price consciousness, that is, for patients to have a true notion of the costs of service and thus be able to make judgements around the price and (possibly) value for money of care received. User charges are often introduced to curb healthcare demand. However, little evidence exists to show that charges produce efficiency savings. In fact, there is evidence to suggest they may deter individuals from seeking appropriate and cost-effective care, especially for those on low incomes (Thomson et al., 2014).

A survey of OECD countries undertaken by Paris et al. (2010) showed that 29 member states had charges or co-payments for pharmaceuticals and 20 countries had some form of out-of-pocket payment for general practice visits. While patient charges are often seen as a method to curtail costs, there is a suggestion that they provide incentives to increase healthcare activity (Carrin and Hanvoravongchai, 2003; Rosenthal et al., 2005; Shomaker, 2010). That is, they reward providers for productivity regardless of need, effectiveness or quality (Shomaker, 2010). In addition, charges for some services can deter patients from accessing services and lead to inefficiencies, with primary care patients presenting at emergency departments and or detection of disease being delayed (Eckermann, 2014).

As patients demand better quality services, including non-clinical services, such as bedside computers, phones, televisions and car parking, the question arises as to where charges should stop. Nutritious food and pleasant surroundings are commonly considered to be essential components of good-quality care, but each system has to make a judgement as to the point at which services are deemed to require an additional payment from users, and if this payment is to be levied on all or just some people according to their ability to pay. Charges and co-payments are therefore criticized for being a regressive means of raising revenue, limiting access to services and discriminating against those on low incomes (Tamblyn et al., 2001). In addition, the cost of administering out-of-pocket payments and charges can be expensive and reduce the net contribution of changes (Mckenna et al., 2017).

How funds are distributed

> *It may thus be less the type of system that matters but rather how it is managed.*
> (OECD Economics Department, 2010 Policy Notes, No. 2)

Countries vary in terms of the methods and mix of systems used to distribute funds around the system and pay providers for the delivery of health services. The main methods include global-based funding, capitation, activity-based funding, outcomes-based funding and bundled payment.

Global-based (or 'block') funding: this involves placing a limit on the amount of money spent on healthcare. A fixed level of payment is agreed in advance of the treatment activity taking place, with a block of money going to healthcare providers. The amount of funding is often based on historical patterns and demographic data. Advantages include cost control mechanisms where capped funding can be applied; certainty of funding; ease and cheapness to administer; and can help improve the planning and coordination of services (Dredge, 2004). The main criticisms of this approach are lack of incentives around production; lack of sensitivity to volume; lack of transparency and fairness; and limits to the notion of the actual cost associated with treatments (Collier, 2008; Berenson et al., 2016).

Capitation funding: a population-based funding model with healthcare providers receiving a fixed payment for each patient enrolled, regardless of the services provided. The capitation formula is often adjusted for age and gender but less for population health status (Barber et al., 2019). Capitation funding is often used to control costs by providing a fixed amount of funding. While this strategy can minimize waste, it may also lead to under-provision of care, particularly for more complex costly cases.

Both global-based and capitation funding involve a one-off payment that is not attached to actual service provision to patients, thus there is limited risk in relation to the type and amount of service provision. However, providers could struggle to maintain financial sustainability if they are unable to accurately manage their costs and revenues.

Activity-based funding: (other names: episode funding; activity-funding; pay for performance, payment by results, case-mix; or diagnosis-related group funding). This approach involves providers being paid for activity. Over recent years there has been a shift towards activity-based funding – this policy direction links to a focus on efficiency savings. One of the notions behind the use of pay for performance was that of incentivizing people and institutions by payment mechanisms. It was felt by many countries that activity-based funding would incentivize efficiency, quality and the opportunity to increase transparency with regard to how the money is being spent in the system (O'Reilly et al., 2012; Ashish, 2013).

Critics suggest that the approach rewards volume, not quality, of service, and that there is a real possibility of hospitals developing cost-cutting strategies that could compromise the quality of services. However, recent studies suggest that activity-based funding has made no real difference in quality of care (Anderson, 2009; Farrar et al., 2009). A recent study comparing waiting times found that they are less of a problem in countries that rely mainly on activity-based funding than those that have mainly fixed budgets. Results suggest a rise in activity leads to shorter waiting times and shorter lengths of stay in hospital (Hurst and Siciliani, 2003; Kjerstad, 2003; Farrar et al., 2007). However, in England reduction in waiting times may be due to the impact of other government policies (Farrar et al., 2007). Norway and Sweden have also seen efficiency savings in relation to productivity, although these have declined over time (Street et al., 2007). In the US, while length of stay decreased, so did the raise in acute illness after discharge and the need for nursing home or home healthcare (Anderson, 2009).

While activity-based funding may help to improve efficiency, it can impact on equity and needs-based funding, focusing on productivity rather than population need. Furthermore, there is no incentive to redirect patients to other services, i.e. from hospital to community-based services. Over recent years we have seen policymakers utilizing other incentives around value and quality and a shift in policy mantra from volume to value.

Outcomes-based funding (value-based funding): is a model focused on payments for performance, with payments being based on the outcomes achieved. The intention of this model is to incentivize providers to focus on the delivery of high-quality outcomes for patients as the financial payment is based on the results of their care. Porter and Thomas (2013) termed the model 'value-based funding', which focuses on maximizing patient value, moving away from supply-driven care systems to one that focuses on a patient-centered model of care. They believe the shift from volume and profitability to patient outcomes will drive down costs while improving outcomes (Porter and Thomas, 2013).

Bundled-payment funding: this is a fixed price agreement that involves a single payment for an agreed service relating to an episode of care – often used for surgery or chronic disease management. The incentive for this model is that providers can more effectively manage the budget and ensure quality (Struijk et al., 2020). Providers are able to keep any cost savings, but also need to cover costs of unexpected health care utilization. There has been an increase in the use of bundled payments, which is largely driven by the notion that giving providers a financial stake in driving value is more effective than activity-based funding and co-payments in reducing health spending (Baicker and Chernew, 2017). The evidence suggests that bundled payments have had a positive effect on health care spending and quality of care, this is irrespective of country, condition or procedure (Struijk et al., 2020).

Expenditure on health

Spending on health is one of the most pressing policy issues for many governments across the world. Drawing on data from the Organisation for Economic Co-operation and Development database, this section wsaill focus on healthcare spending across developed countries.

Figure 9.3 presents figures on the total health spending on healthcare in 2022 across several OECD countries. The OECD median total health spending was $4983.30. The US had

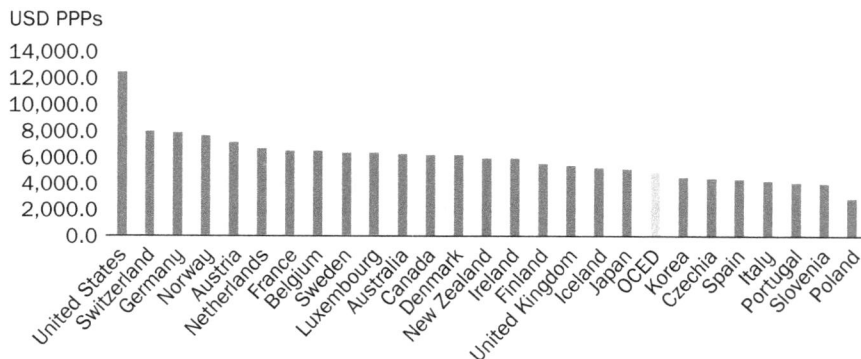

Purchasing power parities (PPPs) are the rates of currency conversion that try to equalize the purchasing power of different currencies, by eliminating the differences in price levels between countries.

Figure 9.3 Total health spending estimates on healthcare in 2022 across OECD countries
Source: Data from OECD (2023a).

the highest healthcare spend per capita ($12,555.30) of all the countries assessed and is well over the average OECD spend (shown in orange). The next biggest healthcare spenders are Switzerland and Germany, which spend around 50 per cent more than the OECD average.

Table 9.2 presents the share of expenditure as a proportion of GDP for a selection of OECD countries. The trend shows a rise in healthcare expenditure in all countries over the last 50+ years. Following the COVID-19 pandemic of 2019, some countries saw a decline in expenditure as a proportion of GDP, which was similar to the economic downturn of 2008. The highest expenditure was in the US, who spent around 16.6 per cent of GDP on healthcare in 2022. France, Germany, Belgium, Austria, Canada, Switzerland and the UK had the next highest percentages, with around 11–12 per cent of GDP spending on health. Allowing for inflation, the UK National Health Service (NHS) in 2004 cost eight-and-a-half times more than in 1949,

Table 9.2 Total expenditure on health as a percentage of GDP in selected OECD countries, 1970–2022

	1970	1980	1990	2000	2010	2015	2016	2017	2018	2019	2020	2021	2022*
Australia	3.7	5.8	6.5	7.6	8.4	10.2	10.1	10.1	10.1	10.2	10.7	10.6	9.6
Austria	4.8	7.0	7.7	9.2	10.2	10.4	10.4	10.4	10.3	10.5	11.4	12.1	11.4
Belgium	3.9	6.2	7.1	8.0	10.2	10.8	10.8	10.8	10.9	10.8	11.2	11.0	10.9
Canada	6.3	6.5	8.4	8.2	10.7	10.7	11.0	10.9	10.9	11.0	13.0	12.3	11.2
Denmark	3.6	8.4	8.0	8.1	10.6	10.3	10.2	10.1	10.1	10.2	10.6	10.8	9.5
Finland	5.0	5.9	7.3	7.1	9.1	9.6	9.4	9.1	9.0	9.2	9.6	10.3	10.0
France	5.2	6.8	8.0	9.6	11.2	11.4	11.5	11.4	11.2	11.1	12.1	12.3	12.1
Germany	5.7	8.1	8.0	9.9	11.1	11.2	11.2	11.3	11.5	11.7	12.7	12.9	12.7
Greece	3.6	5.5	6.1	7.2	9.6	8.2	8.4	8.1	8.1	8.2	9.5	9.2	8.6
Iceland	4.7	5.9	7.4	8.9	7.4	8.1	8.1	8.3	8.4	8.6	9.6	9.7	8.6
Ireland	4.9	7.5	5.6	5.9	8.4	7.3	7.5	7.1	6.9	6.7	7.1	6.7	6.1
Italy	3.6	5.1	7.0	7.6	10.5	8.9	8.7	8.7	8.7	8.7	9.6	9.4	9.0
Japan	4.3	6.1	5.7	7.0	8.9	10.8	10.7	10.7	10.7	11.0	11.0	11.3	..
Netherlands	..	6.5	7.0	7.7	9.1	10.3	10.3	10.1	10.0	10.1	11.2	11.3	..
New Zealand	5.1	5.8	6.7	7.5	10.2	9.3	9.2	9.0	9.0	9.1	9.7	10.1	11.2
Norway	4.0	5.4	7.1	7.7	9.6	10.1	10.5	10.2	10.0	10.4	11.2	9.9	7.9
Spain	3.1	5.0	6.1	6.8	8.9	9.1	8.9	8.9	9.0	9.1	10.7	10.7	10.4
Sweden	5.4	7.7	7.2	7.3	9.1	10.8	10.9	10.8	10.9	10.8	11.3	11.2	10.7
Switzerland	4.8	6.4	7.6	9.1	8.3	10.8	11.0	11.0	10.8	11.1	11.7	11.8	11.3
United Kingdom	4.0	5.1	5.1	7.1	9.9	9.8	9.7	9.6	9.7	10.0	12.2	12.4	11.3
United States	6.2	8.2	11.2	12.5	9.7	16.5	16.8	16.8	16.6	16.7	18.8	17.4	16.6

Legend* OECD estimated

Source: Data from OECD (2023a).

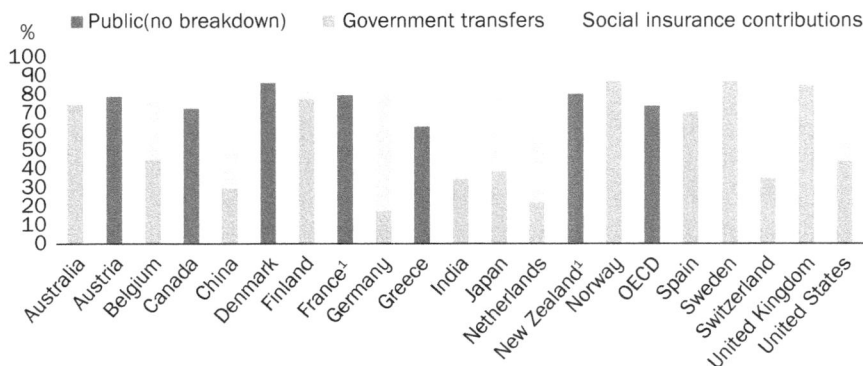

Figure 9.4 Public health funding as a percentage of total healthcare expenditure, 2021
Legend 1 Public is calculated using spending by government schemes and social health insurance.
Source: Data from OECD (2023a).

with the average cost per person rising over seven times above the 1949 level (Klumpes and Tang, 2008). Government spending on health often reflects a country's social priorities, as well as its economic capability. While richer countries tend to spend more on health, there are variations in spending. For example, Japan spends less on health than many other countries, yet people live longer and have a healthier life expectancy.

Figure 9.4 presents the type of financing activity as a percentage of total healthcare expenditure for a selection of countries in 2021. All countries have a mix of mechanisms to raise funds to pay for health. In 2021 the OECD average of government funding was 73 per cent of total healthcare spending. Denmark, Norway, Sweden and the UK have over 80 per cent funding through government transfers. Germany, the Netherlands and Japan have a higher percentage of funding through social insurance contributions. Even in the US, which has one of the largest private expenditures on healthcare (45 per cent), public healthcare expenditure still accounts for 55 per cent of total health expenditure, with all countries having some form of private funding.

Learning activity 9.2

Consider any emergent trends between the type of expenditure (Figure 9.4) and total expenditure on health as a percentage of GDP (Table 9.2). Do countries that rely heavily on general government funds tend to have higher or lower spending than those that rely heavily on social security or private funding? Consider why that might be the case and what that means for funding in your country.

If you are interested in exploring trends in health system expenditure, finance and performance then do take a look at the OECD Data Explorer: https://www.oecd.org/health/health-data.htm

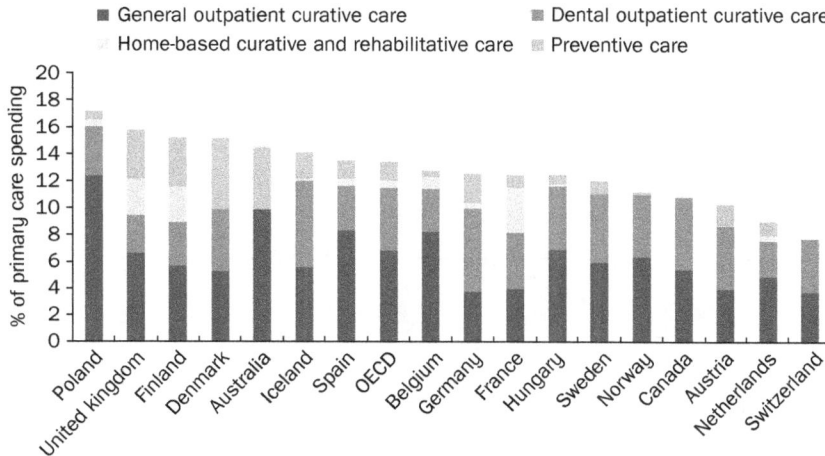

■ General outpatient curative care   ■ Dental outpatient curative care
■ Home-based curative and rehabilitative care   ■ Preventive care

Figure 9.5 Primary care health services spending as a share of health expenditure 2021
Source: Data from OECD (2023a).

The way funds are allocated across the health system varies between countries. Generally, funds are allocated to hospital care, primary care, mental health, preventive care, research and development, infrastructure and administration. While spending on primary care is often seen as the cornerstone of an effective and efficient health system (Hanson et al., 2023), spending on primary care as a share of total health expenditure is 13 per cent across OECD countries (see Figure 9.5). Poland, the UK, Finland and Denmark have the highest spend (above 15 per cent) and the Netherlands and Switzerland have less than 10 per cent. The majority of spending in primary care is on general management and care services, then dental services, then prevention services, with home visits having a smaller share of funding.

Other aspects of efficient funding models relate to administrative efficiency, which refers to how well a system reduces its bureaucratic tasks. This can be achieved by simplifying billing, insurance coverage, and so on. According to the Commonwealth Fund (Schneider et al., 2021) the most administratively efficient systems are Australia, New Zealand, Norway and the UK, with the US ranking last. Despite the introduction of the Affordable Care Act aimed at increasing insurance coverage and subsidies for US citizens, the US is the only high-income country with a substantial portion of the uninsured population, 8.6 per cent in 2021 (Gunja et al., 2023).

The global economic crisis and COVID-19

The global economic crisis of 2008 and the COVID-19 pandemic are two major economic shocks that impacted healthcare funding and delivery. The global economic crisis had a major impact across the world and is considered to have been the worst financial crisis since the 1930s. The impact was felt worst across a number of European countries and the USA, with spending growth maintained in the short term before dipping to just above zero as public measures aimed at curbing spending started to take effect in 2010–12, with all countries seeing a reduction in health spending during that period (see Figure 9.6).

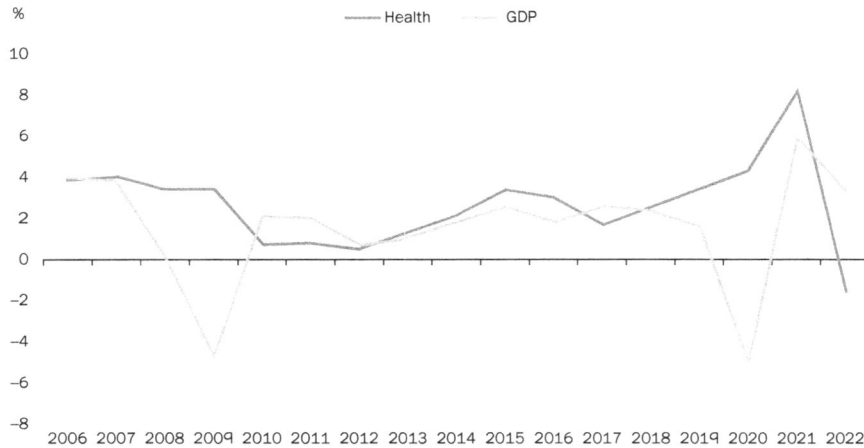

Figure 9.6 Annual real growth rate in per capita health expenditure and GDP, OECD, 2006–22
Source: Data from OECD (2023a).

The reduction in spending was largely driven by cuts in public spending. In Ireland health spending fell by 7.6 per cent in 2010, compared with a growth rate of around 8.4 per cent between 2000–2009. Estonia had seen a growth rate or around 7 per cent year on year from 2000–2009, yet expenditure fell by around 7 per cent in 2010 (OECD, 2012). Governments continued to maintain health spending growth through to 2012 using a variety of policy initiatives including:

- Cuts in wages or fees paid to professionals and reductions in the number of health workers (this was evident in Ireland)
- Cutting Ministry of Health budgets (Bulgaria, Cyprus, Czech Republic, Estonia, Finland, France, Greece, Iceland, Ireland, Italy, Portugal, Romania, Serbia, Slovenia, Spain, UK)
- Efficiency gains pursued through mergers of hospitals or ministries or accelerating the move from in-patient hospitalization towards outpatient care and day surgery
- Negotiation on reduced prices paid to pharmaceutical industries and increase in the use of generic drugs
- Investment plans were put on hold in several countries, including Estonia, Ireland, Iceland and Czech Republic
- Increase in out-of-pocket payments. For example, Ireland increased the share of direct payments by households for prescribed medicines and appliances, while the Czech Republic increased users' charges for hospital stays.

(Adapted from OECD, 2012 and Thomson et al., 2014)

From 2012 until the pandemic there was growth in both healthcare spending and GDP, but the impact of the pandemic, including lockdowns and other public health measures led to a decrease in GDP. While health spending increased from 4 per cent in 2020 to 8 per cent in 2021, this was due to the funding allocated to tackling the pandemic (OECD, 2023a). The funding increase was allocated to funding public health prevention, focused on emergency measures (including testing, surveillance and vaccination programmes), rather than long-term, planned public health programmes (OECD, 2023a). During the COVID-19 pandemic, there was a decline in spending on voluntary insurance due to reduced demand and the post-ponement of elective surgery (Australian Institute of Health and Welfare, 2023).

Economic shocks demonstrate the importance of policy design of healthcare financing. For example, Greece had no 'reserves or countercyclical formulas to compensate the health insurance system for falling revenue from payroll taxes, and Ireland had no countercycli-cal formula to cover a huge increase in the share of the population entitled to means-tested benefits' (Thomson et al., 2014: 229). Furthermore, countries with the highest out-of-pocket expenses had significant gaps in coverage during the economic crisis and tended to have the least potential to cut public spending without having major issues on access to health ser-vices (Thomson et al., 2014).

Funding pressures

There are several pressures that drive healthcare expenditure including changing demo-graphics and disease patterns, and other non-demographic factors related to a variety of aspects including the income of a country (as economies grow so does the spend on health). Other non-demographic aspects include rising prices and technological developments, and climate change, as well as the policy and structure of health systems. For example, hospitals are costly drivers of care and evidence predicts that more efficient systems have a strong pri-mary care function (see Chapter 13 for further discussion on primary care). In addition, the current fragile economic and geopolitical climate and the lingering impacts of COVID-19 are all set to put increased pressure on healthcare costs and spending (OECD, 2024b).

The global pandemic highlighted the need for health system resilience and agility to respond to health shocks. Key areas here include strengthening digital transformation and workforce investment aimed at training and retention, which reflects the benefits of a healthy population that go beyond health system performance and are at the heart of strong and healthy economies (OECD, 2024b).

The success of health systems means people are living longer, and chronic diseases like diabetes and heart disease are increasing, along with some of the associated risk fac-tors, such as being overweight and obese. Community expectations around access and affordability have also increased. On the supply side, there has been a major increase in the use of expensive new technology; while new treatments could be cost-effective, if the prevalence of the condition they treat is high then financial sustainability could be a major concern (OECD, 2017). The rise in expensive technology means that policymakers are under increasing pressure to make efficient use of resources, while ensuring equitable access and provision (see Chapter 10 for further discussion on healthcare economics and Chapter 11 for priority setting).

The increased demand for healthcare means an increase in the workforce capacity for decades to come. The US workforce projections forecast the health and social assistance sectors to see the largest workforce growth than any other sector (BLS, 2023). Current global labour shortages are leading to increased healthcare costs due to the competitive labour market and health services needing to rely on more expensive contract labour to meet staffing demands (Lagasse, 2023).

Other pressures include the impacts of climate change on the population, including the health issues and the devastation caused by extreme weather events and the impacts of high-carbon healthcare and policy around net-zero decarbonization of the health sector (see Chapter 12). The latter will involve funding targeted at infrastructure improvements to healthcare buildings and other assets. A recent audit of nitrous oxide purchasing in Australia indicated that between 70–90 per cent is being leaked from hospital pipes (Murray, 2023). A study by Malik et al. (2018) demonstrated that the majority of healthcare emissions come from supply chains involved in the manufacturing, distribution and provision of healthcare services.

While digitalization of healthcare systems is seen as a mechanism to transform health systems and improve performance and outcomes (OECD, 2023b), there are a number of financial pressures to consider, including infrastructure and staff training costs, as well as potential costs offset to patients.

How can governments and health leaders respond to funding pressures?

At a macro level there is evidence that universal health insurance coverage is important for healthcare performance. The World Bank, OECD and WHO have led a global push for universal health coverage that ensures all individuals have access to good-quality health services without financial hardship (OECD/European Commission, 2024). Most OECD countries have achieved universal or near-universal coverage for a core set of health services (see OECD/European Commission, 2024 for further discussion). When health is funded through taxation, governments do have the option to raise tax to cover increased costs, although this is not often an election winner. We have seen very few instances when countries have changed the predominate funding model; rather countries tend to look at the ancillary methods to either increase funds or curb spending. Examples include increased out-of-pocket payments. France has introduced increased co-payments for individuals who refuse generic drugs and those who do not use the gatekeeping system (Tikkanen et al., 2020b). However, as noted earlier, these can have a negative impact on patients and deter them from seeking care due to increased out-of-pocket payments. Tax incentives for those taking out voluntary insurance is an option to encourage uptake of voluntary insurance, with mixed success in Australia (Duckett and Nemet, 2019) and the UK (McKenna et al., 2017).

Other mechanisms to curb spending include the use of health technology assessment (HTA) to advise on the cost-effectiveness of new technologies and to negotiate prices with the pharmaceutical industry. Countries have mixed application of HTA and their ability to effectively negotiate technology costs with the pharmaceutical industry (see Chapter 10 for more on HTA and health economics). A number of countries have focused on at reducing low-value care as a way to save costs and drive down spending; examples include the Canadian Choosing Wisely Campaign (2024), which is aimed at reducing unnecessary tests and treatments.

Many funding reforms typically concentrate on allocations of funds within the healthcare system. The implementation of activity-based funding is largely focused on encouraging attention to the cost of healthcare activities. However, a system that incentivizes volume and activity may detract from quality and actually increase expenditure and/or decrease a focus on integrated care when payment follows the patient. More recently there has been a shift in focus from volume to value with a focus on value-based financing that emphasizes the focus on patient-centred care. However, operationalizing in practice poses challenges, including defining and measuring value effectively (Zanotto et al., 2021). Other models include blended funding that incorporates both capitation and value-based funding approaches with agreed outcomes and risks shared across organizations (see Schroeder and Cutler, 2021 and Hegde and Haddock, 2019 for further discussion). Value-based funding models require high-quality data for costing and resource usage, patient characteristics to support risk-adjusted funding and relevant outcomes to reward good practice (Schroeder and Cutler, 2021).

In conclusion, there is no perfect funding system, all carry inherent risks and incentivize positive and negative behaviours. As health managers it is important to understand the current funding arrangements at health system and organizational level and consider how these impact on performance. Funding reform is often seen as a mechanism to curb spending, however, before embarking on reform, consideration of other policy levers should be considered.

Learning activity 9.3 Journal club focused on value-based healthcare moving from volume to value

Journal clubs are a great way to read published work and explore views with colleagues. The articles below are focused on value-based healthcare funding and the questions are a guide to aid discussion.

There has been a shift in focus from volume to value with value-based health care, the concept that emphasizes rewarding quality outcomes and cost-effective care, steering away from traditional fee-for-service funding models.

Read the following articles on value-based healthcare and consider the questions posed below:

- Hegde and Haddock (2019) Re-orienting funding from volume to value in public dental health services Deeble issues Brief No 32 https://apo.org.au/node/241086
- Hurst, L. et al., (2019) Defining Value-based Healthcare in the NHS: CEBM report May 2019. https://www.cebm.net/2019/04/defining-value-based-healthcare-in-the-nhs/

Continued

Learning activity 9.3 *Continued*

1   Discuss the challenges and barriers that healthcare providers may encounter when adopting value-based healthcare.
2   Talk to colleagues and share thoughts on implementing value-based healthcare funding approaches and the impact on patient outcomes, care quality and financial sustainability.
3   What would need to change in how services are currently funded?
4   Consider the future of value-based funding and how emerging trends, such as digital technology and environmental challenges, may shape the landscape of healthcare financing.

Write an action plan, identifying potential opportunities for applying value-based concepts, outlining strategies for overcoming challenges, and propose ways to measure the impact of value-based funding on patient care and organizational performance.

Learning resources

The Commonwealth Fund: This New York-based research foundation aims to promote a high-performing healthcare system, particularly for the most vulnerable in society. As such, it has a strong focus the performance of health systems and considers issues around the efficiency and equity of health funding. They also have a section specifically outlining a number of healthcare system profiles that include information on health funding [www.commonwealthfund.org] and [www.commonwealthfund.org/international-health-policy-center/system-profiles].

Organisation for Economic Co-operation and Development (OECD): An excellent resource for healthcare funding information – it collates and analyses data on healthcare funding activity across OECD countries. It provides comparative analysis around expenditure and performance of health systems. It is committed to ensuring that economic and social aspects are taken into account [http://www.oecd.org]. For OECD data go to [https://data.oecd.org].

European Observatory on Health Systems and Policies: The European Observatory European Observatory on Health Systems and Policies is another excellent resource that provides comprehensive information on health system structures and performance including funding. They have country profiles and summaries for most European countries

[https://eurohealthobservatory.who.int/about-us/overview].

World Health Organization: The WHO produces report and analyses on healthcare expenditure and performance [www.who.int/about/en].

World in data: Excellent freely available resource World in Data's mission is to 'publish the *research and data to make progress against the world's largest problems*' [https://ourworldindata.org/financing-healthcare].

References

Australian Institute of Health and Welfare (2023) Governments spent more, individuals spent less, on health care during 2021–22 Australian Institute of Health and Welfare [https://www.aihw.gov.au/news-media/media-releases/2023/2023-october/governments-spent-more-individuals-spent-less-on-health-care-during-2021-22; accessed 4 December 2024].

Australian Medical Association (2023) *The AMA Repeat Prescription for Private Health Insurance* [https://www.ama.com.au/articles/ama-repeat-prescription-private-health-insurance; accessed 4 December 2024].

Abimbola, S., Baatiema, L. and Bigdeli, M. (2019) The impacts of decentralization on health system equity, efficiency and resilience: a realist synthesis of the evidence, *Health Policy Plan*, 34(8): 605–617. https://doi.org/10.1093/heapol/czz055.

Anandaciva, S. (2023) *How does the NHS compare to health care systems of other countries*. The King's Fund [https://www.kingsfund.org.uk/insight-and-analysis/reports/nhs-compare-health-care-systems-other-countries; accessed 4 December 2024].

Anderson, G. (2009) The effects of payment by results, *British Medical Journal*, 339, b3081. https://doi.org/10.1136/bmj.b3081.

Ashish, K. (2013) Time to get serious about pay for performance, *Journal of the American Medical Association*, 309(4): 347–348. doi:10.1001/jama.2012.196646.

Baicker, K. and Chernew, M.E. (2017) Alternative payment models, *Journal of the American Medical Association Internal Medicine*, 177(2): 222–223. doi:10.1001/jamainternmed.2016.8280.

Barber, S.L., Lorenzoni, L. and Ong, P. (2019) *Price setting and price regulation in health care: lessons for advancing Universal Health Coverage*. Geneva: World Health Organization, Organisation for economic Co-operation and Development [https://iris.who.int/bitstream/handle/10665/325547/9789241515924-eng.pdf?sequence=1&isAllowed=y; accessed 4 December 2024].

Berenson, R.A., Upadhyay, D.K., Delbanco, S.F. and Murray, R. (2016) *Payment Methods: How They Work*. Washington, DC: Urban Institute.

BLS (2023) *Occupational employment projections, 2022-32*, U.S. Bureau of Labor Statistics [https://www.bls.gov/emp/; accessed 4 December 2024].

Blümel, M., Spranger, A., Achstetter, K., Maresso, A. and Busse, R. (2020) Germany: health system review, *Health Systems in Transition*, 22(6): 1–273 [https://pubmed.ncbi.nlm.nih.gov/34232120/; accessed 4 December 2024].

Buchmueller, T.C. and Couffinhal, A. (2004) *Private health insurance in France. OECD Working Papers 12*. Paris: Organisation for Economic Co-operation and Development [https://www.oecd.org/en/publications/private-health-insurance-in-france_555485381821.html; accessed 4 December 2024].

Canadian Choosing Wisely Campaign (2024) [https://choosingwiselycanada.org/about/; accessed 4 December 2024].

Carrin, G. and Hanvoravongchai, P. (2003) Provider payments and patient charges as policy tools for cost-containment: how successful are they in high-income countries? *Human Resources for Health*, 1(1): 6. https://doi.org/10.1186/1478-4491-1-6.

Chambers, S. (2020) Why the economic aspects of healthcare are not unique, *Sultan Qaboos University Medical Journal*, 20(2): e165–e172. https://doi.org/10.18295/squmj.2020.20.02.006.

Cheng, T.C. (2014) Measuring the effects of reducing subsidies for private insurance on public expenditure for health care, *Journal of Health Economics*, 33: 159–79. https://doi.org/10.1016/j.jhealeco.2013.11.007.

Collier, R. (2008) Activity-based hospital funding: boon or boondoggle? *CMAJ*, 178(11): 1407–1408. https://doi.org/10.1503/cmaj.080594.

Cylus, J., Papanicolas, I. and Smith, P.C. (2017) *How to make sense of health system efficiency comparisons?* European Observatory on Health Systems and Policies [https://www.ncbi.nlm.nih.gov/books/NBK493379/; accessed 4 December 2024].

Doherty, R.B. (2010) The certitudes and uncertainties of health care reform, *Annals of Internal Medicine*, 152: 679–682 [https://pubmed.ncbi.nlm.nih.gov/20378676/; accessed 4 December 2024].

Dredge, R. (2004) *Hospital global budgeting*, HNP Discussion Paper [https://www.researchgate.net/publication/228646960_Hospital_Global_Budgeting; accessed 4 December 2024].

Duckett, S. and Nemet, K. (2019) *The history and purposes of private health insurance*, Grattan Institute [https://grattan.edu.au/wp-content/uploads/2019/07/918-The-history-and-purposes-of-private-health-insurance.pdf; accessed 4 December 2024].

Eckermann, S. (2014) Avoiding a health system hernia and the associated outcomes and costs, *Australian and New Zealand Journal of Public Health*, 38: 303–305. https://doi.org/10.1111/1753-6405.12277.

European Commission (2016, October) *Joint report on health care and long-term care systems & fiscal sustainability*. Directorate-General for Economic and Financial Affairs [https://data.europa.eu/doi/10.2765/776073; accessed 4 December 2024].

European Observatory (2024) *Country overview*. European Observatory on Health Systems and Policies [https://eurohealthobservatory.who.int/overview; accessed 4 December 2024].

Farrar, S., Sussex, J., Yi, D., Sutton, M., Chalkley, M., Scott, A. et al. (2007) *National Evaluation of Payment by Results*. York: Health Economics Research Unit.

Farrar, S., Yi, D., Sutton, M., Chalkley, M., Sussex, J. and Scott, A. (2009) Has payment by results affected the way that English hospitals provide care? Difference in differences analysis, *British Medical Journal*, 339, b3047 (https://doi.org/10.1136/bmj.b3047).

Fiebig, D.G., Gool, K. van, Hall, J. and Mu, C. (2021) Health care use in response to health shocks: does socio-economic status matter? *Health Economics* (United Kingdom), 30(12): 3032–3050. ISSN: 10991050. doi: 10.1002/hec.4427.

Gundgaard J. (2006) Income-related inequality in utilization of health services in Denmark: evidence from Funen County, *Scandinavian Journal of Public Health*, 34(5): 462–471. doi:10.1080/14034940600554644.

Gunja, M.Z., Gumas, E.D. and Williams R.D (II) (2023) U.S. Health Care from a Global Perspective, 2022: Accelerating Spending, Worsening Outcomes, *Commonwealth Fund* (https://doi.org/10.26099/8ejy-yc74).

Hanson, K., Brikci, N., Erlangga, D., Alebachew, A., De Allegri, M., Balabanova, D., et al. (2023) The Lancet Global Health Commission on financing primary health care: putting people at the centre, *The Lancet Global Health*, 10(5): e715-e772. https://doi.org/10.1016/S2214-109X(22)00005-5.

Health Policy Consensus Group (2005) *Options for Healthcare Funding.* London: Institute for the Study of Civil Society [https://civitas.org.uk/pdf/hpcgSystems.pdf; accessed 4 December 2024].

Hegde, S. and Haddock, R. (2019) Re-orienting funding from volume to value in public dental health services Deeble Institute issues Brief No 32 [https://apo.org.au/node/241086; accessed 4 December 2024].

Holman, H.R. (2020) The relation of the chronic disease epidemic to the health care crisis, *ACR Open Rheumatology*, 2(3): 167–173. https://doi.org/10.1002/acr2.11114.

Hurst, J. and L. Siciliani (2003) *Tackling excessive waiting times for elective surgery: a comparison of policies in twelve OECD countries*, OECD Health Working Papers, No. 6, OECD Publishing, Paris. https://doi.org/10.1787/108471127058.

Institute of Medicine (US) (2001) *Crossing the Quality Chasm: A New Health System for the 21st Century.* Washington, DC: The National Academies Press. https://doi.org/10.17226/10027.

Joumard, I., André, C. and Nicq, C. (2010) *Health care systems: efficiency and institutions*, OECD Economics Department Working Papers, No. 769, OECD Publishing. https://doi.org/10.1787/18151973.

Kjerstad, E.M. (2003) Prospective funding of general hospitals in Norway – incentives for higher production?, *International Journal of Health Care Finance and Economics*, 3(4): 231–251 [https://pubmed.ncbi.nlm.nih.gov/14650078/; accessed 4 December 2024].

Klumpes, P. and Tang, L. (2008) *The cost incidence of the U.K.'s NHS System, Geneva papers on risk and insurance - issues and practice*, 33: 744–767. https://doi.org/10.1057/gpp.2008.29.

Kos, M. (2019) Introduction to healthcare systems, in F. Alves da Costa, J.W.F., van Mil and A. Alvarez-Risco (eds) (2019) *The Pharmacist Guide to Implementing Pharmaceutical Care*, Springer International Publishing.

Lagasse, J. (2023) *Hospitals' labor costs increased 258% over the last three years.* Healthcare Finance HIMSS Media [https://www.healthcarefinancenews.com/news/hospitals-labor-costs-increased-258-over-last-three-years; accessed 4 December 2024].

Malik, A., Lenzen, M., McAlister, S. and McGain, F. (2018) The carbon footprint of Australian health care, *Lancet Planet Health*, 2(1): e27–e35. doi: 10.1016/S2542-5196(17)30180-8. Epub 2018 Jan 9. PMID: 29615206.

McDaid, D. (2003) Who pays? Approaches to funding health care in Europe, *Consumer Policy Review*, 13(5): 166–172 [https://www.proquest.com/trade-journals/who-pays-approaches-funding-healthcare-europe/docview/219277412/se-2; accessed 4 December 2024].

McKenna, H., Dunn, P., Northern, E. and Buckley, T. (2017) *How health care is funded.* The King's Fund [https://www.kingsfund.org.uk/insight-and-analysis/long-reads/how-health-care-is-funded; accessed 4 December 2024].

Mossialos, E., Dixon, A., Figueras, J. and Kutzin, J. (eds) (2002) *Funding Healthcare: Options for Europe.* Maidenhead: Open University Press.

Mossialos, E., Wenz M., Osborn, R. and Anderson, C. (2015) *International profiles of health care systems.* Commonwealth Fund [https://www.commonwealthfund.org/sites/default/files/documents/___media_files_publications_fund_report_2016_jan_1857_mossialos_intl_profiles_2015_v7.pdf; accessed 4 December 2024].

Mueller, M., Hagenaars, L. and Morgan, D. (2017) *Administrative spending in OECD health care systems: Where is the fat and can it be trimmed?*, OECD, Tackling Wasteful Spending on Health, OECD Publishing, Paris. https://doi.org/10.1787/9789264266414-en.

Murray, V. (2023) *Sustainability in healthcare: reflections from advocacy leaders*, AMA Vic DOC Magazine, December 2023.

OECD (2004) *Private health insurance in OECD countries.* OECD, Paris, (15). https://doi.org/10.1787/18152015.

OECD (2012) *Health: growth in health spending grinds to a halt* [https://web-archive.oecd.org/2013-06-27/198647-healthgrowthinhealthspendinggrindstoahalt.htm; accessed 4 December 2024].

OECD (2017*) New health technologies: managing access, value and sustainability.* OECD Publishing, Paris. https://doi.org/10.1787/9789264266438-en.

OECD (2023a) *Health at a glance 2023: OECD indicators*, OECD Publishing, Paris. https://doi.org/10.1787/7a7afb35-en.

OECD (2023b) *Digitalisation of health systems can significantly improve performance and outcomes* [https://www.oecd.org/newsroom/digitalisation-of-health-systems-can-significantly-improve-performance-and-outcomes.htm; accessed 4 December 2024].

OECD (2024a) *OECD data gross domestic product* [https://data.oecd.org/gdp/gross-domestic-product-gdp.htm; accessed 4 December 2024].

OECD (2024b) *Fiscal sustainability of health systems: how to finance more resilient health systems when money is tight?*, OECD Publishing, Paris. https://doi.org/10.1787/880f3195-en.

OECD/European Commission (2024) Population coverage for healthcare, in *Health at a Glance: Europe 2024: State of Health in the EU Cycle*, OECD Publishing, Paris. https://doi.org/10.1787/9e61579e-en.

Or, Z., Gandré, C., Seppänen, A.V., Hernández-Quevedo, C., Webb, E., Michel, M., et al. (2023) France: health system review, *Health Systems in Transition*, 2023; 25(3): i–241**.** [https://iris.who.int/bitstream/handle/10665/371027/9789289059442-eng.pdf?sequence=4].

O'Reilly, J., Busse, R., Häkkinen, U., Or, Z., Street A. and Wiley, M. (2012) Paying for hospital care: the experience with implementing activity-based funding in five European countries, *Health Economics, Policy and Law*, 7(1): 73–101.73101. https://doi.org/10.1017/S1744133111000314.

Paris, V., Devaux, M. and Wei, L. (2010) Health systems institutional characteristics: a survey of 29 OECD countries, in *Health Systems Institutional Characteristics: A Survey of 29 OECD Countries*, OECD Publishing [https://www.oecd.org/content/dam/oecd/en/publications/

reports/2010/04/health-systems-institutional-characteristics_g17a1e51/5kmfxfq9qbnr-en. pdf; accessed 4 December 2024].

Pickett, K. and Wilkinson, R. (2010) *The Spirit Level: Why More Equal Societies Almost Always Do Better*. London, Penguin [https://www.researchgate.net/publication/257664917_Richard_Wilkinson_and_Kate_Pickett_2009_The_Spirit_Level_Why_More_Equal_Societies_Almost_Always_Do_Better_Allen_Lane_London; accessed 4 December 2024].

Ping Yu, C., Whynes, D.K. and Sach, T.H. (2008) Equity in health care financing: the case of Malaysia, *International Journal for Equity in Health*, 7(15). https://doi.org/10.1186/1475-9276-7-15.

Porter, M.E. and Thomas, L.H. (2013) The strategy that will fix health care, *Harvard Business Review*, 91(10): 50–70 [https://hbr.org/2013/10/the-strategy-that-will-fix-health-care; accessed 4 December 2024].

Pulok, M.H., van Gool, K. and Hall, J. (2020) Horizontal inequity in the utilisation of healthcare services in Australia, *Health Policy*, 124(11): 1263–1271. https://doi.org/10.1016/j.healthpol.2020.08.012.

Rosenthal, M.B., Frank, R.G., Li, Z. and Epstein, A.M. (2005) Early experience with pay-for-performance: from concept to practice, *Journal of the American Medical Association*, 294: 1788–1793.

Rotulo, A., Paraskevopoulou, C. and Kondilis, E. (2022) The effects of health sector fiscal decentralisation on availability, accessibility, and utilisation of healthcare services: a panel data analysis, *International Journal of Health Policy Management*, 11(11): 2440–2450. doi: 10.34172/ijhpm.2021.163.

Saltman, R.B. and Dubois, H.F.W. (2004) Individual incentive schemes in social health insurance systems, *Eurohealth*, 10(2): 21–25.

Saltman, R.B., Reinhard, B. and Figueras, J. (eds) (2004) Social health insurance systems in western Europe, in *European Observatory on Health Systems and Policies Series*. Oxford: Oxford University Press.

San Sebastián, M., Mosquera, P.A., Ng, N. and Gustafsson, P.E. (2017) Health care on equal terms? Assessing horizontal equity in health care use in Northern Sweden, *European Journal of Public Health*, Aug 1; 27(4): 637–643. doi: 10.1093/eurpub/ckx031. PMID: 28340208.

Savedoff, W. (2004) *Tax-based financing for health systems: options and experiences*, discussion paper number 4, Geneva, WHO [https://iris.who.int/handle/10665/69022; accessed 4 December 2024].

Schneider, E.C., Shah, S., Doty, M., Tikkanen, R., Fields, K. and Williams II, R.D. (2021) *Mirror, mirror 2021 — reflecting poorly: health care in the U.S. compared to other high-income countries*, Commonwealth Fund [https://www.commonwealthfund.org/publications/fund-reports/2021/aug/mirror-mirror-2021-reflecting-poorly; accessed 4 December 2024].

Schroeder, L. and Cutler, H. (2021) Changing invisible landscapes - financial reform of health and care systems: ten issues to consider, *International Journal of Integrated Care*, Nov 18; 21(4): 21. doi: https://ijic.org/articles/10.5334/ijic.6461. PMID: 34824570; PMCID: PMC8603852.

Shomaker, S.T. (2010) Health care payment reform and academic medicine: threat or opportunity? *Academic Medicine*, 85(5): 756–758. doi: 10.1097/ACM.0b013e3181d0fdfb.

Smith, P.C. and Witter, S.N. (2004) *Risk Pooling in Health Care Financing: The Implications for Health System Performance.* HNP Discussion paper, Washington: World Bank Organization [www.researchgate.net/publication/228590900_Risk_Pooling_in_Health_Care_Financing_The_Implications_for_Health_System_Performance; accessed 26 February 2025].

Street, A., Vitikainen, K., Bjorvatn, A. and Hvenegaard, A. (2007) *Introducing Activity-Based Financing: A Review of Experience in Australia, Denmark, Norway and Sweden.* CHE [https://www.researchgate.net/publication/5004030_Introducing_Activity-based_Financing_A_Review_of_Experience_in_Australia_Denmark_Norway_and_Sweden; accessed 4 December 2024].

Struijk, J.N., de Vries, E.F., Baan, C.A., van Gils, P.F. and Rosenthal, M.B. (2020) Bundled-payment models around the world: how they work and what their impact has been, *Commonwealth Fund.* https://doi.org/10.26099/936s-0y65.

Tamblyn, R.R., Laprise, R., Hanley, J.A., Abrahamowicz, M., Scott, S., Mayo, N., et al. (2001) Adverse events associated with prescription drug cost sharing among poor and elderly persons, *Journal of the American Medical Association*, 285(4): 421–429. doi:10.1001/jama.285.4.421.

Thomson, S., Foubister, T. and Mossialos, E. (2010) Can user charges make health care more efficient?, *British Medical Journal*, 341, c3759. https://doi.org/10.1136/bmj.c3759.

Thomson, S., Figueras, J., Evetovits, T., Jowett, M., Mladovsky, P., Maresso, A., et al. (2014) *Economic crisis, health systems and health in Europe: impact and implications for policy*, Policy summary 12, Denmark, World Health Organization [https://pubmed.ncbi.nlm.nih.gov/28837306/; accessed 4 December 2024].

Tikkanen, R., Osborn, R., Mossialos, E., Djordjevic, A. and Wharton, G.A. (2020a) *International Health Care System Profiles: Denmark*, The Commonwealth Fund [https://www.commonwealthfund.org/international-health-policy-center/countries/denmark; accessed 4 December 2024].

Tikkanen, R., Osborn, R., Mossialos, E., Djordjevic, A. and Wharton, G.A. (2020b) *International Health Care System Profiles: France* [The Commonwealth Fund [https://www.commonwealthfund.org/international-health-policy-center/countries/france; accessed 4 December 2024].

Toth, F. (2021) *Comparative Health Systems: A New Framework.* Cambridge: Cambridge University Press. doi:10.1017/9781108775397.

Van Doorslaer, E., Savage, E. and Hall, J. (2008) Horizontal inequities in Australia's mixed public/private health care system, *Health Policy*, 86(1), 97–108 (https://doi.org/10.1016/j.healthpol.2007.09.018).

Wagstaff, A. (2010) Social health insurance reexamined, *Health Economics*, 19: 503–517. https://doi.org/10.1002/hec.1492.

Wagstaff, A. and van Doorslaer, E. (2000) Equity in healthcare finance and delivery, in A.J. Culyer and J.P. Newhouse (eds). *Handbook of health economics part one*, pp. 1803–1862, Amsterdam: Elsevier.

Wickens, C. and Brown, T. (2023) *The NHS in crisis – evaluating the radical alternatives.* The King's Fund. [https://www.kingsfund.org.uk/insight-and-analysis/long-reads/nhs-crisis-evaluating-radical-alternatives; accessed 4 December 2024].

Wilper, A.P., Woolhandler, S., Lasser, K.E., McCormick, D., Bor, D.H. and Himmelstein, D.U. (2009) Health insurance and mortality in US Adults, *American Journal of Public Health*, 99(12): 1–7. doi: 10.2105/AJPH.2008.157685.

Van der Zee, J. and Kroneman, M.N. (2007) Bismarck or Beveridge: a beauty contest between dinosaurs, *BMC Health Services Research*, 7(94). https://doi.org/10.1186/1472-6963-7-94.

The White House (2024) *Record Marketplace Coverage in 2024: A Banner Year for Coverage.* [https://www.whitehouse.gov/cea/written-materials/2024/01/24/record-marketplace-coverage-in-2024-a-banner-year-for-coverage/; accessed 21 April 2024].

World Health Organization (2021) *Global expenditure on health: public spending on the rise?* Geneva: World Health Organization; 2021. Licence: CC BY-NC-SA 3.0 IGO.

Zanotto, B.S., Etges, A.P.B.D.S., Marcolino, M.A.Z. and Polanczyk C.A. (2021) Value-based healthcare initiatives in practice: a systematic review, *Journal of Healthcare Management*, Jun 29; 66(5): 340–365. doi: 10.1097/JHM-D-20-00283; PMID: 34192716; PMCID: PMC8423138.

Zhang, X., Lin, D., Pforsich, H. and Lin, V.W. (2020) Physician workforce in the United States of America: forecasting nationwide shortages, *Human Resources for Health*, 18(1): 8. doi: 10.1186/s12960-020-0448-3.

The economics of healthcare

Richard Lewis and Matthew Bell

Introduction

Healthcare spending in higher income countries represents a large proportion of gross domestic product (GDP). For most countries in Europe, North America, Australia and New Zealand spending in 2022 was well over 10 per cent of GDP, and in the USA it was around 16.6 per cent of GDP (OECD, 2023). The willingness to pay for improved health in wealthier countries may reflect the priority put on increasing healthy lives once many other needs have been met. Nevertheless, at current levels, the demands for health spending are starting to put significant constraints on household and government spending in other important areas, from education to housing. Furthermore, many of these other areas might have a direct impact on health. For example, investment in improved housing conditions may lead to better health for some.

Aggregate spending on health and choices about how to finance it are discussed in Chapter 9. However, that aggregate amount is made up of millions of individual decisions about what to treat and how much to pay for treatment. Those decisions are shaped by government and, in some systems, insurer policies. The decisions can result in pressure to increase total spending or can help to improve efficiency and outcomes in such a way that pressures on spending are reduced. This chapter focuses on those millions of individual decisions, the role of government and insurers in influencing these resource allocation decisions, and how to determine prices to support an efficient and effective health system.

Economic theory of health and healthcare

In economic textbooks markets 'clear' at the price where supply equals demand: the market price is the point at which all goods produced are sold and suppliers (businesses) have no interest in supplying more, demanders (consumers) have no interest in consuming more. If prices were to rise there would be more production but less demand; if prices were to fall there would be more demand but less production: the market clearing price signals the 'equilibrium' (Varian, 2014).

Implicit in this, simplified characterization of markets is that all sides agree on the quality of the good in question. From staplers to sweaters, apples to automobiles, the price that consumers agree to pay (and businesses to supply) reflects an agreed level of quality. The same product (whether a car or an apple) may have several prices reflecting different levels of quality but consumers will, to a reasonable degree, be able to decide whether to pay more for a higher quality version or less for a lower quality version.

That breaks down when it comes to healthcare (and some other goods, like education). It is very difficult for a typical consumer of healthcare services to judge whether they have received good or bad care. It is more difficult when the care is designed to have an impact over a longer period of time without complete certainty about the result (e.g. to reduce the risk of death from cancer or a heart attack, or to reduce levels of depression compared to what might otherwise have been experienced without the treatment).

The economics of health and healthcare are fundamentally driven by this factor: the difficulty of knowing how well particular treatments work. In some cases, a combination of longstanding experience and speed-of-action make the link between treatment and cure more obvious (e.g. taking an aspirin for a headache). However, in many cases the link between treatment and outcome is sufficiently difficult for the recipient to be sure that they are receiving the quality of treatment they expected. Would someone who dies of cancer have died a year earlier without the treatment they received? Could a mother giving birth have suffered less pain had a different approach been taken by midwives and the wider care team on the day? Did a weight-loss programme prevent a future stroke?

This difference between healthcare as a product and other products that operate in markets was highlighted by Kenneth Arrow (1963), sometimes thought of as the originator of health economics as a discipline. He highlighted, among other things, that the demand function for healthcare as a commodity is unpredictable, that there is considerable uncertainty over the quality of the product and that the behaviour of suppliers may be impacted by considerations such as medical ethics and non-advocacy role. This suggests that standard economic theory may not apply well when considering the healthcare market. A summary of key economic concepts that are used to analyse healthcare in this chapter is provided in Box 10.1.

Box 10.1 Economic concepts used to analyse healthcare systems

Adverse selection: when one participant in the market cannot observe the characteristics of goods or other participants it creates a risk that the wrong (adverse) choices are made.

Creaming: focusing on serving a particular group of patients in order to increase profitability or efficiency. At the extreme, over-provision of services to low-severity patients.

For example, offering insurance only to young adults to avoid the (often) higher costs of children and older people.

Dumping: removal (explicit or implicit) of liability to pay for the procedures of high-cost individuals. For example, insurers or providers refusing to renew coverage for those using a lot of (high-cost) services. (Note: dumping has other meanings outside the health economics literature.)

Externalities: benefits or costs that are not captured in the price. For example, broader well-being improvements from health services that are not reflected in a cost-based price, or the impact of greenhouse gas emissions from the production of medicines that are not reflected in their costs.

Information asymmetry: one participant in the market or exchange has information that another (or others) does not have. For example, patients that do not know or understand the quality of service offered by different providers for the same procedure.

Market failure: when the costs and benefits that are captured in the price of a good or service do not reflect all the costs or benefits of that good or services (e.g. producing a new medicine involves a series of costs included in the price, such as the cost of labour and equipment, but not the greenhouse gas emissions caused by its production).

Moral hazard: situation where one participant in the market or exchange takes on too much risk (or is willing to consume too much of a good) because they do not bear the full cost of the resulting impact(s). For example, those taking out health (or other) insurance then take on too much risk (e.g. participate in high-risk sport) on the basis that the insurance will pay the cost of the consequences.

Payer (also known as payor): the institution paying for health services. This is different in different countries or health systems. In some cases, it is the state, in others it is state-owned bodies and in others it is private insurers, or a mixture of these options.

Skimping: provision of services to patients below the level required to avoid low or negative profitability.

Value (as distinct from cost or price): the value of a service or procedure generally incorporates wider benefits beyond those captured in its (cost-based) price. For example, wider well-being impacts, impacts on the ability to return to work or participate more fully in life. Some approaches to pricing (e.g. based on willingness to pay) might capture some or all of these wider aspects of value. When speaking of value, it is important to define clearly how it is being viewed because it can have different meanings in different contexts.

What are 'prices' in healthcare?

Prices in health systems are often not visible to the consumer of the healthcare services. In many countries people will have paid insurance, which means that the prices of individual procedures are no longer relevant to them (although as we discuss shortly, the insured may face some form of co-payment not directly related to the cost of any treatment). In other countries, the state pays for treatment directly using previously raised taxation and again individuals are not aware of the specific prices. However, demand (and the associated prices) still play an important role in signalling to providers how to allocate their services today, and what investment might be needed to support services in the future.

Where prices are not visible to the consumers (i.e. patients) they may exist and be visible to others, such as insurers (private sector bodies taking on the risks of payments in return for premiums) or commissioners (public bodies who hold the resources for healthcare and contract with providers to deliver them). These bodies (collectively sometimes referred to as 'payers', the term we shall use in this chapter) may pay based on agreed prices once operations or other interventions have been delivered. Even where patients are not aware of the mechanisms by which money flows from payers to providers, those financial flows have real impacts. For example, if the payer has agreed to pay a fixed fee per hip replacement operation, providers will have an incentive to undertake more or fewer hip operations (depending, among other factors, on the return they can earn). Consequently, they could change their behaviour to attract more patients, reduce their costs or take other actions in response to the price signal. Even where prices are not explicitly defined, 'shadow prices' will exist to support 'block payments' (e.g. paying a hospital £50 million a year to maintain an Accident & Emergency department implies a certain price per admission even if that is not defined explicitly). Those shadow prices may also rise or fall depending on levels of demand, efficiency, inflationary pressures and other factors. How prices may (or may not) relate to the costs of providing healthcare is considered in Box 10.2.

Box 10.2 Costs and prices in healthcare

The provision of health services has a cost – such as payments for staff, medicines, equipment and other elements. Who pays that cost and whether (or how) it is reflected in a price differs considerably across health systems.

In systems where individuals or private insurers pay for treatment, there are likely to be prices that (if the market is working effectively) also reflect the cost-of-service provision. In some systems where the state pays for provision, prices may not exist and the state may provide lump sum (or 'block') transfers to health providers to cover their total costs. In other systems where the state pays, prices may be calculated and form part of the method of payment. For example, a price per hip operation or per primary care visit may be calculated (based on identifying the costs of such activity) and then charged back to the state for each procedure or appointment.

In both private and public systems, prices should reflect costs but may not do so if markets are not functioning properly or costs are not calculated accurately. If prices do not reflect costs, there is a risk of inefficiencies in the provision of care: excess profits being earned, or resources being misdirected into the wrong activities. Considerable effort is often required to monitor and verify the link between prices and costs.

In some cases, payers may try to include incentives to make decisions they see as more efficient or to counteract issues created by other parts of the payment system. For example, they may include payments to encourage day surgery rather than inpatient care or, conversely, to agree only to pay a price that discourages particular types of interventions (such as extended lengths of hospital stay).

The relationship between demand, prices and income signals to providers (and payers) how to act; for example, whether to change staffing, invest in new equipment, work harder to prevent illness and so on. Prices, and overall spending, also signal to the ultimate payer whether they are getting value for money and how they should act, potentially including raising insurance premiums or taxes (see Box 10.3). However, the specific characteristics of healthcare markets mean that more elaborate regulatory and other approaches are needed to help meet current and future demand equitably. The rest of this chapter explores how economic factors influence the ability of governments and other funders to achieve the best outcomes in health markets.

Box 10.3   Prices and value in healthcare

Prices are the most common, and effective, way to signal 'value' across all sectors of an economy. In competitive markets, the prices reflect costs of production and the value of the good or service to the person making the purchase.

However, it is well known that this is not always the case. There are many dimensions of value that might not be captured in prices. Most commonly, for example, aspects of pollution (such as greenhouse gas emissions) may not be captured in prices. When it comes to health, the value of someone being healthy to their friends, employers or family may not be fully reflected in the price of care. In these cases, value can be estimated through other means. For example, value might be estimated based on a survey to estimate willingness to pay or a bottom-up calculation that captures the time friends or family spend caring for ill individuals.

In practice, it may be difficult to fully reflect value in prices across healthcare. It is often necessary to understand whether prices are sufficiently reflective or whether other approaches are needed (e.g. moving away from individual prices in some areas of care and covering total costs across many services).

Learning activity 10.1

Write down as many different types of value that might be delivered through health services in your own health system. Are all of these properly 'priced in' or are some of them not taken into account? If so, what measures might you use to fully understand the value created?

Having responded to those questions, discuss with colleagues what 'value' means to them and how you might generate measures to fully understand the value created.

Pricing systems

The consequence of the 'information asymmetry' (where one person has more information than another) between consumers and providers is that prices can only do part of their job of 'clearing the market' for healthcare services (Akerlof, 1970). The difficulty in observing quality creates a risk that prices are too high (resulting in unnecessarily expensive care) or too low (resulting in insufficient or low-quality care). Countries have developed different solutions in response to the challenge of how to allocate healthcare given quality is difficult to observe. The different solutions all have one thing in common: an attempt to replace a relatively uninformed patient with a more informed consumer who is better able to judge the quality of care being received, and thereby the appropriate price to pay. This can be formulated in terms of principal-agent theory in which a principal (e.g. insurer, state) takes some decisions on the part of their agent (the consumer, patient; see Box 10.4). Difficulties can arise where the principal misinterprets or does not know the wishes of the agent (Smith et al., 1997).

These 'better informed' consumers take different forms in different countries. In some countries they are the insurers, in others 'commissioners' of care, and in yet others the Ministry of Health. Any of these can be a part of the public sector, regulated parts of the private sector or some combination of the two. They include Medicare and Medicaid in the US alongside private insurers, various social insurance systems in many European countries and 'commissioners' within integrated care boards in the English system.

Box 10.4   Consumers and patients

Whether or not they pay directly, patients consume the healthcare that is provided. Even where they are not paying directly, they will make choices (e.g. between alternative possible treatments, about timing of treatment and even whether or not to have a recommended treatment) that will reflect their understanding of the information provided to them and a range of other factors (e.g. ease of access to the possible alternatives).

As such, even when patients are not paying directly, they act as a consumer and will influence the final cost of treatment. However, it is also the case that patients will vary greatly in their knowledge and therefore capacity to make informed decisions. This can lead to inequalities in access to care and in outcomes.

Prices still play a role in all of these systems but the aggregation of demand (the purchasing of many procedures by a single insurer or commissioner) creates a better-informed buyer. An insurer/commissioner paying for thousands of cancer treatments or tens of thousands of weight-loss clinical sessions is able to better observe and compare outcomes to decide on the right price, right provider or both, i.e. to act as a principal on behalf of its agents. This does not remove all the challenges (e.g. difficulty of knowing whether some procedures designed to have longer term effects really have the impact suggested), which is why regulation continues to be prevalent in all healthcare systems (e.g. to certify the impact of drugs, to regulate the qualifications of medical professionals, to inspect the quality of hospital services).

Payment models

A range of payment models have been created both across different health systems and within single health systems for different types of care. Some of these guarantee providers a fixed payment per patient's overall care for a period of time ('capitation') and leave providers the freedom to decide what combination of interventions is best. Providers that provide services efficiently or, better still, successfully reduce future health demand for expensive treatments (for example avoiding heart operations by reducing smoking rates) may get to keep more of that payment for themselves. With the right capitation formula everyone could win: payers avoid the costs of expensive treatments, while providers earn more money by avoiding the cost of those treatments and keep a higher share of the guaranteed income (the agreed fee per patient or per head of population) (Emanuel et al., 2021).

In other systems, explicit quality payments may be included in contracts. Providers can earn extra money if patients receive recommended treatments, recover faster from operations or if they promote broader health measures (like smoking cessation or obesity management services). These quality payments help to promote actions by providers that have the effect of reducing the future volume of more expensive interventions. Without these additional quality payments there may be limited incentives on providers to undertake preventative measures because they reduce future demand. However, such payment may have other unintended consequences, such as rewarding physicians primarily in areas where it is easier to set or to achieve quality benchmarks (Mann et al., 2023).

All of these different approaches are an attempt to overcome the previously described information asymmetry that exists because the quality of service offered is difficult for consumers (or patients) to observe. However, they also suffer from disadvantages, or market failures, common to many (non-health) insurance markets: there are risks of 'adverse selection' (only the most ill take out policies, making it difficult for the insurer to spread their risk to healthier or lower-cost patients), and 'moral hazard' (people take less care of their health on the basis that treatment is free when needed) (Keane and Stavrunova, 2014). There are also unintended insurer behaviours that pricing models may create. These are often put under three headings: 'creaming' (over-provision of services to low-severity patients or, at the extreme, only serving relatively healthy, low-cost patients); 'skimping' (under-provision of services to high-severity patients); and 'dumping' (the explicit avoidance of high-severity patients) (Ellis, 1998). (See earlier, Box 10.1 for a summary of these terms.)

Payment models need to be designed with these potential perverse outcomes in mind. Creating currencies and paying based on the volume of each identified operation helps to promote quick, standardized treatments for many people. That might work very well when it comes to cataract surgery but may mean that more complex and less easily defined services are either not done in sufficient quantities or actively avoided because they risk future revenue (e.g. why hurry to discharge patients if you are paid per day spent in hospital – see OECD, 2017).

Capitation systems avoid the desire of providers to drive up volume because they are paid the same per person regardless of the number of operations undertaken. However, they may have the opposite problem of delaying expensive interventions for too long because they use up a significant proportion of the capitated allowance (skimping, creaming or dumping).

Systems may use bespoke quality payments to help moderate some of these risks. In fee-for-service systems these include making additional payments for reducing follow-up appointments or reducing payments for longer than expected inpatient stays. In capitated systems, additional payments may be made for very expensive interventions. These can help but require their own administrative system to clearly define what is being paid for and ensure it is delivered to trigger pay-out. A blended payments approach is often used to combine the advantages of different types of systems. They can combine elements of fee-for-services, quality payments and capitation (for example, see Bell et al., 2021). (See section on 'Primary Care' later for country-specific examples.)

Learning activity 10.2 Finding the optimal payment system

1   Thinking about the payment system operating in your own country's health system:
    a.   Write down the different payment mechanisms that you can identify being used in hospital, community, primary and social care.
    b.   Why do you think that these mechanisms have been selected?
    c.   Does the selection of payment type differ across sector and, if so, why do you think this is?
2   Write down the risks that are inherent in different payment systems (block contracts, fee-for-service, capitation). Can you think of strategies that might be used to counter these risks?

Use of market mechanisms

While many healthcare systems have continued to manage the allocation of resources to healthcare through planning mechanisms organized by government departments or public authorities, there has been increasing interest over the past 30 years in deploying market principles of competition. This has been part of a wider movement known as 'new public management' that evolved particularly in Europe since the 1980s (Hood, 1991). New public management was founded on the belief that unreformed public bureaucracies were inherently inefficient and that efficiency and quality of public services would increase with, among other things, the introduction of private sector management techniques, competition between providers (and sometimes funders) of public services and a reduction in control of services by central government (for example, by disaggregating public sector providers and replacing direct governmental oversight with arms' length regulators).

In the case of healthcare, the principles of new public management were exemplified by:

- Freeing up of providers and purchasers from central government control (e.g. creation of Foundation Trust hospitals in England who had more autonomy over how they spent revenue earned from their treatments).
- Introduction of greater choice for patients over their provider (England over out-of-hospital care, and in Sweden over the choice of general practitioner (GP)).
- Contracting between purchaser and provider to help reach the efficient market equilibrium position described above (e.g. the creation of the purchaser–provider split in the English NHS).
- Choice for patients, in some cases, of their purchasing agent (i.e. an insurer or 'commissioner') to provide incentives to optimize efficiency and quality in the purchasing of care (e.g. choice of insurance provider in the Netherlands or Ireland).

The results of these approaches have been mixed and health systems have often been subject to ongoing reform as governments have sought to alight on the optimal model. Examples of how markets have been applied in practice are given later in this chapter.

Fairness and equity

A final but important consideration for the economics of healthcare systems is how to promote fairness or equity in access to care and in treatment. In private healthcare systems there are usually rules about insurance premiums and accepting new customers that limit discrimination based on health or other status. In public systems, there are usually regulatory measures to try to equalize quality of care between different providers and to mitigate potential inequity between different patient groups. Some elements of payments may also vary explicitly to promote increased quality (e.g. higher salaries for doctors or nurses in more remote, less well-served areas are particularly common in places like Canada with large, thinly populated regions). In the USA, Medicare and Medicaid, among other measures, are designed to support a fairer healthcare system for those without access to insurance. There are many other aspects of fairness that go beyond the scope of this chapter (e.g. individual versus collective responsibility for health in debates, such as whether those who contract cancer from smoking should have to pay for their own care even in taxpayer-funded systems or where to draw the line between cosmetic and health-related procedures in areas like dentistry or weight management).

Putting theory into practice

There are important differences between countries in how they choose to fund the overall provision of health. Those are discussed separately in Chapter 11. In this section we focus on how different countries choose to allocate that funding. As set out in the previous section, the economic principles underpinning efficient resource allocation within healthcare systems are universal. What differs across the globe are the choices made about which of the available tools are selected and who wields them. In this section, we discuss key mechanisms that are an essential part of resource allocation, drawing in particular on examples from the health systems in England (which is organized differently to other parts of the United Kingdom), the Netherlands, the United States of America and Sweden.

Setting currencies and prices

As discussed, prices serve to give signals to providers of care to enable them to develop their service offering. They also inform purchasers of care about the relative cost (and benefit) of different healthcare interventions and of alternative uses of that resource on goods and services outside of the health sector. Hence understanding the price (or costs) of care and developing appropriate currencies to compare between providers is important and has been the subject of considerable work over the last few decades.

In most advanced healthcare systems, hospital-level care has attracted more resources than other care sectors and partly for this reason currencies have been explored earlier and in more depth for hospital care.

Hospital care is high cost and also complex. There are a large number of different procedures with different levels of resource intensity depending on the condition of individual patients. This has led to interest in grouping treatments together to form pricing categories that are similar in clinical management and overall resource use. This trend started in the USA in the 1980s with 'diagnosis-related groups' (DRGs; see Box 10.5) and were later emulated in the UK as healthcare resource groups (HRGs) and in the Netherlands, where they are known as diagnosis treatment combinations (DBCs).

Box 10.5   DRGs

Diagnosis-related groups (DRGs) are a system to categorize patients based on grouping similar diagnoses. It is often done to help determine payments: providers receive the same payment for all patients in the same DRG. They were introduced to help control costs and support more efficient operations; for example, the same payment may be received for treating 'sepsis' regardless of the precise costs of the inputs used to treat each case.

In Sweden DRG-style payments were also introduced in the early 1990s as part of the introduction of market principles to healthcare. However, DRGs have largely been abandoned following an economic crash in 1990–94 and concern over unintended incentives for providers, leading to the subsequent return of hospital planning and global budgeting by regional governments (Janlöv et al., 2023).

By combining related costs of treatment, such as surgery, drugs, inpatient stays and diagnostics among other things, DRG-style prices are intended to prevent cost-inflation through multiple invoicing by providers. Moreover, they provide the opportunity for purchasers to set largely fixed prices based on negotiation or by using a normative approach, such as setting the cost at the sector average.

DRGs therefore have the advantage of setting maximum costs for a given treatment (for example, in the USA, DRGs set costs based on expected treatments replacing a system where hospitals often billed insurers for each day spent in hospital). The cost of the DRG can be market tested – in the Netherlands, the price of many DBCs is negotiable (currently representing about 70 per cent of hospital care) (Kroneman et al., 2016), or they can be determined by the payer based on an assessment of a reasonable cost. In England, for example, prices were introduced based on 'reference costs' that reflected average costs across hospitals adjusted for local factors (such as differences in local property costs or wages). These prices were then adjusted to reflect an expected level of productivity improvement by providers (Appleby et al., 2012).

However, it is notable that in England (as in Sweden), since the mid-2010s, there has been a significant shift away from HRG-based payments as the system has moved from a competitive market towards a more planned and collaborative approach. This has reintroduced 'block contracts' where global budgets are agreed (albeit underpinned by real or indicative activity levels), which perhaps reflects a shift in attention, during the period of austerity of the 2010s, from access to planned care to ensuring that health systems coordinated care to reduce unnecessary hospital admissions through better disease management (Lewis, 2019).

Other examples of a shift to greater focus on managing the health of the population, (or wellbeing of the individual), and away from treating each episode of care on a case-by-case basis, can be seen in the development of 'accountable care organizations' in the USA (Barnes et al., 2014), and the ongoing shift to population health in England and elsewhere. Central to population health management is more focus on prevention and, thereby, on primary care services.

Primary care

Primary care services are generally delivered with no restriction on a patient's ability to see their GP (partly on the basis that primary care is seen as a means to avoid later, more costly illness and because there is no obvious 'gatekeeping' mechanism for first contact care). Chapter 13 discusses primary care and gatekeeping in more detail.

In theory, the lack of restrictions to care allows for unconstrained demand to fall on suppliers and unconstrained costs to fall on purchasers. To manage this risk and to incentivize disease prevention, mixed payment models are often preferred and form a majority of the payment systems in Europe (Kroneman, 2011; Charlesworth et al., 2012).

Payment options for primary care include risk-adjusted capitation together with fees for specific services (such as vaccinations) and target payments (for example, related to the achievement of quality indicators). In many countries GPs are self-employed, but in others, GPs are salaried and therefore paid for their time rather than for specific services (Kroneman, 2011). In England there has been a shift towards a mixed system of self-employment and salaried GPs with the current workforce currently comprising 28 per cent salaried doctors in 2023 compared to 20 per cent in 2015 (NHS Digital, 2023).

As discussed, capitated models of payment for GPs insulate the payer from unexpected costs and are perceived to provide an incentive for providers to manage health and optimize resource use compared to fee-for-service approaches. However, one drawback is that providers may also be incentivized to offer low levels of activity per patient given that payments per patient are fixed (referred to as 'skimping' as previously discussed). Blended payments are intended to act as a delicate balance of provider incentives.

The role of the GP as 'gatekeeper' to other (often higher cost) service provision has also given rise to the delegation of funding for other care sectors to them as a means of improving cost- and clinical effectiveness. In England, from 1990 GP practices were offered hospital inpatient and outpatient and community services budgets with associated incentives related to any underspends (known as GP 'fundholding') (Kay, 2002). This particular model was ended in 1998 but was superseded by new approaches, where GPs serving a defined population and had collective influence or control over purchasing decisions for most population care, albeit with fewer personal incentives (Miller et al., 2016). This approach ended in 2022 when 'clinical commissioning groups' (the final incarnation of mainly GP-led purchasers) were abolished, although there continues to be some spending overseen by GPs or GP networks on shared primary care services (e.g. primary care networks in England).

While examples of wholescale transfer of purchasing responsibility to GPs are rare, there has been a growth (particularly in the USA) since 2000 in the use of 'bundled-payments' (Evans, 2010). This approach has been applied to particular procedures (such as joint replacements), complex treatments (such as for cancer) and for the management of long-term conditions (such as diabetes and chronic obstructive pulmonary disease (COPD)). Here, the aim is to pay for whole episodes of care (or in the case of long-term conditions, specified lengths of treatment). Budgets for this care are given to providers, creating incentives for them to manage resources more effectively than when paid on a fee-for-service basis and to coordinate care across numerous providers. One review of studies of 23 initiatives, involving bundled-payments in high-income countries, suggested that most reported cost-savings on medical spending and more than half recorded some improvements in quality. This included a decrease of 34 per cent in total average medical spending in Sweden's bundled-payment for total hip and knee replacement (Struijs et al., 2020).

In the Netherlands, bundled-payments were implemented in 2010 where 'care groups' (newly created groups of providers focused primarily on GPs) provide integrated care for diabetes, COPD and vascular risk assessment. Care groups receive a single prospective payment for one year of primary care (but also including limited assessment by specialists) with the intention that overall resource use would be less, as a result of greater integration of services across sectoral boundaries, improved quality and reduced need for specialist care (Llano, 2013). However, in practice, a long-term evaluation suggests that the financial aims, at least, were not met, with an increase in expenditure per patients treated by care groups (which was higher still for patients with multi-morbidity) (Karimi et al., 2020).

Co-payments

With patients rarely facing the true cost of their treatment due to insurance or publicly funded healthcare, there is the risk of 'over consumption', often referred to as 'moral hazard' (i.e. that patients will consume more healthcare than they need – the 'worried well'). This would be seen as a market failure as resources are dedicated to producing one form of care when greater benefit might have been derived from investing those resources elsewhere.

To address this, some systems have introduced co-payments as a means of reducing demand for care by patients. Co-payments are relatively common in developed healthcare systems. For example, in the Netherlands, the basic insurance package incorporates a compulsory deductible (at the time of writing €385) for all healthcare except general practice, maternity, home nursing and integrated care for some long-term conditions. Insurance companies may vary the co-payment level to influence patient behaviour (for example, by encouraging them to follow prevention programmes). In addition, a voluntary additional deductible payment (up to a maximum) can be chosen in return for a lower insurance premium (Kroneman et al., 2016). Even systems funded through direct taxation, such as the NHS in the UK, apply co-payments for some care, such as general dental services and pharmaceuticals prescribed by a GP (the latter has been abandoned in Scotland).

Co-payments may have important distributional effects that may run counter to other health policies, such as those related to equity. For example, people with a high need for services are disproportionately affected by co-payments when these are related to service use, unadjusted for income. Alternatively, exempting vulnerable groups from the need to make co-payments shifts the cost of healthcare disproportionately onto the working age population (Kiil and Houlberg, 2014).

The use of co-payments has been studied empirically for its impact. In a landmark, large-scale federal initiative in the USA, the Rand Health Insurance Experiment, patients were assigned to different health insurance plans with different levels of co-payment (varying by percentage of fee paid out-of-pocket by patients and by an upper limit on out-of-pocket expenditure). This study concluded that co-payments reduce the use of healthcare services and that average price elasticity of individuals' demand for health is -0.2 (i.e., a £1 increase in price results in a 0.2 unit decrease in demand) (Manning et al., 1987).

A review of research found that co-payments generally reduce the use of prescription medicine, consultations with GPs and specialists and for ambulatory care (Kiil and Houlberg, 2014). While co-payments may successfully reduce demand, they may have other less desirable consequences. The review found no significant effects of co-payments on the prevalence of hospitalizations which, the authors suggest, 'implies that copayment for this type of treatment mainly shifts the burden of financing from the public coffers to the users rather than reduces demand' (Kiil and Houlberg, 2014: 825).

The question remains as to whether there are significant negative outcomes from co-payments for service users in terms of their health status. Kiil and Houlberg (2014) did not find significant evidence of effects of co-payments on health in the short term (although the evidence was sparse). However, a study of the impact of removing prescription co-payments on a socio-economically deprived population in New Zealand did find reduced statistically significant reductions in levels of hospitalization, admissions for mental health problems and for COPD compared to controls (rates of all-cause mortality and diabetes length of stay were not lower) (Norris et al., 2023).

In theory, by increasing the cost of insurance and therefore treatment, co-payments could encourage patients to invest more heavily in preventative care to stop illness occurring. The relationship between co-payments on the use of preventative services and health-related lifestyle was explored by Rezayatmand and colleagues in a review of research (Rezayatmand et al., 2012). Their findings were inconclusive about the relationship between co-payments generally and prevention but did suggest that when co-payments were applied to preventative services themselves utilization fell because they became more costly.

Choice and competition

Competition and choice have been widely used in healthcare as a means to optimize quality and efficiency of care. Competitive markets can apply to providers, purchasers (e.g. health insurers) or both. As discussed at the start, introducing competition to publicly provided services was a key part of new public management. Competition can come in different forms: competition for the market (e.g. to open a new GP practice or a new secondary care service in a particular area) or competition in the market (e.g. to offer choice of providers to patients). We focus on the latter but note that healthcare systems often procure services through competitive tenders and similar approaches consistent with competition of the market.

Under systems where patients and/or payers are enabled to choose from an array of providers, it is presumed that incentives will be created for providers to improve the quality of their care and the efficiency of production. Competition in this context can be on price, on quality or both. One clear risk of price competition is that it crowds out providers' focus on quality; providers reduce prices to gain or maintain market share and quality falls (Cooper et al., 2011; Gaynor et al., 2012, 2013; Siciliani et al., 2019). This risk is particularly prevalent in health where quality (particularly for an individual with a condition that needs treatment) is hard to observe. Under fixed-price competition, the payer sets or negotiates a price for the activity and providers compete to attract patients. In this model, it is assumed that patients will choose based on quality and that providers will respond by maintaining or improving that quality. Usually this applies to planned care as patients are unlikely to be in a position to make informed choices at the point of emergency care.

One such health system reform was the 'Patient Choice' policy (NHS, 2023) introduced in the NHS (most fully from 2006). The effects of this reform have been much debated (Stevens, 2011; Mays, 2011). Some studies suggested that high levels of competition facing hospitals (known as 'market concentration') were correlated with higher levels of quality as measured by mortality after an admission for acute myocardial infraction (Cooper et al., 2011; Gaynor et al., 2012) and hip fracture (Moscelli et al., 2018).

In Sweden, patient choice and the liberalization of market entry was made mandatory for primary care in 2010 (although had existed prior to this in some regions) (Janlöv et al., 2023).

Analysis of these reforms show that between 2005 and 2013 there was a substantial increase in the entry of new providers in these markets, but that this was accompanied by only modest effects on primary care quality. While small increases to patients' overall satisfaction with care were found, there were no consistently significant effects on avoidable hospitalization or satisfaction with access (Dietrichson et al., 2020). A further study by Dahlgren and colleagues found that while distance from the provider is the most important factor in choosing a GP in the Stockholm region, they also detected a willingness to make a trade-off between distance and quality measures, albeit the effects were marginal (Dahlgren et al., 2021).

While these studies may suggest a weak impact of provider choice along the lines that were hoped for by the authors of the reforms, the mechanism by which it might occur has also been explored. Economic theory would suggest that patients would base their choice of GP provider on an assessment of service quality and that this would stimulate improvements among providers. However, Hoffstedt and colleagues' study (2021) of what information adults used to make their choice of GP does not support the theory. They found that adults in the Stockholm region used mainly basic information (such as location of provider and how to switch). Less than a third searched for information relating to quality of services. The authors concluded that a 'large majority of patients in actual choice situations did not seek information that could potentially form the basis for a well-informed, and thus a rational choice of primary care provider' (Hoffstedt et al., 2021: 13).

Introducing patient choice is unlikely to be a 'silver bullet'. Its effectiveness depends on the objective it is designed to address (e.g. signalling locational preferences versus health outcomes), the architecture supporting choice and its role within broader regulatory measures. Competition alone will not lead to the scale of improvement likely desired; conversely, the actions required to increase choice, and competition may have beneficial impacts even without widespread adoption of competitive mechanisms. For example, the publication of performance data has additional effects unrelated to decisions made by patients. The publication of comparative data can increase quality activity taking place at hospitals even if it doesn't impact greatly on patients themselves (although the evidence on the impact of this is sparse (Fung et al., 2008; Cacace et al., 2011).

Paying for quality

As discussed previously, if healthcare markets operated with total efficiency, then optimal quality would arise as a natural outcome of the matching of demand and supply. But as we have discovered, healthcare as a product varies significantly from other products and consequently healthcare markets need to adapt to avoid market failure (for example, undesirably low levels of quality). One market adaptation is the introduction of specific incentives to focus the minds of providers on particular aspects of service quality. These are often termed 'pay-for-performance' schemes.

In the USA, concerns over insurers' lack of ability to influence the quality of hospital care has led to a growth in pay-for-performance schemes in private and public hospitals. Following the 2010 Affordable Care Act all US acute care hospitals were required to participate in an incentive scheme. It was funded under Medicare (the 'safety net' insurer for older people) but based on performance measures relating to all patients (Werner et al., 2011).

Earlier demonstration projects funded by the Centers for Medicare & Medicaid Services were evaluated and pay-for-performance hospitals showed a larger improvement in all measures of quality compared to controls (who had no incentive but did report publicly on quality). After adjusting for different hospital characteristics, including baseline performance, the incentive scheme was associated with improvements ranging from 2.6 per cent to 4.1 per cent over the 2 years of the demonstration (Lindenauer et al., 2007).

However, a further follow-up study of most of the demonstration project hospitals found that after 5 years their quality scores were virtually identical to those of matched controls, suggesting that, over time, differences in quality diminished. Within the demonstrator group, improvements were largest among hospitals eligible for larger bonuses that were well financed or operated in less competitive markets (Werner et al., 2011). No significant effects were found with Medicare pay-for-performance on the hospital revenues, costs and margins or Medicare payments for patients admitted for acute myocardial infarction (Kruse et al., 2012).

In primary care, the introduction of the Quality and Outcomes Framework (QOF) to all general practices in England in 2004 (Forbes et al., 2017) provides useful insights into how quality payments in this sector have fared. This incentive scheme incorporated a range of clinical process and patient experience quality measures and attached a significant proportion of GP revenue to their achievement. Roland and Campbell (2014: 1944) summarize the research findings thus: 'it is clear that pay for performance can be effective. However, the effects are sometimes only short-term and are often not as large as payors wish'.

The proportion of income at risk as part of an incentive scheme is also important in terms of (positive and negative) outcomes. According to Roland and Campbell (2014: 1944), '…as the proportion of physicians' pay that is tied to performance increases (e.g. above 10 per cent) the effect of the program is likely to increase, but so are the risks of unexpected or perverse consequences'. In the case of the QOF, when introduced, 25 per cent of GP income was subject to the QOF, but this was later reduced due to concerns over unintended consequences related to the size of the payment.

Learning activity 10.3

Identify one country where a quality payment scheme has been introduced in the last 15 years. Search for evidence of its impact in national statistics or published research literature. Think about the impact on:

1   The achievement of the desired indicators
2   Any impacts on measures of quality that were not included within the scheme
3   The cost of the payment scheme compared to its benefits
4   Any other outcomes that were surprising or not considered initially by the scheme's designers

With the information you found, discuss your findings with local purchasers or commissioners of care about how payment schemes for quality could be enhanced.

Conclusions

Healthcare spending around the world has been growing (in total and as a percentage of GDP) for many decades. That has contributed to improved quality and longer lives but has also come at a cost to taxpayers and the population at large. Those costs have reached levels where governments and individuals are increasingly having to trade-off the cost of healthcare against other important priorities (e.g. cost of education, defence, welfare payments and others). Healthcare managers are frequently faced with demands to get greater value from the resources at their disposal.

In many other areas of the economy, market mechanisms are used to help make these choices: to allow people to decide where to spend more or less. The market for improving health is unique. It is a market in which everyone participates – willingly or not – and one that is fraught with poor or missing information and with high levels of uncertainty. As a result, the architecture of such a market is unusually important in determining outputs for population health but also taxpayer and wider population costs, as well as impacts on the economy.

This chapter focused specifically on important elements in the architecture of health provision – with a focus on health systems rather than wider healthcare products (e.g. medicines, pharmaceutical products, broader health and well-being services). It discussed in particular how pricing, choice and competition and payment mechanisms might be used to enhance the efficiency of, and value derived from healthcare. In particular, it demonstrated that many countries have explored the use of similar economic approaches, albeit in different contexts and often with substantively different types of health system organization.

It also demonstrated, however, that there is no simple solution, and, as a consequence, healthcare leaders will need to understand and make trade-offs between different and competing priorities. Health economics, and its associated analytical approaches, offers additional tools for healthcare managers with which to understand performance and to allocate resources most effectively.

Learning resources

The King's Fund: The King's Fund has a range of facts and analysis about NHS costs and spending [https://www.kingsfund.org.uk/insight-and-analysis/data-and-charts/key-facts-figures-nhs].

The Research and Economic Analysis (REAL) Centre, part of The Health Foundation: Provides independent analysis on health, economic and financing issues relating to the NHS and social care in England [https://www.health.org.uk/what-we-do/real-centre].

NHS England: Details of the NHS payment scheme in England can be found on this website [https://www.england.nhs.uk/pay-syst/nhs-payment-scheme/].

The Commonwealth Fund: The Commonwealth Fund has a wealth of independent research on health issues including payment systems and efficiency. Based in the USA but often includes international comparisons [www.commonwealthfund.org].

The European Health Observatory on Health Systems and Policies: A World Health Organization collaboration that provides data and analysis including financing and payment systems [https://eurohealthobservatory.who.int/].

The Congressional Budget Office: The Congressional Budget Office provides independent analysis of budgetary issues in the USA, including those relating to healthcare [https://www.cbo.gov/topics/health-care].

References

Akerlof, G. (1970) The market for 'lemons': quality uncertainty and the market mechanism, *Quarterly Journal of Economics*, 84: 488–500.

Appleby J., Harrison, T., Hawkins, L. and Dixon, A. (2012) Payment by results. How can payment systems help to deliver better care?, The King's Fund [kingsfund.org.uk; accessed 28 March 2024].

Arrow, K.J. (1963) Uncertainty and the welfare economics of medical care, *The American Economic Review*, 53: 5941–73.

Barnes, A.J., Unruh, L., Chukmaitov, A. and van Ginneken, E. (2014) Accountable care organizations in the USA: types, developments and challenges, *Health Policy*, 118(1): 1–7.

Bell, M., Charlesworth, A. and Lewis, R. (2021) The future of the NHS hospital payment system in England REAL Centre Briefing Paper, *The Health Foundation* [https://www.health.org.uk/publications/reports/the-future-of-the-nhs-hospital-payment-system-in-england; accessed 06 December 2024].

Cacace, M., Ettelt, S., Brereton, L., Pedersen, J.S. and Nolte, E. (2011) How health systems make available information on service providers: experience in seven countries, *Rand Health Quarterly*, Mar 1; 1(1): 11. PMID: 28083167; PMCID: PMC4945218.

Charlesworth, A., Davies, A. and Dixon, J. (2012) Reforming payment for health care in Europe to achieve better value. Research Report. London, Nuffield Trust [https://www.nuffieldtrust.org.uk/sites/default/files/2017-01/reforming-payment-for-health-care-in-europe-web-final.pdf; accessed 23 March 24).

Cooper, Z., Gibbons, S., Jones, S. and McGuire, A. (2011) Does hospital competition save lives? Evidence from the English NHS Patient Choice Reforms, *The Economic Journal*, 121(554): F228–F260.

Dahlgren, C., Dackehag, M., Wändell, P. and Rehnberg, C. (2021) Simply the best? The impact of quality on choice of primary healthcare provider in Sweden, *Health Policy*, 125: 1448–1454.

Dietrichson, J., Ellegård, L.M. and Kjellsson, G. (2020) Patient choice, entry, and the quality of primary care: evidence from Swedish reforms, *Health Economics*. Jun; 29(6): 716–730.

doi: 10.1002/hec.4015. Epub 2020 Mar 18. PMID: 32187777. Wiley Online Library [https://onlinelibrary.wiley.com/doi/full/10.1002/hec.4015?msockid=1e65d85a0d7066cb29dbcc0c0c1367ec; accessed 06 December 2024].

Ellis, R.P. (1998) Creaming, skimping and dumping: provider competition on the intensive and extensive margins, *Journal of Health Economics*, Oct; 17(5): 537–555.

Emanuel, E., Mostashari, F. and Navathe, M.D. (2021) Designing a successful primary care physician capitation model, *Journal of the American Medical Association*, 325(20): 2043–2044.

Evans, J. (2010) The Current state of bundled payments, *American Health & Drug Benefits*, Jul–Aug; 3(4): 292.

Forbes, L., Marchand, C., Doran, T. and Peckham, S. (2017) The role of the quality and outcomes framework in the care of long-term conditions: a systematic review, *British Journal of General Practice*, Nov; 67(664): e775–e784. doi: 10.3399/bjgp17X693077.

Fung, C.H., Lim, Y.W., Mattke, S., Damberg, C. and Shekelle, P.G. (2008) Systematic review: the evidence that publishing patient care performance data improves quality of care, *Annals of Internal Medicine*, 148(2): 111–23. doi: 10.7326/0003-4819-148-2-200801150-00006. PMID: 18195336.

Gaynor, M., Moreno-Serra, R. and Propper, C. (2012) Can competition improve outcomes in UK health care? Lessons from the past two decades, *Journal of Health Services Research & Policy*, 17(1_suppl): 49–54.

Gaynor, M., Moreno-Serra, R. and Propper, C. (2013) Death by market power: reform, competition and patient outcomes in the national health service, *American Economic Journal: Economic Policy*, 5(4): 134–166.

Hoffstedt, C., Fredriksson, M. and Winblad, U. (2021) How do people choose to be informed? A survey of the information searched for in the choice of primary care provider in Sweden, *BMC Health Services Research*, 21: 559.

Hood, C. (1991) A public management for all seasons, *Public Administration*, 69: 3–19.

Janlöv, N., Blume, S., Glenngård, A.H., Hanspers, K., Anell, A. and Merkur, S. (2023) Sweden: health system review, *Health Systems in Transition*, 25(4): 1–236. PMID: 38230685.

Karimi, M., Tsiachristas, A., Loorman, W., Stokes, J., van Galen, M. and Rutten-van Mölken, M. (2021) Bundled payments for chronic diseases increased health care expenditure in the Netherlands, especially for multimorbid patients, *Health Policy*, 125: 751–759.

Kay, A. (2002) The abolition of the GP fundholding scheme: a lesson in evidence-based policy making, *British Journal of General Practice*, February; 52(475): 141–144 [https://www.ncbi.nlm.nih.gov/pmc/articles/PMC1314221/; accessed 23 March 2024].

Keane, M. and Stavrunova, O. (2014) Adverse selection, moral hazard and the demand for Medigap insurance, *Nuffield College Working Paper*, 2014–3 [https://www.nuffield.ox.ac.uk/economics/papers/2014/PaperApril2014_3.pdf; accessed 23 March 2024].

Kiil A. and Houlberg K. (2014) How does copayment for health care services affect demand, health and redistribution? A systematic review of the empirical evidence from 1990 to 2011, *European Journal of Health Economics*, 15: 813–828.

Kroneman M. (2011) Paying general practitioners in Europe, *Netherlands Institute for Health Services Research* [https://www.nivel.nl/sites/default/files/bestanden/Rapport-paying-gp-in%20europe.pdf; accessed 23 March 24].

Kroneman, M., Boerma, W., van den Berg, M., Groenewegen, P., de Jong, J. and van Ginneken, E. (2016) Netherlands health system review, *Health Systems in Transition*, 18(2): 1–240.

Kruse, G.B., Polsky, D., Stuart, E.A. and Werner, R.M. (2012) The impact of hospital pay-for-performance on hospital and medicare costs, *Health Services Research*, 47(6): 2118–2136.

Llano, R. (2013) Bundled payments for integrated care in the Netherlands, *Eurohealth Incorporating Euro Observer*, 19(2): 15–16.

Lewis, R.Q. (2019) More reform of the English National Health Service: from competition back to planning?, *International Journal of Health Services*, 49(1): 5–16.

Lindenauer, P.K., Remus, D., Roman, S., Rothberg, M.B., Benjamin, E.M., Ma, A., et al. (2007) Public reporting and pay for performance in hospital quality improvement, *The New England Journal of Medicine*, 356: 486–496.

Mann, O., Bracegirdle, T. and Shantikumar, S. (2023) The relationship between Quality and Outcomes Framework scores and socioeconomic deprivation, *British Journal of General Practice Open*, 7: 4.

Manning, W.G., Newhouse, J.P., Duan, N., Keeler, E.B. and Leibowitz, A. (1987) Health insurance and the demand for health care, *The American Economic Review*, 77(3): 251–277.

Mays, N. (2011) Is there evidence that competition in healthcare is a good thing? No, *British Medical Journal*, 343: d4205. doi:10.1136/bmj.d4205.

Miller, R., Peckham, S., Coleman, A., McDermott, I., Harrison, S. and Checkland, K. (2016) What happens when GPs engage in commissioning? Two decades of experience in the English NHS, *Journal of Health Services Research and Policy*, 21(2): 126–133.

Moscelli, G., Gravelle, H., Siciliani, L. and Santos, R. (2018) Heterogeneous effects of patient choice and hospital competition on mortality, *Social Science and Medicine*, 216: 50–58. doi: 10.1016/j.socscimed.2018.09.009. Epub 2018 Sep 9. PMID: 30265998.

NHS (2023) Your choices in the NHS, 10 May [https://www.nhs.uk/using-the-nhs/about-the-nhs/your-choices-in-the-nhs/; accessed 04 June 2024].

NHS Digital (2023) General practice workforce, 31 December 2023 [https://digital.nhs.uk/data-and-information/publications/statistical/general-and-personal-medical-services/31-december-2023; accessed 23 March 2024).

Norris, P., Cousins, K., Horsburgh, S., Keown, S., Churchward, M., Samarayanaka, A., et al. (2023) Impact of removing prescription co-payments on the use of costly health services: a pragmatic randomised controlled trial, *BMC Health Services Research*, 23: 31.

OECD (2017) Health at a Glance 2017: OECD indicators, average length of stay in hospitals, [https://www.oecd-ilibrary.org/social-issues-migration-health/health-at-a-glance-2017/average-length-of-stay-in-hospitals_health_glance-2017-64-en;jsessionid=WUB6oTNE8OX5lPvqCqS1yveTx_ucYJVvus_JCfhz.ip-10-240-5-15; accessed 06 December 2024].

OECD Health Statistics (2023) [https://web-archive.oecd.org/temp/2024-02-21/78817-health-data.htm; accessed 29 March 24].

Rezayatmand, R., Pavlova, M. and Groot, W. (2012) The impact of out-of-pocket payments on prevention and health-related lifestyle: a systematic literature review, *European Journal of Public Health*, 23: 74–79.

Roland, M. and Campbell, S. (2014) Successes and failures of pay for performance in the United Kingdom, *The New England Journal of Medicine*, 370(20): 1944–1949.

Siciliani, L., Moscelli, G. and Gravelle, H. (2019) Does hospital competition improve efficiency? The effect of patient choice reform in England, *Health Economics*, 28(5): 618–640.

Smith, P., Stepan, A., Valdmanis, V. and Verheyen, P. (1997) Principal-Agent problems in health care systems: an international perspective, *Health Policy*, 41(1): 37–60.

Stevens, S. (2011) Is there evidence that competition in healthcare is a good thing? Yes, *British Medical Journal*, 343: d4136. doi:10.1136/bmj.d4136.

Struijs, J.N., de Vries, E.F., Baan, C.A., van Gils, P.F. and Rosenthal, M.B. (2020) Bundled-payment models around the world: how they work and what their impact has been, Issue Brief, Commonwealth Fund [https://www.commonwealthfund.org/publications/2020/apr/bundled-payment-models-around-world-how-they-work-their-impact; accessed 29 March 2024].

Varian, H.R. (2014) *Intermediate Microeconomics 9th Edition*. New York: WW Norton and Co.

Werner, R.M., Kolstad, J.T., Stuart, E.A. and Polsky, D. (2011) The effect of pay-for-performance in hospitals: lessons for quality improvement, *Health Affairs*, 30(4): 690–698.

Setting and managing priorities for healthcare

Iestyn Williams and Chris Q. Smith

Introduction

Deciding how to allocate resources when planning and providing services is a core function of healthcare management. Financial and other resources are often highly constrained, and decisions are therefore required over which areas of spending to prioritize, and where to set limits (Williams et al., 2012; Berezowski et al., 2023). However, healthcare 'rationing' is a notoriously fraught endeavour, which has escaped simple formulations to guide management practice. Instead, the allocation of resources in healthcare is something of a complex problem, marked by competing claims, political controversy and system constraints (Holm, 1998; Martinus Hauge et al., 2022). In this chapter, we detail the reasons why priority setting is required and the ways in which it is enacted in different contexts. We identify some of the fundamental, and often conflicting, ethical precepts that inform debates over how resources should be used. This is followed by a summary of some of the most prevalent tools and inputs for decision-making, and their limitations, most notably in the face of political and system constraints. The discussion draws on consideration of the differences in resource allocation systems used by a range of countries and puts forward a series of suggestions and recommendations for healthcare managers and leaders.

Setting the scene

The terms 'rationing' and 'priority setting' refer to processes for determining how to allocate limited resources. They are often used interchangeably although can also be used to apply to different stages of resource allocation processes (Klein, 2010). Common to both is the assumption that limits need to be placed on the outflow of healthcare resources like finance, human resources, materials and physical resources such as transplantable organs. In publicly funded systems, the main drivers of demand for healthcare are commonly understood to include (Williams et al., 2012):

- *Changing demographics.* The reduction in size of the economically active as a percentage of the population creates cost pressures, as the overall contributions pool decreases relative to healthcare need/demand.
- *Developments in medicine and technology.* The rate at which new, expensive healthcare interventions come to market has accelerated and this creates pressures on healthcare systems operating with fixed budgets.
- *Patient expectations.* Expectations of what public services can and should provide have changed in line with the broader 'consumerization' of societies. As patients become more expert in understanding their healthcare needs and more empowered to make demands of healthcare providers, they are prepared to tolerate fewer of the discomforts and inconveniences of previous generations.
- *Sustainability.* The growing environmental crisis also has implications for health systems, which typically are heavy energy users and contributors to global warming. This has added another dimension to the resource allocation equation (Ledda et al., 2024).

Of course, priority setting is only one among many approaches to managing such pressures. Alternatives include raising overall resource levels so that all needs can be satisfactorily met. Funding levels for health systems remain much debated (Charlesworth et al., 2021; Al-Janabi et al., 2023) and highly variable across the world (Hopkins, 2010), with spending for OECD countries ranging from 16.6 per cent of GDP in the USA to 2.9 per cent in India (OECD, 2023). Further alternatives include investing in improvements to how services are organized and delivered, and the introduction of market (or quasi-market) mechanisms to drive competition and thereby bring down expenditure. Another common approach has been to set budget 'ceilings' on provider organizations, necessitating in turn further limit-setting strategies at the organizational level. These latter include withholding treatments 'at the bedside' (Danis et al., 2014). Ubel and Goold (1997: 78) provide the following example:

> A neurologist works at a county hospital that does not have a magnetic resonance image (MRI) scanner. The hospital puts money aside each year so that six patients can receive an MRI at a nearby hospital. A physician evaluates a patient who has a "soft indication" for an MRI. The physician could order an MRI for the patient. However, he knows that if he requests an MRI for this patient, he denies an MRI to another patient, who may need it more. Thus, he tells the patient that an MRI is unnecessary.

Other rationing strategies include introducing delays through waiting lists, diluting the quality of services and diverting demand to other parts of the system (Klein, 2010; Williams et al., 2019) (see Box 11.1).

Box 11.1   The seven forms of rationing

1   *Deterrence:* Patients are put off from seeking care by excessive travel, hostile staff, or other factors. Broader system versions include co-payments and demand management policies.
2   *Deflection:* Patients are individually or collectively redirected to alternative health (or social care) providers.
3   *Dilution:* Reducing quality standards to cope with demand, e.g. reduced consultation time, use of second-line treatment and/or less qualified staff.
4   *Delay:* Reducing resource use through imposition of waiting lists and treatment delays.
5   *Denial:* Patients are denied treatment, for example, on grounds of suitability or urgency. At system level, decisions not to reimburse (or 'cover') certain health interventions.
6   *Selection:* Criteria introduced to decide which subgroups of a) patients or b) interventions are deemed eligible for coverage.
7   *Termination:* Deliberate cessation of treatment or care without replacement or redirection elsewhere.

Source: adapted by Williams et al. (2019).

Among these strategies for stemming the flow of resources, priority setting is distinguished by its advocacy of *explicit* decision-making in which the rationale and reasons are made clear. Beyond this, the approach to priority setting adopted in each context will inevitably be influenced by the prevailing model of revenue generation (see Chapter 10), which may include combinations of taxation, insurance (both social and private), and out-of-pocket payments. Tax-funded systems typically create a stronger hand for government bodies to influence distribution of resources, whereas independent payers have a more substantial role to play in systems funded through social or private insurance.

The structure and organization of a country's health system is also critical. Although private insurers can operate as priority setters on behalf of their patient/consumers, more typically, responsibility lies with government bodies or their intermediaries. Decisions can be made at various levels, including national (through government departments and national organizations), local (for example, through health authorities and other purchasers) and at the level of the individual patient and clinician (Williams et al., 2012). Approaches to priority setting also reflect broader civic cultures and societal expectations about the role of government in relation to individuals and communities (Batifoulier et al., 2013).

The main source of divergence in approaches to implementing priority setting is in the relative emphasis on either *technocracy* – i.e. evidence driven decision-making – or *democracy* – i.e. participation of citizens and other stakeholders. This is redolent of the distinction in the classic policy formulation literature between 'rational' and 'pluralistic' models of decision-making (Parsons, 1995). The rational model seeks to derive evidence on investment alternatives and to select those that promise the most benefit. To this end, governments in richer countries have typically set up Health Technology Assessment (HTA) agencies to produce guidance on the efficacy, safety, ethics and costs of healthcare interventions (Miller et al., 2020; Hollingworth et al., 2021). For example, the International Network of Agencies for Health Technology Assessment (INAHTA) includes '55 HTA agencies that support health system decision making that affects over 1 billion people in 35 countries around the globe' (INAHTA, no date). However, the functioning of such bodies also requires resources and expertise that are not readily available in resource-poor settings. For example, Babigumira et al. (2016) surveyed countries including Bangladesh, Dominican Republic, DR Congo, Kenya, Swaziland and Vietnam, and found limited evidence of any formal HTA and no instances of dedicated, independent HTA bodies. In these lower- and middle-income settings, further constraints on decision-making can be imposed by supranational donors, such as NGOs as conditions of endowment (Abimbola et al., 2017).

In England, the National Institute for Health and Care Excellence (NICE) plays a major role in setting priorities for much of the health service, through production of guidance based on evidence-based technology (or treatment) assessment. This is typical of a desire to *delegate* responsibility for the contentious business of priority setting (Löblová, 2018). Despite this, bodies such as NICE have yet to succeed in taking the 'politics' out of resource allocation, or in enabling rationing decisions that are routinely both explicit and politically palatable (Williams, 2024).

This technocratic approach to priority setting contrasts with earlier approaches involving collective discussion on broader priority-setting principles conducted by specially convened panels of stakeholders and experts – notably in Scandinavian countries in the 1990s (Calltorp, 1999; Ham and Robert, 2003). Others have argued for the importance of extending these deliberative processes to include a wider array of citizen, stakeholder and patient input (Steffensen et al., 2022). It is increasingly accepted that priority setting requires incorporation of both evidence and participation in decision-making. However, achieving the ideal balance between adherence to decision rules and encouraging informed deliberation is a constant challenge.

Ethical precepts

In systems funded primarily out of public money it is reasonable to assume that priorities should in some way reflect societal values and deliver demonstrable benefits to the public good (Oswald, 2015). Deciding what we mean by societal values and public good requires us to engage, at least in the first instance, with questions of ethics (Clark and Weale, 2012). Furthermore, in a context of resource scarcity, priority setters need to show that their decisions bring about benefits to the public and that more benefit could not be achieved by using resources in a different way (opportunity cost).

Although these propositions may seem uncontentious, establishing precisely what we mean by the 'public good' in healthcare priority setting remains a considerable challenge. Health economists such as Alan Williams have argued that: 'in health care, "doing good" means improving people's life expectancy and the quality of their life' (2006: 29). From this perspective, successful resource allocation will generate the greatest increase in overall population health. This maximizing principle is based on a utilitarian commitment to the greatest benefit to the greatest number of people. As noted, HTA informed by cost effectiveness analysis has emerged as a key vehicle for choosing between investment options on such grounds (Sorenson and Chalkidou, 2012).

Nonetheless, there are many challenges to this approach. Few if any contemporary commentators would advocate utilitarianism, or HTA, as the single driver of priority setting. The primary ethical objection stems from the need to demonstrate *distributive justice* in the allocation of public resources and therefore the belief that considerations of fairness and equity should not be overridden by the health maximization principle (Barra et al., 2020). For example, an egalitarian perspective might hold that we should all be entitled to an equal proportion of healthcare resources regardless of our capacity to benefit, or, more commonly, that we should all be given equal opportunity to enjoy good health. From this perspective, resource distribution should be linked to levels of need with the 'worse off' receiving greater priority than the relatively healthy.

Various accounts of who might qualify as 'worse off' have been put forward. For example, Eric Nord (2005) proposed a disease severity approach in which severe conditions are granted higher importance, and Alan Williams (1997) advocated a 'fair innings' model in which resources are allocated to distribute the number of healthy years most equitably throughout a population. However, both approaches are controversial, subject to critique (see for example Rivlin, 2000; Rosoff, 2014), and far from being universally accepted.

Patient-level principles also mitigate against imposition of these distributive principles, including notions of individual choice and respect for human dignity (Sandman et al., 2018). A focus on the individual also brings into play other ethical considerations such as the 'rule of rescue', i.e. the imperative to save the lives of individuals where these are endangered (Jonsen, 1986; Charlton, 2022). In healthcare this may take the form of, for example, 'emergency surgery, intensive care, antibiotics for severe infections, transplants or artificial organs, highly active anti-retro-viral therapy (HAART) and life-preserving cancer drugs' (Orr and Wolff, 2015). By prioritizing such treatments we are asserting the importance of saving lives, rather than calculating either cost-effectiveness or equity.

Others have explored the principle of 'moral desert', which is the extent to which an individual or group *deserves* something (Porter, 2020). This might present in the form of de-prioritization of those who engage in personal behaviour that increases their risk of poor health (Brown, 2013). As with collectivist principles of equity and justice, notions of choice, rescue and desert have been heavily criticized and it is to the priority setter that the unenviable task of negotiation between these competing ethical stances falls. It should not surprise us therefore that healthcare resource allocation often appears to reflect a confusion of ethical considerations, or that there is often controversy and contestation over underlying principles (see Box 11.2).

Box 11.2   Ethical standpoints and principles to consider in priority setting

Utilitarianism: The injunction to bring about the maximum level of utility (for example, overall health gain)

Egalitarianism: The ethical foregrounding of collective responsibility for fair distribution of resources

Libertarianism: The ethical foregrounding of individual choice and reward, whereby patients are understood as consumers with rights and choices

Communitarianism: The injunction to allocate resources according to collectively agreed citizen values

Efficiency: The concern to maximize outcomes from within a limited resource

Equity: The principle that equal people should be given equal treatment, and in some cases that those worse off should receive extra resources

Desert: The principle that individuals should be held responsible for their behaviour and that this should influence access to scarce resources

Rule of rescue: The imperative to save human life wherever possible

Fair innings: The ethical principle that resources should be distributed so as to distribute healthy years most evenly across a population

Disease severity: The ethical principle that resources should be weighted towards those in greatest need or with the most severe conditions

Source: Williams and Robinson (2012).

Improving decision-making

Although these ethical debates remain largely unresolved, they are useful in pointing to what the range of inputs into decision-making could and should be. In this respect, they are a necessary precursor to identifying what evidence and information should be applied and which perspectives should be accounted for. This section describes some of the most notable tools and methods that have been developed to shape how decision-making unfolds.

Needs assessment and cost-effectiveness analysis

Evidence that is relevant to the local context of resource allocation can be generated through long-established methods, such as needs assessment (Stevens and Gillam, 1998), and newer applications, such as predictive modelling based on local data. As noted, the inclusion of cost-effectiveness analysis (CEA) within HTAs has become increasingly routine, and prospective economic evaluation of technologies is now also a regular accompaniment to clinical trials. CEA can be defined as information on the inputs or costs and the outputs or consequences associated with alternative healthcare interventions and procedures. HTA and CEA results are typically reported in generic, summary outcome measures that facilitate comparison across intervention areas (Drummond et al., 1997). Summary measures of results include: the incremental cost-effectiveness ratio (ICER), which is the ratio of additional costs to additional health effects associated with a new intervention (e.g. cost per quality-adjusted life years gained (QALYs)); and the net-benefit statistic, which expresses the additional health effects in monetary units by using an estimate of the 'maximum willingness to pay' per unit of health gain, where available.

These techniques are intended to enable interventions to be ranked according to their cost-effectiveness (the league table approach) or to be measured against a 'critical threshold value' (Lord et al., 2004) to determine cost-effectiveness. By contrast, a profile – or cost consequence – approach to reporting results sets out the impact of the intervention on resource use and costs (including specific healthcare service use and costs, and productivity losses) and health outcomes (including disease symptoms, life expectancy and quality of life) in a tabular form, without any attempt to summarize or aggregate them.

The international evidence suggests that use of HTA and economic evaluation is far more prevalent among national, guidance-producing organizations than it is among local decision-makers operating with fixed healthcare budgets (Williams and Bryan, 2015). This disjuncture reflects factors including a lack of the requisite resources and expertise within healthcare organizations. Perhaps more significant, however, is the failure of CEA to capture the range of factors that influence priority-setting decisions at local levels, such as: budgets; service structures and arrangements; organizational practices and norms; and social and political considerations. The aims of priority setting (as we have seen) are likely to be multiple, and, to be appropriate, decisions need to reflect local population characteristics and trends, as well as being compatible with systems and structures.

Programme budgeting and marginal analysis

Programme budgeting and marginal analysis (PBMA) is another approach based on economic principles that offers a more practical set of steps to enable decision-makers to maximize use of resources (Gibson et al., 2006). 'Programme budgeting' enables decision-makers to analyse current expenditure and 'marginal analysis' enables comparison of the costs and outcomes of programmes (Mitton and Donaldson, 2004). The emphasis is on the identification of areas where more impact could be achieved from within a finite resource to inform future allocation decisions. Typically, PBMA involves an expert panel that draws upon local knowledge and evidence and operates according to economic principles of maximization and opportunity cost.

The benefits of such processes are invariably acknowledged by decision-makers that adopt them. Even so, the costs of taking such evidence-based approaches to decision-making are considerable when measured in terms of the time, resources and expertise involved.

Furthermore, the optimal division of responsibility for evidence generation and analysis – for example, between internal and external, national and local bodies – will vary from context to context. The challenge for local planning is to achieve the ideal trade-off between local specificity and appropriate economies of scale.

Multi-criteria decision tools

Multi-criteria decision analysis (MCDA) has been defined as 'an umbrella term to describe a collection of formal approaches which seek to take explicit account of multiple criteria in helping individuals or groups explore decisions that matter' (Belton and Stewart, 2002: 2). The common feature of these approaches is the aim to structure decision-making problems using an explicitly identified set of criteria. MCDA involves deciding on aims and criteria to build an initial decision-making model, before interrogating the resulting decision recommendations through discussion and deliberation. The level of complexity of MCDA tools varies significantly, from simple checklists and score cards to computer-based modelling. As with PBMA, the use of multi-criteria frameworks has generally been positively evaluated but without becoming normalized into routine management practice (Seixas et al., 2021). Reasons may again include the paucity of reliable and robust data to populate models, and the extensive time and resource required for their implementation. Critique has also centred on the limits of 'checklists' in capturing the dynamics of decision-making processes in which rhetoric and emotion can be powerful influences (de Graaff et al., 2021).

Public involvement

In explicit priority-setting processes, public engagement has been found to improve decision-making and to increase awareness of the challenges that decision-makers face (Mooney, 1998; Manafò et al., 2018). This is often underpinned by principles of communitarianism and a commitment to citizen dialogue over the means and ends of public services. Communitarian citizen engagement requires those involved to take on the 'veil of ignorance' (Rawls, 1972), thereby shedding all considerations of personal interest when deliberating on priorities and trade-offs.

Public involvement can provide important benefits for priority setters. When done well, it can help generate the knowledge required to ensure all those who need a service can access it (equal access) or that resources are directed towards those with the greatest need (equal outcomes) (Hunter et al., 2016). It can also generate instrumental benefits through enabling appropriate resource allocation decisions, which are aligned with the values and preferences of the public (Williams et al., 2012; Hunter et al., 2016). Additionally, public involvement can improve democratic legitimacy and accountability, while educative gains can be made through showing why a prioritization decision is needed and the trade-offs that will be involved (Williams et al., 2012; Hunter et al., 2016).

The public can be involved in several different types of decision. This includes decisions as to what types of services, medicines and procedures to offer (service coverage); decisions on who should be eligible to receive services (eligibility); and questions as to how – and to what extent – services should be funded (overall funding) (Lomas, 1997; Weale et al., 2016). There are also many different methods for engagement that priority setters can draw upon to involve the public. In their systematic rapid review of research on patient and public involvement in priority setting, Manafò et al. (2018) identify two tiers of engagement: deliberative and consultative (see Box 11.3). The former typically involves a deeper level of engagement designed to transform the perspectives of both parties, and can include activities such as citizens' juries, citizens' panels, consensus conferences and deliberative polling. In contrast, consultative engagement focuses on the public providing information to decision-makers in an advisory capacity, and can include focus groups, responses to consultation documents, advisory panels/patient representatives, referenda, questionnaires and opinion polling.

Box 11.3   Deliberative involvement methods

Citizens' juries 12–24 citizens deliberate over a decision over a period of several days.

Citizens' panels A similar number of citizens meet over a longer period to reach decisions.

Consensus conferences Citizens meet in small groups to discuss scientific or technical issues. A second meeting assembles experts, media and the public to draw together observations and conclusions.

Deliberative polling Deliberative processes are incorporated into opinion polling through follow-up discussions with respondents.

Source: Adapted from Abelson et al. (2003).

Although public involvement promises to offer much to the rationing enterprise – helping to resolve disputes over substantive aims, increasing democratic accountability and raising awareness of the difficulties faced by decision-makers – caution is required. The evidence base for the impacts of deliberative methods in priority setting remains scarce (Conklin et al., 2015). Furthermore, commentators have cautioned against the assertion that deliberative engagement can or should be viewed as a panacea for the difficulties of priority setting (Abelson et al., 2003) or that decision-makers are always prepared to authentically share responsibility (Daniels et al., 2018).

Citizen engagement is invariably costly and complex and deliberative approaches tend to be small-scale and do not equate to a democratic mandate for action (see Box 11.4). It is also important that the consensus-seeking facilitated by deliberative engagement is not pursued at the cost of respect for diversity and recognition of genuine differences where these exist. Finally, the logic of involvement requires that decisions are genuinely open to be shaped by public preferences. This would suggest that plans need to be in place to integrate these with other decision inputs, and that engagement should be avoided when decisions are subject to strong government direction.

Box 11.4 Case study – community involvement in priority setting in Tanzania

In Tanzania, community participation has been advocated in healthcare planning and decision-making at district levels. A study in Mbarali district considered how citizens were engaged by the Council Health Management Team (CHMT) in development of local population health plans (Kamuzora et al., 2013). Despite good intentions, the CHMT initially dropped their community involvement plans. Reasons given for this included a perceived lack of requisite knowledge and expertise within the community, fears that the engagement might jeopardize government approval of the plan and lack of funds to cover costs of engagement activities. Subsequently, engagement plans were revived and implemented. As a result, the CHMT felt that engagement had improved the priority-setting process and increased openness. However, it was acknowledged that the process was somewhat rushed and under-resourced, with little community feedback on subsequent decisions and actions.

Learning activity 11.1 Involving patients and the public

Identify a priority-setting process from within your health system and devise a plan for how best to involve patients and the public in this process. Consider the following questions:

Question 1: Which of the following types of decision do you want to involve the public in?

- *Service coverage*
- *Eligibility for services*
- *Overall funding* (Weale et al., 2016).

Question 2: What benefit(s) do you want to achieve through the involvement?

- *Equity benefit* - Achieving more equitable decisions. E.g. decisions that lead to equal access, equal outcomes, equal use of services etc.
- *Democratic benefit* - Increasing democratic involvement and legitimacy.
- *Educative benefit* - Educating the public on demands and trade-offs of providing services.
- *Instrumental benefit* - Achieving a better link between priority decision and the values of the public (Hunter et al., 2016).

Question 3: Based on your answers, which method(s) of engagement would help you best achieve your public involvement goals? This could include:

- Deliberative forms of engagement - E.g. citizens' juries, citizens' panels, consensus conferences, deliberative polling etc.

- *Consultative forms of engagement* – E.g. consultation document, focus groups, advisory panels/patient representatives, a referendum, an opinion poll/survey etc. (Manafò et al., 2018).

Question 4: What barriers could there be to achieving your goals? How can you best overcome these?

Accountability for reasonableness

The communitarian commitment to procedural (as opposed to substantive) justice is behind Daniels and Sabin's framework 'Accountability for Reasonableness' (A4R) (Daniels and Sabin, 2008). They argue that social value pluralism is irreducible and therefore priority setters should set their sights on achieving decision-making *processes* that stakeholders will consider to be fair. This fairness, they claim, can be measured by performance against four conditions (see Box 11.5).

Box 11.5   The four conditions of Accountability for Reasonableness (A4R)

1	*Publicity*	Decisions taken over the allocation of healthcare resources should be made accessible to the public.
2	*Relevance*	Decisions should be influenced by evidence that fair-minded people would consider relevant.
3	*Appeals*	There should be mechanisms for challenge and review of decisions reached and for resolving any resulting disputes.
4	*Enforcement*	There should be effective mechanisms for ensuring the other three conditions are implemented.

Through the development of a consistent approach to resource allocation decision-making, Daniels and Sabin (2008) argue that it becomes possible for a body of case law to emerge that both constrains and informs future decisions and protects decision-makers against unreasonable challenge. In this way, A4R seeks to address the legitimacy deficits of rationing, as well as the challenges posed by ethical pluralism and poorly developed decision processes. Although A4R has proven useful to decision-makers operating in a variety of settings (Kapiriri et al., 2009) it is not without its critics, including for its failure to capture all procedural dimensions of decision-making (Dale et al., 2023). Ultimately, A4R cannot entirely substitute for engagement (and public engagement in particular) on the ethical trade-offs involved in rationing as the notion of 'relevance' remains inherently subjective and therefore contested (Friedman, 2008).

Given the failure of A4R to entirely 'proceduralize' decision-making, some analysts have sought to nest within it an element of explicit criteria-based decision-making. For example, Baltussen et al. (2016) advocate for 'evidence-informed deliberative processes' involving application of multi-criteria decision analysis within decision-making processes that otherwise adhere to the A4R conditions. However, the conditions required for such an approach to be adopted are not always observed in practice, especially in resource poor settings (Kapiriri et al., 2020).

Learning activity 11.2 Applying the A4R framework

Processes for setting priorities for the allocation of healthcare resources can be assessed using the four conditions of A4R set out in Box 11.5.

- Using media reports or other sources, identify a priority-setting decision from your country, such as a decision to introduce a new cancer drug or to restrict provision of an expensive surgical procedure. Using these sources, assess how the process performs in terms of: publicity, relevance, appeals and enforcement.
- Based on your analysis, identify how such decisions might be handled differently in the future.

Politics

A common point of critique for each of these tools and frameworks is their vulnerability to misuse or neglect in real-world settings. Both rational and pluralistic models risk naivety in their inattention to the role that unequal relationships of power can play in resource allocation. As well as responding to formal authorities, priority setters must also contend with a plethora of sectional and cause-based interest groups employing strategies of horse-trading, 'log-rolling' and even coercion in pursuit of partisan agendas (Williams, 2024). At national levels, these interest groups can act as more amorphous 'epistemic communities' or 'networks of the like-minded', including for example coalitions of senior health managers, industry representatives or the clinical community (Löblová, 2018).

Major healthcare spending decisions invariably take place against a backdrop of media scrutiny and disagreement over what health services should fund (Williams, 2015). Unsurprisingly, therefore, the best laid rationing plans have been damaged by lack of support from government, the public, key stakeholders or a combination of all of these (Jacobs et al., 1998; Sibbald et al., 2009). In the case of the US state of Oregon, the legislature sought to develop a list of core services to be funded through Medicaid but saw ongoing political revisions to the plan to the extent that the original objective of rationalizing the process of technology coverage became largely lost (Jacobs et al., 1998).

As we have seen, the response of Daniels and Sabin is to attempt to tie such stake-holders into formalized processes so that the 'fall-out' from tough decisions can be minimized. However, this assumes that the fundamental premise of priority setting – i.e. that resources are scarce and must therefore be allocated between valid claims for investment – is commonly accepted. In practice, stakeholder contributions often reflect a rejection of the entire foundation of rationing (Bhatia, 2020). Therefore, while A4R can help us choose between investment options and can reduce undue influence from interest groups, it does not in itself rescue the overall enterprise from the threat of backlash and disengagement.

It is not easy to determine what the role of external parties in priority setting ought to be. A key issue is the extent of delegation or devolution of responsibility away from government and the subsequent relationship between appointed bureaucrats and democratically elected representatives. As noted at the outset of this chapter, the extent to which local autonomy is possible and desirable will vary according to broader political structures and the relative responsibility afforded to elected and non-elected public sector functions (Landwehr, 2015). However, international experience suggests that governments will not hesitate to intervene where they feel the actions of subordinates threaten their own interests (Mbau et al., 2023). For example, Yeo et al. (1999) found that the attempts of a Canadian provincial health board to adopt a rules-based approach to priority setting were undermined by political instability and government intrusion. This was a clear illustration of how the democratic authority of governments can be exercised in ways that run counter to locally determined processes and priorities (Robinson et al., 2012). Ingram and Schneider (2005) argue that decision-making in public policy should work to secure 'the democratic promise for all people' (p. 2) and Gibson et al. (2005) propose 'empowerment' as an added condition to those put forward by Daniels and Sabin in their criteria for defensible decision-making.

Box 11.6 Case study from Argentina

Gordon et al. (2009) report from a case study of priority setting in an acute care public hospital in Buenos Aires, Argentina using the A4R framework as an evaluation tool. Respondents in their study consistently cited the influence of the Government Department of Health in shaping priorities. Government interventions were considered to be primarily 'political and personal' rather than driven by a response to perceived need (p. 188). Decision-making was also considered to be influenced by historical spending patterns and relationships and, in the absence of compelling evidence, the process was prey to 'union whims, prestige and uninformed biases' (Gordon et al, 2009: 188). The authors noted that these unwelcome influences were made possible by transparency deficits and the absence of an appeals mechanism.

Learning activity 11.3 Mapping the authorizing environment

Identify a priority-setting process from within your healthcare system. Try to map and appraise the relationship between your priority-setting process and the authorizing environment through the following activities.

Stage 1: Address the following questions:

- Apart from those actively involved, whose support is required for the priority-setting process to be considered legitimate?
- What other aspects of context (e.g. local events, politics and demographics) might affect support for the priority-setting process?
- What are the key media bodies that influence perceptions of healthcare locally?

Stage 2: Draw up a list of external groups and add to these: government (e.g. national or provincial) and the public. Answer the following questions for each group to help you to understand the relationship between the priority-setting process and its authorizing environment:

- How could this group influence the priority-setting process?
- How – if at all – does this group currently influence the priority-setting process?
- Do you actively engage this group? If so, how?
- Does this group currently have a high level of awareness of the priority-setting process? What is their perception of those making decisions?
- Could they be involved in the priority-setting process?
- Are they involved in the priority-setting process?
- What is the nature of the relationship between this group and other parts of the authorizing environment?
- Has this group criticized decisions in the past?
- Are this group's interests threatened by a particular decision?

Source: Williams (2015).

Implementation

Until now this chapter has depicted priority setting as a series of decisions and/or decision processes. In practice, formal decisions to cover (i.e. fund) health interventions are a necessary, but not the only, element of priority setting, and equal focus is required to the subsequent enactment of these decisions within healthcare delivery systems. Much of the priority-setting literature concentrates on decisions about allocating resources and fails to draw insights from disciplines, such as implementation science and organizational studies. Nevertheless, existing research suggests some key areas of consideration for those implementing priority-setting systems at local levels of healthcare.

The first of these is the need to connect priority-setting activities to actual resource allocation processes (including budget setting and finance). Where these links are weak – i.e. priority setters make recommendations that may or may not be actioned – the priority-setting enterprise runs the risk of losing 'clout' and being circumvented by other drivers and pressures (Williams and Bryan, 2007). Where ties are stronger (for example, decision-makers have veto over entry onto a formulary list), the priority-setting function is likely to be subject to greater levels of internal and external scrutiny, requiring processes that are highly robust to challenge.

A second area of importance is the relationship between priority setting and other aspects of strategic planning, performance measurement and so on. Arguably, priority setting should suffuse each of these activities. However, embedding decision-making in this way requires greater clarity over roles, responsibilities and relationships than is often evident in local healthcare systems (Kieslich et al., 2023).

A third area of concern is the lack of attention paid to the implementation of priority-setting decisions, with decision-making often considered a satisfactory endpoint in itself. A wealth of literature developed in other arenas supports the claim that healthcare systems tend to be complex – involving multiple interactions between groups across boundaries – and it therefore appears naïve to assume that the introduction and withdrawal of healthcare interventions can proceed in a simple, mechanistic fashion. Sophisticated implementation and improvement strategies are required if priority-setting decisions are to be fully adopted and adapted into practice.

Implementation barriers take on even greater significance when the priority-setting enterprise turns to 'disinvestment' (or 'decommissioning') of obsolete practices (Williams et al., 2021; Black et al., 2022). Previous studies have found that explicit priority setting tends to have an additive effect on overall spending (Sabik and Lie, 2008) suggesting that for priority setting to become an effective tool for reducing overall activity and spend, more work needs to be done.

Insights from the broader public policy literature suggest that implementation is most challenging when decisions are surrounded by high levels of ambiguity and conflict (Matland, 1995; Robert et al., 2014). This may help to explain some of the difficulties priority setters face. We have seen that the ethical complexity of rationing heightens the sense of decision ambiguity (i.e. what are we trying to achieve?). Furthermore, the highly politicized context of healthcare resource allocation increases the likelihood of conflict ensuing from decisions to invest and disinvest. In these circumstances, implementation of priority-setting decisions will be more vulnerable to the interplay of coalitions of local interest groups – including those involved in the provision and receipt of healthcare. Addressing these barriers can therefore be understood as an attempt to *reduce* ambiguity and conflict surrounding decision-making.

Learning activity 11.4 Planning for implementation

Select one of the following hypothetical decisions:

1 Decision to remove a drug from a hospital formulary.
2 Decision to locally implement national guidance on treatments for cancer.
3 Decision to cease funding for a specific surgical procedure.
4 Decision not to renew a contract with a charity providing specialist health/ social care services.
5 Decision to make all treatments available according to strict considerations of cost-effectiveness.
6 Decision to close the emergency department of a local hospital.

Consider the implementation responsibilities and potential impediments to implementation and how these might be addressed:

- Has responsibility for putting the decision into practice been allocated and accepted?
- Have you assessed the readiness of your organization(s) to implement the decisions?
- Have internal and external groups been engaged in the process?
- Have sufficient implementation resources been identified?
- Has support from senior leaders and other opinion formers been obtained?
- Are mechanisms in place to feedback information following the implementation process?

Key messages for healthcare managers

Although there is no blueprint for successful priority setting, there are some key 'ingredients' that decision-makers should consider:

- The first requirement is to explore and debate the ethical underpinnings of resource allocation: even though resolution of the tensions involved may not be possible, this will help to make explicit the moral concerns informing decisions.
- Managers and decision-makers should involve the public in these discussions. Although engaging citizens is difficult, it is essential if decisions over resource allocation are to be considered legitimate. Public engagement can also help to raise awareness of the challenges and trade-offs decision-makers face.
- There is a need to attend to the procedural dimensions of decision-making. For example, adopting process-based models (such as A4R) can improve quality, consistency and legitimacy of decisions.
- Priority setters should also draw on the evidence base, albeit decision analysis cannot be expected to fully replace debate and deliberation. Recent work has sought to

create a structure and process for combining the plethora of substantive, procedural and participative elements of decision-making (Kleinhout-Vliek et al., 2022).

- There is a need to clarify the remit of decision-making bodies, the roles and responsibilities of those involved, the budgets implicated in determinations, and the link to other organizational strategies and priorities.
- Finally, some management of the authorizing environment is required. Many of the above strategies can help garner legitimacy for the priority-setting enterprise. However, as rationing remains a highly politicized activity, those involved should deploy all available means to maximize public trust and stakeholder commitment and to create a coalition of support for the decision-making processes of resource allocation.
- This implies that local decision-makers require the skills to manage multiple accountabilities and a potentially hostile external environment (Waring et al., 2023). High profile public engagement and a strong media and communications strategy would seem to be prerequisites of a process in which leadership, political acumen and change management expertise are also likely to be beneficial.

Conclusions

Explicit approaches to priority setting and rationing are increasingly advocated as an alternative or supplement to other cost containment strategies. However, explicit approaches require attention to a range of factors if they are to be successful. This chapter has summarized some key themes from the literature on resource allocation and priority setting in healthcare, focusing mainly on the management function. As research, policy and practice in this area have matured, there has been an increasing acceptance that a single prescription (whether ethical, analytical or structural) is unlikely to emerge as a solution for all the problems priority setters face. Priority-setting methodologies are increasingly intensive and process-heavy and are perhaps unsurprisingly not always adopted by managers grappling with imperfect implementation systems and an inclination to avoid controversy. Characterized by ever-changing political and social tensions, the challenges of rationing are adaptive and therefore require skills in areas of profile and relationship management, as well as decision analysis and policy implementation (Heifetz and Laurie, 2001). More controversially, it could be argued that 'pragmatism' should be added to 'principles' and 'processes' in prescriptions for effective priority setting in as much as this denotes the flexibility and judgement required to assess, respond to and shape the prevailing authorizing environment in pursuit of longer-term public sector goals.

Learning resources

International Society for Priorities in Health: This resource contains a repository of papers and other resources on priority setting [www.prioritiesinhealth.org].

Continued

Learning resources *Continued*

World Health Organization: Contains information and resources on progress towards the Sustainable Development Goal of Universal Health Coverage [www.who.int/news-room/fact-sheets/detail/universal-health-coverage-(uhc)].

NICE: Provides guidance on the clinical and cost-effectiveness of new and existing medicines, treatments and procedures [www.nice.org.uk].

Social Care Institute for Excellence (SCIE): An independent charity, funded by the DH (in England). Identifies and disseminates the knowledge base for good practice in social care [www.scie.org.uk].

The Centre for Reviews and Dissemination (CRD): Based at the University of York and is part of the National Institute for Health Research. Undertakes systematic reviews that evaluate the effects of health and social care interventions. It also is the home to the following databases – Database of Abstracts of Reviews of Effects (DARE), HTA AND NHS Economic Evaluation Database (EED), which provide details on economic reviews and health technology assessments [www.york.ac.uk/inst/crd].

Health information resources (formerly the National Library for Health): Provides extensive access to studies conducted in health and social care [www.library.nhs.uk].

Personal Social Services Research Unit (PSSRU): Provides data on the unit costs of health and social care, which can be used in economic evaluations [www.pssru.ac.uk].

References

Abelson, J., Forest, P., Eyles, J., Smith, P., Martin, E. and Gauvin, F. (2003) Deliberations about deliberative methods: issues in the design and evaluation of public participation processes, *Social Science & Medicine*, 57: 239–51.

Abimbola, S., Negin, J., Martiniuk, A.L. and Jan, S. (2017) Institutional analysis of health system governance, *Health Policy and Planning*, 32(9): 1337–1344.

Al-Janabi, H., Williams, I. and Powell, M. (2023) Is the NHS underfunded? Three approaches to answering the question, *Journal of the Royal Society of Medicine*, 116(12): 409–412.

Babigumira, J.B., Jenny, A.M., Bartlein, R., Stergachis, A. and Garrison, L.P. (2016) Health technology assessment in low-and middle-income countries: a landscape assessment, *Journal of Pharmaceutical Health Services Research*, 7(1): 37–42.

Baltussen, R., Jansen, M.P., Mikkelsen, E., et al. (2016) Priority setting for universal health coverage: we need evidence-informed deliberative processes, not just more evidence on cost-effectiveness, *International Journal of Health Policy and Management*, 5(11): 615–618.

Barra, M., Broqvist, M., Gustavsson, E., Henriksson, M., Juth, N., Sandman, L. and Solberg, C.T. (2020) Severity as a priority setting criterion: setting a challenging research agenda, *Health Care Analysis*, 28(1): 25–44.

Batifoulier, P., Braddock, L. and Latsis, J. (2013) Priority setting in health care: from arbitrariness to societal values, *Journal of Institutional Economics*, 9(1): 61–80.

Belton, V. and Stewart, T. (2002) *Multiple Criteria Decision Analysis: An Integrated Approach.* Dordrecht: Springer Science & Business Media.

Berezowski, J., Czapla, M. and Ross, C. (2023) Rationing in healthcare—a scoping review, *Frontiers in Public Health*, 11. https://doi.org/10.3389/fpubh.2023.1160691.

Bhatia, N. (2020) We need to talk about rationing: the need to normalize discussion about healthcare rationing in a post COVID-19 era, *Journal of Bioethical Inquiry*, 17: 731–735.

Black, G.B., Wood, V.J., Ramsay, A.I., Vindrola-Padros, C., Perry, C., Clarke, C.S. et al. (2022) Loss associated with subtractive health service change: the case of specialist cancer centralization in England, *Journal of Health Services Research & Policy*, 27(4): 301–312.

Brown, R.C.H. (2013) Moral responsibility for (un)healthy behaviour, *Journal of Medical Ethics*, 39(11): 695–698.

Calltorp, J. (1999) Priority setting in health policy in Sweden and a comparison with Norway, *Health Policy*, 50: 1–9.

Charlesworth, A., Anderson, M., Donaldson, C., Johnston, P., Knapp, M., McGuire, A. et al. (2021) What is the right level of spending needed for health and care in the UK?, *The Lancet*, 397: 2012–2022.

Charlton, V. (2022) Does NICE apply the rule of rescue in its approach to highly specialised technologies? *Journal of Medical Ethics*, 48(2): 118–125.

Clark, S. and Weale, A. (2012) Social values in health priority setting: a conceptual framework, *Journal of Health Organization and Management* 26(3): 293–316.

Conklin, A., Morris, Z. and Nolte, E. (2015) What is the evidence base for public involvement in health-care policy? Results of a systematic scoping review, *Health Expectations*, 18(2): 153–165.

Dale, E., Peacocke, E.F., Movik, E., Voorhoeve, A., Ottersen, T., Kurowski, C., et al. (2023) Criteria for the procedural fairness of health financing decisions: a scoping review, *Health Policy and Planning*, 38(Suppl 1): i13.

Daniels, N. and Sabin, J. (2008) *Setting Limits Fairly: Learning to Share Resources for Health.* Oxford: Oxford University Press.

Daniels, T., Williams, I., Bryan, S., Mitton, C. and Robinson, S. (2018) Involving citizens in disinvestment decisions: what do health professionals think? Findings from a multi-method study in the English NHS, *Health Economics, Policy and Law*, 13(2): 162–188.

Danis, M., Hurst, S.A., Fleck, L., Forde, R. and Slowther, A. (eds) (2014) *Fair Resource Allocation and Rationing at the Bedside.* Oxford: Oxford University Press.

de Graaff, B., Kleinhout-Vliek, T. and Van de Bovenkamp, H. (2021) In the works: patient and public involvement and engagement in healthcare decision-making, *Health Expectations*, 24(6): 1903–1904.

Drummond, M.F.B., O'Brien, G., Stoddart, G. and Torrance, G. (1997) *Methods for the Economic Evaluation of Healthcare Programmes.* Oxford: Oxford University Press.

Friedman, A. (2008) Beyond accountability for reasonableness, *Bioethics*, 22(2): 101–12.

Gibson, J., Mitton, C., Martin, D., Donaldson, C. and Singer, P. (2006) Ethics and economics: does programme budgeting and marginal analysis contribute to fair priority setting? *Journal of Health Services Research and Policy*, 11(1): 32–37.

Gibson, J.L., Martin, D.K. and Singer, P.A. (2005) Priority setting in hospitals: fairness, inclusiveness, and the problem of institutional power differences, *Social Science & Medicine*, 61(11): 2355–2362.

Gordon, H., Kapiriri, L. and Martin, D.K. (2009) Priority setting in an acute care hospital in Argentina: a qualitative case study, *Acta Bioethica*, 15(2): 184–192.

Ham, C. and Robert, G. (eds) (2003) *Reasonable Rationing: International Experience of Priority Setting in Health Care*. Maidenhead: Open University Press.

Heifetz, R.A. and Laurie, D.L. (2001) The work of leadership, *Harvard Business Review*, Reprint R0111.

Hollingworth, S., Fenny, A.P., Yu, S.Y., Ruiz, F. and Chalkidou, K. (2021) Health technology assessment in sub-Saharan Africa: a descriptive analysis and narrative synthesis, *Cost Effectiveness and Resource Allocation*, 19(1): 39.

Holm, S. (1998) Goodbye to the simple solutions: the second phase of priority setting in health care, *British Medical Journal*, 317: 1000–1002.

Hopkins, S. (2010) Health expenditure comparisons: low, middle and high income countries, *The Open Health Services and Policy Journal*, 3: 21–27.

Hunter, D.J., Kieslich, K., Littlejohns, P. Staniszewska, S., Tumilty, E., Weale, A, et al. (2016) Public involvement in health priority setting: future challenges for policy, research and society, *Journal of Health Organization and Management*, 30(5): 796–808. doi: 10.1108/JHOM-04-2016-0057.

INAHTA (n.d.) Welcome to INAHTA. [https://www.inahta.org/; accessed 22 May 2024).

Ingram, H.M. and Schneider, A.L. (2005) Introduction: public policy and the social construction of deservedness, in A.L. Schneider and H.M. Ingram (eds) *Deserving and Entitled: Social Constructions and Public Policy*. New York: State University of New York Press.

Jacobs, L.R., Marmor, T. and Oberlander, J. (1998) *The Political Paradox of Rationing. The Case of the Oregon Health Plan*. The Innovations in American Government Program. John F. Kennedy School of Government, Harvard University, Occasional Paper 4.

Jonsen, A.R. (1986) Bentham in a box: technology assessment and health care allocation, *Law, Medicine and Health Care*, 14(3): 172–174.

Kamuzora, P., Maluka, S., Ndawi, B., Byskov, J. and Hurtig, A.K. (2013) Promoting community participation in priority setting in district health systems: experiences from Mbarali district, Tanzania, *Global Health Action*, 6(1): 22669.

Kapiriri, L., Baltussen, R. and Oortwijn, W. (2020) Implementing evidence-informed deliberative processes in health technology assessment: a low income country perspective, *International Journal of Technology Assessment in Health Care*, 36(1): 29–33.

Kapiriri, L., Norheim, O.F. and Martin, D.K. (2009) Fairness and accountability for reasonableness: do the views of priority setting decision makers differ across health systems? *Social Science & Medicine*, 68: 766–773.

Kieslich, K., Coultas, C. and Littlejohns, P. (2023) How reforms hamper priority-setting in health care: an interview study with local decision-makers in London, *Health Economics, Policy and Law*, 1–16.

Klein, R. (2010) Rationing in the fiscal ice age, *Health Economics, Politics and Law*, 5(4): 389–396.

Kleinhout-Vliek, T.H., De Bont, A.A. and Boer, A. (2022) Under careful construction: combining findings, arguments, and values into robust health care coverage decisions, *BMC Health Services Research*, 22(1): 756.

Landwehr, C. (2015) Democratic Meta-Deliberation: towards reflective institutional design, *Political Studies* 63(S1): 38–54.

Ledda, V., George, C., Glasbey, J. Labib, P., Li, E., Lu, A., et al. (2024) Uncertainties and opportunities in delivering environmentally sustainable surgery: the surgeons' view, *Anaesthesia*, 79(3): 293–300.

Löblová, O. (2018) When epistemic communities fail: exploring the mechanism of policy influence, *Policy Studies Journal*, 46(1): 160–189.

Lomas, J. (1997) Reluctant rationers: public input to health care priorities, *Journal of Health Services Research & Policy*, 2(2): 103–111.

Lord, J., Laking, G. and Fischer, A. (2004) Health care resource allocation: is the threshold rule good enough? *Journal of Health Services Research & Policy*, 9(4): 237–245.

Manafò, E., Petermann, L., Vandall-Walker, V. and Mason-Lai, P. (2018) Patient and public engagement in priority setting: a systematic rapid review of the literature, *PLOS one*, 13(3): e0193579.

Martinus Hauge, A., Otto, E.I. and Wadmann, S. (2022) The sociology of rationing: towards increased interdisciplinary dialogue – A critical interpretive literature review, *Sociology of Health & Illness*, 44(8): 1287–1304.

Matland, R.E. (1995) Synthesising the implementation literature: the ambiguity-conflict model of policy implementation, *Journal of Public Administration Research and Theory*, 5(2): 145–157.

Mbau, R., Oliver, K., Vassall, A., Gilson, L. and Barasa, E. (2023) A qualitative evaluation of priority-setting by the Health Benefits Package Advisory Panel in Kenya, *Health Policy and Planning*, 38(1): 49–60.

Miller, F.A., Lehoux, P., Rac, V.E., Bytautas, J.P., Krahn, M. and Peacock, S. (2020) Modes of coordination for health technology adoption: health technology assessment agencies and group procurement organizations in a polycentric regulatory regime, *Social Science & Medicine*, 265: 113528.

Mitton, C. and Donaldson, C. (2004) Health care priority setting: principles, practice and challenges, *Cost Effectiveness and Resource Allocation*, 2(3). doi: 10.1186/1478-7547-2-3.

Mooney, G. (1998) 'Communitarian claims' as an ethical basis for allocating health care resources, *Social Science & Medicine*, 4(9): 1171–180.

Nord, E. (2005) Concerns for the worse off: fair innings versus severity, *Social Science & Medicine*, 60: 257–263.

OECD (2023) Health at a Glance 2023: OECD Indicators. Paris: OECD Publishing. doi: 10.1787/7a7afb35-en.

Orr, S. and Wolff, J. (2015) Reconciling cost-effectiveness with the rule of rescue: the institutional division of moral labour, *Theory and Decision*, 78: 525–538.

Oswald, M. (2015) In a democracy, what should a healthcare system do? A dilemma for public policymakers, *Politics, Philosophy & Economics*, 14(1): 23–52.

Parsons, W. (1995) *Public Policy: An Introduction to the Theory and Practice of Policy Analysis*. Edward Elgar Publishing Ltd (UK).

Porter, L.B. (2020) Harm reduction and moral desert in the context of drug policy, *Health Care Analysis*, 28(4): 362–371.

Rawls, J. (1972) *A Theory of Justice*. Oxford: Oxford University Press.

Rivlin, M.M. (2000) Why the fair innings argument is not persuasive, *BMC Medical Ethics*, 1: 1.

Robert, G., Harlock, J., Williams, I. (2014) Disentangling rhetoric and reality: an international Delphi study of factors and processes that facilitate the successful implementation of decisions to decommission healthcare services, *Implementation Science*, 9: 123.

Robinson, S., Williams, I., Dickinson, H., Freeman, T. and Rumbold, B. (2012) Priority-setting and rationing in healthcare: evidence from the English experience, *Social Science & Medicine*, 75(12): 238623–238693.

Rosoff, P.M. (2014) *Rationing Is Not a Four-Letter Word: Setting Limits on Healthcare.* Cambridge, MA: MIT Press.

Sabik, L.M. and Lie, R.K. (2008) Priority setting in health care: lessons from the experiences of eight countries, *International Journal for Equity and Health*, 7: 4.

Sandman, L., Davidson, T., Helgesson, G. and Juth, N. (2018) The ethical problems in limiting the role for cost-effectiveness, *Lakartidningen*, 115: E4EH.

Seixas, B.V., Regier, D.A., Bryan, S. and Mitton, C. (2021) Describing practices of priority setting and resource allocation in publicly funded health care systems of high-income countries, *BMC Health Services Research*, 21: 1–15.

Sibbald, S.L., Singer, P.A., Upshur, R. and Martin, D.K. (2009) Priority setting: what constitutes success? A conceptual framework for successful priority setting, *BMC Health Services Research,* 9(43), doi:10.1186/1472-6963-9-43.

Sorenson, C. and Chalkidou, K. (2012) Reflections on the evolution of health technology assessment in Europe, *Health Economics, Policy and Law*, 7(1): 24 -45.

Steffensen, M.B., Matzen, C.L. and Wadmann, S. (2022) Patient participation in priority setting: co-existing participant roles, *Social Science & Medicine*, 294. doi: 10.1016/j. socscimed.2022.114713.

Stevens, A. and Gillam, S. (1998) Needs assessment: from theory to practice, *British Medical Journal*, 316: 1448–1452.

Ubel, P.A. and Goold, S. (1997) Recognizing bedside rationing: clear cases and tough calls, *Annals of Internal Medicine*, 126(1): 74–80.

Waring, J., Bishop, S., Clarke, J., Exworthy, M. and Hartley, J. (2023) Healthcare leadership with political astuteness, in N. Chambers (ed.) *Research Handbook on Leadership in Healthcare.* Cheltenham: Edward Elgar Publishing.

Weale, A., Kieslich, K., Littlejohns, P., et al. (2016) Introduction: priority setting, equitable access and public involvement in health care, *Journal of Health Organization and Management*, 30(5): 736–750.

Williams, A. (1997) Intergenerational equity: an exploration of the 'fair innings' argument, *Health Economics*, 6(2): 117–132.

Williams, A. (2006) Economics, QALYs and Medical Ethics: A Health Economist's Perspective, in S. Dracopolou (ed.) *Ethics and Values in Healthcare Management* (2nd edn.) Abingdon: Routledge.

Williams, I. (2015) Receptive rationing: reflections and suggestions for priority setters in health care, *Journal of Health Organization and Management*, 29(6): 701–710.

Williams, I. (2024) Decision Making and Policy Formulation: The Case of Health Care Coverage, in M. Powell, M., T.I. Agartan, and D. Béland, (eds) *Research Handbook on Health Care Policy* (pp. 30–45). Gloucestershire, UK: Edward Elgar Publishing.

Williams, I. and Bryan, S. (2007) Cost-effectiveness analysis and formulary decision making in England: findings from research, *Social Science & Medicine*, 65(10): 2116–2129.

Williams, I. and Bryan, S. (2015) Lonely at the top and stuck in the middle? The ongoing challenge of using cost-effectiveness information in priority setting, *International Journal of Health Policy and Management*, 4(3): 185–187.

Williams, I. and Robinson, S. (2012) Decision Making and Priority Setting, in J. Glasby (ed.) *Commissioning for health and well-being*. Bristol: Policy Press.

Williams, A. (1997) Intergenerational equity: an exploration of the 'fair innings' argument, *Health Economics*, 6(2): 117–132.

Williams, I., Allen, K. and Plahe, G. (2019) Reports of rationing from the neglected realm of capital investment: responses to resource constraint in the English National Health Service, *Social Science & Medicine*, 225: 1–8.

Williams, I., Dickinson, H. and Robinson, S. (2012) *Rationing in Health Care: The Theory and Practice of Priority Setting*. Bristol: Policy Press.

Williams, I., Harlock, J., Robert, G., Kimberly, J. and Mannion, R. (2021) Is the end in sight? A study of how and why services are decommissioned in the English National Health Service, *Sociology of Health & Illness*, 43(2): 441–458.

Yeo, M., Williams, J.R. and Hooper, W. (1999) Incorporating ethics in priority setting: a case study of a rational health board in Canada, *Health Care Analysis*, 7: 177–194.

Chapter 12

Climate change and sustainability

Chris Naylor and Hayley Pinto

Introduction

Climate change is a major risk for health and health systems. The climate crisis has entered a phase in which broad-based leadership is needed from all sectors and industries, including healthcare. Healthcare managers can play a vital role both by reducing the environmental impact of healthcare systems and by ensuring services are resilient to the current and future effects of climate change.

This chapter describes what healthcare managers need to know and how they can have the greatest impact. It explains why environmental sustainability is important for healthcare management and how, using the tools and frameworks we describe, this can be embedded into existing work and align with other healthcare priorities. We consider how managers can lead a culture change to accelerate the necessary transformation towards sustainable healthcare and we offer illustrative examples from around the world

We argue that sustainability creates an additional impetus for changing models of care in ways that could also deliver benefits in terms of cost, quality of care and population health. Carbon reduction goals are unlikely to be met without a shift towards more preventative, person-centred care that reduces avoidable or low-value activity. The drive for sustainability across all sectors of the global economy is creating a stimulus for innovation, and by playing a leading role in this the healthcare sector can accelerate progress towards its core strategic goals.

Why is environmental sustainability important for healthcare management?

The health sector is both vulnerable to – and a major contributor to – the impacts of climate change and wider environmental degradation (e.g. plastic and pharmaceutical pollution).

In this section we consider four reasons why environmental sustainability is important for healthcare management (see Box 12.1).

Box 12.1   Four reasons to prioritize sustainability

1   Climate change has multiple health impacts now and in the future.
2   Action to mitigate climate change can also bring public health benefits.
3   Climate change poses direct risks to healthcare service delivery.
4   Health systems are themselves significant contributors to climate change.

Health impacts of climate change

The World Health Organization (WHO) estimates that more than 13 million deaths occur each year due to environmental causes and describes the climate crisis as 'the single biggest health threat facing humanity' (World Health Organization, 2022a). Even countries accustomed to more temperate weather are already experiencing multiple and increasing health impacts of climate change (UK Health Security Agency, 2023). The 2023 Lancet Countdown (Romanello et al., 2023) monitors and reports on global and regional health impacts including:

- **Air pollution**. Primarily caused by the burning of fossil fuels, air pollution increases the risk of a wide range of physical and mental health conditions throughout the lifespan (Royal College of Physicians, 2016; Bourdrel et al., 2017; Doiron et al., 2019). Ninety-nine per cent of the global population are exposed to air which exceeds WHO pollution limits, contributing to 6.7 million premature deaths per year (World Health Organization, 2022b), 26,000 to 38,000 in the UK (Department of Health and Social Care (DHSC), 2022). Many more people live with chronic disease as a result of this exposure.
- **Heatwaves**. Globally, heat-related deaths in over 65s have increased by 85 per cent in 20 years (Romanello et al., 2023). Children, pregnant women and people with serious mental health conditions are also more vulnerable as they are less able to regulate their body temperatures (Page et al., 2012; Giudice et al., 2021). In pregnancy, excess heat is associated with increased risk of low birthweight, preterm birth, congenital abnormalities and other complications (Giudice et al., 2021).
- **Vector-borne diseases**. Heat increases the geographical range and months of suitable conditions for mosquitoes, ticks and other vectors that spread diseases, such as Malaria, Dengue fever, Zika Virus and Lyme's disease (Ma et al., 2022).
- **Water-borne diseases**. Warmer water increases the geographical range of pathogens responsible for diseases, such as cholera, liver fluke and schistosomiasis (Donnelly and Talley, 2023).
- **Storms and flooding**. Immediate risks include death or injury and contamination of water supplies. Longer-term risks include waterborne and respiratory infections

and significantly increased prevalence of PTSD, anxiety and depression (Waite et al., 2017).
- **Water shortages**. Changes to the water cycle are increasing drought worldwide. The World Bank predicts a two thirds reduction in water availability for cites globally by 2050 (World Bank, 2016).
- **Food security.** Heat, drought, storms, wildfires, soil degradation and the loss of pollinators is already affecting agriculture worldwide. The risk of simultaneous crop failure in major food-producing regions is increasing and would lead to abrupt increases in food prices worldwide, with potential to destabilize social and economic systems (Gaupp et al., 2019).
- **Conflict and migration.** Food and water insecurity are driving conflicts and migration in many parts of the world, as well as population displacement due to sea-level rises. Some analyses predict as many as 1.2 billion climate refugees by 2050 (European Parliament, 2023).

As well as the direct health impacts, many of the above will have significant social and economic consequences globally, and these are in turn likely to affect health and health inequalities in ways that cannot be fully foreseen. Disdvantaged groups, whether through income, health status, gender, age or race are often more exposed to climate impacts, such as living in areas at risk of flooding (Environment Agency, 2022), are more vulnerable to these impacts, for example, due to living in buildings more likely to overheat (CDP, 2023) and have poorer access to resources, such as insurance, that allow them to recover (Islam and Winkel, 2017) – leading to vicious cycles of deprivation.

Public health benefits of climate action

Many of the actions that would reduce carbon emissions and wider environmental damage could have enormous benefits for public health and well-being and help to address health inequalities.

Shifting dietary behaviours is one of the biggest opportunities to align climate action with health improvement. The Lancet Commission described the global food system as 'the single strongest lever to optimise human health and environmental sustainability on Earth' (Swinburn et al., 2019). Diets high in meat and dairy, in addition to ultra-processed foods high in fats, salt and sugar are linked to epidemics of obesity and undernutrition causing diabetes, heart and liver disease, and cancer (Swinburn et al., 2019). Changing diets to increase the proportion of wholegrains, legumes, fruit, vegetables and nuts could dramatically improve our health and make a significant contribution to addressing the climate crisis (EAT-Lancet Commission, 2019).

Making it easier for people to cycle, walk or use public transport instead of private vehicles would deliver reductions in greenhouse gas emissions alongside considerable health benefits through increasing physical activity and reducing social isolation. This could also significantly reduce road traffic accidents and air pollution – even over a relatively short time-period, reduced car use during the COVID-19 pandemic led to immediate reductions in hospital

How Climate Action Improves Health and Reduces Social Inequality

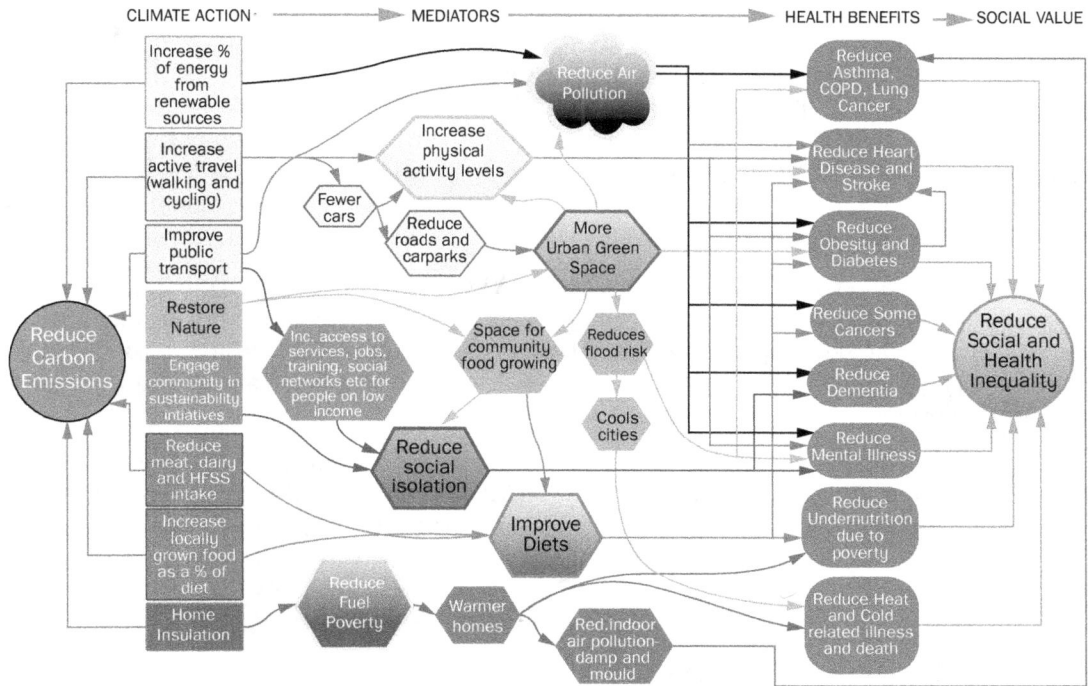

Figure 12.1 Mechanisms that show how climate action can improve health and reduce social inequality
Source: The Centre for Sustainable Healthcare.

admissions for asthma (Singh et al., 2024). Long-term, this also has potential to reduce a wide range of chronic physical and mental health conditions as described above.

A large and growing body of research demonstrates the breadth of positive impacts of green space for physical and mental health (Twohig-Bennett and Jones, 2018). Protecting and enhancing existing green spaces, as well as creating new ones and increasing public access, can therefore deliver population health benefits as well as assisting climate change mitigation.

Figure 12.1 shows how these and other actions to tackle the climate and ecological emergencies have potential to reduce the prevalence of many chronic conditions.

Risks to healthcare delivery posed by environmental change

Climate change poses a significant threat to the functioning of healthcare services. For example, between April 2021 and March 2022 there were 176 flooding incidents at NHS sites in the UK (Jeffrey, 2023). Ten per cent of hospitals in the UK are currently assessed as being at risk from flooding, with the risk increasing as climate change worsens (Climate Change

Committee, 2021). Hospital wards, other clinical areas and key infrastructure, such as IT systems and medication storage, are also at risk of overheating during heatwaves.

For example, the 2022 heatwave in the UK led to 5,554 reported cases of clinical areas exceeding 26°C, triggering risk assessments (Watkins et al., 2023). This was an increase of 86 per cent in such incidents since 2016 when the data were first available. High temperatures can negatively affect cognitive functioning for staff, increasing risks of clinical error (Mazloumi et al., 2014). Many hospitals also struggled with overheating of IT systems, scanners and medicine storage areas (Quadri, 2022). Other concerns caused by heatwaves include the risk of legionella in cold water systems.

Extreme weather events may also disrupt critical infrastructure, including transport networks, power and water supplies locally. Complex global supply chains for medication, medical equipment and other supplies add to this vulnerability (Masters, 2021). Local supply chains may be more resilient to global climate impacts, as well as being associated with lower transport emissions.

Extreme weather can also result in abrupt increases in demand, compounding problems related to healthcare system functioning. Official data shows that heatwaves in the UK were associated with higher admission rates from 2010–2020 (Office for National Statistics, 2022). Injuries, mental health disorders and cardiovascular-related deaths were the biggest contributors.

Environmental impact of healthcare

The health sector is a significant contributor to climate change, responsible for around 5 per cent of carbon emissions globally. If the global health sector were a country, it would be the fifth-largest emitter on the planet (Health Care Without Harm, 2019). Healthcare also contributes to pollution, particularly through plastics and pharmaceutical waste (Rizan et al., 2020). Addressing the sector's contribution to the problems and health impacts outlined above represents part of the duty of care that healthcare systems have to the populations they serve.

To focus efforts effectively it is helpful to understand where carbon emissions come from within the healthcare system. While the exact figures will vary for each health system, it is instructive to examine the breakdown conducted for the NHS in England, as illustrated in Figure 12.2 (NHS England, 2020). A number of important observations can be taken from this analysis.

First, 62 per cent of carbon emissions attributable to the NHS in England relate to its supply chain (medicines, equipment and other procured goods). Given this, a major part of any healthcare organization's efforts to reduce carbon emissions needs to involve reducing the volume of goods procured (for example, through more efficient stock management, reduced use of low-value items, increased use of reusable equipment, better prescribing and medicines management), as well as exerting influence on suppliers and assessing sustainability as part of procurement decisions. The approach to this taken by Newcastle University Hospitals NHS Trust illustrates what can be achieved through structured engagement with suppliers and consistent leadership (see Box 12.2).

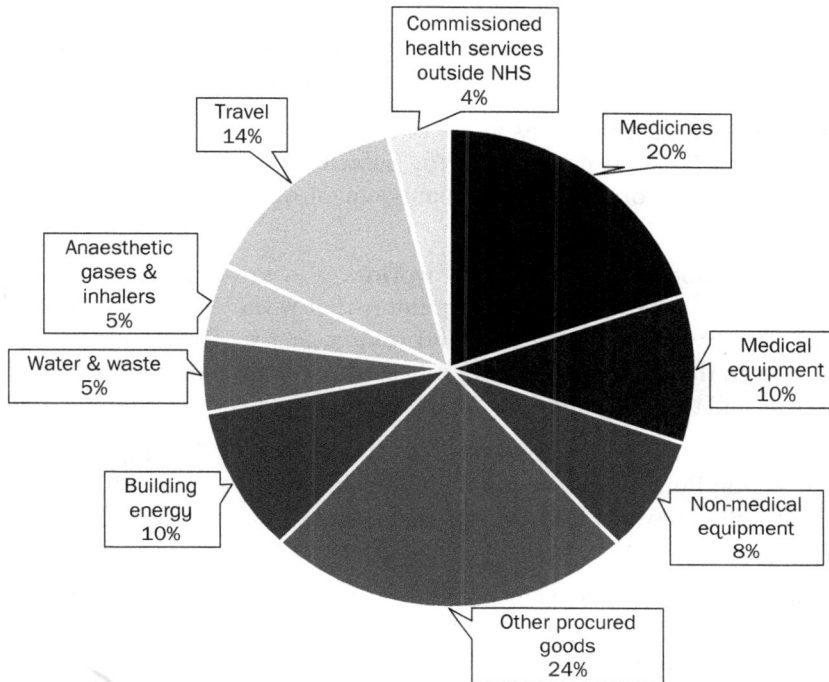

Figure 12.2 Sources of greenhouse gas emissions attributable to the NHS in England
Source: Adapted from NHS England (2020).

Box 12.2 Newcastle University Hospitals NHS Foundation Trust: Embedding sustainability at organizational level

Newcastle University Hospitals (NUH) has benefited from strong senior leadership on sustainability over a number of years. The organization declared a climate emergency in 2019, and the following year published a Climate Emergency Action Strategy setting out its ambition to be a global leader in sustainable healthcare delivery, including achieving net-zero carbon emissions several years before the national targets set for the NHS as a whole. This began a comprehensive programme of activity known as the Shine programme.

Staff engagement is a major part of the strategy. Staff wanting to get more deeply involved can become 'Green Champions +' – this involves completing online training, attending regular meetings and development sessions, and implementing small-scale sustainability projects in their areas of work. Over 300 members of staff have signed up to become Green Champions and are supported in this role by a Sustainability Team. The organization also provides funding for a small number of clinicians to take part in Sustainability Fellowships, with half or more of their time dedicated to quality-improvement activities related specifically to environmental sustainability.

Training is available at various levels of intensity – from 30 minutes introductory courses through to a 5-day programme for Sustainability Ambassadors. The organization's Board of Directors and senior management group have all received climate education.

Over 1,000 members of staff (out of a workforce of around 16,000) have signed up to 'Shine Rewards' – a staff benefits programme that rewards staff for saving energy, reducing waste, travelling sustainably and taking part in other sustainable actions. Staff take part in the programme using a bespoke website and app. Benefits include monthly prizes and team charity donations.

Any member of staff can apply for small amounts of funding from a Climate Emergency Action Fund to get sustainability projects off the ground. Projects can be submitted for a Shine Award and are added to a bank of case studies for others in the organization to learn from.

The Shine programme is seen as one of the means through which NUH can deliver its broader aim to enable staff to flourish and realize their full potential. In this way, a deliberate connection has been made between the organization's work on sustainability and its work on staff well-being and morale.

Procurement is one of the areas in which NUH has made particular progress. The organization has developed a five-step process to proactively engage and support all suppliers. This includes giving suppliers support in the form of webinars, events and other resources, and requiring them to enrol in an online SmartCarbon Calculator tool where they can calculate and report their carbon emissions. This practical 48-minute video outlines the approach taken to supplier engagement: [https://vimeo.com/883922511?share=copy].

NUH is also actively collaborating with key partners in its local system and more broadly. For example, it has worked with Newcastle City Council, the North of Tyne Combined Authority, the North East and North Cumbria Integrated Care Board and others to develop an integrated regional approach towards clean air, with support from the environmental charity Global Action Plan.

More information on the Shine programme is available at:]https://www.newcastle-hospitals.nhs.uk/about/sustainable-healthcare/].

Second, most of the carbon footprint is shaped directly by clinical decisions and the way patient care is provided. Figure 12.2 also shows that 20 per cent is attributable to medicines, 10 per cent to medical equipment, and 5 per cent to anaesthetic gases and inhalers (NHS England, 2020). Beyond this, how buildings are used, travel requirements, quantities of waste generated and water used are also largely determined by clinical pathways and activities. This makes it clear that healthcare systems cannot achieve net-zero without significant transformation to the way care is provided. Non-clinical teams of course also play a vital role – for example, retrofitting and design of healthcare buildings and facilities can help to reduce the carbon footprint attributable to building energy use (heating, lighting and other electricity use) – but as this only accounts for 10 per cent of the overall carbon footprint (NHS England, 2020) providing the same care within more efficient buildings will not be sufficient.

Third, there are some carbon 'hot spots' where efforts to reduce emissions can have a particularly significant and rapid impact. Anaesthetic gases (notably desflurane and nitrous oxide) and the propellants used in metered dose inhalers are greenhouse gases in their own right, with some having a larger climate impact than others (Sulbaek Andersen et al., 2023). Similarly, some forms of care, such as kidney dialysis, have a particularly large carbon footprint (Connor et al., 2010). Identifying carbon hot spots such as these can help healthcare managers to think where best to focus their efforts. These priorities will vary by sector and setting, for example, in primary care the most impactful areas to focus on are medicines prescribing and inhaler use, which together contribute 65–90 per cent of primary care emissions (British Medical Association, 2020).

Learning activity 12.1

What do you think are the most compelling arguments for sustainability being a core concern for healthcare managers? Imagine you were emailing colleagues to persuade them that sustainability should be a top priority – what would you say, and what action would you ask for? As an exercise, write an email setting out your concerns and the potential benefits of taking action. Consider who you could send this to in practice.

Tools and frameworks to help incorporate sustainability in healthcare management

Having outlined why sustainability is important for healthcare management, we now turn to some of the tools and frameworks available to help managers better understand the range of actions they can take, measure the impact of these actions and engage clinical teams to take ownership of the sustainability agenda.

Principles of sustainable healthcare

At the broadest level, there are two ways healthcare systems can reduce their environmental impact. The first is to reduce the amount of healthcare activity, and the second is to reduce the environmental impact of activity that needs to persist. The five principles of sustainable healthcare developed by the Centre for Sustainable Healthcare indicate what can be done within these two broad categories. These five principles can be presented as a driver diagram (as in Figure 12.3) to stimulate specific change ideas.

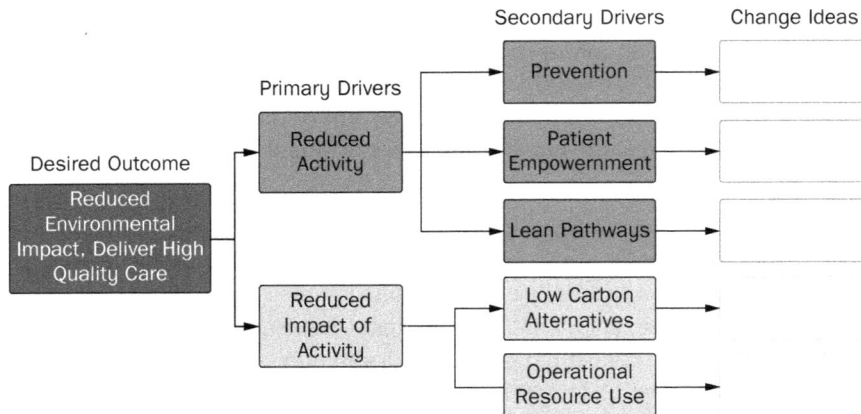

Figure 12.3 Five principles of sustainable healthcare – driver diagram
Source: The Centre for Sustainable Healthcare.

Prevention

The most powerful approach is to reduce the need for healthcare activity by improving pop-ulation health, hence reducing demand. The approach with the broadest potential benefits is primary prevention. This means working with wider system partners, such as local and national governments, community organizations and the general public. These interventions are most effective when they target the wider socio-economic and environmental determi-nants of health, for example, through local strategies to improve public and active transport, which in turn reduces air pollution and greenhouse gas emissions while also promoting phys-ical activity and accessibility of transport options for low-income groups. An example of this was the earlier case study of Newcastle University Hospitals NHS Foundation Trust that worked with partners to develop an integrated clean air initiative with a focus on reducing emissions and mitigating health inequalities (see Box 12.2).

Prevention also includes early identification and intervention to avoid development of chronic conditions and complications, reducing the need for more complex and carbon-intensive healthcare interventions down the line.

Patient empowerment

Empowering patients to self-monitor and manage their health and health conditions can streamline healthcare activity and associated greenhouse gas emissions by minimizing the need for routine checks and appointments and reducing low-value interventions and those which the patient is unlikely to actively engage with. Additionally, it could enable patients to seek help promptly before their condition deteriorates. Shared decision-making is a key aspect of this approach. Digital technology provides new opportunities for increased self-monitoring and self-management, particularly for more vulnerable populations or people with chronic conditions (see Box 12.3). Involving people with lived experience of the condi-tion is vital to the success of these projects and helps mitigate the risk of digital exclusion.

> ## Box 12.3 Remote monitoring hub in Northwest England
>
> This service was developed for patients with diabetes, chronic cardiovascular and respiratory diseases that were identified as a priority using local population health data. Patients measure their vital signs at home and upload these using a phone app: 4G-enabled devices are provided for those who do not have one. The uploaded information is digitally assessed at the hub and alerts are sent to the clinical team when readings lie outside personalized preset thresholds. The multidisciplinary team can then assess the situation and decide the most appropriate course of action – ranging from a phone or video call to an in-person review.
>
> For patients in the service this has reduced emergency admissions by 22.3 per cent and use of health and care services by 40 per cent. Staff report improved effectiveness of time management and improved partnership working across primary, secondary and social care.
>
> For further information see: [https://www.merseycare.nhs.uk/our-services/liverpool/telehealth-health-technology-service].

Lean pathways

A lean pathway is one that delivers effective care in the right place at the right time and eliminates unnecessary steps to achieve that goal (see Chapter 3 on quality improvement). There are many opportunities to improve care pathways so that all activity delivers maximum benefit to patients. In many healthcare systems there is evidence of unwarranted clinical variation and provision of tests and procedures that are of limited clinical value (Wennberg, 2002). There is also widespread evidence of duplication, waste and inefficiency as a result of barriers to information sharing, inefficient referral pathways and lack of joint working between services. Lean pathways are designed to maximize efficiency, stripping out wasteful or low-value activity, thereby reducing both costs and carbon emissions, while also improving patient experience, increasing the effectiveness of services and minimizing the risk of avoidable harm from unnecessary interventions.

It is vital to involve patients in the design of lean pathways to ensure that activities that may appear of low value from a process perspective, but which are highly valued by patients, are not lost. For example, activities that involve human contact and therapeutic relationship-building may result in greater engagement and trust, improving outcomes and efficiency.

Low-carbon alternatives

Low-carbon alternatives include technologies, pharmaceuticals and devices with lower environmental impacts that can replace currently used products often without significantly changing care pathways. Well-known examples include dry powder inhalers (as an alternative to metered-dose inhalers) and sevoflurane, total intravenous anaesthesia (TIVA) or regional anaesthesia (as an alternative to more polluting anaesthetic gases such as desflurane).

Switching from single-use to reusable medical equipment is another example that has the potential to reduce the carbon footprint (and long-term costs) of these products considerably (Brighton and Sussex Medical School et al., 2023). Items such as textiles, laryngoscopes, sharps bins, speculums, tourniquets and surgical instruments can be decontaminated and safely reused (Sherman et al., 2018; Grimmond et al., 2021; Drayton et al., 2023). For example, Liverpool University Hospitals NHS Foundation Trust achieved savings of over £53,000 over 3 years, alongside reduced emissions and waste by switching from single-use theatre caps to reusable caps embroidered with staff members' names and roles (NHS England, 2022).

Maximizing the environmental and financial benefits of switching to reusable equipment requires creating or expanding local infrastructure for cleaning and sterilization to avoid additional emissions due to transportation and potentially expensive external contracts.

Operational resource use

Finally, we consider potential carbon-emissions savings to be made relating to buildings, energy use (and generation) and other physical infrastructure. An important aspect of this is transitioning away from fossil fuels by increasing energy efficiency, purchasing renewable energy and (where possible) incorporating renewable energy generation on hospital sites (see Box 12.4). Doing so provides opportunities for financial as well as carbon savings – for example, NHS England estimates that switching to 100 per cent LED lighting could save £3 billion over 30 years, while more efficient heating, cooling and ventilation could save £250 million per year (NHS England, 2020).

Box 12.4   Saving lives with solar

University Hospitals of North Midlands NHS Trust funded the installation of rooftop solar panels on hospital buildings by selling community bonds to local people and businesses with a 4.5 per cent rate of return. Income generated through feed-in tariff payments were re-invested in a local charity (Beat the Cold) which provides support for people experiencing fuel poverty [https://www.england.nhs.uk/midlands/2022/12/29/university-hospitals-of-north-midlands-supports-local-people-living-in-fuel-poverty-while-reducing-its-carbon-footprint/#:~:text=The%20University%20Hospitals%20of%20North,are%20living%20in%20fuel%20poverty].

Learning activity 12.2

Use the driver diagram of the 'five principles of sustainable healthcare' from Figure 12.3 to generate your own ideas for improving sustainability. Try to list at least two to three specific, achievable ideas for each of the five principles. What information would you need to develop these ideas further? Who would you need to speak to?

Measuring sustainability impact

Measurement is crucial for identifying prime areas to target for emission reductions ('carbon hotspots') and monitoring and showcasing progress towards sustainable transformation. There are some key concepts relating to measurement of environmental metrics that healthcare managers should have an understanding of, specifically: carbon footprinting, life-cycle assessment (LCA) and 'Triple Bottom Line' accounting.

Carbon footprinting

Carbon footprinting estimates the combined greenhouse gas emissions (not just carbon dioxide) for an item, activity or organization. It does not account for wider environmental impacts, such as pollution or water use, but it is a logical place to start and is an area where much work has been done to develop measurement methodologies. There are two main approaches to carbon footprinting. 'Top-down' approaches estimate carbon emissions by making plausible assumptions based on existing (often financial) data about energy, water and other products consumed and multiplying this by emission factors for those items in existing databases. This approach lacks the accuracy of full 'bottom-up' methods that involve calculating the footprint of a product or service by breaking it down into its constituent parts or processes and using reference data on the carbon emissions typically associated with each of these components. In practice, top-down and bottom-up methodologies are often combined to give a pragmatic balance of the two. For example, when assessing the carbon footprint of a service or intervention, a top-down approach might be used for energy use emissions based on meter readings, while a bottom-up approach might be used to identify the emission associated with a specific piece of surgical equipment.

Life-cycle assessment

Life-cycle assessment (LCA) to attempts to understand the environmental impact of a product (for example, a pharmaceutical product or medical device) across its entire life cycle, including extraction of raw materials, manufacturing, use and disposal. This can be measured in terms of carbon emissions or including a broader set of environmental impacts, such as water consumption and various aspects of environmental pollution. Standardized approaches to this, such as those produced by the International Organisation for Standardization (e.g. ISO 14040), are available but this complex methodology is primarily for use in research environments, rather than, for example, healthcare procurement teams. Having a basic understanding of the principles, however, is useful for those assessing the validity of manufacturers' claims. Increasingly, there are existing, peer-reviewed life-cycle analyses for medical products, for example, single-use vs. reusable laryngoscopes (Sherman et al., 2018) that healthcare managers can draw on.

Triple bottom-line accounting

Triple bottom-line accounting involves measuring costs in terms of environmental, social and financial impact. This is an approach that has been used in a range of industries (Kenton, 2024). The 'sustainable value' equation illustrated below (Figure 12.4) applies this principle

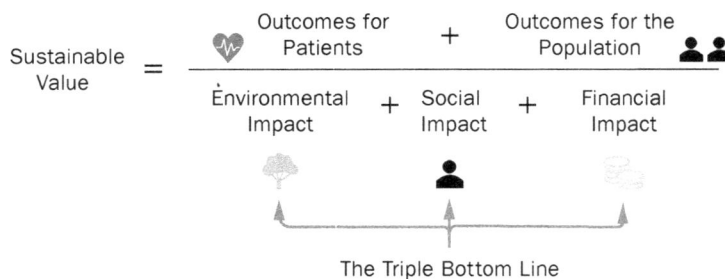

Figure 12.4 The sustainable value equation
Source: The Centre for Sustainable Healthcare.

to healthcare, incorporating the requirement to maintain or improve quality of care. This approach to measuring the impacts of healthcare activity broadens the focus from individual clinical outcomes and financial costs (cost-effectiveness) to include the impact on the wider population, social impacts (e.g. accessibility of services, time off work or education for patients, staff well-being) and environment impacts.

This is not intended as a mathematical equation to calculate value numerically, but rather an approach to evaluating alternative options that can be used as part of routine decision-making at clinical and management levels.

Embedding sustainability in quality improvement

A practical way of applying the five principles and the sustainable value approach as described above is to use them as a way of stimulating and refining ideas for service improvement as part of quality improvement (QI) processes. As described in Chapter 3, QI methodologies provide a powerful set of tools that support clinical teams, service managers and others to identify opportunities to improve the quality and efficiency of care processes, test these change ideas in practice, measure the results and then adapt and refine the original ideas through an iterative improvement process.

Embedding environmental sustainability into existing QI processes is one way that healthcare managers can ensure that environmental challenges are addressed routinely, making it part of the core business of a health system rather than a peripheral concern. The Sustainability in Quality Improvement (SusQI) framework provides a toolkit for incorporating sustainability principles in the planning and assessment of quality improvement projects, designed to be integrated into existing QI approaches (Mortimer et al., 2018). The framework explains how to apply sustainability at four key steps in the QI process:

1 Setting goals for improvement activities.
2 Studying how the system currently works using process mapping or similar tools.
3 Identifying change ideas for testing.
4 Selecting measures through which the impact of these ideas will be assessed.

Embedding sustainability in each of these four stages ensures that environmental impacts are considered alongside patient outcomes, patient experience, social impacts and financial costs. It also provides a way of engaging clinical teams in implementing the sustainability agenda (see Box 12.5), rather than it being seen as only relevant primarily to estates and facilities teams.

Box 12.5   Sustainable quality improvement in HIV care

Having used the SusQI tool to identify and assess opportunities for improvement in the care pathway for people living with HIV, Northamptonshire Healthcare NHS Foundation Trust reduced the frequency of routine blood testing for stable patients from 6 monthly to 12 monthly. This change was made possible by improved treatment effectiveness and tolerability. The measured benefits included:

- Improved convenience for patients and less time off work.
- Staff time released to focus on unstable patients with higher needs.
- Potential financial savings of £45,000 per year.
- Potential carbon savings of 26,000 kgCO2e per year.

The free-to-access SusQI website provides a step-by-step guide to SusQI and a range of practical resources and case studies of implementation in practice (see 'Learning resources' at the end of the chapter).

Leading for sustainability in the health sector

To act as effective leaders on sustainability, there are five areas that healthcare managers will need to give particular attention to:

1   Providing visible leadership
2   Building capacity
3   Scaling and spreading successful projects
4   Collaborating internally and externally
5   Measuring progress

Visible leadership

The first task for healthcare managers is to demonstrate, through their own behaviours, is that sustainability is an important organizational objective. This means talking about it at every opportunity and working with peers to consider how to embed sustainability as part of business as usual.

If sustainability does not currently have a high profile within an organization, it can be helpful to instigate an initial consultation and education package to engage relevant stakeholders, including staff, patient and carer groups, and key partners in the local community e.g. local government. This can help to ensure the initiative has broad support and relevant groups know how they can contribute. A communications drive may be needed initially to raise awareness and recruit participants to engage in the consultation (see Box 12.6).

Box 12.6   Communicating effectively about climate change

The following approaches can help healthcare managers to communicate about sustainability in a compelling way that changes attitudes and behaviours.

1   **Find shared values** with the people you seek to influence, and then join the dots between these values and climate change. Highlight the various ways in which action on climate change can help healthcare systems to deliver their core objectives. Outline explicitly the links to existing priorities, such as quality of care, health inequalities or financial and staffing pressures.

2   **Use human stories and make it local.** People are more motivated by issues likely to affect them or those they care for. For example, draw attention to examples of how extreme weather is already affecting people and/or services in the local area.

3   **Tell the story of why you care.** Authentic emotion is impactful – people remember how you made them feel more than the detail of what you said. Social contagion can be powerful. Highlight how other people in the organization or the broader healthcare sector are worried about climate change.

4   **Balance gloom with hope.** Be honest about the threats but highlight how acting on climate change could improve health and well-being and deliver other benefits. Describe a positive vision of a sustainable future to give your audience something to work towards.

5   **Give people something to do.** Be clear about how people can contribute. Getting involved helps people feel more empowered and less fatalistic, creating a virtuous circle.

To make sustainability a part of 'business as usual', it needs to be included in organizational values and mission statements. Healthcare managers should look for ways of embedding sustainability within the functioning of their organization, such as including it in meeting agendas, on the risk register and in business case criteria, decision-making frameworks and other tools. It may be helpful to organize regular communications showcasing local successes; to engage the broadest audience, include information on the impacts on quality of care, social and financial benefits as well as reduction in environmental impacts.

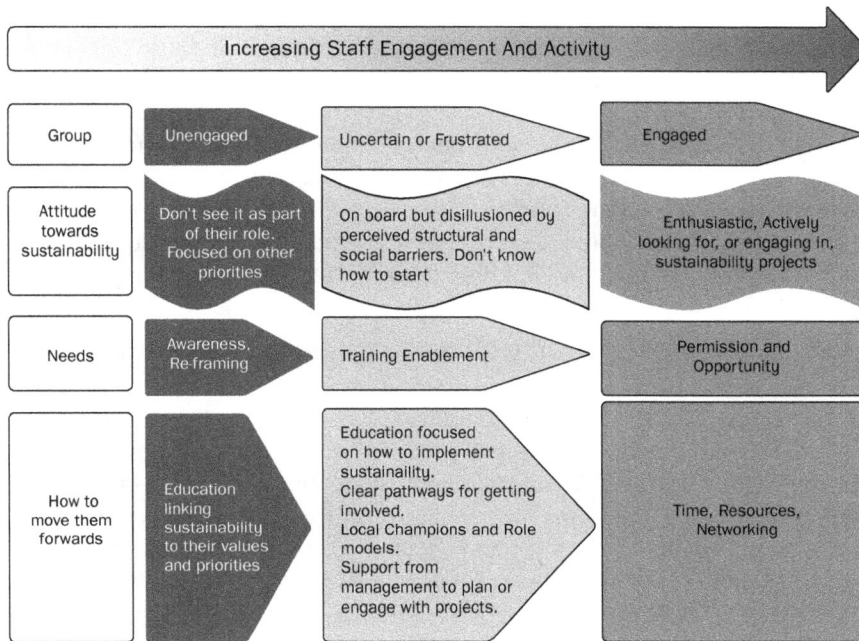

Figure 12.5 Strategies to increase engagement in sustainability
Source: The Centre for Sustainable Healthcare.

Building capacity

A common situation in healthcare organizations internationally is that efforts to promote sustainability are being driven by a few passionate individuals trying to fit this around their day jobs and/or by isolated sustainability leads, where these roles exist. This reliance on enthusiasts and volunteers is not sustainable or sufficient (McGeoch et al., 2023). In any organization, staff on the ground know how the system works and have the expertise to innovate or to block change, so getting them involved is crucial. A range of strategies are needed for people at different levels of motivation and engagement (see Figure 12.5).

Learning activity 12.3

Thinking of staff you have worked with or encountered in the health sector, where do you think they lie on the spectrum illustrated in Figure 12.5 – are they unengaged, uncertain/frustrated or engaged? What about yourself? List ideas for specific strategies that would help to move yourself or your colleagues to the right. Try putting some of these strategies into practice with two or three individuals and take note of what approaches prove most effective.

Training and education for staff is a vital component of this capacity building. The focus and depth of this training can be adapted to the needs of the individual or their role. Ideally the entire staff base should have a basic awareness. In the UK there is a free e-learning for health online module 'Building a Net-Zero NHS' that is available to anyone with an NHS email and outlines the basics of a sustainable approach to healthcare. Given the significant impacts on health and healthcare delivery there is a strong argument for making basic training on this subject mandatory for staff. Some roles require more in-depth training, tailored to their role, to support embedding sustainable practice. These include members of quality improvement teams, middle and senior management, clinical leads and procurement teams (see 'Learning resources').

It can be more effective to work with the willing rather than relying on formal hierarchies. This means identifying motivated staff and giving them the support, training and permission they need to drive the sustainability agenda forward. Many staff may already have improvement ideas that could benefit patients at the same time as reducing environmental damage. To harness these ideas, they need protected time, access to resources, senior project sponsors to help them overcome barriers and opportunities to network and feed into decision-making. An example of this is Newcastle University Hospitals NHS Foundation Trust, which employed junior doctors in three specialities with half or more of their time dedicated to quality improvement activities related specifically to environmental sustainability (see earlier, Box 12.2).

Scaling and spreading

To make changes on the scale needed within the time available, healthcare managers need to ensure there are structures in place to share learning within and between organizations, so that small-scale but successful sustainability projects can be replicated. This could involve setting up a dedicated team to identify projects suitable for replication and to oversee local implementation (see Box 12.7). Research on the successful spread of innovation identifies several key factors that can help, including the use of peer networks to allow learning to be shared (Horton et al., 2018).

Box 12.7   Spreading and scaling good practice in the Royal National Orthopaedic Hospital

The Royal National Orthopaedic Hospital NHS Trust in London has a team responsible for seeking out and prioritizing successful sustainability projects from elsewhere to replicate, such as the 'Gloves are off' project to reduce unnecessary use of non-sterile gloves and the 'Nix the Nitrous' project to reduce waste emissions of nitrous oxide. A dedicated sustainability page on the Trust website includes an email for staff to submit ideas and feedback [https://www.england.nhs.uk/atlas_case_study/the-gloves-are-off-campaign/] and [https://sustainablehealthcare.org.uk/what-we-do/sustainable-specialties/anaesthetics/nitrous-oxide-project.

The CEO is the sustainability lead and there are leads for each area of focus in their Green Plan who meet quarterly to review progress. Progress is also evaluated in an annual impact report.

Collaborating on sustainability

Change management theory often stresses the importance of building a coalition of people with a shared commitment (Appelbaum et al., 2012), and sustainability is no exception to this. To foster this coalition within their own organization, healthcare managers can set up events and forums to engage staff and patients; create green champion groups to share learning and successful projects; develop routes for staff to present ideas (e.g. through a social media group); or organize 'lunch and learn' sessions to facilitate peer learning. One of the goals should be to encourage cross-disciplinary communication and collaboration, for example, between clinicians, procurement and facilities teams. It was this kind of cross-disciplinary exchange of information that formed the basis of the Nix the Nitrous project referred to in Box 12.7, which identified that over 90 per cent of nitrous oxide in one hospital was wasted through leaks (Chakera, 2020).

Healthcare managers can have an impact on a broader scale by collaborating with other local organizations and sectors. For example, the climate change team in the West Yorkshire and Harrogate Health and Care Partnership has worked with local government and other agencies to influence transport planning decisions about the future of public transport and active travel schemes, supporting health improvement and carbon reduction at the same time (Swinton, n.d.). Local or regional partnerships also offer an opportunity to consider what could be done once across larger geographies – for example, through procurement teams working together on identifying sustainable products and using bulk ordering to reduce costs.

Working collaboratively with partners, such as local government and community organizations, requires healthcare managers to develop a different set of skills and competencies, as it involves bringing about change through 'soft power' and influence rather than through formal hierarchy and authority (Walsh and de Sarandy, 2023).

Measuring progress

A further important role for healthcare managers is to ensure the system is sufficiently capable of measuring and demonstrating progress. This will often involve strengthening local expertise in environmental metrics and methodologies, such as those described above. Measures of progress in relation to sustainability should be included in annual reports and other key documents. It is also helpful to share results more widely using regional and national networks, journals and other channels – for example, Newcastle University Hospitals NHS Trust produces an annual 'SHINE' report which shares their progress towards their net-zero goals (see earlier, Box 12.2).

Learning activity 12.4

Find out about the processes and structures being used to drive sustainability in your health organization, or one you are familiar with.

- Do you have a sustainability lead on the board?
- What expertise is there within the organization to measure greenhouse gas emissions and wider environmental impacts?
- How is this information presented to the board and wider audiences?
- Does it form part of your annual review and if so, what actions have been taken in response to the data?
- Does the organization have a road map to reach net zero?
- What actions could you take to ensure effective governance on this issue?
- What are your peers doing in other organizations?

Examples of sustainable healthcare initiatives

Sustainable healthcare is a rapidly growing field being driven by a growing number of organizations at global, national and local level.

Internationally, the World Health Organization has a programme of work on environmentally sustainable health systems and has produced a number of guidance documents, including an operational framework for building climate-resilient and low-carbon health systems (World Health Organization, 2023) and a toolkit for health professionals on communicating on climate change and health (World Health Organization, 2024). International non-governmental organizations also play an important role. For example, Health Care Without Harm supports networks of health organizations and professionals in all global regions, such as the Global Green & Healthy Hospitals network, which includes hospitals in over 80 countries that have committed to reduce their environmental footprint and promote public and environmental health (Health Care Without Harm, n.d.).

At national level, a growing number of health systems have introduced policies and targets in relation to environmental sustainability, a prominent example being the English NHS: in 2020 it became the first national health system to set specific targets for reaching net-zero carbon emissions (see Box 12.8). In Scandinavia, the Nordic Centre for Sustainable Healthcare has supported knowledge sharing, including through an online platform based on Grönnköpingki∂ University Hospital – a fictional new hospital showcasing cutting-edge solutions for improved environmental performance, all of which are based on products and services that are on the market and already in use in healthcare facilities across the Nordic countries (Nordic Centre for Sustainable Healthcare, n.d.).

Box 12.8   The Greener NHS programme in England

The NHS in England has had a carbon-reduction strategy since 2009. In 2020 it launched a Greener NHS programme including a new plan for reaching net zero carbon emissions (NHS England, 2020). The headline goals in this plan are to reach net zero by 2040 for the emissions the NHS controls directly, and by 2045 for emissions it can influence (including emissions related to supply chains).

These targets mean that the NHS is required to reduce its carbon footprint dramatically over the next 15–20 years. Similar targets have also been introduced by the NHS in Wales (NHS Wales, 2021) and Scotland (NHS Scotland, 2022).

In addition to these headline targets there are a number of specific requirements for NHS organizations in England, including to do the following:

- Publish a Green Plan setting out how the organization will reduce its carbon footprint in line with national targets.
- Appoint a board-level lead responsible for net-zero and the organization's Green Plan.
- Report annually on carbon emissions.
- Purchase 100 per cent renewable energy (or have plans to do so as soon as possible).
- Phase out the use of the anaesthetic gas desflurane.
- Develop plans for switching to lower carbon inhalers where clinically appropriate.
- Ensure that new facilities deliver gains in biodiversity through creating better quality natural habitats.
- Consider social and environmental impacts when buying goods or services.

To support emissions reductions in the wider supply chain, the Greener NHS programme also introduces requirements and resources for organizations supplying goods and services to the NHS. This includes the NHS Net Zero Supplier Roadmap that sets requirements, which become increasingly exacting over the next few years. By April 2027, all suppliers to the NHS will be required to have carbon reduction targets aligned to the overall NHS targets, and to report progress against these publicly.

Academic institutions are also increasingly active in sustainable healthcare. For example, the National University of Singapore has launched a Centre for Sustainable Medicine aiming to accelerate Singapore's transition to net-zero healthcare and to train future healthcare leaders (National University of Singapore, 2023).

At service level, there is a wealth of examples of clinical teams and services that have conducted projects leading to improved clinical and environmental outcomes (for example, see the case studies described on the Sustainable Healthcare Networks Platform in 'Learning resources'). So far there are fewer examples of healthcare organizations that have successfully embedded sustainability across all of their services. Newcastle University Hospitals NHS Foundation Trust provides one good example of an organization that has taken significant steps in this direction (see earlier, Box 12.2).

Conclusion

Time is often precious in healthcare and sustainability can sometimes be seen as just one of a long list of important issues to which healthcare managers need to give their attention. Framing it this way is unhelpful and risks leaving people feeling overwhelmed. This chapter has offered an alternative way of understanding the relationship between health and sustainability. The climate emergency gives new life and urgency to some of the most important strategic shifts that healthcare managers have been attempting to bring about for many years. It calls for an approach to health that is more preventative, more personalized and less wasteful, in which there is a determined focus on providing the interventions that create most value for patients and populations. It also makes it more important than ever that health systems take full advantage of the opportunities created by new technologies and innovation.

Finally, sustainability creates an opportunity for healthcare staff to reconnect with their values and sense of mission. People working in the health sector often have to live with the discomfort of taking steps in their home lives to reduce their environmental impact but feeling that they must shut their eyes to unsustainable practices at work. Offering the chance to work in a proactive, innovative environment that aligns with their values has the potential to improve staff well-being and aid retention and recruitment. In this way, sustainable healthcare can be better for staff as well as for patients and planet.

Learning resources

World Health Organization toolkit: Communicating on climate change and health [https://www.who.int/publications/i/item/9789240090224].

Greener NHS campaign toolkit: To assist development of communication strategies [https://campaignresources.dhsc.gov.uk/campaigns/for-a-greener-nhs/campaign-toolkit/].

Greener NHS guidance: On producing a green plan for your organization [england.nhs.uk/greenernhs/wp-content/uploads/sites/51/2021/06/B0507-how-to-produce-a-green-plan-three-year-strategy-towards-net-zero-june-2021.pdf].

Centre for Sustainable Healthcare: Overview of sustainability training courses for healthcare managers and clinicians [https://sustainablehealthcare.org.uk/courses].

Sustainable Healthcare Networks Platform: Supports healthcare professionals to connect with others and share learning, including case studies of impactful sustainable healthcare projects [https://networks.sustainablehealthcare.org.uk/].

Sustainability in Quality Improvement (SusQi): Website provides a step-by-step guide, resources, templates and case studies on embedding sustainability in quality improvement processes: https://www.susqi.org/

Institute of Environmental Management and Assessment (IEMA): Guidance offers practical advice for non-executive directors of healthcare organizations on how sustainability can be incorporated into their role [https://www.iema.net/resources/blog/2022/10/24/launch-of-iema-guidance-on-sustainability-for-nhs-non-executive-directors-ned].

Greener Practice: Website that provides networks and resources on sustainability in primary care settings [https://www.greenerpractice.co.uk/].

Green Impact: A United Nations programme designed to support environmentally and socially sustainable practices in a wide range of organizations [https://greenimpact.nus.org.uk/].

References

Appelbaum, S.H., Habashy, S., Malo, J. and Shafiq, H. (2012) Back to the future: revisiting Kotter's 1996 change model, *Journal of Management Development*, 31(8): 764–782. https://doi.org/10.1108/02621711211253231.

Bourdrel, T., Bind, M.A., Béjot, Y., Morel, O. and Argacha, J.F. (2017) Cardiovascular effects of air pollution, *Archives of Cardiovascular Diseases*, 110(11): 634–642. https://doi.org/10.1016/j.acvd.2017.05.003.

Brighton and Sussex Medical School, Centre for Sustainable Healthcare, and UK Health Alliance on Climate Change (2023) Green surgery: reducing the environmental impact of surgical care (v1.1). London: UKHACC. [https://ukhealthalliance.org/sustainable-healthcare/green-surgery-report/; accessed 20 February 2025].

British Medical Association (2020) Sustainable and environmentally friendly general practice report. [https://www.bma.org.uk/advice-and-support/gp-practices/gp-premises/sustainable-and-environmentally-friendly-general-practice-report; accessed 20 February 2025].

CDP (2023) Building local resilience. [https://www.cdp.net/en/articles/citiesannouncements/those-on-low-income-and-elderly-most-vulnerable-to-uk-climate-change; accessed 3 December 2024].

Chakera, A. (2020) *Reducing the Impact of Nitrous Oxide Emissions within Theatres to Mitigate Dangerous Climate Change*, Evidence-Based Policy Brief Dissertation, University of Edinburgh.

Climate Change Committee (2021) UK Climate Risk Health and Social Care Sector Briefing [https://www.ukclimaterisk.org/publications/health-and-social-care-sector-briefing/; accessed 3 December 2024].

Connor, A., Lillywhite, R. and Cooke, M.W. (2010) The carbon footprint of a renal service in the United Kingdom, *QJM: Monthly Journal of the Association of Physicians*, 103(12): 965–975. https://doi.org/10.1093/qjmed/hcq150.

Department of Health and Social Care (DHSC) (2022) Chief Medical Officer's annual report 2022: air pollution [https://www.gov.uk/government/publications/chief-medical-officers-annual-report-2022-air-pollution; accessed 3 December 2024].

Doiron, D., de Hoogh, K., Probst-Hensch, N., Fortier, I., Cai, Y., De Matteis, S. et al. (2019) Air pollution, lung function and COPD: results from the population-based UK Biobank study, *The European Respiratory Journal*, 54(1): 1802140. https://doi.org/10.1183/13993003.02140-2018.

Donnelly, M.C. and Talley, N.J. (2023) Effects of climate change on digestive health and preventative measures, *Gut*, 72: 2199–2201.

Drayton, R., Smith, H. and Ratnappuli, A. (2023) Sustainable practice: switching to reusable vaginal speculums, *The BMJ*, (Clinical research ed.), 383: e075779. https://doi.org/10.1136/bmj-2023-075779.

EAT-Lancet Commission (2019) EAT-Lancet Commission Summary Report. [https://eatforum.org/eat-lancet-commission/eat-lancet-commission-summary-report/; accessed 20 February 2025].

Environment Agency (2022) Social deprivation and the likelihood of flooding [https://www.gov.uk/government/publications/social-deprivation-and-the-likelihood-of-flooding; accessed 3 December 2024].

European Parliament (2023) The concept of 'climate refugee': towards a possible definition [https://www.europarl.europa.eu/RegData/etudes/BRIE/2021/698753/EPRS_BRI(2021)698753_EN.pdf; accessed 3 December 2024].

Gaupp, F., Hall, J., Mitchell, D. and Dadson, S. (2019) Increasing risks of multiple breadbasket failure under 1.5 and 2 °C global warming, *Agricultural Systems*, 175: 34–45. https://doi.org/10.1016/j.agsy.2019.05.010.

Giudice, L.C., Llamas-Clark, E.F., DeNicola, N., Pandipati, S., Zlatnik, M.G., Decena, D.C.D., et al. (2021) The FIGO Committee on Climate Change, Toxic Environmental Exposures. Climate change, women's health, and the role of obstetricians and gynecologists in leadership, *International Journal of Gynecology & Obstetrics*, 155: 345–356. https://doi.org/10.1002/ijgo.13958.

Grimmond, T.R., Bright, A., Cadman, J., Dixon, J., Luddit, S., Robinson, C. and Topping, C. (2021) Before/after intervention study to determine impact on life-cycle carbon footprint of converting from single-use to reusable sharps containers in 40 UK NHS trusts, *BMJ Open*, 11(9): e046200. https://doi.org/10.1136/bmjopen-2020-046200.

Health Care Without Harm (2019) Health care's climate footprint. How the health sector contributes to the global climate crisis and opportunities for action. [https://noharm-global.org/documents/health-care-climate-footprint-report; accessed 20 February 2025].

Health Care Without Harm (n.d.) Global Green and Healthy Hospitals website [https://greenhospitals.org/; accessed 3 December 2024].

Horton, T., Illingworth, J. and Warburton, W. (2018) The spread challenge, *The Health Foundation* [https://www.health.org.uk/publications/the-spread-challenge; accessed 4 December 2024].

Islam, N. and Winkel, J. (2017) Climate change and social inequality. United Nations Department of Economic and Social Affairs [https://www.un.org/en/desa/climate-change-and-social-inequality; accessed 3 December 2024].

Jeffrey, J. (2023) NHS underwater. Analysis of increasing flooding events in the NHS and its impact on patients [https://socialspark1.co.uk/uploads/files/ROW-NHS-UNDERWATER-REPORT-MARCH23-FINAL.pdf; accessed 20 February 2025].

Kenton, W. (2024) Triple bottom line. *Investopedia* [https://www.investopedia.com/terms/t/triple-bottom-line.asp; accessed 3 December 2024].

Ma, J., Guo, Y., Gao, J., Tang, H., Xu, K., Liu, Q, et al. (2022) Climate change drives the transmission and spread of vector-borne diseases: an ecological perspective, *Biology*, 11(11): 1628. https://doi.org/10.3390/biology11111628.

Masters, J. (2021) Suez Canal shutdown shows the vulnerability of the global economy to extreme events, *Yale Climate Connections*. [https://yaleclimateconnections.org/2021/03/suez-canal-shutdown-shows-vulnerability-of-global-economy-to-extreme-events/; accessed 20 February 2025].

Mazloumi, A., Golbabaei, F., Mahmood Khani, S., Kazemi, Z., Hosseini, M., Abbasinia, M., et al. (2014) Evaluating effects of heat stress on cognitive function among workers in a hot industry, *Health Promotion Perspectives*, 4(2): 240–246.

McGeoch, L., Hardie, T., Coxon, C. and Cameron, G. (2023) Net zero care: what will it take? *The Health Foundation* [https://www.health.org.uk/publications/long-reads/net-zero-care-what-will-it-take; accessed 3 December 2024].

Mortimer, F., Isherwood, J., Wilkinson, A. and Vaux, E. (2018) Sustainability in quality improvement: redefining value, *Future Healthcare Journal*, Jun; 5(2): 88–93.

National University of Singapore (2023) NUS Medicine sets up new Centre for Sustainable Medicine. [https://news.nus.edu.sg/new-centre-for-sustainable-medicine/; accessed 20 February 2025].

NHS England (2020) Delivering a 'Net Zero' National Health Service. https://www.england.nhs.uk/greenernhs/wp-content/uploads/sites/51/2020/10/delivering-a-net-zero-national-health-service.pdf.

NHS England (2022) Case study – Switching to Reusable Theatre Caps. [https://www.england.nhs.uk/north-west/greener-nhs/case-studies-greener-nhs/case-study-switching-to-reusable-theatre-caps/; accessed 20 February 2025].

NHS Scotland (2022) NHS Scotland climate emergency and sustainability strategy: 2022-2026. [https://www.gov.scot/publications/nhs-scotland-climate-emergency-sustainability-strategy-2022-2026/; accessed 20 February 2025].

NHS Wales (2021) NHS Wales Decarbonisation Strategic Delivery Plan. [https://www.gov.wales/nhs-wales-decarbonisation-strategic-delivery-plan; accessed 20 February 2025].

Nordic Centre for Sustainable Healthcare (n.d.) Grönnköpingkið Hospital – World's Greenest Hospital. [https://worldsgreenesthospital.org/; accessed 3 December 2024].

Office for National Statistics (2022) Climate-Related Mortality and Hospital Admissions, England and Wales: 2001 to 2020. [https://www.ons.gov.uk/peoplepopulationandcommunity/birthsdeathsandmarriages/deaths/articles/climaterelatedmortalityandhospitaladmissionsenglandandwales/2001to2020; accessed 3 December 2024].

Page, L., Hajat, S., Kovats, S. and Howard, L. (2012) Temperature-related deaths in people with psychosis, dementia and substance misuse, *British Journal of Psychiatry*, 200: 485–490.

Quadri, S. (2022) IT systems at two of London's biggest hospitals 'shuts down' due to heatwave. *The Standard* [https://www.standard.co.uk/news/london/london-guy-s-st-thomas-hospital-london-it-heatwave-weather-b1015699.html; accessed 3 December 2024].

Rizan, C., Mortimer, F., Stancliffe, R. and Bhutta, M.F. (2020) Plastics in healthcare: time for a re-evaluation, *Journal of the Royal Society of Medicine*, 113(2): 49–53. https://doi.org/10.1177/0141076819890554.

Romanello et al. (2023) The 2023 report of the Lancet Countdown on health and climate change: the imperative for a health-centred response in a world facing irreversible harms, *Lancet Countdown*, 402(10419): 2346–2394. [https://www.thelancet.com/journals/lancet/article/PIIS0140-6736(23)01859-7; accessed 20 February 2025].

Royal College of Physicians (2016) Every Breath We Take: The Lifelong Impact of Air Pollution. Report of a Working Party. London: RCP. [www.rcp.ac.uk/improving-care/resources/every-breath-we-take-the-lifelong-impact-of-air-pollution/; accessed 20 February 2025].

Sherman, J.D., Raibley, L.A., 4th and Eckelman, M.J. (2018) Life cycle assessment and costing methods for device procurement: comparing reusable and single-use disposable laryngoscopes, *Anesthesia and Analgesia*, 127(2): 434–443. https://doi.org/10.1213/ANE.0000000000002683.

Singh, A., Morley, G.L., Coignet, C., Leach, F., Pope, F.D., Thomas, G.N., et al. (2024) Impacts of ambient air quality on acute asthma hospital admissions during the COVID-19 pandemic in Oxford City, UK: a time-series study, *BMJ Open*,14: e070704. doi:10.1136/bmjopen-2022-070704; accessed 3 December 2024.

Sulbaek Andersen, M.P., Nielsen, O.J. and Sherman, J.D. (2023) Assessing the potential climate impact of anaesthetic gases, *The Lancet. Planetary Health*, 7(7): e622–e629. https://doi.org/10.1016/S2542-5196(23)00084-0.

Swinburn, B.A., Kraak, V.I., Allender, S., Atkins, V..J., Baker, P.I., Bogard, J.R., et al. (2019) The Global Syndemic of Obesity, Undernutrition, and Climate Change. *The Lancet Commission Report*. [https://www.thelancet.com/commissions/global-syndemic; accessed 20 February 2025].

Swinton, F. (n.d.) West Yorkshire and Harrogate Climate Change Team: A Year of Sustainable Achievements. Centre for Sustainable Healthcare. [https://sustainablehealthcare.org.uk/blog/west-yorkshire-and-harrogate-climate-change-team-year-sustainable-achievements; accessed 3 December 2024].

Twohig-Bennett, C. and Jones, A. (2018) The health benefits of the great outdoors: a systematic review and meta-analysis of greenspace exposure and health outcomes, *Environmental Research*, 166: 628–637. https://doi.org/10.1016/j.envres.2018.06.030.

UK Health Security Agency (2023) Health Effects of Climate Change in the UK: State of the Evidence 2023. [https://assets.publishing.service.gov.uk/media/659ff6a93308d200131fbe78/HECC-report-2023-overview.pdf; accessed 3 December 2024].

Waite, T.D., Chaintarli, K., Beck, C.R., Bone, A., Amlôt, R., Kovats, S., et al. (2017) The English national cohort study of flooding and health: cross-sectional analysis of mental health outcomes at year one, *BMC Public Health*, 17(1): 129. https://doi.org/10.1186/s12889-016-4000-2.

Walsh, N. and de Sarandy, S. (2023) The Practice of Collaborative Leadership across Health and Care Services. London: The King's Fund. [https://www.kingsfund.org.uk/insight-and-analysis/reports/practice-collaborative-leadership; accessed 20 February 2025].

Watkins, A., Williams, B. and Wattiau, R. (2023) Climate change insights, health and well-being, UK: May 2023. Office for National Statistics [https://www.ons.gov.uk/economy/environmentalaccounts/articles/climatechangeinsightsuk/may2023; accessed 3 December 2024].

Wennberg, J.E. (2002) Unwarranted variations in healthcare delivery: implications for academic medical centres, *The BMJ*, Oct 26; 325(7370): 961–964.

World Bank (2016) High and Dry: Climate Change, Water, and the Economy. [https://www.worldbank.org/en/topic/water/publication/high-and-dry-climate-change-water-and-the-economy; accessed 3 December 2024].

World Health Organization (2022a) World Health Day 2022. [https://www.who.int/campaigns/world-health-day/2022; accessed 3 December 2024].

World Health Organization (2022b) Ambient (Outdoor) Air Pollution. [https://www.who.int/news-room/fact-sheets/detail/ambient-(outdoor)-air-quality-and-health; accessed 3 December 2024].

World Health Organization (2023) Operational Framework for Building Climate Resilient and Low Carbon Health Systems. [https://www.who.int/publications/i/item/9789240081888; accessed 3 December 2024].

World Health Organization (2024) Communicating on Climate Change and Health: Toolkit for Health Professionals. [https://www.who.int/publications/i/item/9789240090224; accessed 3 December 2024].

Primary care

Manbinder Sidhu and Judith Smith

Introduction

Primary care is central to a modern-day healthcare system dealing with the growing prevalence of multimorbidity, often-widening health inequalities and over-stretched workforces delivering care with limited resources. Throughout this chapter, we draw on international examples of research and practice to understand how primary care is distinctive from the community, acute and tertiary health sectors; the contribution made towards self-care; emerging models of online support; and primary care organizations, and the specific challenges of managing primary care services.

The chapter will explore the introduction of new roles in primary care as part of multidisciplinary teams and the challenges this aims to address alongside the work of the generalist primary care physician. Further, we examine new models of primary care that attempt to better manage and coordinate the care of people with long-term and complex conditions, which also encompass end of life care; and explore the increasingly widespread use of digital, telephone and video technology as part of triage, diagnosis, consultations and follow-up treatment in primary care.

We consider strategic planning and management for stronger and more extensive primary care that broadens the capabilities of primary care, including what this means for healthcare management roles. Case studies are used to illustrate and analyse the latest developments in the organization and management of primary care, drawing out common themes across nations, and using these to identify the particular challenges for healthcare managers.

Nature and role of primary care

Primary care (also known as primary healthcare), embraces principles of 'social justice, equity, self-reliance, appropriate technology, decentralization, community involvement, intersectoral collaboration, and affordable cost' (World Health Organization, 1978).

The defining moment in contemporary history of primary healthcare is generally considered to have been the declaration, at a World Health Organization (WHO) conference in 1978, of what primary healthcare should provide to people in communities and nations. This declaration, known as the Declaration of Alma-Ata after the name of the town, Almaty, where the conference took place, set out the following statement about the nature of primary healthcare:

> Primary health care addresses the main health problems, providing preventive, curative, and rehabilitative services accordingly . . . but will include at least: promotion of proper nutrition and an adequate supply of safe water; basic sanitation; maternal and child care, including family planning; immunization against the major infectious diseases; education concerning basic health problems and the methods of preventing and controlling them; and appropriate treatment of common diseases and injuries.
>
> (World Health Organization, 1978: Section VII)

Primary healthcare comprises pragmatic and evidence-based care, which at times is supported by technology-enabled tools, made accessible to individuals and families, via a private or publicly funded model (World Health Organization, 2023). Primary healthcare is central to a country's healthcare system and fundamental to the social and economic prosperity of a given population. It is the first point of contact for individuals and carers, delivered close to where communities live and often leads to navigating further health treatments more widely across healthcare sectors (World Health Organization, 2023).

There is no single model for the universal implementation of primary healthcare policy and associated services. Primary healthcare can encompass disease-focused prevention – including immunizations and vaccinations – and self-management for the long-term management of chronic diseases, as well as supporting behavioural change. The successful implementation and delivery of primary healthcare services acutely depend on the availability of trained lay and professional health service providers to support models of care relevant to resource allocation, working under the management of government policymakers (Rifkin, 2018).

There is significant variation internationally in the policy focus and implementation of primary healthcare. Rajan et al. (2024), reflecting on a WHO global report on primary care, draw attention to the proven importance of primary care for cost-effective and health-promoting health systems, yet note the often-wavering political reticence to invest and support this sector. For instance, Thailand implements a primary healthcare policy of universal health coverage (Sakboonyarat et al., 2022); India employs a model using a large-scale delivery of community health worker programmes (Gaitonde et al., 2017); while Brazil has created Family Health Teams, comprising multidisciplinary teams of physicians, nurses and community health workers, similar to models more recently adopted in the United Kingdom (Perry, 2016). Models of primary healthcare delivery are typically designed to address the challenges associated with the inverse care law (Hart, 1971), for example, enabling and sustaining accessible care to disadvantaged communities. Hence, healthcare managers should consider how primary healthcare accounts for the complexity of health equity and promotes access for individuals and families in most need (Rifkin, 2018).

Management for primary care within a health system

The growing prominence of primary healthcare, especially given the challenges of addressing global public health concerns as outlined in Chapter 4 (Public health and global inequalities), has led to the management of such services becoming complex. There are several distinctive aspects of primary care development that have driven this increased complexity: the role of primary care in coordinating a wide range of services; ensuring equitable access to primary care; collaborating across the local health system; embracing technology and self-care; and strategic planning and management for stronger and more extensive primary care (see pages 290–294 for more detail on these).

The management of primary care typically receives significant policy attention as many lay and clinical practitioner communities interpret primary healthcare as the main locus for seeking to improve the coordination and quality of care for an ageing population, those living with multiple chronic diseases, with diverse needs and hence a key priority within health system reform (e.g. Smith and Goodwin, 2006; Edwards et al., 2013; Kringos et al., 2013a, 2013b).

Such strengthening of primary healthcare has seen the emergence of many new models of primary care provision, often at significant scale. These developments form a particular focus of this chapter given their call for more sophisticated, senior and experienced management arrangements, tailored to the specific needs and nature of primary healthcare services, professionals and multidisciplinary relationships.

Management of primary care organizations

According to the WHO European Observatory on Health Systems and Policies, organizational models of primary healthcare, which are conducive to integration with public health, can provide a useful checklist for integration attempts at either national or regional levels. Yet, the nature of the model and which factors play a key role will depend on the context and the organizational set-up of primary healthcare in each country (Rechel, 2020).

For example, in most European countries, policymakers have developed organizational models that are conducive to integration across primary, secondary and tertiary health sectors. The report from OECD, Realising the Potential of Primary Healthcare (OECD, 2020), discusses how to make healthcare systems more sustainable and efficient. Authors identified three key characteristics for the successful organization of primary healthcare. First, models of organization need to move away from single-handed physicians responding to acute episodes of illness, without a wider network of support to deliver nuanced care. This would result in a model that comprises a network of providers, to better serve patients with complex needs and can improve access for disadvantaged groups in society. Second, economic incentives are needed for primary healthcare providers to work as part of networks. For example, in England, general practitioner (GP) practices work as part of primary care networks to deliver community, social care, mental health and pharmacy services local to where communities live (see Box 13.1).

Box 13.1   Key characteristics of primary care networks: a model of the organization of primary healthcare in England

- Delivery of primary care services that enable healthcare clinicians and managers to deliver more coordinated and integrated health and social care for people closer to home.
- Typically serving between 30,000 to 50,000 people (with some networks being much smaller or larger). Benefit from economies of scale through better collaboration between GP practices and others in the local health and social care system.
- Led by clinical directors who may be a GP, general practice nurse, clinical pharmacist or other clinical professional working in general practice.
- In 2019, the Additional Roles Reimbursement Scheme was introduced, whereby PCNs can claim reimbursement for the salaries of 18 new roles within the multidisciplinary team:

  - Clinical/senior pharmacist
  - Pharmacy technician
  - Social prescribing link worker
  - Health and well-being coach
  - Care coordinator
  - First contact physiotherapist
  - Paramedic
  - Occupational therapist
  - Podiatrist
  - Dietitian
  - Nursing associate
  - Trainee nursing associate
  - Adult mental health practitioner
  - Children and young people's mental health practitioner
  - Physician associate
  - General practice assistant
  - Digital and transformation lead
  - Advanced practitioner

Source: NHS England, 2022 [https://www.england.nhs.uk/primary-care/primary-care-networks/ and https://www.england.nhs.uk/gp/expanding-our-workforce/].

Third, organizational models of primary healthcare should include patient and community voice in the design and implementation of services. This is pertinent giving the increasing application of digitally enabled technology. For instance, Estonia, Finland, Norway and Sweden have developed patient portals giving patients increased opportunity to access their health data, which can ultimately improve their communication with healthcare professionals (Kujala et al., 2024). However, generic patient portals can lead to considerable variation in usability depending on patient preferences, including, but not limited to, accessing appointments, reviewing clinical decisions, or renewing and viewing prescriptions (Fennelly et al., 2020).

Service provision in primary care

While care coordination is understood as a key element of family medicine and primary care, analysis of patient experiences in many countries often tell a different story (Sarnak and Ryan, 2016). Hence, small family medicine or general practices cannot undertake full responsibility for the full range of care coordination for people with a range of complex needs due to lack of resource and/or the limited availability of clinical expertise in primary care, despite increasing coordination with third sector and other providers.

More recently, the scope of primary healthcare has broadened to include end of life (palliative) care. Reports from WHO (2014) and a European expert panel on primary care (De Maeseneer, 2015) have stated the need to include palliative care at a primary healthcare level due to inadequate integration of palliative care in current health and social care systems, which further exacerbate the lack of equitable access to such care. To address this deficiency in care, the WHO recommends that the coordination of care needs to be supported by the provision of in-service training. To summarize, we provide a list of core activities delivered in primary care in Box 13.2.

Box 13.2   Categorization of core activities in primary care

Primary care services provide the first point of contact in a healthcare system and can include general practice, community pharmacy, dental and optometry (eye health) services. Primary care services will broadly cover the following:

- Diagnostic services
- Treatment and follow-up care
- End of life care
- Medical technical procedures
- Prevention and health promotion
- Mother, child and reproductive healthcare

Primary healthcare providers may deliver a broader scope of services in countries with more single-handed practices, although this may be a function of demographics; for example, in remote areas, practitioners are more likely to work without the support of networks and offer a fuller range of services.

Source: Wilson et al. (2015).

The seminal work of Barbara Starfield (1994; 1998) identified four essential features of effective primary care provision, which she suggested as an organizing framework for analysis of health systems (see Box 13.3).

Box 13.3   Starfield's four Cs as an organizing framework

1   Point of first **contact** – a system of primary care gatekeeping, a single point of access to most services provided by the health system.
2   Person-focused **continuous care** over time – enrolment of patients with a single primary care practitioner or practice.
3   **Comprehensive care** for all common needs – multidisciplinary primary care and community health services that can assess, diagnose and treat common conditions.
4   **Coordination of care** provided elsewhere – role as the individual's advocate and guide through the wider health system, including the guardian of overall patient information.

Source: Adapted from Starfield (1994; 1998).

These 'four Cs' were used by Starfield to assess the effectiveness of a country's primary care system. Indeed, Starfield's research into the quality and nature of primary healthcare in an international context suggested a link between the strength of a country's primary care system (as measured against the four Cs) and its likely greater cost-effectiveness, and improved levels of health outcomes achieved for the population (Starfield, 1994; 1998; Macinko et al., 2003).

More recent analyses of the relationship between primary care systems and population health (e.g. Kringos et al., 2015) have produced more nuanced conclusions. This work has shown that while strong primary healthcare appears to be associated with improved population health, it is also related to higher levels of health spending, at least in the short to medium term. There does, however, seem to be a link in Kringos and colleagues' analyses between comprehensive primary healthcare provision and slower overall growth in healthcare expenditure, making it a sound bet for countries considering how best to invest health resources over the long term in a context of financial austerity and rising demand for health services, especially post-pandemic.

In addition, further comparison could be made with the conceptual framework presented by Hogg et al. (2008) that has two domains: structure and performance. According to Hogg et al. (2008: 308) 'the structural domain describes the health care system, practice context and organization of the practice in which any primary care organization operates. The performance domain includes features of health care service delivery and technical quality of clinical care'. Despite this, recognizing the importance of the 4 Cs articulated by Starfield and the importance of the patient–provider relationship including appreciation of a patient's culture, Hogg et al. (2008) propose a further element – trust – and its role in promoting patient satisfaction and adherence to clinical advice.

Learning activity 13.1

Have a conversation with a clinician or manager working in primary care, exploring with them how this sector of healthcare works in your country, along with its strengths and weaknesses. If you cannot have such a conversation directly, use online resources to explore what primary care physicians and managers are reporting about their experiences of service organization and provision.

- Based on this discussion, write a brief analytical memo setting out your thoughts, ideas and questions about what you have just learnt.
- Use this analysis to set out how the primary care orientation of your country's health system seems to measure up in relation to Starfield's 'four Cs'.
- Conclude your analytical memo by considering where there is scope for improvement in your health system's ability to provide well-integrated primary care services for people with complex chronic health needs.

Primary care within health systems

Patient registration

Globally, the registration of patients with a single primary care practice or practitioner is viewed by public health practitioners and policymakers as central to the maintenance and improvement of individual and overall population health and well-being. Yet, new models of primary healthcare have often prioritized patient choice or emphasized choice and access over continuity of care (Salisbury et al., 2009). Traditionally, patient registration allowed for individuals to develop long-term relationships with a particular family physician (or medical practice), with the physician establishing an overview of a patient's medical history, taking account for socioeconomic context, including family situation, employment status, housing provision and education. In more recent years, increasing demands on general practice have made it increasingly difficult for physicians in some countries to provide designated family medicine support. In part, this struggle to ensure a personal primary care physician is inversely related to expanding the choice of services available in primary care, as well as trying to assure access to such services, especially in rural and remote areas (Natarajan et al., 2023).

Patient registration or enrolment provides managers in a health system with key health data (e.g. age, sex, any chronic ill-health problems, family situation, health service utilization) and is fundamental to delivering population-focused health interventions, such as health screening, vaccinations programmes, child health surveillance and health monitoring associated with specific age categories. In countries where there has not been a tradition of having to be 'signed up' with a regular primary healthcare provider, a registration or enrolment system can still have benefits as shown in Aotearoa New Zealand with people enrolling with primary health organizations following health reforms announced in a Primary Health Care Strategy in 2001 (Irurzun-Lopez et al., 2021). In the United States, patients with access to a regular primary healthcare physician have lower overall healthcare costs than those without one, improved health outcomes and fewer hospitalizations (Savoy et al., 2017).

Primary care gatekeeping

Researchers, evidence users and policymakers consider primary care gatekeeping as central to the effective management of a healthcare system, with respect to both clinical delivery and cost containment (Starfield et al., 2005). Gatekeeping is the identification of a single point of access to the health system for most of the health needs that people experience, and in many nations this takes the form of a general practice or clinic staffed by family doctors and their teams. Within a system of primary care gatekeeping, patients typically cannot access hospital specialists or associated diagnostic services unless they have first consulted their family doctor and then been referred appropriately. Yet, some countries have taken a more nuanced approach to gatekeeping, such as France, where patients retain the right to consult a specialist directly even where they are enrolled with a general practitioner (Dumontet et al., 2017). The strength of such a system based on primary care gatekeeping is considered to be the ability of the family doctor to take a holistic view of a person's care, ensuring that only appropriate referrals are made to more specialist services, and thus avoiding unnecessary expensive and possibly invasive tests and care in hospital settings.

However, the effectiveness of gatekeeping in controlling expenditure in secondary care is open to conjecture. Gatekeeping is a function typically associated with mainly tax-funded health systems, such as those in the UK, Denmark, Italy and Sweden. Notably, expenditure as percentage of gross domestic product (GDP) on health does not differ significantly between countries with and without primary care gatekeeping (Greenfield et al., 2016).

Critics of gatekeeping assert that it limits patients' rights and choices within a health system and its impact on health-related and patient-related outcomes (Sripa et al., 2019). In the UK, the reliance on GP gatekeeping has been suggested as a possible contributory reason for poorer survival rates for breast, colorectal and lung cancers compared with other European countries, in part caused by delayed diagnoses (Cancer Research UK, 2024). Analysis of child healthcare across six European countries has similarly pointed to a reliance on generalism as a factor that may be compromising the quality and outcomes of such care (Zdunek et al., 2019).

In recent years, some new models of care delivery have provided patients with opportunities to bypass traditional primary care provision through community health centres, specialists visiting places of employment, locating GPs in hospital emergency rooms, patient advice lines (telephone and internet), as well as telehealth and telecare. Primary care gatekeeping requires a health system to systematically coordinate and manage a diverse range of healthcare providers, while trying to develop and improve primary care (this is explored further in the 'Managing in primary care' section of this chapter). This is a complex organizational and management challenge.

In summary, we have shown the importance of effective primary care gatekeeping, which involves how best to achieve cost-containment in a health system, developing patient pathways that avoid unnecessary investigations and treatments, enhance care coordination and delivery of a holistic approach to care. In parallel, effective gatekeeping needs to be understood against a backdrop of the challenges associated with access and the increasing complexity of delivering primary healthcare.

Primary care organizations

Internationally, and specifically (but not exclusively) in Western democracies, a broad range of primary care organizations have been established to manage and develop healthcare services to both improve population health and enable effective and high-quality general practice provision (Smith and Goodwin, 2006; Edwards et al., 2013; Kringos et al., 2015). Primary care organizations are a manifestation of the move towards a more managed and extensive primary care in a number of health systems and represent a managerial solution to the dilemma of how to draw together often diverse and autonomous general practices and other community services into a coherent local network or organization for improving health.

The scale and scope of primary care organizations varies country to country, with stand-alone clinics run by single-handed doctors being typical in some countries, and large health centres run by multidisciplinary teams being the norm in others (Gumas et al., 2023). This variation results from factors, such as the sociopolitical context of a country (for example, a focus on municipality-based health centres in some Scandinavian countries and a history of polyclinics in some Eastern European nations); the method of remuneration of family doctors (for example, independent contractor status driving traditionally small practices in the UK and the Netherlands); and the degree of self-organization among groups of doctors (for example, independent practitioner associations that have morphed into care networks in California, the United States and Aotearoa New Zealand).

There is considerable variation in the nature and structure of primary care organizations, their scope of service provision and individuals or roles involved. In the following sections we explore several types of primary care organization.

Corporate chains in primary care

Corporate chains in primary care are now becoming increasingly visible players in healthcare systems in high- and middle-income countries globally and their growth has been fuelled by the increasing commercialization of healthcare and private equity finance (Hunter and Murray, 2019). Furthermore, international expansion of healthcare industry financial institutions, such as the World Bank's International Finance Corporation, are increasingly highlighting primary healthcare as a potentially profitable venture (Hunter and Murray, 2019). Relatively little is yet known about the number and scale of corporate chains providing primary healthcare and international research on their impact on care delivery and health outcomes is yet to emerge.

According to Swerissen et al. (2018), Australia's three largest corporate chains currently manage around 5 per cent of practices and employ about 15 per cent of GPs. It is often assumed that the introduction of greater competition in primary care will in return lead to increased patient choice, more efficient delivery of services, as well as improving the quality of care provided; however, the increased use of corporate chains in primary care can mean policymaking becomes less effective and government control over health policy is diminished (Swerissen et al., 2018).

Super-partnerships or independent physician associations

How GP practices can best work together at scale to deliver effective and equitable care has been the subject of much debate in recent years (Smith et al., 2013; Pettigrew et al., 2019). Super-partnerships and physician associations are where GP practices merge important functions, such as managing finances and contracts (Rosen et al., 2016), and the term generally applies to those who choose to work as a single entity. Some of the largest super-partnerships in the UK contain over 100 partners and provide care for over a quarter of a million patients (Pettigrew et al., 2019).

The key benefits that can arise from working within a super-partnership or physician association can include alleviating clinicians from some of the administrative burden faced as a small or sole practice owner (Thorlby et al., 2012). In addition, by working as a single entity, larger organizations can offer a more diverse range of services to patients and provide staff (both clinical and non-clinical) with a more diverse portfolio of career opportunities. Yet, there are some notable challenges (Smith et al., 2013; Pettigrew et al., 2019). GP partners of medical practices need to feel fully engaged in the leadership and operational delivery of a super-partnership (see Box 13.4) and remain focused on what is important for the delivery of care for patients registered to their specific practice (Rosen, 2012). There needs also to remain close working with primary care funders or commissioners to ensure practices continue to fulfil governmental contracts that provide sources of income and assure achievement of quality and other performance metrics.

Box 13.4   Example of a super-partnership in the UK: Our Health Partnership

Our Health Partnership (OHP), a super-partnership formed by the merger of 33 Practices with 42 surgeries; 176 GP partners and around 80 salaried GPs in OHP serve around 300,000 patients.

OHP also supports 10 primary care networks with a combined footprint of 450,000 enrolled patients. Due to their size, OHP has created peer networks for learning for clinical directors, primary care network managers and people working in newly introduced additional roles in general practice, to help support learning and development alongside a dedicated resource for population health management.

At a larger scale, OHP supports locality-based care and teams, has formed partnerships with community diagnostics centres, launched a research hub to mainstream primary care evaluation and continues to test innovative health-based solutions to shape the future of primary care.

Contact: https://www.ourhealthpartnership.com/

Community health organizations

In some countries and with specific communities, such as the Aotearoa New Zealand Māori and Canadian Inuit populations, tribally or community owned organizations are central to the delivery of primary healthcare, including public health awareness and delivering health promotion interventions. These organizations form part of the tradition of 'community oriented primary care' (Kark, 1981: 61) and can be defined as 'a continuous process by which primary healthcare is provided to a defined community on the basis of its assessed health needs, by the planned integration of primary care practice and public health'. Often, local health workers and nurses play a large role in the delivery of care, alongside GPs (Boulton et al., 2013).

Community health organizations, also sometimes described as polyclinics or community health centres, are often made up of multiple practices in a network in a single locality. In other cases, they may comprise a single, large health centre or clinic that serves as a hub for a locality and its community and primary healthcare. They seek to combine patient-centredness with a strong population orientation and often have an ownership model that includes significant public and community involvement. Examples include the Hokianga Health Enterprise Trust in Aotearoa New Zealand, which is owned and run by the local community (www.hokiangahealth.org.nz); and Community Health Centre Botermarkt in Belgium (see Box 13.5), which is a not-for-profit organization focusing on patient empowerment, social cohesion and local participation (www.wgcbotermarkt.be).

Box 13.5   Community Health Centre Botermarkt

The Community Health Centre Botermarkt is a not-for-profit organization set up in 1978 in Ledeberg, a socioeconomically disadvantaged area in the city of Ghent. The primary care team is composed of family physicians, nurses and social workers and other staff, including receptionists, health promoters, dieticians, ancillary staff, dentists and oral hygienists. The centre takes care of 6,400 patients, from over 95 different countries. All patient information is coordinated in an integrated, interdisciplinary electronic patient health record.

The centre aims to deliver integrated primary care focusing both on individuals and families, and on the population. Central to their approach is their 'goal-oriented' model of care, starting from the life goals of the patient. Service delivery focuses on accessibility (with no financial, geographical or cultural barriers) and quality, using a comprehensive eco-bio-psycho-social frame of reference. The focus is on empowerment of patients and contribution to social cohesion. Patients are registered on a list (enrolment). The range of services provided includes health promotion and prevention; screening; curative care; palliative; and rehabilitative services (consultations and home visits); integrated home care by an interdisciplinary team; nursing services; nutrition services; social work; and dental care. More recently, primary care psychologists joined the team.

The centre is financed through contracts with health insurance companies that include a monthly capitation payment for every citizen on the list. Since 2013, there has been an integrated, mixed, needs-adjusted capitation funding formula for the centre that takes into account social variables, morbidity, age, sex, functional status and income of the patient. Cooperation agreements are established between the centre and secondary care providers, physiotherapists, specialized palliative home care services and specialized social services, to contribute to comprehensive approaches.

In 1986, the health centre created a local intersectoral platform of primary care providers, local schools, local police, civil society organizations and representatives of the community, including organizations of ethnic cultural minorities. This multidisciplinary team meets every three months to undertake 'community diagnosis' and enhance interprofessional and inter-sectoral cooperation, as well as engaging in advocacy to address the upstream causes of ill health (e.g. social determinants of health).

Contact: www.wgcbotermarkt.be and the International Federation of Community Health Centres [https://www.ifchc.org/].

The community health organization model is typically found in underserved and economically challenged areas, and there is often a strong focus on one or more marginalized groups, such as refugees, homeless people, the unemployed or those with severe, enduring mental health problems. Brazil's family healthcare teams are one such prominent example illustrating that the approach has had a significant impact on improving child health indicators (Bastos et al., 2017). However, the relationship between family healthcare teams' coverage and hospitalizations remains unclear.

Primary care provider networks

General medical practice is often organized on the basis of independent self-employed doctors working in small groups (or individually) and contracting with local health authorities to provide services to a (usually but not always) registered local population. These collaborations range from informal networks to formal multi-site practice organizations (Smith et al., 2013; Pettigrew et al., 2019). These collaborations can have varied aims, including improving care at a local level and delivering new services to patients, strengthening the resilience of general practice and supporting better management in primary care, including improved financial stability (Smith and Goodwin, 2006; Smith et al., 2013; Pettigrew et al., 2019). This system operates in the UK, the Netherlands, Denmark and Canada, among many other countries. In other countries, namely Aotearoa New Zealand, Australia and the USA, doctors similarly work in independent practices that sometimes group together into provider networks, but levy fees directly from users for some services or groups of patients. These patients may be able to seek reimbursement of some or all of these fees from their state or private health insurance, depending on the particular jurisdiction and its service arrangements.

There has been a gradual move towards a more networked delivery of local primary care, with smaller practices and medical groups in many countries forming networks or federations. Akin to primary care organizations, primary care provider networks usually share responsibility for back-office functions, training and education, safety and clinical governance, after-hours care, or specialized and extended clinical services, such as diabetes, maternity and child health (Pettigrew et al., 2019). Notably, they are often founded on shared goals and motivations and a structure whereby each practice within a network has a voice, as well as being organized to be able to execute predefined tasks to meet local population needs. Examples include primary care networks in England (Parkinson et al., 2021; Goff et al., 2024), primary health organizations in Aotearoa New Zealand (Cumming, 2022a, 2022b) (see Box 13.6) and community care teams in the Netherlands.

Box 13.6 Tu Ora Compass Health, Aoetearoa New Zealand

Tu Ora Compass Health, through their Kapiti Community Health Network (KCHN), brings health providers in a geographical area together, whereby priorities or work streams are set by the partnership with *mana whenua* (Indigenous people) in the area, the Crown entity (The Whatu Ora) and the agency leading the implementation (Tū Ora). This is then reflected by the makeup of the governance group which is *iwi* (Māori people) led and has community voices guiding the development of the work.

KCHN engages with groups of providers under different work streams to promote cohesion between healthcare providers; for example, working with mental health providers under the *whānau* (collective group of people) with complex care needs, as part of older person work.

KCHN also supports community engagement by employing a local, existing disability advocate to develop a meaningful engagement plan for the community as a whole, where the advocate leads the piece of work to develop the capacity, capability and leadership within the community to support future service design opportunities.

Examples of work that have been completed include:

- Mental health teams joining practice multidisciplinary team meetings – developing links between services, improving connections and quality of care.
- Enabling paramedics to refer people who have fallen but are safe to be left at home to the Whatu Ora Older Person Rehabilitation service, where they will be seen the next day to avoid unnecessary emergency department attendances.
- Linking Whatu Ora Physiotherapy services to a specialist youth provider to break down barriers to access for a group that underutilizes physiotherapy services.
- Working with a community pharmacy to fund consultations, ensuring medication is optimized and developing links with clinical pharmacists in practices.
- Supporting the set-up of a health clinic for a boarding house with a high-priority population and linking other agencies with vulnerable populations, such as Women's Refuge and Salvation Army, to general practices.

Contact: https://tuora.org.nz/

Public health-based primary care

Internationally, policymakers have called for greater integration of public health and primary care (World Health Organization, 2018); however, in practice there are often many challenges preventing closer integration. Such challenges include systemic factors (funding and resource; national health policy; meeting local needs), organizational factors (lack of a common vision; lack of information sharing; managerial burden) and interactional factors (effective communication and decision-making strategies) (Rechel, 2020). Public health-based primary care is focused on developing a community-based approach as set out in the Declaration of Alma-Ata (World Health Organization, 1978), assuring delivery of equity-focused healthcare; addressing broader determinants of health; and the development of an integrated health promotion approach. Such an approach can be based on a multidisciplinary team model and requires highly skilled and committed staff to deliver a range of services in local communities.

Independent practices

Denmark is a tax-payer funded, universal healthcare system, its uniqueness being a comprehensive primary care system, where independent GPs act as coordinators and health advisors for patients and work closely with secondary care providers of care for individuals who require acute or complex care, and with local government or other social care providers to support elderly patients following discharge from hospitals (European Observatory on Health Systems and Policies, 2022).

As of July 2022, Denmark has formed 21 health clusters centred on emergency departments (see Box 13.7). These are cross-sectoral in their composition (with representatives from the regions, the municipalities and general practice) and constructed to support and enhance integrated care (European Observatory on Health Systems and Policies, 2022). Health clusters are seen to be central to better preventative services being designed and implemented, as well as improving quality of care.

Box 13.7   Danish health clusters

Health clusters focus on solving local health challenges, including strengthening coherence with better treatment and rehabilitation care pathways for those citizens who receive treatment across regions, municipalities and general practice. Health clusters are also envisaged as being a driving force for enhanced prevention, quality and bringing the healthcare system closer to citizens.

The health clusters involve contributions from stakeholders across the health system including emergency departments, primary and secondary care. To support health clusters, the Danish government has proposed the creation of 21 local health centres delivering services traditionally provided in both primary and secondary care to deliver treatment closer to patients' homes.

Source: European Observatory on Health Systems and Policies (2022).

Despite the varying nature and context of primary care organizations developed and implemented internationally, they share many strengths and challenges. However, primary care organizations continue to face challenges of coordinating care amid staff shortages. We will explore the challenges of managing primary care in the next section.

Learning activity 13.2

Undertake a SWOT analysis (to identify the Strengths, Weaknesses, Opportunities and Threats) of an example of a primary care organization in the country in which you live, with reference to its ability to provide well-integrated services for people with complex chronic health needs living in areas of deprivation. It may help to have a conversation with a manager or clinician who leads this primary care organization or, if this is not possible, to examine their website and strategy documents.

Drawing on this SWOT analysis:

- What do you consider to be the particular issues requiring attention by healthcare managers and policymakers in your country as they seek to further improve the primary care system?
- What policy and organization changes would need to take place for such an improved system to be created?
- What would be the role of the primary care organization within this improved system?

Managing in primary care

There are five distinctive aspects of primary care development that have driven this increased range and complexity of the management task: the role of primary care in coordinating a wider range of services; ensuring equitable access to primary care; collaborating across the local health system; embracing technology and self-care; and the strategic planning and management for stronger and more extensive primary care.

Coordinating a wide range of services

Given the need to manage financial resources to provide a strong primary healthcare orientation to a health system, and its importance for local public health, it is striking that relatively little has been written about the management (as opposed to the delivery) of primary care, especially when compared with the amount of analysis accorded to the management of hospital services. This is likely linked to the dominance of acute care and its leadership within debates and policy on health management and leadership, a point made by Fisher and Smith (2022) about the NHS in England. The management of primary care has, however, received greater prominence in recent years as the full range of functions and services, including health promotion and disease prevention, diagnosis, treatment, ongoing support, maternal and child health, mental health, and end of life care, have increasingly been viewed as core primary care work (e.g. Smith and Goodwin, 2006; Edwards et al., 2013; Kringos et al., 2013a, 2013b).

For example, in Slovenia collaborations between GPs and nurses in separate care units are funded and encouraged in an attempt to deliver more integrated preventative local primary care (Hämel and Vössing, 2017). The varying nature of governance, funding and structural mechanisms used in healthcare systems can have a considerable impact on the coordination and organization of primary care. For example, the respective share of public and private providers may affect a health system's ability to coordinate care and will likely influence the types of contracts and ownership models ('hard governance') or regulatory and payment mechanisms ('soft governance'), which in turn may impact the accessibility and comprehensiveness of care provided (Wendt et al., 2013).

Employing more staff in new clinical and support roles, as part of multidisciplinary teams in primary care, has been proposed as a solution to improve care coordination. However, evidence from England has shown that the introduction of new roles is not always complementary to existing ones (e.g. GPs) and will likely entail significant time on the part of GPs and nurses to supervise these new categories of staff and develop and operate new care pathways (Nelson et al., 2018; Gibson et al., 2023; Hutchinson et al., 2023). This skill-substitution work may therefore increase workforce capacity on the face of it, yet it might lead to unexpected increases in some health system costs while potentially reducing patient satisfaction and quality (Francetic et al., 2022). This experience points to the importance of having senior and experienced healthcare management support alongside such service changes, to ensure that planning and implementation of what are major changes to how teams work can be carefully supported, evaluated and modified as necessary (Fisher and Smith, 2022; Smith, 2024).

Ensuring equitable access to primary care

Following the COVID-19 pandemic there has been considerable growth in the routes available to patients to access primary care services, which have developed at pace since early 2020 (Sidhu et al., 2022b). This growth has been supported by the increase in remote consulting in countries with established primary care health systems (Murphy et al., 2021). However, there is emerging consensus that there is a need to balance the provision of remote consulting and face-to-face consultations against the growing number of tools used for triage and how patients can communicate with staff in primary care (e.g. automated triage algorithms, structured questionnaires or free-text submissions with clinician review) (Marshall et al., 2018; Greenhalgh and Rosen, 2021; Rosen et al., 2022). Such adoption of technology has implications for how primary care teams work and managing patient expectations when receiving care. Greenhalgh et al. (2017) and their development of the non-adoption, abandonment, scale-up, spread, and sustainability (NASSS) framework can help healthcare managers better understand the outcomes of adopting technology in primary care settings, taking into consideration a clinical team's capacity and readiness for adoption and organizational resilience, as well as acknowledging wider sociocultural factors when meeting the need of patients.

Yet, some groups remain marginalized from accessing mainstream primary care services (Rosen et al., 2022). For example, English GP practices struggle to provide primary healthcare provision for homeless people. A study by Crane et al. (2023), with 363 homeless people in England, found traditional models of primary care were ill-equipped to serve their needs (e.g. substance misuse, mental health problems, dental needs) and only in locations where specialist provision was provided, using drop-in clinics and increased collaboration with community-based outreach teams, did patients feel their needs were being addressed. In Scotland, the Scottish Deep End project explored the inverse care law (Tudor-Hart, 1971) in general practice and examined the impact of primary healthcare polices since 2000 regarding the support provided to those living in the most deprived areas of the country (Blane et al., 2024). The authors found that patients living in the most deprived areas had access to fewer GPs while staff were under increased burden trying to treat those with complex long-term needs.

Collaborating across the local health system

The fragmented nature of many health systems remains important to those who manage primary care, navigating differing priorities, metrics, outcomes and budgets across a local health system, while trying to enable effective, safe and timely delivery of equitable primary care. To address such challenges, some healthcare systems internationally are exploring the potential benefits of vertical integration, whereby acute or specialist secondary care providers acquire general practices and either directly employ physicians or develop commercial organizational entities in their own right to manage and deliver primary care (Sidhu et al., 2022a). The merging of general practice and hospital services is present in some areas of Spain, the UK, the United States, Aotearoa New Zealand and Denmark (Sidhu et al., 2022a). Examples of the different types of models used in England are presented in Box 13.8.

Box 13.8 Different models of vertical integration in England: Wolverhampton and Somerset

The Royal Wolverhampton NHS Trust, a large acute and community health services provider, currently has nine integrated general practices. The trust has established links between its community health services and GP practices, for example, creating a rapid intervention team intended to improve health in the area and reduce unnecessary demand for emergency care services. Working in partnership with integrated practices, the trust has developed and implemented new triage and cloud-based telephony systems. GP practices operated by the trust also have access to a daily dashboard showing their patients' contacts with acute, primary and community services.

Contact: https://www.royalwolverhampton.nhs.uk/privacy-notice/our-services/primary-care-services.html

In Somerset, the acute hospital trust owns a limited company, an 'arm's length' subsidiary called Symphony Healthcare Services (Symphony), which run GP services for a group of 20 practices covering a total registered population of approximately 122,000 patients. The Symphony Board reports directly to Somerset NHS Foundation Trust Board. The Trust uses practice data to assign each patient a score for how complex their health needs are and monitors their well-being and risk for potential hospitalization. Symphony has also implemented centralized hubs to manage medication requests, data and document workflow across the Symphony practices, in addition to centralizing HR and finance. Symphony is working closely with the Trust to develop Integrated Neighbourhood Teams and intermediate care services.

Contact: https://www.symphonyhealthcareservices.com/

Embracing technology and self-care

Another factor influencing the complexity, scope and management of primary care is the increasing engagement of individuals in their own care, in part because of technological developments since the COVID-19 pandemic. In addition to the internet as a frequent source of initial health advice – which is, of course, primary care in the strictest sense of the word – primary care services are now often delivered with the support of text or email reminders using online platforms, mobile apps for booking appointments and with supportive online information resources for chronic disease management (e.g. Accurx, eConsult, askmyGP).

Some countries have been much earlier adopters of digitally enabled technology (both analogue and online) than others (e.g., Singapore) (Tan et al., 2022). Standard primary care services are increasingly being delivered in new ways, for example, with telephone, web-based, video and Short Messaging Service (SMS) platforms used to engage with a range of primary care-based clinicians, largely physicians and nurses. Such developments are often enabled through the use of integrated electronic health records and, in some countries, these are now fully accessible to – and even able to be written onto by – patients, for example, Sweden. The widespread use of digitally enabled technology is seen as necessary for the successful coordination of healthcare to patients, but there remain challenges with regard to levels of digital literacy among patients to engage with technology and organizations having the necessary data governance arrangements to support technology roll out (Greenhalgh et al., 2017; Rosen, 2020). These developments are also significant for professional staff, as they can lead to changes in care pathways and context, and even the sense of what it is to be a primary care clinician (Burn et al., 2021, 2022).

Digitally enabled technology was used in some nations to mitigate the spread of COVID-19 during the early stages of the pandemic. In Taiwan, mobile phone-based 'electronic fencing' used telephone signals to monitor self-isolation compliance; and in Singapore, the rollout of the TraceTogether app helped health authorities to identify close contacts of those who tested positive (Ritchie et al., 2020). What has seemed to happen as nations emerged from the pandemic is the continued adoption of digitally enabled technology within broader care pathways that also offer other modalities of consultation and treatment. Healthcare managers need to consider carefully the necessary governance and clinical arrangements that need to be put in place, such as adaptation of care pathways, updating staff training, management of risk, and engagement with patients and carers to understand, manage and meet such demand.

Strategic planning and management for stronger and more extensive primary care

Primary healthcare can only continue to evolve by broadening its capabilities and with the support of skilled and experienced healthcare managers alongside clinical leaders (Figueroa et al., 2019). As this book demonstrates, demand for healthcare is rising worldwide as the population ages and health needs become more complex. In part, this is a result of the increased scaling-up of screening and vaccination rollout undertaken by primary healthcare staff in community settings, along with increased capacity to offer minor surgery, locally based diagnostics and end of life treatment and support delivered locally with primary care teams undertaking care coordination.

Primary healthcare management roles have become more complex given the diversity of services being delivered, yet often without the operational, tactical and strategic demands of managing more multifaceted primary healthcare organizations being adequately considered by those who fund and offer management development and training. The more involved healthcare managers become in the long-term development of primary care organizations and practice (i.e. strategic input), the more this can create challenges for the ability of physicians to manage their managers' performance (Fisher and Smith, 2022). There is a need for collaborative management and leadership between healthcare managers and clinicians in primary care, something that is well-documented for clinical leadership more generally (Dickinson et al., 2013).

Conclusion

Health systems increasing seek to coordinate and manage a diverse range of providers of primary care, try to develop and improve these services and ensure overall better integration of care for improved health outcomes. The desire on the part of many countries is to have less of a biomedical and more of a holistic healthcare system based on strong primary care. Yet, some of the major challenges healthcare providers face is the lack of collective power and influence of primary care (supported by excellent and sustained healthcare management) to respond to local needs that may not align with national policies.

Thus, there is a paradox whereby much is expected of primary care, yet it is so often organizationally fragile (Saltman et al., 2006). Some of the main challenges facing healthcare managers working in primary care include how to enable previously small-scale clinics and practices to form larger networks or organizations; ensuring that primary care plays its part within work to develop better integrated care (see Chapter 15 Integrated care); maximizing the opportunities presented by a diverse multidisciplinary workforce; and balancing the needs and priorities of local professional and community innovation with those of the wider regional and national health system. The challenge for primary healthcare managers is to be able to plan, manage and support health professionals, funders and citizens so that they can collectively secure the opportunities sought for primary care by each nation's policymakers.

Learning resources

Primary Health Care Research and Information Service (PHCRIS): Based at Flinders University in Adelaide, South Australia, PHCRIS offers a weekly electronic bulletin with links to newly published articles, reports and blogs on primary care from around the world. It also holds a wide range of primary care research syntheses, accessible via a tailored search filter [www.phcris.org.au].

European Forum for Primary Care: This multi-professional forum aims to improve the health of populations by promoting strong primary care and supporting primary care research. Members of the forum are sent a weekly bulletin of primary care resources, and there is an annual conference [www.euprimarycare.org].

Commonwealth Fund: This New York-based research foundation aims to promote a high-performing healthcare system, particularly for the most vulnerable in society. As such, it has a strong focus on primary care, chronic disease and complex conditions, and research into new models of care for these groups. It also carries out highly respected international comparative work, including of primary care services [www. commonwealthfund.org].

Nuffield Trust: This London-based independent health research foundation undertakes research and policy analysis, and primary care is a particular focus of its work, including study of new 'at scale' organizations. Extensive data and charts are available on their website, analysing healthcare activity and performance [www.nuffieldtrust. org.uk].

World Health Organization: WHO continues to advocate for strong primary care systems across the world and produces reports and analyses on many related topics [https://www.who.int/docs/default-source/primary-health/vision.pdf]. Its regional websites and offices produce detailed analysis of comparative health data, such as the European office [https://who-sandbox.squiz.cloud/en/data-and-evidence].

Health New Zealand | Te Whatu Ora: Te Whatu Ora is the primary publicly funded healthcare system of Aotearoa New Zealand. It was established by the New Zealand Government to replace the country's 20 district health boards on 1 July 2022. Information about primary health care subsidies and services delivered through primary health organizations can be found on their website [https://www.tewhatuora.govt.nz/ for-health-providers/primary-care-sector/subsidies-and-services/].

The Organisation for Economic Co-operation and Development (OECD): An international organization that works to build better policies for better lives. Their goal is to shape policies that foster prosperity, equality, opportunity and well-being for all. More information about their work in improving primary care can be found on their website [https://www.oecd.org/health/primary-care.htm].

Continued

Learning resources *Continued*

The Health Foundation: An independent charity and think tank for healthcare for people in the UK. The organization's aim is a healthier population, supported by high-quality healthcare that can be equitably accessed [https://www.health.org.uk/].

Canadian Institute for Health Information: An independent, not-for-profit organization that provides essential information on Canada's health systems and the health of Canadians [https://www.cihi.ca/en].

References

Bastos, M.L., Menzies, D., Hone, T., Dehghani, K. and Trajman. A. (2017) The impact of the Brazilian family health strategy on selected primary care sensitive conditions: a systematic review, *PLOS One*, 12: e0182336. doi: 10.1371/journal.pone.0182336.

Blane, D., Lunan, C., Bogie, J., Albanese, A., Henderson, D. and Mercer, S. (2024) Tackling the inverse care law in Scottish general practice: policies, interventions and the Scottish Deep End Project. University of Glasgow, University of Edinburgh [https://www.gla.ac.uk/media/Media_1063909_smxx.pdf; accessed 14 April 2024].

Boulton, A., Tamehana, J. and Brannelly, T. (2013) Whānau-centred health and social service delivery in New Zealand, *MAI Review*, 2(1).

Burn, E., Locock, L., Fisher, R. and Smith, J.A. (2021) The impact of COVID-19 on primary care practitioners: transformation, upheaval and uncertainty, in J. Waring, J.-L. Denis, A. Reff Pederson and T. Tebensel (eds) *Organising Care in a Time of COVID-19 Organizational Behaviour in Healthcare.* doi: 10.1007/978-3-030-82696-3_9.

Burn, E., Smith, J.A., Fisher, R., Locock, L. and Shires, K. (2022) Practising in a pandemic: a real time study of primary care practitioners' experience of working through the first year of COVID-19, *Frontiers in Medical Sociology*, 6 October 2022. https://doi.org/10.3389/fsoc.2022.959222.

Cancer Research UK (2024) Cancer survival statistics [https://www.cancerresearchuk.org/health-professional/cancer-statistics/survival; accessed 14 April 2024].

Crane, M., Joly, L., Daly, B.J.M., Gage, H., Manthorpe, J., Cetrano, G., et al. (2023) Integration, effectiveness and costs of different models of primary health care provision for people who are homeless: an evaluation study, *Health and Social Care Delivery Research*, 11(16).

Cumming, J. (2022a) *Aotearoa New Zealand's Primary Health Care Strategy: Equity Enhancing in Policy and in Practice?* [https://www.lshtm.ac.uk/media/59831; accessed 14 April 2024].

Cumming, J. (2022b) *New Zealand Health System Review.* New Delhi: World Health Organization Regional Office for South-East Asia [https://apo.who.int/publications/i/item/9789290210122; accessed 14 April 2024].

De Maeseneer, J. (2015) European Expert Panel on effective ways of investing in health: opinion on primary care, *Primary Health Care Research & Development*, 16(2): 109–110. doi:10.1017/S1463423615000067.

Dickinson, H., Ham, C., Snelling, I. and Spurgeon, P. (2013) Are we there yet? Models of medical leadership and their effectiveness: an exploratory study. Final Report, NIHR Service Delivery and Organisation programme.

Dumontet, M., Buchmueller, T., Dourgnon, P., Jusot, F. and Wittwer, J. (2017) Gatekeeping and the utilization of physician services in France: evidence on the Médecin traitant reform, *Health Policy*, Jun; 121(6): 675–682. doi: 10.1016/j.healthpol.2017.04.006. Epub 2017 Apr 28. PMID: 28495205.

Edwards, N., Smith, J.A. and Rosen, R. (2013) *The Primary Care Paradox: New Designs and Models*. London: KPMG International and the Nuffield Trust.

European Observatory on Health Systems and Policies (2022) New reform package reorganizes primary and secondary care by introducing 'health clusters' and 'proximity hospitals' [https://eurohealthobservatory.who.int/monitors/health-systems-monitor/analyses/hspm/denmark-2012/new-reform-package-reorganizes-primary-and-secondary-care-by-introducing-health-clusters-and-proximity-hospital; accessed 14 April 2024].

Fennelly, O., Cunningham, C., Grogan, L., Cronin, H., O'Shea, C., Roche, M., et al. (2020) Successfully implementing a national electronic health record: a rapid umbrella review *International Journal of Medical Informatics*, 144, Article 104281, 10.1016/j.ijmedinf.2020.104281.

Figueroa, C.A., Harrison, R., Chauhan, A. and Meyer, L. (2019) Priorities and challenges for health leadership and workforce management globally: a rapid review, *BMC Health Services Research*, 19, 239. https://doi.org/10.1186/s12913-019-4080-7.

Fisher, R. and Smith, J.A. (2022) The Messenger Review: a missed opportunity for primary care, *The BMJ*, 377: o1427. [https://www.bmj.com/content/377/bmj.o1427; accessed 14 April 2024].

Francetic, I., Gibson, J., Spooner, S., Checkland, K. and Sutton, M. (2022) Skill-mix change and outcomes in primary care: longitudinal analysis of general practices in England 2015–2019, *Social Science & Medicine*, Sep; 308: 115224. doi: 10.1016/j.socscimed.115224. Epub 2022 Jul 19. PMID: 35872540.

Gaitonde, R., San Sebastian, M., Muraleedharan, V.R. and Hurtig, A.-K. (2017) Community action for health in India's national rural health mission: one policy, many paths, *Social Science & Medicine*, 188: 82–90. doi: 10.1016/j.socscimed.2017.06.043.

Gibson, J., McBride, A., Checkland, K., Goff, M., Hann, M., Hodgson, D., et al. (2023) General practice managers' motivations for skill mix change in primary care: results from a cross-sectional survey in England, *Journal of Health Services Research & Policy*, Jan; 28(1): 5–13. doi: 10.1177/13558196221117647. Epub 2022 Aug 17. PMID: 35977066; PMCID: PMC9850398.

Goff, M., Jacobs, S., Hammond, J., Hindi, A. and Checkland, K. (2024) Investigating the impact of primary care networks on continuity of care in English general practice: analysis of interviews with patients and clinicians from a mixed methods study, *Health Expectations*, Apr; 27(2): e14032. doi: 10.1111/hex.14032. PMID: 38556844; PMCID: PMC10982586.

Greenfield, G., Foley, K. and Majeed, A. (2016) Rethinking primary care's gatekeeper role, *The BMJ*, 354: i4803.

Greenhalgh, T. and Rosen, R. (2021) Remote by default general practice: must we, should we, dare we?, *British Journal of General Practice*, 71(705): 149–150. doi: 10.3399/bjgp21X715313.

Greenhalgh, T., Wherton, J., Papoutsi, C., Lynch, J., Hughes, G., A'Court, C., et al. (2017) Beyond adoption: a new framework for theorizing and evaluating nonadoption, abandonment, and challenges to the scale-up, spread, and sustainability of health and care technologies, *Journal of Medical Internet Research*, 19(11): e367. doi: 10.2196/jmir.8775.

Gumas, E.D., Gunja, M.Z., Shah, A. and Williams II, R.D. (2023) Overworked and Undervalued: Unmasking Primary Care Physicians' Dissatisfaction in 10 High-Income Countries: Findings from the 2022 International Health Policy Survey. Commonwealth Fund, Aug. https://doi.org/10.26099/t0y2-6k44.

Hämel, K. and Vössing, C. (2017) The collaboration of general practitioners and nurses in primary care: a comparative analysis of concepts and practices in Slovenia and Spain, *Primary Health Care Research and Development*, 18(5): 492–506. doi: 10.1017/S1463423617000354.

Hart J.T. (1971) The inverse care law, *The Lancet*, 1: 405–412. doi:10.1016/S0140-6736(71)92410-X pmid:4100731.

Hogg, W., Rowan, M., Russell, G., Geneau, R. and Muldoon, L. (2008) Framework for primary care organizations: the importance of a structural domain, *International Journal for Quality in Health Care*, Oct; 20(5): 308–313. doi: 10.1093/intqhc/mzm054. Epub 2007 Nov 30. PMID: 18055502; PMCID: PMC2533520.

Hunter, B.M. and Murray, S.F. (2019) Deconstructing the financialization of healthcare, *Development and Change*, 50: 1263–1287. doi: 10.1111/dech.12517.

Hutchinson, J., Lau, Y.S., Sutton, M. and Checkland, K. (2023) How new clinical roles in primary care impact on equitable distribution of workforce: a retrospective study, *British Journal of General Practice*, 73(734): e659–e666. doi: 10.3399/BJGP.2023.0007.

Irurzun-Lopez, M., Jeffreys, M. and Cumming, J. (2021) The enrolment gap: who is not enrolling with primary health organizations in Aotearoa New Zealand and what are the implications? An exploration of 2015–2019 administrative data, *International Journal for Equity in Health*, 20(93). https://doi.org/10.1186/s12939-021-01423-4.

Kark, S.L. (1981) *The Practice of Community Oriented Primary Health Care*. New York: Appleton-Century-Crofts.

Kringos, D.S., Boerma, W.G.W., Hutchinson, A. and Saltman, R.B. (eds) (2015) Building primary care in a changing Europe [Online]. Copenhagen (Denmark): *European Observatory on Health Systems and Policies*. PMID: 29035488.

Kringos, D.S., Boerma, W.G.W., Van der Zee, J. and Groenewegen, P.P. (2013a) Europe's strong primary care systems are linked to better population health, but also to higher health spending, *Health Affairs*, 32(4): 686–94.

Kringos, D.S., Boerma, W.G.W., Bourgueil, Y., Cartier, T., Dedeu, T., Hasvold, T., et al. (2013b) The strength of primary care in Europe: an international comparative study, *British Journal of General Practice*, 63 (616): e742–50.

Kujala, S., Simola, S., Wang, B., Soone, H., Hagström, J., Bärkås, A., et al. (2024) Benchmarking usability of patient portals in Estonia, Finland, Norway, and Sweden, *International Journal of Medical Informatics*, 181: 105302. doi: 10.1016/j.ijmedinf.2023.105302. Epub 2023 Nov 19. PMID: 38011806.

Macinko, J., Starfield, B. and Shi, L. (2003) The contribution of primary care systems to health outcomes within Organisation for Economic Co-operation and Development countries, 1970–1998, *Health Services Research*, 38(3): 831–865.

Marshall, M., Shah, R. and Stokes-Lampard, H. (2018) Online consulting in general practice: making the move from disruptive innovation to mainstream service, *The BMJ*, 360: k1195. doi: 10.1136/bmj. k1195.J.

Murphy, M., Scott, L.J., Salisbury, C., Turner, A., Scott, A., Denholm, R., et al. (2021) Implementation of remote consulting in UK primary care following the COVID-19 pandemic: a mixed-methods longitudinal study, *British Journal of General Practice*, 25; 71(704): e166–e177. doi: 10.3399/BJGP.2020.0948.

Natarajan, A., Gould, M., Daniel, A., Mangal, R. and Ganti, L. (2023) Access to healthcare in rural communities: a bibliometric analysis, *Health Psychology Research*, Dec 9; 11: 90615. doi: 10.52965/001c.90615. PMID: 38089642; PMCID: PMC10712557.

Nelson, P., Martindale, A.M., McBride, A., Checkland, K. and Hodgson, D. (2018) Skill-mix change and the general practice workforce challenge, *British Journal of General Practice*, 68 (667): 66–67. doi: 10.3399/bjgp18X694469.

NHS England (2019) The NHS long term plan. Available: https://www.longtermplan.nhs.uk/publication/nhs-long-term-plan/ [Accessed 14 April 2024]

NHS England (2022) Primary care networks. [https://www.england.nhs.uk/primary-care/primary-care-networks/; accessed 14th April 2024].

OECD (2020) Realising the Potential of Primary Health Care, OECD Health Policy Studies, OECD Publishing, Paris. https://doi.org/10.1787/a92adee4-en.

Parkinson, S., Smith, J. and Sidhu, M. (2021) Early development of primary care networks in the NHS in England: a qualitative mixed-methods evaluation, *BMJ Open*, 11: e055199. doi: 10.1136/bmjopen-2021-055199.

Perry, H.B. (2016) A comprehensive description of three national community health worker programs and their contributions to maternal and child health and primary health care: case studies form Latin America (Brazil), Africa (Ethiopia) and Asia (Nepal). [https://www.exemplars.health/-/media/files/egh/resources/community-health-workers/ethiopia/perrychwprogramsinbrazilethiopiaandnepal2016.pdf; accessed 18 December 2024].

Pettigrew, L.M., Kumpunen, S., Rosen, R., Posaner, R. and Mays, N. (2019) Lessons for 'large-scale' general practice provider organisations in England from other inter-organisational healthcare collaborations, *Health Policy*, Jan; 123(1): 51–61. doi: 10.1016/j.healthpol. 2018.10.017. Epub 2018 Nov 10. PMID: 30509873.

Rajan, D., Jakab, M., Schmets, G., Azzopardi-Muscat, N., Winkelmann, J., Peiris, D., et al. (2024) Political economy dichotomy in primary health care: bridging the gap between reality and necessity, *The Lancet Regional Health - Europe*, 2024, 100945, ISSN 2666-7762. https://doi.org/10.1016/j.lanepe.2024.100945.

Rechel, B. (2020) How to enhance the integration of primary care and public health? Approaches, facilitating factors and policy options, *European Observatory on Health Systems and Policies. Policy Brief* [https://iris.who.int/bitstream/handle/10665/330491/Policy-brief-34-1997-8073-eng.pdf?sequence=7; accessed 14 April 2024].

Rifkin, S.B. (2018) Alma Ata after 40 years: Primary Health Care and Health for All—from consensus to complexity, *BMJ Global Health*, 3: e001188.

Ritchie, H., Ortiz-Ospina, E., Beltekian, D., Mathieu, E., Hasell, J., Macdonald, B., et al. (2020) Coronavirus (COVID-19) Cases - Statistics and Research. Our World in Data. (2020-07-30). [https://ourworldindata.org/covid-cases; accessed 14 April 2024].

Rosen, R. (2012) 'GP super-partnerships: a route to integrated care?'. Nuffield Trust comment, 22 November 2012. [https://www.nuffieldtrust.org.uk/news-item/gp-super-partnerships-a-route-to-integrated-care; accessed 14 April 2024].

Rosen, R. (2020) 'A digital general practice: what have we found out so far?', Nuffield Trust. [https://www.nuffieldtrust.org.uk/news-item/a-digital-general-practice-what-have-we-found-out-so-far; accessed 14 April 2024]

Rosen, R., Kumpunen, S., Curry, N., Davies, A., Pettigrew, L. and Kossarova, L. (2016) Is bigger better? Lessons for large-scale general practice. Nuffield Trust. [https://www.nuffieldtrust.org.uk/research/is-bigger-better-lessons-for-large-scale-general-practice; accessed 14th April 2024].

Rosen, R., Wieringa, S., Greenhalgh, T., Leone, C., Rybczynska-Bunt, S., Hughes, G., et al. (2022) Clinical risk in remote consultations in general practice: findings from in-COVID-19 pandemic qualitative research, *BJGP Open*, 6(3): BJGPO.2021.0204. doi: 10.3399/BJGPO.2021.0204.

Rosen, R., Wieringa, S., Greenhalgh, T., Leone, C., Rybczynska-Bunt, S., Hughes, G., et al. (2022) Clinical risk in remote consultations in general practice: findings from in-COVID-19 pandemic qualitative research, *BJGP Open* 2022, 6(3): BJGPO.2021.0204. https://doi.org/10.3399/BJGPO.2021.0204.

Sakboonyarat, B., Mungthin, M., Hatthachote, P., Srichan, Y. and Rangsin, R. (2022) Model development to improve primary care services using an innovative network of homecare providers (WinCare) to promote blood pressure control among elderly patients with non-communicable diseases in Thailand: a prospective cohort study, *BMC Primary Care* 23, 40. https://doi.org/10.1186/s12875-022-01648-4.

Salisbury, C., Sampson, F., Ridd, M. and Montgomery, A.A. (2009) How should continuity of care in primary health care be assessed?, *British Journal of General Practice*, Apr; 59(561): e134–41. doi: 10.3399/bjgp09X420257. PMID: 19341548; PMCID: PMC2662124.

Saltman, R., Rico, A. and Boerma, W. (eds) (2006) *Primary Care in the Driver's Seat?* Maidenhead: Open University Press.

Sarnak, D. and Ryan, J. (2016) *How High Need Patients Experience the Health Care System in Nine Countries.* New York: The Commonwealth Fund.

Savoy, M., Hazlett-O'Brien, C. and Rapacciuolo, J. (2017) The role of primary care physicians in managing chronic disease, *Delaware Journal of Public Health*, Mar 22; 3(1): 86–93. doi: 10.32481/djph.2017.03.012. PMID: 34466902; PMCID: PMC8352465.

Sidhu, M., Pollard, J. and Sussex, J. (2022a) Vertical integration of GP practices with acute hospitals in England and Wales: rapid evaluation, *Health and Social Care Delivery Research*, 10(17).

Sidhu, M.S., Ford, G.A., Fulop, N.J. and Roberts, C.M. (2022b) Learning networks in the pandemic: mobilising evidence for improvement, *The BMJ*, 379: e070215. doi:10.1136/bmj-2022-070215.

Smith, J.A. (2024) Commissioning and contracting of general practice: a paper for the Health Foundation Symposium on the future of general practice. London: Health Foundation. [https://www.health.org.uk/sites/default/files/2024-07/General%20practice%20sympo sium%20-%20Commissioning%20and%20contracting%20of%20general%20practice%20 -%20Professor%20Judith%20Smith.pdf; accessed 18 December 2024].

Smith, J.A. and Goodwin, N. (2006) *Towards Managed Primary Care: The Role and Experience of Primary Care Organizations.* Aldershot: Ashgate.

Smith, J.A., Holder, H., Edwards, N., Maybin, J., Parker, H., Rosen, R., et al. (2013) *Securing the Future of General Practice: New Models of Primary Care.* London: the Nuffield Trust and the King's Fund.

Sripa, P., Hayhoe, B., Garg, P., Majeed, A. and Greenfield, G. (2019) Impact of GP gatekeeping on quality of care, and health outcomes, use, and expenditure: a systematic review, *British Journal of General Practice,* May; 69(682): e294-e303. doi: 10.3399/bjgp19X702209.

Starfield, B. (1994) Is primary care essential?, *The Lancet,* 344: 1129–1133.

Starfield, B. (1998) *Primary Care: Balancing Health Needs, Services and Technology.* Oxford: Oxford University Press.

Starfield, B., Shi, L. and Macinko, J. (2005) Contribution of primary care to health systems and health, *Milbank Quarterly,* 83(3): 457–502. doi: 10.1111/j.1468-0009.2005.00409. x. PMID: 16202000; PMCID: PMC2690145.

Swerissen, H., Duckett, S. and Moran, G. (2018) *Mapping Primary Care in Australia.* Grattan Institute.

Tan, Y.W.B., Tan, E.R., Sin, K.Y., AshaRani, P.V., Abdin, E., Roystonn, K., et al. (2022) Acceptance of healthy lifestyle nudges in the general population of Singapore, *BMC Public Health,* 22: 1297. doi: 10.1186/s12889-022-13668-x.

Thorlby, R., Smith, J.A., Barnett, P. and Mays, N. (2012) *Primary Care for the 21st Century: Learning from New Zealand's Independent Practitioner Associations.* London: The Nuffield Trust.

Wendt, C., Agartan, T.I. and Kaminska, M.E. (2013) Social health insurance without corporate actors: changes in self-regulation in Germany, Poland and Turkey, *Social Science & Medicine,* 86: 88–95.

Wilson, A., Windak, A., Oleszczyk, M., Wilm, S., Hasvold, T. and Kringos, D. (2015) The Delivery of primary Care services, in D.S. Kringos, W.G.W. Boerma, A. Hutchinson and R.B. Saltman (eds). *Building Primary Care in a Changing Europe.* Copenhagen (Denmark): European Observatory on Health Systems and Policies; 2. (Observatory Studies Series, No. 38.) 3.

World Health Organization (WHO) (1978) Declaration of Alma-Ata. Geneva: WHO.

World Health Organization (WHO) (2014) Strengthening of palliative care as a component of comprehensive care throughout the life course. [https://apps.who.int/gb/ebwha/pdf_files/ WHA67/A67_R19-en.pdf?ua=1&ua=1; accessed 14th April 2024].

World Health Organization (WHO) (2018) Technical series on primary health care. Geneva. Primary health care: Closing the gap between public health and primary care through integration. [https://www.who.int/publications-detail/primary-health-care-closing-the-gap-between-public-health-and-primary-care-through-integration; accessed 14 April 2024].

World Health Organization (WHO) (2023) Transformation of primary health care in Kazakhstan: moving towards a multidisciplinary model. Primary health care policy paper series. Copenhagen: WHO Regional Office for Europe. Licence: CC BY-NC-SA 3.0 IGO.

World Health Organization (WHO) and the United Nations Children's Fund (UNICEF) (2022), Primary health care measurement framework and indicators: monitoring health systems through a primary health care lens. Geneva: Licence: CC BY-NC-SA 3.0 IGO.

Zdunek, K., Schröder-Bäck, P., Alexander, D., Rigby, M. and Blair, M. (2019) Contextual determinants of CHILDREN'S health care and policy in Europe, *BMC Public Health*, 19, 839. https://doi.org/10.1186/s12889-019-7164-8.

Acute care

Nigel Edwards and Louella Vaughan

Introduction

Acute care is generally understood as 'time-sensitive, diagnostic and curative actions whose primary purpose is to improve health' (Hirshon et al., 2013). The Organisation for Economic Cooperation and Development (OECD) describes the principal aims of acute care as:

> to manage obstetric labour; to cure illness or provide definitive treatment of injury; to perform surgery; to relieve symptoms of injury or illness (excluding palliative care); to reduce severity of illness or injury; to protect against exacerbation and/or complication of an illness or injury that could threaten life or normal functions; and to perform diagnostic and therapeutic procedures.
>
> (OECD, 2023)

This involves complex inter-related sets of services and functions, usually characterized by being labour intensive and having high, fixed costs. Acute care is usually, but not exclusively, provided in the hospital setting, although various types of pre-hospital care, including ambulance and other services, are critical parts of the system. Hospitals may also provide non-acute services, such as rehabilitation and long-term care, and so are not necessarily synonymous with acute care.

Policymakers face different challenges in designing and providing services, depending on how developed the health system is. For instance, in high-income countries (HICs), financial pressures stemming from growing demand, ageing populations and expensive new technologies are increasingly shaping the nature of provision (McKee et al., 2020). In lower-income countries (LICs), limited access particularly for women and children, poor outcomes for treatable conditions, a greater disease burden and poorer infrastructure resulting from low spending and very low numbers of staff are a challenge (Kruk et al., 2018). Some problems are universal, such as the global shortage of doctors, although context determines appropriate solutions. It should not be assumed, however, that different systems have nothing to learn from each other, especially as low- and middle-income countries (LMICs) have pioneered innovative approaches to delivering services to large populations at low cost (Skopec et al., 2019).

In this chapter, we consider trends in the size and structure of the sector and how it is responding to changes in healthcare and the wider environment.

Nature and role of acute care

Acute care systems are generally considered to have two key components – hospitals, where the bulk of care is provided, and a pre-hospital component, which in most countries is provided by ambulance services.

Hospitals

The term 'hospital' encapsulates a wide range of institutions: from those that might have 10 beds providing basic inpatient care, to a highly specialized organization with thousands of beds and cutting-edge technology. They provide much more than inpatient care, including diagnostics, outpatient care and home care; they are an important source of resources, education, training and knowledge and are often the focal point for healthcare in a community (World Health Organization, 2023).

Historically, hospitals have been the dominant provider of acute care since their emergence in modern form in the late nineteenth century. The drivers for the growth of hospitals have been primarily technical – such as the recognition of the requirement for dedicated clean spaces for surgery, diagnostic equipment (laboratories and radiology suites) and the need to co-locate staff with different types of expertise. Innovation has increased the need for more specialized care and facilities, for example, in intensive care, cancer treatments, gastroscopy, 3D-imaging and non-surgical invasive procedures (Healy and McKee, 2002). More recently, however, the increase in long-term conditions, coupled with the way some acute conditions that once required long inpatient stays can now be managed outside the hospital, has resulted in a growing imperative for acute care to forge closer links with other parts of the health system.

Hospital levels

In many LMICs, hospitals tend to be stratified (Editorial, 2018), with varying levels of formality, into different levels (McCord et al., 2015) as set out in Box 14.1 below.

Box 14.1 Hospital levels

First level, district or referral hospitals: have few specialties – usually internal medicine, obstetrics and gynaecology, paediatrics and general surgery. They may have some general practice physicians or nonphysician clinicians providing some primary care. They have basic laboratory and radiology services.

Second level, regional or provincial hospitals: have more specialties and diagnostic services. Typically, they have 200–800 beds.

Third level, national or university hospitals: have more specialized staff and technical equipment – for example, cardiology, intensive care unit and specialized imaging units – and will carry out teaching. Typically, they have 300–1500 beds.

Patients tend to be referred 'up' levels for more specialized care and 'stepped down' for rehabilitation closer to home.

Many LMICs have seen rapid growth in their hospital sectors through both private and public sector investment. However, many hospitals have relatively low levels of equipment and staffing and access to intensive care, blood transfusions and specialist care is limited. This reflects often low levels of spending on health both as a percentage of gross domestic product (GDP) and in absolute terms (Ortiz-Ospina and Roser, 2023). While improving and increasing hospital resources seems logical, expanding primary care is often more cost-effective (Editorial, 2018).

A similar pattern of hospital levels or categories is found in HICs, with the emphasis on 'general' hospitals being able to meet the bulk of the local population's needs for acute care. However, outside of very rural areas, the smallest hospitals have increasingly stopped providing acute inpatient care and focused on rehabilitation, long-term care and lower intensity work, including outpatient care and minor procedures. Some countries have hospitals that specialize in planned procedures that allow economies of scale from high volume and also reduce the risk of disruption by surges in demand for emergency care (Box 14.2).

Box 14.2   Standalone planned treatment hospitals

Coxa Hospital for joint replacement in Tampere ('International Case Study: Coxa', 2010), Finland, is on the University Hospital campus but in a separate facility and does over 3000 joint replacements a year (COXA, 2024).

South West London Elective Orthopaedic Centre (swleoc, 2024) is located on a general hospital site but also in a separate building. This undertakes around 6300 procedures a year, of which 4000 are joint replacements.

Aravind Eye Hospitals (Avarind Eye Care System, 2023) are a group of 14 specialist ophthalmology hospitals providing surgery and eye care across Tamil Nadu and part of Andhra Pradesh in India. Over 700,000 procedures are undertaken annually.

Hospital ownership

Models of ownership of hospitals differ significantly between countries and hospitals are operated by a mix of public, private for-profit and private non-profit providers. The evidence about the link between the model of ownership and financial performance and quality of care is mixed. Not-for-profit hospitals may be more prepared to offer unprofitable services (Horwitz and Nichols, 2022) but many studies point in different directions as contextual factors, such as patient selection and the payment and regulatory environment, seem to have a significant impact on outcomes and these are often not well controlled for in the research (Tynkkynen and Vrangbæk, 2018).

A further issue is that ownership categories are not discrete or homogenous; for example, there seem to be different outcomes between traditional private sector providers and those run by margin-focused private equity owners (Kannan et al., 2023). Similarly, not-for-profit providers performance may pay more attention to their wider social mission and this can be influenced by ownership, for example, whether they are church owned (Zare and Gabow, 2023).

Different models of ownership can affect coordination and cooperation for delivering care, particularly where different providers have incentives that are not aligned. For example, attempts to develop the role of primary care in managing chronic conditions can be undermined if outpatient care is reimbursed on a fee-for-service basis. Regulation, payment design and the approach taken by purchasers can help to damp down any adverse effects of the ownership model and so in some systems ownership is not seen as a critical issue (Duckett, 2001).

Learning activity 14.1

What are the advantages and disadvantages of having acute services owned by private, public or third sector (e.g. universities, charities or churches) entities?

How might ownership change their priorities?

What implications might these have for healthcare managers?

What steps can policymakers take to deal with and dysfunctional consequences of these different models?

Ambulance services

Ambulance services are an integral part of any acute care system. Timely transport to hospital, especially in the event of an accident or life-threatening situation, saves lives and reduces morbidity (Holmén et al., 2020; Alharbi et al., 2021).

Historically, there has been a division between USA/UK 'load and go' and the Franco-German 'stay and stabilize' models (Lansiaux et al., 2024). The latter relies on mobile medical doctors who can often refer patients directly into hospital specialties and avoid the emergency department (ED) (Sagan and Richardson, 2015). Evidence is limited and sometimes contradictory (see, for example (Westafer, 2020; Waalwijk et al., 2022) on which of these is the more effective model in terms of outcomes and cost-effectiveness, although there appears to be some convergence between them with ambulance services increasingly using paramedics (Bos et al., 2015).

The interface between the ambulance and the hospital is understood to be critical to patient safety and the smooth running of the system (Bost et al., 2010). However, there remains substantial challenges in effectively managing this, particularly with regards to the transfer of patient information between systems.

In LICs, there are multiple barriers to the effective operation of ambulance services, including road infrastructure, appropriate vehicles and equipment, providing training for staff and community based first responders, and access for patients to the emergency care system (Kironji et al., 2018).

Pressures on acute care

The demand for acute care has been rising year on year over the past three decades. Here we explore the patient-related and other factors impacting on acute care.

Patient-related factors

Ageing population

The rapid ageing of the population in many countries has significant implications for acute care. Inpatient admissions and ED use per capita by patients in their 80s is twice as great as for patients in their 40s (Tillmann et al., 2021). Length of stay is also closely associated with age due to longer recovery times being needed and a higher probability that the patient will require rehabilitation and more complex after-care arrangements that take time to put in place. Many countries are also now struggling to meet the increasing demands for social care, leading to delays in discharge, increasing lengths of stay and pressures on beds (Connon, 2022; see Figure 14.1).

Multimorbidity

Linked to the problem of ageing is that of multimorbidity, which is defined as the presence of two or more long-term conditions, which is an independent driver of demand (Valderas et al., 2009). Many chronic conditions share common risk factors that are largely preventable or treatable, such as smoking, obesity and insufficient physical activity, which in turn are underpinned by social and environmental factors, particularly socioeconomic class. It has been posited that some of the growth in multimorbidity has been driven by screening programmes, such as for hypertension and diabetes, although this could reduce demand for more extensive treatment in the long term. Other factors are also at play, such as the

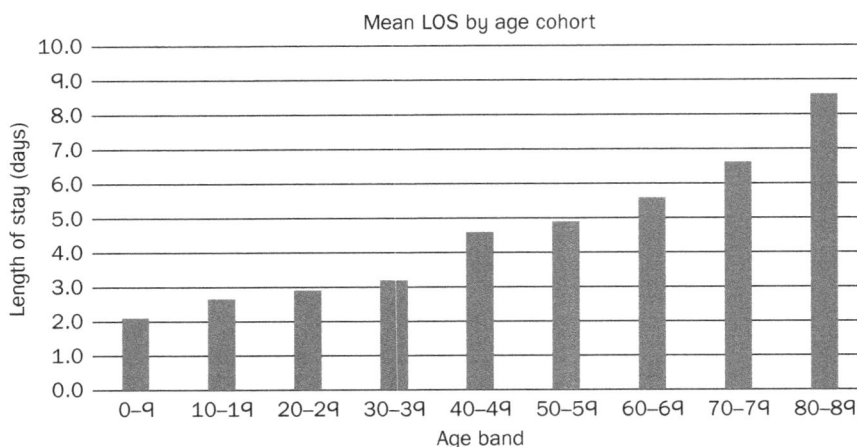

Figure 14.1 Mean length of stay by age cohort
Source: Hospital Episode Statistics England (2016) (authors' analysis).

survival of patients from previously fatal conditions, like myocardial infarction (Laudicella et al., 2018). Long Covid also appears to have created a new cohort of patients who are at higher risk of admission for their cluster of complex issues (Altmann and Pagel, 2023). Many LICS are particularly challenged as they are experiencing a rapid growth in non-communicable diseases while infectious diseases are still a major concern (Chowdhury et al., 2023). The increasing complexity of patients impacts on staff workload and the use of resources (Naik et al., 2024).

Other patient-related factors

Demand has also increased in a number of key subgroups, unrelated to age or multimorbidity. Adolescents and younger adults have been using ambulance services and/or emergency departments in ever greater numbers over the past two decades. Some of this international trend (EUSEM, 2020) reflects changing patterns of trauma care and conditions but some reflect real or perceived barriers to accessing primary care (Behrens et al., 2023). The latter is also reflected in the fact that adults also often default to the emergency department if they perceive a need for urgent diagnostics. The percentage of patients, for example, whose cancer diagnosis is made in the ED has been steadily rising across many HICs (Delamare Fauvel et al., 2023). The number of 'frequent attenders', defined as patients who have five or more ED visits in a year, has also been rising. While this comprises a relatively small percentage of the overall population (2–10 per cent of attendees), they consume a disproportionate amount of resources and have poorer than average outcomes (Shannon et al., 2020).

Other factors affecting acute care

Changes in demand are just one of the pressures facing hospitals. They also have to adapt to a number of other environmental, policy and technological challenges. These include:

Technology

Technological advances have vastly increased the number of treatments able to be provided to patients, such as immune and DNA therapies for diseases that once had limited treatment options. They have also allowed patients who are older and/or frailer to receive treatments, such as the shift from open heart surgery for aortic stenosis to transcatheter aortic valve implantation (TAVI), which allows patients who would not have been able to survive the open procedure to be treated. However, these advances also mean that the number of patients receiving treatments and requiring follow-up is increasing and there is the spectre that many patients may end up suffering from yet more disease, such as secondary cancers caused by therapies for the primary tumour.

Technological change is not, however, an unalloyed good. In a sample of hospital plans we examined we found an assumption that 0.5–1.5 per cent growth in activity would be driven by new technology (Dunn and Edwards, 2022). While technology can increase efficiency of expansion in the scope of care that can be provided, it may simultaneously increase total costs. New technologies also frequently require reconfigurations of hospital space, new engineering or other features that were not originally designed into the hospital building (NHS England, 2013). During the COVID-19 pandemic, for example, the lack of isolation facilities and difficulty in retrofitting these was a significant issue. Similarly, new surgical techniques using robot-assisted surgery can be difficult to accommodate in traditional theatre designs and require other changes to the way that teams work (Randall et al., 2019).

Digital technology

The use of digital technology to assist in the delivery of acute care has accelerated over the past decade, especially in the wake of the COVID-19 pandemic. This has been accompanied by a shift from the use of individual technologies (such as standalone systems for recording of diagnostic imaging) as they develop, to an ambition for hospitals to become 'fully digital' in order to improve clinician efficiency and patient safety (Canfell et al., 2024). This includes:

- A comprehensive electronic medical record (EMR)
- Remote monitoring of patients (both inside and outside of the hospital)
- Point of care diagnostics
- Telehealth

Despite record levels of investment in digital health (globally US$26.5 billion), most hospitals in most jurisdictions still have some way to go. Not only do many still rely on paper for critical functions, but where digital technologies are used, hospitals tend to employ multiple systems, each for a specific task, which are not inter-operable. Further systems are often poorly designed and implemented. These factors mean that digital technologies and electronic patient records have not been shown to automatically improve care or efficiency and have, in some cases, been shown to have a negative impact on the job satisfaction of clinicians (Wachter, 2016).

Learning activity 14.2

What are the main opportunities offered by digitalization in hospitals? Identify two to three examples from your experience and consider:

- What were the main obstacles to achieving these?
- What risks in implementing this technology did managers need to consider?

Workforce

The global workforce crisis (Boniol et al., 2022; Project Hope, 2022) (see also: Chapter 20, The healthcare workforce), has been made worse by the pandemic and is a major challenge (Zapata et al., 2023). Acute care has seen a number of significant changes in the shape of the workforce in response to this and other factors. In the UK and North America, and a lesser extent elsewhere, there has been some substitution of roles usually undertaken by doctors with these being done by other types of staff, such as nurses and allied health professionals. This may include diagnosis, ordering tests and prescribing. However, the debate goes on about the scope of such task substitution, what training and regulation is necessary to protect the public and whether this really economical in the longer term (Maier et al., 2022).

Almost all countries also suffer from a maldistribution of staff, with practitioners of all kinds preferring overall to work in major urban centres. This raises questions about which mechanisms are most effective in encouraging staff to work in non-urban areas. Rural and remote providers have been particularly badly affected by workforce shortages and in recent years a large number of smaller hospitals internationally have closed (Vaughan and Edwards, 2023).

Rurality

As well as the problems of recruiting and retaining staff, rural areas suffer from a number of other specific problems delivering acute care. The demographics of rural areas are not only different but changing. In many places, younger people often leave for urban areas for educational and economic opportunities, leaving behind a dichotomized population (more aged <18 and >65 than those of working age). In some countries, there is a trend for older people to move out of bigger cities into rural and coastal towns, which are often cheaper, further exacerbating the demographic imbalances (Public Health England, 2019). These issues, combined with the increasing trend of centralization and the requirement for larger hospitals, are creating serious problems for care delivery. This is exacerbated by the fact that many service models for hospitals, regulatory standards and the rules for approving training posts tend to be set using the standards of large urban centres (Vaughan et al., 2021). The provision of maternity and paediatric services is particularly problematic – local services end up being expensive and relatively inefficient, while longer travel distances to specialist services can result in increased risk to patients and more inconvenience for their families (Hoang et al., 2014).

Payment mechanisms

Hospital care is costly and has increased over the decades due to the emergence of new diagnostic modalities and treatments, leading to efforts to control the costs of acute care and improve hospital efficiency. In many countries there has been a shift from budgets based on lines of service, including salaries or equipment, to payment models based on activity. Typically, these use diagnostic-related groups (DRGs) or some similar method to group similar types of activity to which a cost is ascribed. The hospitals are reimbursed according to a set price list. There are multiple variants on the model, which historically originated in the desire of payers to encourage provider efficiency, control costs and provide a more transparent and controllable approach to payment (see Chapter 10, The economics of healthcare).

Quality and regulation

There has been an increasing emphasis on quality and safety, often backed up with legislative or regulatory requirements, in many health systems (Chapter 8, Global health governance in a new geopolitical era). These have taken a variety of forms, such as:

- Hospital accreditation systems (e.g. USA, Canada, Spain, France)
- Targets for key hospital functions, such as waiting times in emergency departments (UK, Australia, New Zealand, Ireland) and waiting times for cancer treatments (UK)
- National patient registries (eg. Sweden, Denmark)
- National audit programmes (e.g. Healthcare Improvement Partnership, UK; National Agency for Supporting the Performance of Health and Medico-Social Establishment, France)

A systematic review of the impact of accreditation found a negative impact on employee stress but a consistent positive effect on safety culture, process-related performance measures, efficiency and the patient length of stay. The impact on other important measures was more mixed or uncertain (Hussein et al., 2021). Accreditation is increasingly used as a tool for improving hospitals in LMICs but making this work in resource-constrained environments is challenging (Mansour et al., 2020). Similarly, while there is some evidence that both targets and national audit programmes/registries can drive improvements in performance and outcomes, the former are liable to gaming and driving perverse behaviours, while the latter are often time-consuming, expensive and unreliable (Staib et al., 2016; Willis et al., 2022).

A growing area of regulatory pressure is the requirement to reduce the substantial environmental impact of hospitals both in terms of the embodied carbon in the building and the operation of the hospital (World Health Organization, 2020) (see Chapter 12, Climate change and sustainability). In addition to the usual environmental issues associated with operating large buildings, hospitals have particular challenges related to water, waste, the impact of anaesthetic gases and the significant carbon footprint from single use items. The COVID-19 pandemic and growing problems of antimicrobial resistance have also focused attention on the need for improved infection prevention and control measures, which has implications for the design and working practices in hospitals.

Changes to hospital systems

Overall trends

There has been an overall trend to reduce lengths of stay, convert surgery to day cases, consolidate smaller hospitals and to increase efficiency. This is reflected in Table 14.1, which shows reductions in acute beds across many countries. This has been caused by a number of changes in how care is provided, which are examined in more detail below.

Changes in medicine and surgery

As a result of the drivers previously discussed, patterns of acute medical and surgical care have changed markedly over the past few decades, with subtle but important differences between medicine and surgery.

As part of the push for greater efficiency, and as a result on improvements in technology, internal processes, the development of day surgery and increased provision of out-of-hospital care, there has also been a significant reduction in lengths of hospital stay over the last 30 years in almost all HICs (McKee et al., 2020). Alongside this has been a shift to much elective surgery and some diagnostic medical procedures out of acute hospitals into freestanding ambulatory centres, which are not necessarily co-located with inpatient hospitals. In the USA, there were 34.7 million ambulatory surgery visits in 2006, of which 14.9 million occurred in freestanding ambulatory centres – an increase of around 300 per cent over a 10-year period (Cullen et al., 2009). While there was rapid growth of these centres up to 2008 (5–10 per cent per annum) this has slowed to 1 per cent or less since then (Munnich and Richards, 2022) although the volume of procedures is still increasing (Kumar and Parthasarathy, 2020). These centres also enable providers to increase efficiency and lower costs while also improving the quality of care for patients (Lemos et al., 2006). These changes have allowed for large reductions in the number of beds in many countries particularly in the countries of the former USSR and eastern Europe (OECD, 2011).

With regard to emergency care, patients admitted to both medical and surgical services are increasingly older and have more co-morbidities. In surgery, management is more likely to be conservative in this older group, the result being an overall reduction in the number of emergency surgeries over the past decades (Wohlgemut et al., 2020). In medicine, older and/or co-morbid patients have a longer length of stay and require a focus on nursing and rehabilitative care (Mooney et al., 2023), which has led to the rise of a 'multidisciplinary' approach to care.

The development of emergency departments

One of the key changes to acute care has been the development of emergency departments (EDs) over the past 50 years. They emerged in the USA in the post-war period and offer triage, diagnostics and basic to advanced resuscitation services (Zink, 2005). Approximately 70–80 per cent of hospital admissions constitute emergencies, with the majority being channelled through EDs in applicable countries (EUSEM, 2020).

Table 14.1 Acute beds per 1000 population

Time period		2015		2016		2017		2018		2019		2020		2021		2022
Reference area																
Care type: Somatic care																
Australia		3.4		3.42												
Austria		6.8		6.67		6.62		6.55		6.5		6.36		6.2		5.99
Belgium		4.44		4.39		4.31		4.28	B,D	4.17	D	4.14	D	4.09	D	4.05
Canada		2.27		2.25		2.19		2.19		2.16		2.18		2.21		2.17
Chile		2.04		2.02		2.01		1.91		1.89		1.87		1.82		1.79
Colombia		1.65		1.72		1.73		1.7		1.69		1.62				
Costa Rica		0.98		0.98		0.97		0.96		0.94	B	1.02		1.11	E	1.02
Czechia		5.76		5.76		5.74		5.74		5.7		5.66		5.76		5.61
Denmark				2.2		2.14		2.13		2.08		2.07		2		1.95
Estonia		4.3		4.18		4.09		4.02		4.02		3.97		3.89		3.73
Finland	E	3.66	E	3.39	E	3.22	E	3.07	E,B	2.75	E	2.39	E	2.43	E	2.31
France		5.28		5.21		5.14		5.07		5		4.92		4.83		4.73
Germany		6.86		6.79		6.72		6.69		6.61		6.52		6.45		6.35
Greece		3.51		3.49		3.47		3.46		3.46		3.52		3.56		3.62
Hungary		6.12		6.13		6.15	B	6.1		6.06		6.01		6.01		5.9
Iceland		2.68		2.7		2.69		2.51		2.44		2.48				
Ireland	B	2.58		2.62		2.64		2.64	B	2.56		2.58		2.58		2.61
Israel		2.61		2.57		2.61		2.58		2.57		2.53		2.53		2.62
Italy		3.13		3.11		3.12		3.08		3.08		3.1		3.04		3.01
Japan		10.52		10.47		10.41		10.35		10.22		10.06		10.04		10.02
Korea														11.5		11.54
Latvia		4.43		4.44		4.32		4.27		4.23		4.16		4.06		3.94
Lithuania		5.94		5.69		5.57		5.46		5.37		5.14		5.17		4.85
Luxembourg		4.16		4.03		3.91		3.76	B	3.45		3.4		3.35		3.2
Mexico		0.96		0.96		0.95		0.94		0.92		0.96		0.97		0.97
Netherlands		2.5		2.44		2.34		2.32		2.22		2.12	B	1.83		1.66
New Zealand		2.47		2.42		2.4		2.3		2.23		2.18		2.31		2.24
Norway		2.62		2.58		2.53		2.47		2.45		2.39		2.39		2.35
Poland		5.91		5.91		5.9		5.85	B	5.48		5.51		5.6		5.52
Portugal		2.73		2.74		2.75		2.79		2.86		2.84		2.85	P	2.84
Slovak Republic		4.94		4.97		5.01	B	4.89		4.95		4.88		4.88		4.89

(continued)

Table 14.1 (*continued*)

Time period	2015	2016	2017	2018	2019	2020	2021	2022
Slovenia	3.84	3.83	3.84	3.78	3.78	3.65	3.61	3.5
Spain	2.62	2.61	2.62	2.61	2.59	2.61	2.61	P 2.59
Sweden	2	1.91	1.79	1.72	1.66	1.65	1.6	1.5
Switzerland	3.8	3.76	3.72	3.7	3.67	3.55	3.48	3.43
Türkiye	2.63	2.69	2.76	2.8	2.83	2.96	2.98	3.04
United Kingdom	2.2	2.18	2.15	E 2.13	E 2.1	E 2.09	E 2.09	E 2.1
United States			2.55	2.51	2.49	2.42	2.42	2.4
Non-OECD economies								
• Bulgaria	6.55	6.71	6.87	7	7.17	7.25	7.35	7.64
• Croatia	4.63	4.57	4.6	4.69	4.74	4.74	4.82	4.88
• Romania	5.94	5.99	6.04	6.11	6.2	6.27	6.34	6.42

E = Estimated value
B = Time series break
D = Definition differs
P = Provisional value

This dataset provides data on the number of total hospitals beds **by function of healthcare** (*ie.* curative (acute) care beds, rehabilitative care beds, long-term care beds, other hospital beds) and by **type of care** (*ie.* somatic or psychiatric care)

Total hospital beds are all hospital (HP.1) beds which are regularly maintained and staffed and immediately available for the care of admitted patients. They are the sum of the following categories:

Curative care (acute care) beds in hospitals (HP.1) are hospital beds that are available for curative care (HC.1 in the SHA classification).

Rehabilitative care beds in hospitals (HP.1) are hospital beds that are available for rehabilitative care (HC.2 in the SHA classification).

Long-term care beds in hospitals (HP.1) are hospital beds accommodating patients requiring long-term care (HC.3 in the SHA classification)

All **other beds in hospitals** (HP.1) not elsewhere classified.

Bed numbers according to these functional categories are also broken down between somatic care and psychiatric care.

Somatic care beds in hospitals are hospital beds that are available for care relating to the body, as distinguished from psychiatric/mental care.

Psychiatric care beds in hospitals are hospital beds accommodating patients with mental health problems.

Measure: Hospital beds

Topic: Health > Healthcare resources and equipment

Number of unfiltered data points: 18060
Last updated: July 12, 2024 at 3:23:48 PM

Source: OECD (2024).

As EDs are a relatively new innovation, not all countries operate them. Instead, patients are admitted directly to individual hospital services (such as medicine or surgery), either via the outpatient setting or directly to the ward. The benefits of assessing patients, especially the critically ill, in a single, dedicated space are such that most, if not all countries, are transitioning to models of acute care that include EDs and are putting in place appropriate infrastructure.

Models of ED care are not consistent across jurisdictions. In some countries, for example, in Germany and a number of Eastern European Countries, their primary task is to triage and signpost patients to specialty services. These models tend to be associated with pre-hospital care administered by doctors. In places where ambulance services are provided by paramedics and emergency medical technicians, such as the UK, the focus is on providing a first medical review and appropriate initial investigation, with those patients needing admission being referred to inpatient services. Regardless of the model, a substantial amount of work in all EDs is providing care for patients who require urgent care, but not inpatient hospital admission (Tadesse et al., 2023).

Emergency medicine as a distinct medical specialty has emerged alongside the development of EDs. The maturity of emergency medicine as a specialty varies internationally – Denmark and Germany, for example, only recognized emergency medicine as a specialty in 2018 and many countries still do not, including China and Russia (Sarbay, 2019). In countries that do not recognize emergency medicine as a distinct specialty, EDs are staffed by specialists from across a mixture of disciplines – surgery, medicine and paediatrics.

Learning activity 14.3

Consider which pressures and system factors affect your local acute healthcare providers.

What mechanisms might policymakers and healthcare managers in your area use to mitigate the effect of these pressures?

Refer to any local examples you know of where healthcare managers and policymakers have sought to address pressures facing the local acute healthcare system, considering what appears to have worked or not.

Responses to challenges and change

The burgeoning costs of acute care and the emphasis on the development of primary care in international health policy (see Chapter 13) has seen attempts by payers and policymakers to shift the share of healthcare resources away from acute care and hospitals and/or search for efficiencies within the hospital setting. This has had a major impact on the shape of services at local, regional and, in some cases, national level.

Centralization

A major trend over the past three decades in many countries has been the centralization of acute services (Ferguson et al., 1996; Vaughan and Browne, 2023). This has taken three forms (examples in Box 14.3):

1 The reconfiguration of service lines from multiple to fewer sites.
2 The closure of whole hospitals.
3 The merger of neighbouring organizations with redistribution of services across sites with co-location of similar services on a single site (e.g. two acute hospitals becoming one hot and one cold site).

Box 14.3   National reconfigurations of acute care

Several European countries have embarked on national reconfigurations of acute care.

In Denmark, following a structural reform creating new regions in 2007, the number of acute care hospitals was reduced from around 40 in 2006 to 21 in 2015. That goal was primarily based on an assumption that a catchment area of between 200,000 and 400,000 was needed in order to secure quality and allow for economic staffing (European Observatory, 2024).

Estonia undertook a hospital rationalization programme 1993–2001. The number of hospitals was reduced from 115 to 67, hospital beds from 14,400 to 9,200 and average stay declined from 15.4 to 8.7 days. This was accompanied by improvements in primary care and family medicine and regulatory and payment system reforms. A further programme followed in 2015, and the number of acute hospitals was further reduced, and other hospitals changed their role to ambulatory or long-term care.

Between 2010 and 2020, Finland saw a reduction of 23 per cent in the number of hospitals, Latvia 16 per cent, Lithuania 32 per cent, Belgium 16 per cent and Germany 10 per cent (OECD, 2024) By contrast, Korea and Japan have continued to maintain highly hospital-centric models of care delivery.

The impetus for centralization stems from two main drivers. The first has been workforce shortages and the difficulty of providing highly technical care in very small hospitals. This has led to either hospital closure or redesignation of many of these organizations into long-term care or ambulatory facilities.

The second driver has been the belief that higher volumes drive better patient outcomes and reduce the costs per patient, as many centralized services rely on sophisticated and expensive infrastructures, such as 24/7 CT scanning and access to an interventional suite and there may be learning effects and other benefits of scale (Ferguson et al., 1996; Sowden and Sheldon, 1998; Urbach and Baxter, 2004; Mesman et al., 2015). This has been coupled with a concern that care in smaller hospitals is, by default, poorer (Vaughan et al., 2021). While there is no doubt that the centralization of services that require hyper-specialist, time-critical interventions, such as primary coronary angiography for myocardial infarction and thrombolysis/thrombectomy for stroke, and the centralization of very complex surgery and high-technology care has produced improvements in morbidity and mortality, there is little or no evidence for a correlation between hospital size and outcomes for many types of hospital care (Ferguson et al., 1996; Vaughan and Browne, 2023).

Networks

An alternative response to the centralization of entire services has been to create networks of hospitals that can offer a tiered response, which allows both local access and then rapid escalation to more specialized services elsewhere if required. Initially networks were developed around the pragmatics of delivering care, recognizing that while certain aspects of a clinical service could only be delivered in a major hospital, much care could be delivered safely closer to home. Many cancer services, for example, are now configured along these lines, with local hospitals providing initial investigation, chemotherapy and palliative services, and the larger sites providing more complex diagnostic modalities, major surgery and radiotherapy.

Subsequently, the focus has shifted towards networks as being a way to bring about 'greater market influence, economies of scale and scope, reduced duplication of resources, more effective training and improved efficiency in the provision of services' (Nolte et al., 2014). How networks have been shaped, however, has depended on underlying market structures. Networks in France, Germany and the USA are usually formed between organizations within a single, for-profit provider group. By contrast, Poland, the Netherlands and England have all been developing different models of network collaboration for service planning and in England for sharing some services. In Denmark, hospitals have been formed into clusters with primary care to concentrate on addressing challenges, such as improving coordination for citizens requiring care across different regions, municipalities and general practices. Additionally, they are expected to play a significant role in promoting prevention, ensuring quality and making healthcare services more accessible to citizens (European Observatory, 2024). In many places, network formation has been facilitated by specific policies and regulatory changes, such as the relaxation of staffing structure requirements in the USA.

Networks seem to be an effective mechanism to improve care (Brown et al., 2016) although they do present some novel management challenges. While the drivers for network development are framed as being 'clinical' or 'technical', networked care depends on the quality of relationships between clinicians and managers across organizations (Fraser et al., 2022). These are more difficult when network members are not part of the same overarching provider (Goodwin et al., 2004) or during the formation of new network relationships, which requires time to build trust, especially if this has come at the expense of breaking pre-existing collaborations. Mechanisms for the assurance of quality, such as audit and governance and other 'back-office functions', need to align, which again can be a time-consuming and costly process.

Governance and autonomy

Beyond high-level regulation, there has been an increasing emphasis on the governance of acute providers in an attempt to create systems to improve quality and efficiency through more local oversight. This can be seen as part of a general trend to the application of management methods to the provision of care. Improvements in governance have often been associated with policies to grant more autonomy to hospitals and in some cases to change their legal status (Saltman et al., 2011). This has the effect of limiting the intervention powers of ministries, but also reflects the longer-term trend towards hospital management being less about administration and oversight of routine tasks and more about a proactive role in identifying problems and solutions and managing staff, including holding them to account for performance.

Diverting patients away from acute care

The issue of whether patients, especially those with low acuity problems, should be accessing acute care rather than primary care for any given issue is a longstanding one, born of the concern that inappropriate use of emergency services (in particular) leads to overcrowding of EDs and increased cost (Murphy, 1998). The evidence on the impact of 'inappropriate attendances' is mixed, but nevertheless much effort has been made to divert patients away from them wherever possible. These range from local measures (e.g. telephone advice lines for GPs) through to national initiatives. In Norway and Denmark, for example, patients can only access EDs via general practice or ambulance services, with walk-in access actively deterred. A number of countries in Europe have established national or regional hotlines to signpost them to the most appropriate service. Unfortunately, none of these interventions have been shown to consistently show reductions in ED usage at system level. Indeed, some interventions, such as telephone advice lines, have been shown in some instances to actually increase ED usage (Rushton et al., 2019; Boggan et al., 2020). Interventions seem to be more successful if they involve experienced medical or nursing staff (Turner et al., 2021), but this increases implications for cost and raises the question of how resources should be deployed to benefit the largest number of patients.

Alternative places for first assessment

Alongside attempts to reduce attendances, there has been an international trend towards diverting patients from the ED into new spaces or departments that also provide first assessment and treatment but for specific patient subgroups. In some cases, these new units also can also provide inpatient care for the first portion of the hospital stay. This has included units/services such as acute medical units (AMUs), frailty units, geriatric EDs, same-day emergency care (SDEC), ambulatory care units, mental health crisis services, and so on (Mace, 2017; Southerland et al., 2020). There is some evidence that these services can improve morbidity and mortality for the specific patient groups targeted, as well as improve system-level efficiency (e.g. reduce length of stay). However, the multiplication of parallel services at the front door can be challenging, as they require more resources (staff, space, equipment), more managerial oversight and can increase risk (Vaughan et al., 2021).

Shifting services to the community

Technological advances, such as the ability to remotely monitor patient's vital signs and other physiological parameters (such as blood sugar), have led to a growth in hospital-type services being delivered within the patient's own home. These have included:

- **Hospital at home**: A model found in a growing number of high-income countries. The model provides nursing and other care to prevent admission to hospital, allow early discharge or to provide palliative or end of life care. A review of research has found that these models are safe and generally cost effective (Edgar et al., 2024), but they should not be assumed to be cheaper than hospital care (Shepperd and Iliffe, 2001).
- **Virtual wards**: These use remote monitoring to manage patients who might require admission if their condition deteriorates (Norman et al., 2023). The model was used extensively in Germany to deal with COVID-19 to prevent the risk of spread of infection when patients are admitted. It has also been adopted in Denmark and France (Donnelly, 2024).
- **Support to care homes**: Helping care homes to manage their patients more effectively. This can include telemedicine support (NHS England, 2019).
- **Nursing staff and other professionals increasingly delivering complex services:** These can include chemotherapy, IV fluids and many other services outside the hospital or in patients' homes that traditionally would have been done in hospital.

In addition, there has been increased interest in developing more integration between hospital, community, primary and social care (see Chapter 15, Integrated care). However, this has not translated into significant change in most countries beyond attempts to bundle payments for some treatments to include rehabilitation and, more promisingly, the development of shared guidelines for disease management between specialists and GPs.

Unresolved issues/inflection point

At the time of writing this chapter, acute care is under greater strain than ever before. Emergency departments internationally are dangerously overcrowded, with patients being held in ambulances outside hospitals (Australia, New Zealand, UK, Japan, Italy) or in corridors (UK, China) or being cared for in inappropriate areas on wards (USA, Canada). Many cancer and surgical services have still not recovered to pre-pandemic levels, with patients experiencing longer waits for diagnosis and treatment. Medical and nursing staff are striking over pay and conditions in multiple jurisdictions (UK, USA, Italy, France, Spain, Canada, New Zealand, South Korea), with levels of staff absenteeism and leaving reaching historical peaks (Vaughan and Edwards, 2023). While the antecedents of these problems do differ markedly across countries and are contingent on local context, the current problems with acute care can be seen as a result of the previous solutions having been taken past the point of providing benefit and instead producing negative impacts on the system.

Funding for acute care

In OECD countries there was a sharp fall in the proportion of health expenditure spent on inpatient care between 1990 and 2000 but since then the share has remained at around 28–29 per cent (OECD, 2011, 2021). Some of this has been driven by other elements of health spending, particularly outpatient care. However, the increasing costs of acute care mean that funding to the sector has fallen in real terms.

Despite long-standing commitments by governments to promote the role of primary care (World Health Organization, 1978), primary care and other forms of care in the community remain relatively underfunded. An investigation by the King's Fund, for example, into the failure of the NHS to provide adequate care in the community found a long history of resource allocation not aligning to the policy rhetoric (Baird et al., 2024). The political power and visibility of the hospital sector and the tendency for long-term investment to be derailed by urgent short-term priorities have played an important part in this.

Decision-making about funding is even more complex in lower- and middle-income countries. People in these countries are also living for longer with more chronic diseases. However, with many such countries still struggling with high levels of communicable disease and poor infrastructure, this has led to major complexities with regard to where investments should be made. For example, while improvements in drug treatment have impacted on the morbidity and mortality of patients with malaria, still endemic in many sub-Saharan countries, it has been calculated that increasing the coverage of core malaria control measures is a more effective and cost-efficient mechanism to reduce overall levels of harm (Camponovo et al., 2017). Similarly, while it might seem self-evident to introduce advanced diagnostics, such as CT scanning, and technical interventions, into urban hospitals, these resources are inevitably restricted by geography and income, thereby widening the health inequalities experienced by poorer and more rural populations (Dawkins et al., 2021).

Reductions in hospital beds

Bed closures have been previously seen as desirable, with the evidence suggesting that some beds could be safely removed from systems without impacting on patient outcomes and reducing cost (McKee, 2004). However, there are now signs that some countries (e.g. UK, Australia, Ireland, rural USA, Canada) may now no longer have enough beds. In Australia, for example, the rate of decline in the mean hospital length of stay has slowed considerably, especially in the older age groups. In those 75 or older, the proportion of admissions and the number of bed days has increased, leading the authors to the conclusion that continuing to remove beds from the system cannot produce any further benefits (Reid et al., 2023). Although most of the reductions in bed numbers have come through reductions in length of stay for surgical procedures, there is evidence of rising demand for surgical beds due to the increasing number of operations on older patients. While many of these patients have excellent outcomes, more patients are needing longer lengths of stay and the rate of readmissions for the management of complications is rising (Wohlgemut et al., 2020).

This reversal of the long-term trend for reducing inpatient beds has implications across the system and now may be manifesting in various forms of system strain, such as overcrowding in the emergency department and on the wards, the inability to admit patients for routine procedures and staff struggling to deliver routine care. These, in turn, impact on patient morbidity and mortality and can lead to de facto rationing of services (McKee, 2004). This all suggests that the strategy to use reductions in the number of beds to manage demand in acute care and lower costs has now reached the limits of utility.

Learning activity 14.4

The evidence suggests that although removing beds from the system might reduce costs, the savings are never as great as expected.

- What might be the mechanisms for this finding?
- What implications might this have for service provider and policymakers?

Limits of reconfiguration

Related to the issue of reduction in bed numbers is that of reconfiguration, especially when it comes to whole hospital and emergency department closure, and whether this has also reached the limits of utility in many places. Two large studies of well-planned, national reconfigurations of emergency services (Republic of Ireland and Denmark) failed to show improvements in mortality and found evidence of poorer hospital performance (Browne, 2020; Flojstrup et al., 2023). Other international studies (Burns and Pauly, 2023; Vaughan and Browne, 2023) have shown that mortality increases in remaining hospitals when emergency services in an index hospital are closed. Several mechanisms have been suggested: patients have longer distances to travel increasing the risk of a poorer outcomes for time-sensitive conditions; the creation of conditions of overcrowding, which itself increases mortality; 'speed up', whereby remaining hospitals seek to process patients more quickly and seem to miss critical steps in care. Other reviews have failed to find consistent evidence of other putative benefits from the merger of organizations, such as efficiencies, synergies, improvements in organization culture or community benefits (Burns and Pauly, 2023; Vaughan and Browne, 2023).

Generalism versus specialism

While the increasing numbers of older and multi-morbid patients has suggested, for decades, that doctors will need more generalist skills and holistic approaches to care, medicine itself has tended towards ever greater specialism, with services and practitioners focusing on ever smaller groups of patients with highly specific needs (Schroeder, 1992). In the USA and Canada, for example, there are near-critical shortages of doctors in generalist disciplines, such as family medicine, paediatrics, emergency medicine, internal medicine and psychiatry, yet these are the least popular choices for doctors entering into training programmes (Dall et al., 2024).

Surgery has also seen a move towards increasing specialization, with fewer general surgeons and more specialists each performing only a limited number of procedures. This has made it more difficult for any other than the largest hospitals to provide a full range of surgical services.

There has been some rethinking already of the acute workforce in response to this, with the development of newer forms of generalist physician, such as hospitalists in the USA and acute physicians in the UK, over the past 20 years (Wachter and Bell, 2012). Similarly, the USA and Australia are developing rural general surgery as a distinct specialty in its own right (Long and Sweeney, 2023; Paynter et al., 2024). Other jurisdictions are attempting to re-engineer workforce through either incentives for training in certain specialties/areas of need (e.g. Australia, UK) or restricting doctors from setting up new practices in areas that are viewed as being over-serviced (e.g. France, Switzerland) (Vaughan and Edwards, 2023). While these developments might be helpful, whether this will be sufficient to match future patient need is yet to be seen.

Implications for managers

Most of the resources used in hospitals and acute care are committed as a result of decisions made by clinicians and the clinical processes that arise from these. This means that managers in acute care need to have a high level of understanding of how decisions are made and the methods for creating efficient and effective processes. The non-clinical parts of hospitals are also highly complex, and managers need a similarly high level of proficiency in these areas. This includes:

- The ability to understand the complexities of the system and to diagnose the root causes of dysfunctions.
- Being able to involve staff in developing solutions.
- The skills to manage the sometimes difficult relational and emotional elements of change.

Many of the most significant opportunities for improvement in efficiency, outcomes and patient experience are likely to come from changes to internal processes and ways of working. This includes:

- The automation of many routine administrative procedures.
- The development of pathways and guidelines to allow standardization. This can reduce the inefficiency created by variations in flow and through standardizing the use of equipment to reduce storage and create economies by increasing the opportunities for bulk purchasing. See, for example, the work of the NHS Getting It Right First Time (https://gettingitrightfirsttime.co.uk/) initiative in the UK.
- Reorganizing work and the mix of skills in the workforce.
- The deployment of digital technology.

These changes are difficult to implement and while there has been some success with improvement methods, such as Lean, there are aspects of acute care that make the application of generic improvement methods difficult, and they need to be adapted to fit the complex context (Smith et al., 2020).

The interconnected nature of hospitals and acute care more generally, the wide range of staff who may have differing values and objectives and the overall complexity mean that in addition to the skills and knowledge required for day-to-day management, a wider range of skills in change management is also very important. The fact that hospitals are part of a wider healthcare system increasingly requires managers to have a good understanding of the wider system in which the hospital is situated and of how the hospital relates to this. The ability to develop productive relationships and cooperative working with other organizations in the system, including other hospitals in the network, primary care, local authorities and other providers, is an increasingly important part of the role of hospital managers.

Learning activity 14.5

Thinking about a change initiative in your hospital, consider why change in a hospital setting is so difficult.

- What are the factors that unlocked change and allowed progress?
- What are the reasons why different constituencies might be resistant to change, even those that appear to be positive?

Conclusions

There is something of a tradition in predicting 'the end of the hospital'. However, the logic of healthcare tends to require the amalgamation of specialized inter-related functions, including research and education, that has meant that this prediction has failed. Indeed, some of the long-term trends that have been the main drivers of change in acute care, and that have underpinned these predictions, may be reaching an inflection point and there are new challenges that the sector will need to respond to.

The COVID-19 pandemic illustrated the pivotal importance of hospitals in the system but also their weaknesses. It highlighted the potential for more homecare, the shortage of intensive care and oxygen capacity, the fragility of the supply chain, the inadequacy of many buildings and the risks to staff of such high-intensity work.

Better prevention, long-term condition management, high-quality primary care, well-developed end of life care and a functioning social care system can all reduce the need for acute hospital care. New technologies can reduce the need for patients to travel to hospital. Technology will change the hospital; its activities have been constantly evolving but there is no reason to suppose that predictions about the end of the hospital are any truer now than they were when they were first being made in the 1970s.

Learning resources

Baier, N., et al. (2019) Emergency and urgent care systems in Australia, Denmark, England, France, Germany and the Netherlands – Analysing organization, payment and reforms. Health Policy, 123(1), 1–10.

[https://www.sciencedirect.com/science/article/pii/S0168851018306390]

Dash, P., et al. (2019) The Hospital is Dead, Long Live the Hospital. https://www.mckinsey.com/industries/healthcare/our-insights/the-hospital-is-dead-long-live-the-hospital

McKee, M., et al. (2020) *The Changing Role of the Hospital in European Health Systems*. Cambridge: Cambridge University Press.

[https://eurohealthobservatory.who.int/publications/m/the-changing-role-of-the-hospital-in-european-health-systems]

Commonwealth Fund: This New York-based research foundation aims to promote a high-performing healthcare system, particularly for the most vulnerable in society, encompassing issues such as accountable care organizations, patient data and payment systems that are relevant in a hospital context [www.commonwealthfund.org].

European Observatory on Health Systems and Policies: As part of the World Health Organization, the European Observatory promotes and supports evidence-based policymaking through analysis of the dynamics of health systems in Europe [https://eurohealthobservatory.who.int/home].

References

Alharbi, R.J., Shrestha, S., Lewis, V. and Miller, C. (2021) The effectiveness of trauma care systems at different stages of development in reducing mortality: a systematic review and meta-analysis, *World Journal of Emergency Surgery*, 16(1): 38. https://doi.org/10.1186/s13017-021-00381-0.

Altmann, D.M. and Pagel, C. (2023) Long covid: where are we, what does it say about our pandemic response, and where next?, *British Medical Journal*, 383: 2972. https://doi.org/10.1136/bmj.p2972.

Aravind Eye Care System (2023) Activity Report 2022–2023. [https://online.pubhtml5.com/idml/xvjq/; accessed 1 July 2024].

Baird, B., Fenney, D., Jefferies, D. and Brooks, A. (2024) Making care closer to home a reality. *The King's Fund*. [www.kingsfund.org.uk/insight-and-analysis/reports/making-care-closer-home-reality; accessed 22 February 2025].

Behrens, D.A., Morgan, J.S., Krczal, E., Harper, P.R. and Gartner, D. (2023) Still looking in the wrong place: literature-based evidence of why patients really attend an emergency department, *Socio-Economic Planning Sciences*, 90. https://doi.org/10.1016/j.seps.2023.101707.

Boggan, J.C., Shoup, J.P., Whited, J.D., Van Voorhees, E., Gordon, A.M., Rushton, S. et al. (2020) Effectiveness of acute care remote triage systems: a systematic review, *Journal of General Internal Medicine*, 35(7): 2136–2145. https://doi.org/10.1007/s11606-019-05585-4.

Boniol, M., Kunjumen, T., Nair, T.S., Siyam, A., Campbell, J. and Diallo, K. (2022) The global health workforce stock and distribution in 2020 and 2030: a threat to equity and 'universal' health coverage?, *BMJ Global Health*, 7(6): e009316. https://doi.org/10.1136/bmjgh-2022-009316.

Bos, N., Krol, M., Veenvliet, C. and Plass, A. (2015) Ambulance care in Europe Organization and practices of ambulance services in 14 European countries. Nivel. [https://www.nivel.nl/sites/default/files/bestanden/Rapport_ambulance_care_europe.pdf; accessed 22 February 2025].

Bost, N., Crilly, J., Wallis, M., Patterson, E. and Chaboyer, W. (2010) Clinical handover of patients arriving by ambulance to the emergency department - a literature review, *International Emergency Nursing*, 18(4): 210–220. https://doi.org/10.1016/j.ienj.2009.11.006.

Brown, B.B., Patel, C., McInnes, E., Mays, N., Young, J. and Haines, M. (2016) The effectiveness of clinical networks in improving quality of care and patient outcomes: a systematic review of quantitative and qualitative studies, *BMC Health Services Research*, 16(1): 360. https://doi.org/10.1186/s12913-016-1615-z.

Browne, J.P. (2020) The drivers and impact of emergency care reconfiguration in Ireland: results from a large mixed-methods research programme, *Future Healthcare Journal*, 7(1): 33–37. https://doi.org/10.7861/fhj.2019-0065.

Burns, L.R. and Pauly, M.V. (2023) Big Med's Spread, *The Milbank Quarterly*, 101(2): 287–324. https://doi.org/10.1111/1468-0009.12613.

Camponovo, F., Bever, C.A., Galactionova, K., Smith, T. and Penny, M.A. (2017) Incidence and admission rates for severe malaria and their impact on mortality in Africa, *Malaria Journal*, 16(1): 1. https://doi.org/10.1186/s12936-016-1650-6.

Canfell, O.J., Woods, L., Meshkat, Y., Krivit, J., Gunashanhar, B., Slade, C., et al. (2024) The impact of digital hospitals on patient and clinician experience: systematic review and qualitative evidence synthesis, *Journal of Medical Internet Research*, 26. https://doi.org/10.2196/47715.

Chowdhury, S.R., Das, D.C., Sunna, T.C., Beyene, J. and Hossain, A. (2023) Global and regional prevalence of multimorbidity in the adult population in community settings: a systematic review and meta-analysis, eClinicalMedicine, 57. https://doi.org/10.1016/j.eclinm.2023.101860.

Connon, I. (2022) Literature Review of International Models of Social Care: Lessons for Social Care Delivery, Sustainability and Funding in Scotland. Scottish Government. [https://www.parliament.scot/-/media/files/committees/health-social-care-and-sport-committee/full-report-international-models-of-social-care.pdf; accessed 22 February 2025].

COXA (2024) [https://www.coxa.fi/en/seeking-treatment/why-choose-coxa/; accessed 7 January 2024].

Cullen, K., Hall, M. and Golosinskiy, A. (2009) Ambulatory surgery in the United States, 2006, *National Health Statistics Reports*, 28(11): 1–15.

Dall, T., Reynolds, R., Chakrabarti, R., Ruttinger, C., Zarek, P. and Parker, O. (2024) *The Complexities of Physician Supply and Demand: Projections from 2021 to 2036*. New York City: Association of American Medical Colleges.

Dawkins, B., Renwick, C., Ensor, T., Shinkins, B., Jayne, D. and Meads, D. (2021) What factors affect patients' ability to access healthcare? An overview of systematic reviews, *Tropical Medicine & International Health*, 26(10): 1177–1188. https://doi.org/10.1111/tmi.13651.

Delamare Fauvel, A., Bischof, J.J., Reinbolt, R.E., Weihing, V.K., Boyer, E.W., Caterino, et al. (2023) Diagnosis of cancer in the Emergency Department: a scoping review, *Cancer Medicine*, 12(7): 8710–8728. https://doi.org/10.1002/cam4.5600.

Donnelly, T. (2024) Virtual wards: we are in danger of being eclipsed by our European neighbours, *Digital Health*, 17 April. [https://www.digitalhealth.net/2024/04/virtual-wards-we-are-in-danger-of-being-eclipsed-by-our-european-neighbours/; accessed 2 July 2024].

Duckett, S. (2001) Does it matter who owns health facilities?, *Journal of Health Services Research & Policy*, 6(1): 59–62. https://doi.org/10.1258/1355819011927107.

Dunn, S. and Edwards, N. (2022) Analysis of hospital development business cases. Unpublished. Nuffield Trust.

Edgar, K., Iliffe, S., Doll, H.A., Clarke, M.J., Gonçalves-Bradley, D.C., Wong, E. et al. (2024) Admission avoidance hospital at home, *Cochrane Database of Systematic Reviews* [Preprint], (3). https://doi.org/10.1002/14651858.CD007491.pub3.

Editorial (2018) The Astana Declaration: the future of primary health care?, *The Lancet*, 392(10156): 1369. https://doi.org/10.1016/S0140-6736(18)32478-4.

European Observatory (2024) Denmark - Health Systems and Policy Monitor. [https://eurohealthobservatory.who.int/monitors/health-systems-monitor/countries-hspm; accessed 12 May 2024].

EUSEM (2020) European Emergency Medicine in Numbers: Emergency Medicine Epidemiology Series. [https://eusem.org/images/European_EM_in_numbers.pdf; accessed 22 February 2025].

Ferguson, B., Rice, N., Sykes, D., Aletras, V., Eastwood, A., Sheldon, T. et al. (1996) Hospital volumes and health care outcomes, costs and patient access, *Bulletin on the Effectiveness of Health Service Interventions for Decision Makers*, 2(8).

Flojstrup, M., Bogh, S.B.B., Bech, M., Henriksen, D.P., Johnsen, S.P. and Brabrand, M. (2023) Mortality before and after reconfiguration of the Danish hospital-based emergency healthcare system: a nationwide interrupted time series analysis, *BMJ Quality & Safety*, 32(4): 202–213. https://doi.org/10.1136/bmjqs-2021-013881.

Fraser, A., Jones, L., Lorne, C. and Stewart, E. (2022) 'Attending to Collaboration' in major system change in healthcare in England: a response; comment on 'Attending to History' in major system change in healthcare in England: specialist cancer surgery service reconfiguration, *International Journal of Health Policy and Management*, 12(1): 1–3. https://doi.org/10.34172/ijhpm.2022.7661.

Goodwin, N., Perri 6, Peck, E., Freeman, T. and Posaner, R. (2004) Report to the National Co-ordinating Centre for NHS Service Delivery and Organisation R & D (NCCSDO) January 2004. [https://www.birmingham.ac.uk/Documents/college-social-sciences/social-policy/HSMC/research/diverse-networks-2004.pdf; accessed 26 March 2024].

Healy, J. and McKee, M. (2002) *Hospitals in a Changing Europe*. Buckingham: Open University Press [https://eurohealthobservatory.who.int/docs/librariesprovider3/studies--external/hospitals-in-a-changing-europe.pdf; accessed 22 February 2025].

Hirshon, J.M., Risko, N., Calvello, E.J., Stewart de Ramirez, S., Narayan, M., Theodosis, C. et al. (2013) Health systems and services: the role of acute care, *Bulletin of the World Health Organization*, 91(5): 386–388. doi: 10.2471/BLT.12.112664.

Hoang, H., Le, Q. and Terry, D. (2014) Women's access needs in maternity care in rural Tasmania, Australia: a mixed methods study, *Women and Birth*, 27(1): 9–14. https://doi.org/10.1016/j.wombi.2013.02.001.

Holmén, J., Herlitz, J., Ricksten, S., Strömsöe, A., Hagberg, E., Axelsson, C. et al. (2020) Shortening Ambulance Response Time Increases Survival in Out-of-Hospital Cardiac Arrest, *Journal of the American Heart Association*, 9(21): e017048. https://doi.org/10.1161/JAHA.120.017048.

Horwitz, J.R. and Nichols, A. (2022) Hospital service offerings still differ substantially by ownership type, *Health Affairs*, 41(3): 331–340. https://doi.org/10.1377/hlthaff.2021.01115.

Hussein, M., Pavlova, M., Ghalwash, M. and Groot, W. (2021) The impact of hospital accreditation on the quality of healthcare: a systematic literature review, *BMC Health Services Research*, 21(1), p. 1057. https://doi.org/10.1186/s12913-021-07097-6.

'International Case Study: Coxa' (2010) [https://assets.publishing.service.gov.uk/media/5a80e340ed915d74e6231039/Appendix_B_Coxa_International_Case_Study.pdf; accessed 9 January 2025]

Kannan, S., Bruch, J.D. and Song, Z. (2023) Changes in hospital adverse events and patient outcomes associated with private equity acquisition, *The Journal of the American Medical Association*, 330(24): 2365–2375. https://doi.org/10.1001/jama.2023.23147.

Kironji, A.G., Hodkinson, P., Stewart de Ramirez, S., Anest, T., Wallis, L., Razzak, J., et al. (2018) Identifying barriers for out of hospital emergency care in low and low-middle income countries: a systematic review, *BMC Health Services Research*, 18(1): 291. https://doi.org/10.1186/s12913-018-3091-0.

Kruk, M.E., Gage, A.D., Arsenault, C., Jordan, K., Leslie, H.H., Roder-DeWan, S. et al. (2018) High-quality health systems in the Sustainable Development Goals era: time for a revolution, *The Lancet Global Health*, 6(11): e1196–e1252. https://doi.org/10.1016/S2214-109X(18)30386-3.

Kumar, P. and Parthasarathy, R. (2020) Walking Out of the Hospital. McKinsey & Company. [https://www.mckinsey.com/industries/healthcare/our-insights/walking-out-of-the-hospital-the-continued-rise-of-ambulatory-care-and-how-to-take-advantage-of-it; accessed 6 May 2024].

Lansiaux, E., Cozzi, N., Wacht, O., Travers, S., Drouin, E. and Wiel, E. (2024) Scoop and treat: from an historical controversy to the emergency future, *Frontiers in Disaster and Emergency Medicine*, 2. https://doi.org/10.3389/femer.2024.1340348.

Laudicella, M., Martin, S., Li Donni, P. and Smith, P.C. (2018) Do reduced hospital mortality rates lead to increased utilization of inpatient emergency care? A population-based cohort study, *Health Services Research*, 53(4): 2324–2345. https://doi.org/10.1111/1475-6773.12755.

Lemos, P., Jarrett, P. and Philip, B. (2006) Day Surgery Development and Practice. International Association for Ambulatory Surgery. Report 2006. [https://theiaas.net/wp-content/uploads/2022/06/DaySurgery.pdf; accessed 9 January 2025].

Long, B.A. and Sweeney, M.J. (2023) Examining the Growing Demand for Surgical Care in Rural Communities and Novel Approaches to Achieving a Sustainable Surgical Workforce: A Narrative Review, *Cureus* [Preprint]. https://doi.org/10.7759/cureus.43817.

Mace, S. (ed.) (2017) *Observation Medicine: Principles and Protocols*. Cambridge: Cambridge University Press.

Maier, C., Kroezen, M., Busse, R. and Wismar, M. (eds) (2022) *Skill-mix Innovation, Effectiveness and Implementation: Improving Primary and Chronic Care.* Cambridge: Cambridge University Press.

Mansour, W., Boyd, A. and Walshe, K. (2020) The development of hospital accreditation in low- and middle-income countries: a literature review, *Health Policy and Planning*, 35(6): 684–700. https://doi.org/10.1093/heapol/czaa011.

McCord, C., Ozgediz, D., Beard, J.H. and Debas, H.T. (2015) Table 4.1, Definitions of levels of hospital care. The International Bank for Reconstruction and Development/The World Bank. [https://www.ncbi.nlm.nih.gov/books/NBK333506/table/ch04.sec1.table1/; accessed 4 January 2024].

McKee, M. (2004) Reducing hospital beds: What are the lessons learned? *European Observatory on Health Systems and Policies.* [https://iris.who.int/bitstream/handle/10665/107615/WHO-EURO-2004-654-40389-54118-eng.pdf?sequence=8&isAllowed=y; accessed 10 January 2025].

McKee, M., Merkur, S., Edwards, N. and Nolte, E. (2020) *The Changing Role of the Hospital in European Health Systems.* Cambridge: Cambridge University Press.

Mesman, R., Westert, G.P., Berden, B.J.M.M. and Faber, M.J. (2015) Why do high-volume hospitals achieve better outcomes? A systematic review about intermediate factors in volume–outcome relationships, *Health Policy*, 119(8): 1055–1067. https://doi.org/10.1016/j.healthpol.2015.04.005.

Mooney, A., Keith, J., Marszalek, K., Stafford, M., Gardner, T. and Tallack, C. (2023) What's Driving Increasing Length of Stay in Hospitals Since 2019? - The Health Foundation. [https://www.health.org.uk/publications/long-reads/what-s-driving-increasing-length-of-stay-in-hospitals-since-2019; accessed 1 April 2024].

Munnich, E.L. and Richards, M.R. (2022) Long-run growth of ambulatory surgery centers 1990–2015 and Medicare payment policy, *Health Services Research*, 57(1): 66. https://doi.org/10.1111/1475-6773.13707.

Murphy, A. (1998) 'Inappropriate' attenders at accident and emergency departments I: definition, incidence and reasons for attendance, *Family Practice*, 15(1): 23–32. https://doi.org/10.1093/fampra/15.1.23.

Naik, H., Murray, T.M., Khan, M., Daly-Grafstein, D., Liu, G., Kassen, B.O., et al. (2024) Population-Based Trends in Complexity of Hospital Inpatients, *JAMA Internal Medicine* [Preprint]. https://doi.org/10.1001/jamainternmed.2023.7410.

NHS England (2013) Health Building Note 00-01: General design guidance for healthcare buildings. https://www.england.nhs.uk/publication/designing-health-and-community-care-buildings-hbn-00-01/; accessed 9 January 2025].

NHS England (2019) Implementation of telemedicine at Airedale NHS Foundation Trust. [https://www.england.nhs.uk/atlas_case_study/implementation-of-telemedicine-at-airedale-nhs-foundation-trust/; accessed 28 November 2023].

Nolte, E., Pitchforth, E., Miani, C., and McHugh, S. (2014) The changing hospital landscape: An exploration of international experiences. Santa Monica, CA: RAND Corporation. [https://www.rand.org/pubs/research_reports/RR728.html; accessed 9 January 2025].

Norman, G., Bennett, P. and Vardy, E.R.L.C. (2023) Virtual wards: a rapid evidence synthesis and implications for the care of older people, *Age and Ageing*, 52(1), afac319. https://doi.org/10.1093/ageing/afac319.

OECD (2011) Health at a Glance 2011: OECD Indicators. Paris: Organisation for Economic Co-operation and Development. [https://www.oecd-ilibrary.org/social-issues-migration-health/health-at-a-glance-2011_health_glance-2011-en; accessed 28 March 2024].

OECD (2021) Health at a Glance 2021: OECD Indicators. OECD (Health at a Glance). https://doi.org/10.1787/ae3016b9-en; accessed 22 February 2025].

OECD (2023) OECD Health Statistics 2023 Definitions, Sources and Methods. [https://www.oecd.org/content/dam/oecd/en/data/datasets/oecd-health-statistics/214497-Table-of-Content-Metadata-OECD-Health-Statistics-2023.pdf/_jcr_content/renditions/original./214497-Table-of-Content-Metadata-OECD-Health-Statistics-2023.pdf; accessed 22 February 2025].

OECD (2024) OECD Health Statistics 2024 [https://www.oecd.org/en/data/datasets/oecd-health-statistics.html; accessed 22 February 2025].

Ortiz-Ospina, E. and Roser, M. (2023) 'Healthcare Spending', Our World in Data [Preprint]. [https://ourworldindata.org/financing-healthcare; accessed 9 January 2024].

Paynter, J., Qin, K.R., Brennan, J., Hunter-Smith, D.J. and Rozen, W.M. (2024) The provision of general surgery in rural Australia: a narrative review, *Medical Journal of Australia*, 220(5): 258–263. https://doi.org/10.5694/mja2.52232.

Project Hope (2022) The global healthcare worker shortage: 10 numbers to note. [https://www.projecthope.org/news-stories/story/the-global-health-care-worker-shortage-10-numbers-to-note/; accessed 9 January 2024].

Public Health England (2019) An evidence summary of health inequalities in older populations in coastal and rural areas. Public Health England. [https://assets.publishing.service.gov.uk/media/5d517ce3ed915d7646dea423/Health_Inequalities_in_Ageing_in_Rural_and_Coastal_Areas-Full_report.pdf; accessed 22 February 2025].

Randell, R., Honey, S., Alvarado, N., Greenhalgh, J., Hindmarsh, J., Pearman, A., et al. (2019) Factors supporting and constraining the implementation of robot-assisted surgery: a realist interview study, *BMJ Open*, 9(6): e028635. https://doi.org/10.1136/bmjopen-2018-028635.

Reid, N., Gamage, T., Duckett, S.J. and Graye, L.C. (2023) Hospital utilisation in Australia, 1993–2020, with a focus on use by people over 75 years of age: a review of AIHW data, *Medical Journal of Australia*, 219(3): 113–119. https://doi.org/10.5694/mja2.52026.

Rushton, S., Boggan, J.C., Lewinski, A.A., Gordon, A.M., Shoup, J.P., Van Voorhees, E. et al. (2019) Effectiveness of Remote Triage: A Systematic Review. Washington (DC): Department of Veterans Affairs (US) (VA Evidence-based Synthesis Program Reports). [http://www.ncbi.nlm.nih.gov/books/NBK553039/; accessed 18 October 2023].

Sagan, A. and Richardson, E. (2015) The challenge of providing emergency medical care, *Eurohealth*, 21(4): 3–5.

Saltman, R., Durán, A. and Dubois, H. (2011) Governing Public Hospitals: Reform Strategies and the Movement Towards Institutional Autonomy. WHO. [https://iris.who.int/handle/10665/326425; accessed 22 February 2025].

Sarbay, I. (2019) Countries Recognize Emergency Medicine as a Specialty. International Emergency Medicine Project, 13 May. [https://iem-student.org/2019/05/13/countries-recognize-emergency-medicine/; accessed 12 June 2024].

Schroeder, S.A. (1992) The troubled profession: is medicine's glass half full or half empty?, *Annals of Internal Medicine*, 116(7): 583–592. https://doi.org/10.7326/0003-4819-116-7-583.

Shannon, B., Pang, R., Jepson, M., Williams, C., Andrew, N., Smith, K. et al. (2020) What is the prevalence of frequent attendance to emergency departments and what is the impact on emergency department utilisation? A systematic review and meta-analysis, *Internal and Emergency Medicine*, 15(7): 1303–1316. https://doi.org/10.1007/s11739-020-02403-2.

Shepperd, S. and Iliffe, S. (2001) Hospital at home versus in-patient hospital care, *The Cochrane Database of Systematic Reviews*, (3): CD000356. https://doi.org/10.1002/14651858. CD000356.

Skopec, M., Issa, H. and Harris, M. (2019) Delivering cost effective healthcare through reverse innovation, *British Medical Journal*, 367. https://doi.org/10.1136/bmj.l6205.

Smith, I., Hicks, C. and McGovern, T. (2020) Adapting Lean methods to facilitate stakeholder engagement and co-design in healthcare, *British Medical Journal*, 368. https://doi.org/10.1136/bmj.m35.

Southerland, L.T., Lo, A.X., Biese, K., Arendts, G., Banerjee, J., Hwang, U. et al. (2020) Concepts in practice: geriatric emergency departments, *Annals of Emergency Medicine*, 75(2): 162–170. https://doi.org/10.1016/j.annemergmed.2019.08.430.

Sowden, A. and Sheldon, T. (1998) Does volume really affect outcome? Lessons from the evidence, *Journal of Health Services Research & Policy*, 3(3). https://doi.org/10.1177/135581969800300311.

Staib, A., Sullivan, C., Griffin, B., Bell, A. and Scott, I. (2016) Report on the 4-h rule and National Emergency Access Target (NEAT) in Australia: time to revie', *Australian Health Review*, 40(3): 319. https://doi.org/10.1071/AH15071.

swleoc (2024) South West London Orthopaedic Centre. [https://www.eoc.nhs.uk/; accessed 10 January 2025].

Tadesse, L., Abdullah, N.H., Awadalla, H.M.I, D'Amours, S., Davies, F., Kissoon, N., et al. (2023) A global mandate to strengthen emergency, critical and operative care, *Bulletin of the World Health Organization*, 101(04): 231–231A. https://doi.org/10.2471/BLT.23.289916.

Tillmann, B.W., Fu, L., Hill, A.D., Scales, D.C., Fowler, R.A., Cuthbertson, B.H. and Wunsch, H. (2021) Acute healthcare resource utilization by age: a cohort study, *PLOS ONE*, 16(5): e0251877. https://doi.org/10.1371/journal.pone.0251877.

Turner, J., Knowles, E., Simpson, R., Sampson, F., Dixon, S., Long. J. et al. (2021) Impact of NHS 111 Online on the NHS 111 telephone service and urgent care system: a mixed-methods study, *Health Services and Delivery Research*, 9(21): 1–148. https://doi.org/10.3310/hsdr09210.

Tynkkynen, L.-K. and Vrangbæk, K. (2018) Comparing public and private providers: a scoping review of hospital services in Europe, *BMC Health Services Research*, 18(1): 141. https://doi.org/10.1186/s12913-018-2953-9.

Urbach, D.R. and Baxter, N.N. (2004) Does it matter what a hospital is 'high volume' for? Specificity of hospital volume-outcome associations for surgical procedures: analysis of administrative data, *British Medical Journal*, 328(7442): 737–740. https://doi.org/10.1136/bmj.38030.642963.AE.

Valderas, J.M., Starfield, B., Sibbald, B., Salisbury, C. and Roland, M. (2009) Defining comorbidity: implications for understanding health and health services, *The Annals of Family Medicine*, 7(4): 357–363. https://doi.org/10.1370/afm.983.

Vaughan, L. and Browne, J. (2023) Reconfiguring emergency and acute services: time to pause and reflect, *BMJ Quality & Safety*, 32(4): 185–188. https://doi.org/10.1136/bmjqs-2022-015141.

Vaughan, L., Bardsley, M., Bell, D., Davies, M., Goddard, A., Imison, C. (2021) Models of generalist and specialist care in smaller hospitals in England: a mixed-methods study, *Health Services and Delivery Research*, 9(4): 1–158. https://doi.org/10.3310/hsdr09040.

Vaughan, L. and Edwards, N. (2023) Emergency hospital services are closing because of staff shortages, *British Medical Journal*, 383: e078766. https://doi.org/10.1136/bmj-2023-078766.

Waalwijk, J.F., Van der Sluijs, R., Lokerman, R., Fiddelers, A., Hietbrink, F., Leenen, L., et al. (2022) The impact of prehospital time intervals on mortality in moderately and severely injured patients, *The Journal of Trauma and Acute Care Surgery*, 92(3): 520–527. https://doi.org/10.1097/TA.0000000000003380.

Wachter, R.M. (2016) Making IT Work: Harnessing the Power of Health Information Technology to Improve Care in England, *Making IT Work* [Preprint].

Wachter, R.M. and Bell, D. (2012) Renaissance of hospital generalists, *British Medical Journal*, 344: e652. https://doi.org/10.1136/bmj.e652.

Westafer, L. (2020) 'Stay and Play' Versus 'Scoop and Run' for Out-of-Hospital Cardiac Arrest. [https://www.jwatch.org/na52460/2020/09/23/stay-and-play-versus-scoop-and-run-out-hospital-cardiac; accessed 1 July 2024].

WHO (1978) Declaration of Alma-Ata. World Health Organization. [https://iris.who.int/bitstream/handle/10665/347879/WHO-EURO-1978-3938-43697-61471-eng.pdf?sequence=1; accessed 22 February 2025].

Willis, T.A., Wright-Hughes, A., Weller, A., Alderson, S.L., Wilson, S., Walwyn, R. et al. (2022) Interventions to optimise the outputs of national clinical audits to improve the quality of health care: a multi-method study including RCT, *Health and Social Care Delivery Research*, 10(15), pp. 1–284. [https://doi.org/10.3310/QBBZ1124].

Wohlgemut, J.M., Ramsay, G. and Jansen, J.O. (2020) The changing face of emergency general surgery: a 20-year analysis of secular trends in demographics, diagnoses, operations, and outcomes, *Annals of Surgery*, 271(3), p. 581. [https://doi.org/10.1097/SLA.0000000000003066].

World Health Organization (2020) WHO guidance for climate resilient and environmentally sustainable health care facilities. [https://www.who.int/publications-detail-redirect/9789240012226; accessed 13 March 2024].

World Health Organization (2023) Hospitals. [https://www.who.int/health-topics/hospitals; accessed 19 March 2024].

Zapata, T., Muscat, N.A., Falkenbach, M. and Wismar, M. (2023) From great attrition to great attraction: countering the great resignation of health and care workers, *Eurohealth*, 29(1): 6–10. [https://iris.who.int/handle/10665/372887; accessed 10 January 2025].

Zare, H. and Gabow, P. (2023) Influence of not-for-profit hospital ownership type on community benefit and charity care, *Journal of Community Health*, 48(2): 199–209 https://doi.org/10.1007/s10900-022-01159-4.

Zink, B.L. (2005) *Anyone, Anything, Anytime. A History of Emergency Medicine.* St Louis: Mosby.

Integrated care

Robin Miller and Viktoria Stein

Introduction

Collaboration between different professionals and services has been a greater or lesser component of health and care since support became more formalized and structured. Key transitions, such as crisis care, leaving hospital and entering rehabilitation programmes, involve professionals from different backgrounds working together and progressively handing care onto another set of clinicians and practitioners, whatever the overall funding and organizational arrangements. In some contexts, how to integrate between traditional and complementary medicine, and 'Western' styles of diagnosis and treatment have also been a longstanding issue (World Health Organization, 2019). More intense inter-professional collaborations have been common for some time to support populations with more complex health and care needs, such as those who are homeless, people with profound learning and physical disabilities and children who have been abused (Miller et al., 2016).

In more recent times, integrated care is being seen as a core dynamic of health and care systems (Farmanova et al., 2019). This is due to people's poor experiences of fragmented care, resources being wasted due to duplication, and increasing population numbers with multiple long-term conditions (Farmanova et al., 2019). These demands are forcing most health and care systems to think how to support people before they move into crisis and better coordinate specialists who traditionally focus on one aspect of a person's health and well-being. These demands are often exacerbated by the fragmented systems currently in place, which react to recurring emergencies and tie up considerable resources in hospital-based care rather than proactively prevent progression or enabling service users to better manage their own needs (OECD, 2020). Further pressure arises from a decreasing and exhausted workforce with high staff turnovers in many countries, which calls for redesign of how health and care systems are organized and managed (World Health Organization, 2016).

This chapter will largely focus on implementation of integrated care as the aspect most relevant to healthcare managers. It is important though to first consider the definition and purpose of integrated care as the foundation for implementation. Definitions focus on the structures, processes, contributors and outcomes of integration dependent on the focus of interest (Hughes et al., 2020) and two examples are set out in Box 15.1.

Box 15.1 Examples of definitions of integrated care

System definition: 'health services that are managed and delivered so that people receive a continuum of health promotion, disease prevention, diagnosis, treatment, disease-management, rehabilitation and palliative care services, coordinated across the different levels and sites of care within and beyond the health sector, and according to their needs throughout the life course' (World Health Organization, 2024: 1)

Person-centred definition: 'I can plan my care with people who work together to understand me and my carer(s), allow me control, and bring together services to achieve the outcomes important to me' (National Voices, 2013: 3)

In relation to the purpose of integrated care, there has been a coalescence around what are known as the Quadruple Aim: better experience of those accessing services; improved efficiency in resource usage; reduced inequalities across populations; and greater well-being for the health and care workforce (Bodenheimer and Sinsky, 2014). The extent to which integrated care achieves these outcomes is debatable due to complexity of attribution, the changing economic and social environments in which integrated care operates, and a plethora of interventions being associated under the banner of integration (Baxter et al., 2018).

Advocates of integration have at times overstated the case with governments desperate to believe that they can see substantially improved outcomes through better organization of existing resources. That said, evidence does support improved people's experience, more timely discharges from hospital and some potential impact on hospital admissions (e.g. Damery et al., 2016; Lewis et al., 2021). When managed well, better integrated care supports staff satisfaction and retention, and a better collaboration between hospitals, primary care and voluntary and community sector organizations (Barraclough et al., 2021). The operating term here is 'when managed well', and this chapter will outline some of the key topics that managers need to be aware when trying to implement integrated care successfully.

Managing levels of integration

While there may not be consensus on the impact or definition of integrated care, there is agreement on the challenges of its implementation. Evidence syntheses and learning from numerous national and regional programmes in both high- (HMICs), and low- and middle-income countries (LMICs), outline that integrated care cannot be achieved to any meaningful

Table 15.1 Dimensions of integration

Dimension	Definition
Systemic integration	This dimension of integrated care refers to the ability of the care system in providing an enabling platform for integrated care at an organizational, professional and clinical level (e.g. through the alignment of key systemic factors, such as regulation, financing mechanisms, workforce development and training).
Organizational integration	This dimension of integrated care refers to the ability of different providers to come together to enable joined-up service delivery (that helps to then support professional and clinical integration).
Professional integration	This dimension of integrated care refers to the existence and promotion of partnerships between care professionals that enable them to work together (e.g., in teams or networks) and so promote better care coordination around the needs of the service user.
Functional integration	This dimension of integrated care refers to the capacity to communicate data and information effectively within an integrated care system
Normative integration	This dimension of integrated care relates to the extent to which different partners in care have developed a common frame of reference (i.e. of vision, norms and values) in support of the aims and objectives of care integration.
Service integration	This dimension of integrated care refers to how care services are coordinated and/or organized around the needs of service users.
Person-centred integration	This dimension reflects the perspective of improving someone's overall well-being – not focusing solely on a particular condition/disease – through the active engagement of service users (patients, carers, etc.) as partners in care.

Source: Adapted from Calciolari et al., 2021.

extent or be sustained in the long term through focusing on an isolated element or single intervention, and that change will instead be required at different levels of the health and care system (Mounier-Jack et al., 2017). The dimensions of implementation were outlined and defined through Project Integrate, a major four-year European programme that explored the management and delivery of integrated care (for more details of the overall project see: Borgermans and Devroey, 2017) (Table 15.1). This included surveys, evidence reviews, case studies of best practice and policy and practitioner workshops.

In the following sections each level of integration set out in Table 15.1 will be explored in more detail, focusing on what is most relevant from a managerial perspective and illustrating implementation with international examples. Person-centred integration has not been covered as related management issues are outlined in Chapter 21.

Systemic integration

Integrated care must be developed within the context of national and local health and social care systems (World Health Organization, 2024). Systems may have components that provide helpful building blocks for person-centred and coordinated care, but which are based around traditional divisions, such as primary care, hospitals and social care. These sectors will have been developed over time in response to needs within society and within themselves have considerable complexity. Their distinct boundaries based on finances, staffing, account-ability, objectives and traditions limit their collective ability to respond holistically to changing demands. For example, a study in the UK of the experiences of people with complex needs leaving hospital found that a major barrier to care integration was securing suitable physical accommodation in which care could be provided. There were often major disputes between health, social care and housing providers as to who was responsible for identifying properties, undertaking necessary adaptations and meeting any gaps in tenancies (Glasby et al., 2024). Integrated care therefore requires systems to develop new ways of bridging these boundaries or introducing new configurations in which these barriers no longer exist.

Policy

National (or regional in more devolved health and care systems) policies set an overall purpose for health and social care and outline what is expected from the constituent parts of the system (Miller et al., 2021). Policy intentions are converted into legislation that creates the rules under which the system operates, guidance of how rules should be inter-preted and accountability processes to enforce these rules and guidance. Financial flows are also based on prioritization of policy with organizations and in some cases, profession-als, being incentivized to focus on specific activities. If policy emphasizes that a sector's sole responsibility is the quality and financial health of their services, then this can dis-suade organizations from sharing resources with other sectors.

For example, if policy states that hospitals' responsibilities effectively stop when a patient is discharged and funding ceases when the person is medically assessed as no longer needing treatment, then hospitals are likely to be reluctant to give time for the patient to consider all potential options and for individual packages of care to be created. In countries that have developed long-term care arrangements in which many older people are cared for in large, congregate institutions, such as care homes, a common consequence is that older patients move into such settings to free up hospital capacity. This can lead to a poorer quality of life than returning to their own homes, and longer-term financial burdens on them and/or the part of the state responsible for such costs. Similarly, if social care's responsibilities finish once someone is admitted to hospital, social care may be less keen to invest resources in maintain-ing people with complex needs in the community. Policy that gives hospitals, primary and social care services a shared responsibility to meet the needs of the population will likely encourage them to collaborate more effectively.

Professional practice

Disciplines, such as medicine, nursing, therapy and (in some instances) social work, have a set of responsibilities that fall within their professional scope and that other professions must not undertake. Connected knowledge and skills are gained through established quali-fications and are required for professional registration. Like policy, if these competences focus exclusively on the technical aspects that fall to each profession, then this can dissuade professionals from holistically working alongside the patient and other services. Depending on the scope outlined within connected legislation, professions may not legally be able to take on or delegate responsibilities that could now be more effectively delivered by a different professional. Traditional roles set out for professionals are also part of their identity and perceived value and there can be resistance to share tasks with others as this could lead to a lessening of their profile and status.

Governance

While the many challenges connected with the implementation of new policies and professional regulation should not be overlooked, it is also true that if configured correctly then policies and regulation can provide a more supportive context to encourage more integrated working (Nolte et al., 2016). A common approach for this is for national or regional governments to introduce new governance approaches in which there is shared responsibility for managing the finance, quality and future planning of health and care services. Alongside legal mandates, active participation in care integration can be encouraged through decreased external interference from national bodies, greater local flexibility in how resources are used and access to additional funding. Replacing performance metrics based on the activities and responsibilities of individual organizations and professions with measures that reflect the outcomes for individuals and populations across care delivery bodies can further encourage better collaboration. Similarly, clear policy expectations regarding the involvement of people with lived experience and communities embeds this important enabler of integrated care (see Chapter 21, Service user perspectives, experiences and involvement). An example of systemic care integration is found in Alaska, in which a previously fragmented approach to healthcare was replaced by one grounded in the expectations and cultures of local Native communities. The system includes multidisciplinary teams co-located in primary care centres, complementary medicine and traditional healing, and interventions to address social issues such as domestic violence. The system is coordinated by a single healthcare organization, Southcentral Foundation, which manages acute, primary and wider well-being services (Gottlieb, 2013; Collins, 2015).

Organizational integration

Translating shared governance and accountability from the overall system to the local organizational level is concerned with pooling resources, sharing physical and technological assets and establishing multidisciplinary teamwork across services and organizations, including professionals from primary care, social care and community services to manage a specific population, such as older people with multimorbidity (Barry et al., 2021; Miller, 2022). For managers, it can prove very challenging to agree on shared outcomes across organizations to assess shared performance, or pool budgets to provide the services necessary for an agreed population (Miller and Stein, 2020). For such integration intra- and inter-organizational planning and implementation need to explicitly address the governance and accountability mechanisms as the basis for sharing resources and working collaboratively (Auschra, 2018). The guiding coalition (which can take many forms) that brings all the stakeholders together plays a key role in ensuring that each organization individually and collectively provides their employees with the time, flexibility and support systems to implement integrated care in practice.

Depending on the country context, these guiding coalitions may take the form of networks with or without a lead organization, legal entities (such as foundations, management organizations or accountable care organizations) or looser arrangements based on memoranda of understanding. While this may suggest that a higher level mandate is a prerequisite of orga-nizational integration as happened, for example, in Scotland (Thompson et al., 2021, https://www.gov.scot/policies/social-care/health-and-social-care-integration/) or the Basque country (Nuño-Solinís, 2021), the majority of international examples were initiated at the organiza-tional level. This was because local needs and organizational pressures brought stakeholders together to look for innovative ways of improving services, while simultaneously using resources more effectively and efficiently.

Managing up, across and down

A key challenge in organizational integration is the need to take a multi-directional approach. On the one hand, a common understanding and necessary infrastructure need to be imple-mented *within* an organization to prepare structures, processes and people for integrated care. On the other hand (and at the same time), organizational integration *between* organiza-tions needs to create the rules, roles and responsibilities across the stakeholders participating in the initiative. *Managing up* towards the system or a higher management level, across stakeholder organizations or departments, and downwards – within each organization and teams – requires additional competences from all levels of management and must include a capacity for managing complexity and uncertainty (Miller and Stein, 2020; Mitterlechner and Bilgeri, 2021). Identifying the right people for the job, including having the role of integrated care management included in job descriptions, along with supportive management and lead-ership training from the earliest stages, is crucial. Shared leadership, collaborative leadership and co-leadership are among the many leadership concepts that can support this process (Klinga, 2021; Curry et al., 2022).

Budgets and performance measures

Aligning or pooling budgets also means incentivizing collaboration rather than service frag-mentation and agreeing on shared measures and outcomes to monitor and evaluate integrated care (Tsiachristas, 2016). A shared performance measurement framework ensures transpar-ency and emphasizes the common goals but also demonstrates to partner organizations that everyone has a stake in the game and a vital role to play. Common measures and outcomes in turn can support the development of a learning environment within each organization and across the coalition, which enables the workforce to come together, receive and give feed-back and embark on a joint programme of service improvement and integration.

An example of how a local initiative of organizational integration can be successfully scaled up is the Foundry model from British Columbia, Canada (https://foundrybc.ca). This started out as the Granville Youth Health Centre in 2015 in downtown Vancouver. It was designed to provide integrated primary care, as well as mental health, substance use and peer support services in a welcoming space designed with young people under 24 years of age. This grew into the Foundry provincial network, which is in operation throughout British Columbia today, providing a range of services to young people from early intervention and peer support, primary care and social services. The model of organizational integration is the same for every Foundry centre, where a lead organization brings together local partners, service providers and families and young people including through a Youth Advisory Com-mittee (TransForm, 2021a, 2021b).

Professional integration

Health and social care professionals are central to enabling a better understanding of people's challenges and conditions and delivering and coordinating suitable treatments and supports. Their distinctive knowledge and skills are important in enabling a thorough response to the diversity of people's needs and conditions. However, these differences in training, roles and perspective can also result in fragmented care if professionals are not accustomed or willing to engage in constructive dialogue with others. Likewise, they may not necessarily have the skills, influence or interest in coordinating their professional input with that of other disciplines.

Multidisciplinary teams

Organizing professionals within teams is a common approach to encouraging better collaboration between disciplines (Jelphs et al., 2016). These may be designed around a geographical area, patients with similar long-term conditions or specific transitional processes, such as hospital discharge (Miller, 2022). There is generally a shared service entry point through which people are referred into a team with common assessment processes to understand their needs, and collectively discuss, plan and enact support options. Teams can be effective in enabling professionals to learn more of their colleagues' practices and coordinate supportive care around an individual and their family. They can also provide a forum in which professionals constructively challenge each other and perhaps create new service offers to address gaps between their traditional forms of care.

To achieve their potential, however, teams must be skilfully led with no one profession dominating and alternative perspectives respected within practice discussions (West and Lyubovnikova, 2012). There is also a danger that team processes can become ineffective through tying up resources that would be more effectively spent providing direct care or not delaying decisions unnecessarily. Patients can find this particularly frustrating if they sense that their care is being decided by a group that they know very little about, and the multidisciplinary team (MDT) can then seem a distant yet mysterious body with considerable influence over their treatment and care (Miller, 2022). Shared team objectives and metrics can help to provide focus and identify opportunities to strengthen practical service collaboration. An example of MDTs in action are Community Health Centres in Canada that aim to improve access to healthcare for marginalized populations (Box 15.2).

Inter-professional education

It is vital that health and social care professionals graduate with the core competences to safely deliver their practice, but it is also important that they have the skills to successfully work in collaboration with other disciplines. This has been recognized internationally as a major issue that reflects the uni-professional nature of much health and care qualifying education (Thistlethwaite, 2012). One approach to helping gain these skills is inter-professional education (IPE) in which students learn not only alongside but also from one another (Miller et al., 2019). IPE is often action-orientated in its approach to highlight differences in students' interpretations of a situation and to find opportunities to create a common way forward. Activities can include discussing case examples of people with cross-disciplinary needs, undertaking joint projects, and working together within an integrated health and care clinic (Miller et al., 2019). Planning and delivering IPE can be challenging for professional educators who may only have experience of teaching within the boundaries of their own discipline and may therefore not be confident in facilitating learning across a wider professional range. Most research into IPE has focused on its use within qualifying programmes, such as undergraduate medicine, nursing and social work, but it can also be effectively applied within postgraduate courses or continuing professional development.

Box 15.2   Community Health Centres, Canada

Community Health Centres (CHC) were initially introduced in the 1970s within the Province of Ontario and have grown steadily in number so that there are now over 70 in total. They are set up within localities that face multiple deprivation and are governed by community-elected boards.

At the heart of CHCs are multidisciplinary primary care teams that contain a higher proportion of non-medical professionals than general primary care teams, including nurse practitioners, social workers, psychologists and other roles, such as system navigators. A crucial element of the model is that doctors are employed directly by the CHC rather than being independent practitioners funded through fee-for-service payments. Around the teams are community development and preventative care activities designed to strengthen local people's ability to improve its collective health.

Evaluations report that CHCs enhance patient satisfaction, make a positive contribution to addressing of health inequalities, and demonstrate lower costs of care (Collins et al., 2014; Bhuiya et al., 2020).

For more details see: About Us | Alliance for Healthier Communities (allianceon.org)

Learning activity 15.1

Identify two professions of relevance to your area of health or social care responsibility or interest and undertake desktop research on their underpinning professional standards and overall scope of practice.

- To what extent are the principles of integration reflected in their standards and how do these compare?
- If you were developing an integrated service involving these two professions, how could you communicate its potential benefits and each profession's contribution to encourage participation in new collaborative ways of working?

Functional integration

Functional integration focuses primarily on operational and administrative integration, such as decision support tools, shared care records, appropriate and interoperable information and communication technology (ICT), and streamlining processes to improve efficiency and effectiveness (Gray, 2021). Appropriate and user-friendly ICT does not always have to be high tech – its importance lies in the transparent and accessible transmittance of information to everyone in the system requiring it, including the individual and family. In addition, eHealth (e.g. electronic records), mHealth (e.g. wearables and apps) and other technological solutions (e.g. teleconsultations via online platforms, webinars, etc.) support easy access to the right level of care for professionals and service users alike, assist in self-management and can, in some circumstances, be an indispensable tool to enable people to stay at home on their own terms (Steele Gray, 2021).

Digital health literacy and co-design

It is important to provide different channels of information and communication and not rely on digital alone, as related literacy and connectivity vary. It is also essential to explore the willingness and competence of professionals and service users who need to access the information and provide training on the effective use of such tools (LaMonica et al., 2020). Not involving end users, which include both professionals and patients, results in designs of technology that are not fit for purpose in everyday practice and thus do not get used (Sanz et al., 2021). However, if implemented well, technology may increase access for patients and family caregivers, assist in signposting and coordinating otherwise inaccessible services, and therefore help to coordinate care. Examples include online platforms to book and renew services, the use of wearables and digital devices to monitor and transfer live data on people's health, or the offer of online consultations ranging from specialist advice to a simple social welfare check-in (Baltaxe et al., 2019).

Access to and use of data

Data sharing and analysis are among the most challenging issues for integration of care across sectors (Kozlowska et al., 2018; Baltaxe et al., 2019; Steele Gray, 2021). Successful examples include the four early adopter schemes from the European Union Joint Action on the implementation of digitally enabled integrated person-centred care (JADECARE): the Basque country, Catalonia, the 'Healthy Kinzigtal' in southwest Germany and the region of Southern Denmark [https://www.jadecare.eu/structure/transfer-good-practices/]. Apart from the (often misused) data protection and legal aspect, ensuring technical interoperability or shareability of data can be a major stumbling block. Workarounds, such as creating a Health Information Exchange Platform (e.g. in Catalonia), into which professionals can upload their own data, is one viable option, as is data collation from different information systems as part of a multidisciplinary team (e.g. Catalonia and Basque country) (Cano et al., 2015; Baltaxe et al., 2019; Blijleven et al., 2022).

Integrated care pathways are another example of functional integration, where service providers for a particular patient or user group can access summaries of the latest evidence-based guidelines, information about previous treatments and other services involved. Ideally, they can also document care provided and be alerted to issues, such as possible contraindications for medication. However, these care pathways usually only work effectively when they are designed and used for a tightly specified group of people over a well-defined period of time (Vrijhoef et al., 2017).

Normative integration

Health and social care practice is undertaken within the context of organizational and professional cultures (Miller et al., 2016). These are the often informal rules, expectations and established patterns of behaviour that outline what is acceptable, and what is not, in relation to the behaviours of individuals and teams. Such norms build over time as people are socialized into them and may not even explicitly realize how they influence their thinking. Such cultures can therefore provide a considerable barrier to the successful introduction of integrated care, as they may not support a professional taking on a new task, if this is outside their previous responsibilities, or resist developments that are seen to reduce professional autonomy or status. The converse is also true – where a culture that embraces collaboration through shared values is fostered then this can result in new and innovative approaches emerging (Zonneveld et al., 2018).

Cultural artefacts

While the importance of culture to quality and innovation has been long recognized, the process of understanding the mosaic of local cultures is complex (Mannion, 2022). Within an organization, for example, there may be some aspects of culture that are shared across its members, but other co-existent cultures may vary between teams and professions. Schein's cultural model seeks to make sense of this complexity (Schein, 1995). It contains three elements – the *espoused values* that the senior management promotes, *artefacts* that reflect the actual culture within the organization, and the *assumptions* that underpin those artefacts being present. Artefacts can be practical symbols, such as branding, titles or uniforms, or established patterns of behaviours. For example, the common tendency to have doctors as the chair of MDTs could be taken to imply that they have a higher status than other professions. Similarly, if a team has separate refreshment funds between disciplines, this could imply that they are not in a position where they trust others to use resources responsibly. Creating new artefacts that reflect more integrated working can also help nudge cultures in this direction. For example, opening up MDT leadership roles to all disciplines can be seen to indicate that no one profession is seen as inherently more skilled to take on such roles.

Culture change

Changing culture is notoriously difficult (Mannion and Davies, 2016). As outlined in Chapter 3, leadership can make a strong contribution through creating a common team or organizational vision to which people are willing to commit their support. Within integrated care, this is often communicated through developing an accessible narrative about how care would be better for a fictional person if there were to be greater collaboration (Thistlethwaite, 2011). Multidisciplinary teams, inter-professional training and building in processes for shared reflection on what is working and what could be improved can all play a part (Miller et al., 2016). Using the values that have been identified as underpinning integrated care can similarly generate helpful discussion about which cultures and behaviours are currently present and which ones require further attention (Zonneveld et al., 2018).

Creating opportunities whereby professionals and managers can meet with people with lived experience can also help to strengthen common values. A commitment to improve the quality of life and address underlying inequalities is at the heart of much professional practice and what motivates people to initially undertake such careers. Such engagement opportunities can help to amplify this shared aspiration and help professionals to see beyond their differences and historical tensions. One example of normative integration being built into a programme is the 'Wigan Deal' in the UK, in which local health and local government leaders sought to reinvent fundamental assumptions about the role of and relationship between public services and communities (Box 15.3).

Box 15.3   Wigan Deal, UK (Naylor and Wellings, 2019)

Wigan is an area of North-West England, UK that has experienced many challenges including unemployment, obesity, homelessness and other complex social issues. Faced with the need to make major savings, local government leaders decided that as well as reducing spending on some services, they would seek efficiencies by redesigning services and investing in new ways of working. Fundamentally, it was giving frontline staff more agency to make changes to services to better reflect the specific needs and strengths of local individuals and communities. This began with social care working with people differently to better understand their aspirations and how services could complement their personal and community resources.

This 'asset based' approach became the underpinning ethos for the Council ('The Wigan Deal') based on reciprocity and trust between the organization and the communities ('our part, your part'). To embed into cultures, leaders made themselves more accessible and accountable to staff, gave permission to innovate through promoting stories of change, recruited on basis of values reflecting the 'Deal', and provided training on asset-based working. Health organizations also adopted the principles of the Wigan Deal and these were built into shared objectives and monitoring processes.

For more details see: Lessons from the Wigan Deal

Learning activity 15.2

Identify and describe a cultural artefact connected with integrated care practice in your organization or partnership, or one that you have read about locally or encountered during your student placement.

- How far is this artefact consistent with the adopted values of the organization or integrated care scheme?
- What do you consider would be the assumptions of different stakeholder groups in relation to this artefact, and why do they matter?

Service integration

It is in service integration that the foundations set within the other levels of the health and care system come to fruition – supporting MDTs (professional integration), implementing culture change and creating a common language (normative integration), and defining processes and information flows along the care continuum (functional integration). In contrast to professional integration, which focuses on the interaction and collaboration between different professions, service integration focuses on the interaction between professionals and service users. It refers to the coordination and delivery of various services across different providers, sectors and settings to ensure seamless and efficient person-centred care. Some authors suggest (e.g. Goodwin et al., 2021; Nolte and McKee, 2008) that this is the level that matters most, because it is in the day-to-day actions that integrated care will either fail or prevail.

Care coordination and related terms

There is a core set of elements that should be considered in designing and managing service integration. Care coordination is defined as the deliberate organization of care activities among interdependent participants across different settings, sharing of necessary information among all the participants concerned, including the patient and family, with the final aim to provide appropriate, safe and effective care (Schultz and MacDonald, 2014). This only happens when it is a clearly defined task either performed by a dedicated person or as part of the role of an MDT. The intensity of care coordination differs depending on the needs of the person and is supported by a shared care plan, a map of care or an integrated care pathway.

Continuity of care ensures that service users receive the right care, at the right time, in the right setting, and by the right people (AHQR, 2018). Ideally, this is defined along an evidence-based integrated care pathway, which describes the roles and responsibilities, information-sharing requirements and accountability at each transition of care (AHQR, 2018). In combination with proactively managed care transitioning, this can also ensure that no person stays in hospital longer than necessary, as both admission and discharge are planned well ahead with the patient, their carers and community service providers. Taking a life-course approach means that care needs are not seen as episodic, isolated and unrelated short-term events but that a person's needs are understood to progress and change over the course of their life. Taken together, these concepts constitute important tools to support the integration of care, and they form an integral part of the examples provided in this chapter. However, they do not necessarily lead to integrated care in the sense that they do not automatically lead to professional, organizational or system integration (Nolte and McKee, 2008; Curry and Ham 2010). Integrated care needs to be managed; it does not come naturally (Goodwin et al., 2021).

Community participation and co-design

Service user and community participation prioritizes the needs and preferences of people, carers and communities, involving them as active participants in the design, implementation and management of their care (see Chapter 21). It emphasizes patient engagement, shared decision-making, and personalized care planning to promote better health outcomes and patient satisfaction. As many conditions and situations require active participation, self-management and changes on the part of the person, their carer or community to improve the overall outcomes, their inclusion as members of the care team and decision-makers on their own terms is crucial for success. It implies a long-term relationship between people, professionals and organizations where information, decision-making and service delivery become shared. Thus, co-production emphasizes the shift to designing and managing services locally, as municipalities; local service providers and communities know best, what the local needs and assets are (Lara Montero et al., 2016). As a healthcare manager, it is also important to involve employees and service providers in these co-design efforts to ensure that they understand their existing and new roles and responsibilities and provide them with the necessary training to be able to work in a more collaborative way (Miller and Stein, 2020).

In summary, service integration in healthcare involves the coordinated delivery of comprehensive, patient-centred care across multiple providers, settings and disciplines to improve patient outcomes, enhance patient experience and optimize healthcare delivery. There are many successful examples of service integration available in the literature and in practice, such as the PACE programme (Program of All-Inclusive Care for the Elderly) in the USA. This programme, offered by Medicaid and Medicare, covers all health and social services required by an individual, according to a longstanding integrated care model based around a multidisciplinary PACE team, which determines the care plan and coordinates the services for the older person (https://www.medicaid.gov/medicaid/long-term-services-supports/program-all-inclusive-care-elderly/index.html). The National PACE Association (NPA, https://www.npaonline.org/about-npa) ensures a cohesive quality, programme standards and continuous programme development, provides education and training for PACE teams and advocates for the rights of older people in the USA.

The challenge for managers

Management of integrated care undoubtedly builds on the skills and knowledge required for the general delivery of health and care services but poses additional complexities and uncertainties (Miller and Stein, 2020). It requires working across a greater range of agencies and professions, and to be effective the manager must take time to understand their parameters, motivations and possible frustrations. Only by doing so will their potential concerns be recognized and measures to address these built into the development process. Along with the greater diversity of stakeholders, integrated care does not always have a clear set of accountabilities and established rules to inform decision-making. This can result in considerable negotiation being required to secure resources and agree how responsibility might be allocated. An integrated care manager therefore needs to be a skilled diplomat and boundary spanner who can represent the benefits of new collaborative arrangements while not alienating those who may have been responsible for previous practice (Mitterlechner, 2020).

As will have been apparent from the overview given in this chapter, integrated care sits within the wider system of health and social care policy, practice and governance. Some of these may be explicitly changed as part of national or regional initiatives, but in many cases integrated care is developed on top of or alongside existing practices, processes and traditions. Managers must be skilled and trained to understand the potential tensions inherent within this wider context to anticipate where there are likely to be challenges to more person-centred and coordinated care. It will not be possible to influence all these locally, but recognizing these helps to clarify what can be changed and what needs to be worked around. Communicating these structural challenges to others, who may not have had the time or interest to do so themselves, can help to explain why previous attempts may not have been successful.

A particular problem for integrated care is sustaining improvements beyond pilots when dedicated funding and spotlight of interest have dissipated – a more honest recognition of the existing context may lead to less ambitious but ultimately more realistic plans (Lewis et al., 2021). The examples provided in the boxes throughout this chapter illustrate the various ways of how sustainability may ultimately be achieved: whether it is through the deliberate set up of a new system or to address a very clear and local challenge, all of the examples ultimately achieved a lasting system change. Dedicated and determined managers, who knew how to lead and navigate any opposition to change, were one key element of success in these examples.

An integrated care toolbox

Despite the considerable complexity inherent in managing for integrated care, there are approaches that can be used to support integration and where there is a considerable evidence base. Managers do therefore have a set of tools that they can potentially draw upon, and many of them have been highlighted throughout this chapter. As ever with implementation, it is important to connect the opportunity with the intervention and be clear about why this approach could work within the context in question. The process of implementation will be as important as the model – for example, on paper multidisciplinary teams can look very similar, but it is the way they are developed, deployed and reviewed that will make the difference between more and less successful teams. Providing opportunities for different stakeholders to contribute to the process will both enable the important nuances to be heard and be a demonstration of the culture of respect for alternative perspectives. This requires considerable skill and confidence on the part of managers, as they must be able to facilitate discussion, respond positively to conflict and identify a pragmatic way to maintain progress (Miller and Stein, 2020; Curry et al., 2022).

Finally – and in many ways most importantly – managers should constantly seek to put people with lived experience at the heart of integrated care (see Chapter 21). This relates to strategic planning as much as it does to direct practice. Connecting with relevant lived experience groups, or indeed supporting the creation of a bespoke one to reflect the needs of the patient population to be served, will be time well spent. Not only is there the likelihood of invaluable insights into what matters to people, but such a network can be a powerful ally for managers in wider discussions with funders, senior managers and professionals. Being clear about the role that people would potentially play, and putting in the relevant supports and infrastructure, will help to maximize their contribution and help ensure that they find the process rewarding. Being aware of the diversity of the population and positively seeking opportunities to be inclusive will also be important enablers.

Learning activity 15.3

Use the dimensions of integrated care outlined in Table 15.1 to consider an opportunity to develop more integrated care within your local health and care system.

Identify the likely enablers and barriers with the different layers on integration and consider how as a manager you could build on the strengths and overcome the likely challenges.

- Which stakeholders would have potential to change the factors with your influence and how would you encourage them to do so?
- Which stakeholders could support the changes necessary and how would you encourage them to do so?

Conclusion

Integrated care can only happen when all levels of the health and care system and its stakeholders are actively involved in the design, management, implementation and evaluation of the initiatives. Thus, there needs to be a parallel top-down and bottom-up approach. For a sustainable implementation of integrated care this process needs to be part of the day-to-day activities of managers on every level of the system, and not an afterthought. Integrated care needs to be nurtured, led, coordinated and actively managed, which in turn necessitates a clear buy-in from policymakers and decision-makers. It requires continuous and active engagement of people and professionals, stakeholders and communities, to create, reinforce and adapt a common understanding, language and values according to the needs of the local context. Managers need to be able to handle the complexity, flexibility and uncertainty that integration requires, as models, processes and activities adapt to the needs of the community and the professionals involved.

Crucially, integrated services must be organized around the needs of the people, not the providers or the institutions. This necessitates the bridging of gaps between health, social and other services to provide the care necessary for people and communities. This requires consideration of social determinants of health and the continuum of care. At the core lies the bio-psycho-social approach to health, which views the person holistically and not by disease or deficiency. A key element therefore is a comprehensive look at the data available to analyse the outcomes, identify needs and define priorities. This analysis provides the foundations for change highlighting, for example, lack of resources, inadequate access or below-average health outcomes. It also provides the basis for a clear narrative about what needs to change, plans and measurable objectives. There are many examples of integration from which to learn, but ultimately integrated care needs not only to be adapted to the local context but developed by the local communities and providers to guarantee ownership, accountability and relevance.

Learning resources

International Journal of Integrated Care (IJIC): The leading international journal on the impact and implementation of integrated care [www.ijic.org].

Emerald Insight: The leading UK based journal on the practice of integrated care: *Journal of Integrated Care* [https://www.emerald.com/insight/publication/issn/1476-9018)] and

EU funded research projects considering implementation integrated care in Europe [Project Integrate] https://ijic.org/collections/project-integrate-lessons-for-policy-management-and-implementation-of-integrated-care-in-europe [Sustain] https://sustain-eu.org/ [Selfie] https://www.selfie2020.eu/.

NIHR Policy Innovation and Evaluation Policy Research Unit (PIRU): Long-term evaluation of national integrated care programme in UK [https://piru.ac.uk/projects/current-projects/integrated-care-pioneers-evaluation.html].

Social Care Institute for Excellence (SCIE): Practical approaches and resources to support implementation of integrated care [Integrated care - SCIE].

International Foundation for Integrated Care (IFIC): International network to support the understanding and implementation of integrated care [The International Foundation for Integrated Care (integratedcarefoundation.org)].

WHO Integrated Care for Older People (ICOPE): Toolkit and resources [Ageing and Health unit (who.int)].

Nuffield Trust: Overview of integrated care in the UK and associated resources [Integrated care explained | Nuffield Trust].

Integrated People-Centred Health Services (IPCHS): World Health Organization global platform of resources and practices featuring examples from every WHO region [https://www.integratedcare4people.org/practices/].

EPIC Learning Health System: Resource contains practical tools and guidance on integrated primary care [The EPIC Learning Health System | Alliance for Healthier Communities (allianceon.org)].

Integrated Health Systems in Latin America and the Caribbean (IHSLAC): Was a project funded by Canada and PAHO from 2016–2019, strengthening maternal, newborn, child and adolescent health in 11 countries [https://www.paho.org/en/canada/integrated-health-systems-latin-america-and-caribbean-ihslac].

References

AHQR (2018) Care Coordination. Content last reviewed August 2018. *Agency for Healthcare Research and Quality*, Rockville, MD; [https://www.ahrq.gov/ncepcr/care/coordination.html; accessed 12 June 2024].

Auschra, C. (2018) Barriers to the integration of care in inter-organisational settings: a literature review, *International Journal of Integrated Care*, 18(1).

Baltaxe, E., Czypionka, T., Kraus, M., Reiss, M., Askildsen, J.E., Grenković, R., et al. (2019) Digital health transformation of integrated care in Europe: overarching analysis of 17 integrated care programs, *Journal of Medical Internet Research*, 21(9):e14956.

Barraclough, F., Smith-Merry, J., Stein, V. and Pit, S. (2021) Workforce development in integrated care: a scoping review, *International Journal of Integrated Care*, 21(4).

Barry, S., Fhallúin, M.N., Thomas, S., Harnett, P.J. and Burke, S. (2021) Implementing integrated care in practice – learning from MDTs driving the integrated care programme for older persons in Ireland, *International Journal of Integrated Care*, Mar 18; 21(1):15. doi: 10.5334/ijic.4682.

Baxter, S., Johnson, M., Chambers, D., Sutton, A., Goyder, E. and Booth, A. (2018) The effects of integrated care: a systematic review of UK and international evidence. *BMC Health Services Research*, 18(1): 350.

Bhuiya, A.R., Scallan, E., Alam, S. and Sharma, K. (2020) Identifying the Features and Impacts of Community Health Centres. McMaster University Health Forum [https://www.mcmasterforum.org/docs/default-source/product-documents/rapid-responses/identifying-the-features-and-impacts-of-community-health-centres.pdf?sfvrsn=234559d5_3; accessed 16 December 2024].

Blijleven, V., Hoxha, F. and Jaspers, M. (2022) Workarounds in Electronic health record systems and the Revised Sociotechnical Electronic Health Record Workaround Analysis Framework: scoping review, *Journal of Medical Internet Research*, 24(3):e33046.

Bodenheimer, T. and Sinsky, C. (2014) From triple to quadruple aim: care of the patient requires care of the provider, *The Annals of Family Medicine*, 12(6): 573–576.

Borgermans, L. and Devroey, D. (2017) A policy guide on integrated care (PGIC): lessons learned from EU project integrate and beyond, *International Journal of Integrated Care*, 17(4).

Calciolari, S., González Ortiz, L., Goodwin, N. and Stein, V. (2021) Validation of a conceptual framework aimed to standardize and compare care integration initiatives: the project INTEGRATE framework, *Journal of Interprofessional Care*, 2021. doi: 10.1080/13561820.2020.1864307.

Cano, I., Alonso, A., Hernandez, C., Burgos, F., Barberan-Garcia, A., Roldan, J. et al. (2015) An adaptive case management system to support integrated care services: lessons learned from the NEXES project, *Journal of Biomedical Informatics*, Jun; 55:11–22.

Collins, B. (2015) Intentional whole health system redesign Southcentral Foundation's 'Nuka' system of care. London: Kings Fund [https://assets.kingsfund.org.uk/f/256914/x/941ab2be02/intentional_whole_health_system_design_southcentral_nuka_november_2015.pdf; accessed 16 December 2024].

Collins, P.A., Resendes, S.J. and Dunn, J.R. (2014) The untold story: examining Ontario's community health centre" initiatives to address upstream determinants of health, *Healthcare Policy*, 10(1): 14.

Curry, L., Ayedun, A., Cherlin, E., Taylor, B., Castle-Clarke, S. and Linnander, E. (2022) The role of leadership in times of systems disruption: a qualitative study of health and social care integration, *BMJ Open*, 12:e054847. doi: 10.1136/bmjopen-2021-054847.

Curry, N. and Ham, C. (2010) Clinical and service integration. The route to improved outcomes. The King's Fund, London, UK.

Damery, S., Flanagan, S. and Combes, G. (2016) Does integrated care reduce hospital activity for patients with chronic diseases? An umbrella review of systematic reviews. *BMJ Open*, 6(11): e011952.

Farmanova, E., Baker, G.R. and Cohen, D. (2019) Combining integration of care and a population health approach: a scoping review of redesign strategies and interventions, and their impact, *International Journal of Integrated Care*, 19(2): 5. https://doi.org/10.5334/ijic.4197.

Glasby, J., Miller, R., Glasby, A.M., Ince, R. and Konteh, F. (2024) Why are we stuck in hospital? Barriers to people with learning disabilities/autistic people leaving 'long-stay' hospital: a mixed methods study, *Health and Social Care Delivery Research*, 2(3).

Goodwin, N., Stein, K.V. and Amelung, V.E. (2021) What is Integrated Care?, in V.E. Amelung, K.V. Stein, N. Goodwin, E. Suter, E. Nolte and R. Balicer (eds) *Handbook Integrated Care, 2nd edn.* Cham: Springer Publishing.

Gottlieb, K. (2013) The Nuka System of Care: improving health through ownership and relationships, *International Journal of Circumpolar Health*, 72(1): 21118.

Gray, C.S. (2021) Integrated care's new protagonist: the expanding role of digital health, *International Journal of Integrated Care*, 21(4).

Hughes, G., Shaw, S.E. and Greenhalgh, T. (2020) Rethinking integrated care: a systematic hermeneutic review of the literature on integrated care strategies and concepts, *The Milbank Quarterly*, 98(2): 446–492.

Jelphs, K., Dickinson, H. and Miller, R. (2016) *Working in Teams* (2nd edn.). Bristol: Policy Press.

Klinga, C. (2021) Co-leadership—A facilitator of health- and social care integration, in V.E. Amelung, K.V. Stein, N. Goodwin, E. Suter, E. Nolte and R. Balicer (eds) *Handbook Integrated Care, 2nd edn.* Switzerland: Springer Publishing.

Kozlowska, O., Lumb, A., Tan, G.D. and Rea, R. (2018) Barriers and facilitators to integrating primary and specialist healthcare in the United Kingdom: a narrative literature review, *Future Healthcare Journal*, 5(1): 64–80. doi: 10.7861/futurehosp.5-1-64.

LaMonica, H.M., Milton, A., Braunstein, K., Rowe, S.C., Ottavio, A., Jackson, T., et al. (2020) Technology-enabled solutions for Australian mental health services reform: impact evaluation, *JMIR Formative Research*, 2020 Nov 19; 4(11): e18759.

Lara Montero, A., van Duijn, S., Zonneveld, N., Minkman, M. and Nies, H. (2016) Integrated Social Services in Europe. European Social Network, Brighton.

Lewis, R.Q., Checkland, K., Durand, M.A., Ling, T., Mays, N., Roland, M. and Smith, J.A. (2021) Integrated care in England – what can we learn from a decade of national pilot programmes?. *International Journal of Integrated Care*, 21(4).

Mannion, R. (2022) *Making Culture Change Happen.* Cambridge: Cambridge University Press.

Mannion, R. and Davies, H. (2016) Culture in Health Care Organization in E. Ferlie, K. Montogomery and A.R. Pederson, *The Oxford Handbook of Health Care Management.* Oxford: Oxford University Press.

Miller, R. (2022) *Multidisciplinary Teams: Integrating Care in Places and Neighbourhoods.* London: Social Care Institute for Excellence.

Miller, R. and Stein, K.V. (2020) The odyssey of integration: is management its Achilles' heel?, *International Journal of Integrated Care*, 20(1):7. doi: https://doi.org/10.5334/ijic.5440.

Miller, R., Brown, H. and Mangan, C. (2016) *Integrated Care in Action: A Practical Guide for Health, Social Carer and Housing Support*. London: Jessica Kingsley.

Miller, R., Glasby, J. and Dickinson, H. (2021) Integrated health and social care in England: ten years on, *International Journal of Integrated Care*, 21(4).

Miller, R., Scherpbier, N., van Amsterdam, L., Guedes, V. and Pype, P. (2019) Inter-professional education and primary care: EFPC position paper, *Primary Health Care Research & development*, 20: e138.

Mitterlechner, M. (2020) Leadership in integrated care networks: a literature review and opportunities for future research, *International Journal of Integrated Care*, 20(3):1–14.

Mitterlechner, M. and Bilgeri, A.S. (2021) Perspectives on governing integrated care networks, in V.E. Amelung, K.V. Stein, N. Goodwin, E. Suter, E. Nolte and R. Balicer (eds) *Handbook Integrated Care* (2nd edn.). Switzerland: Springer Publishing.

Mounier-Jack, S., Mayhew, S.H. and Mays, N. (2017) Integrated care: learning between high-income, and low-and middle-income country health systems, *Health Policy and Planning*, 32(suppl_4):iv6-iv12.

National Voices and Think Local Act Personal (2013) A narrative for person-centred coordinated care. [https://www.nationalvoices.org.uk/publication/narrative-person-centred-coordinated-care/; accessed 26 February 2024].

Naylor, C. and Wellings, D. (2019) A citizen-led approach to health and care. Lessons from the Wigan Deal. London: Kings Fund.

Nolte, E. and McKee, M. (2008) *Caring for People with Chronic Conditions: A Health System Perspective*. Maidenhead: McGraw-Hill Education.

Nolte, E., Frölich, A., Hildebrandt, H., Pimperl, A., Schulpen, G.J. and Vrijhoef, H.J. (2016) Implementing integrated care: a synthesis of experiences in three European countries, *International Journal of Care Coordination*, 19(1–2): 5–19.

Nuño-Solinís, R. (2021) Building an integrated health ecosystem during the Great Recession: the case of the Basque strategy to tackle the challenge of chronicity, in V.E. Amelung, K.V. Stein, N. Goodwin, E. Suter, E. Nolte and R. Balicer (eds) *Handbook Integrated Care* (2nd edn.). Switzerland: Springer Publishing.

OECD (2020) Realising the potential of primary health care, *OECD Health Policy Studies*, https://doi.org/10.1787/a92adee4-en.

Sanz, M.F., Acha, B.V. and García, M.F. (2021) Co-design for people- centred care digital solutions: a literature review, *International Journal of Integrated Care*, 21(2): 16.

Schein, E. (1995) *Understanding Organisational Culture*. San Francisco, CA: Jossey Bass.

Schultz, E.M. and McDonald, K.M. (2014) What is care coordination?, *International Journal of Care Coordination*, 17(1–2): 5–24.

Steele Gray, C (2021) Integrated care's new protagonist: the expanding role of digital health, *International Journal of Integrated Care*, 21(4).

Thistlethwaite, J. (2012) Interprofessional education: a review of context, learning and the research agenda, *Medical Education*, 46(1):58–70.

Thistlethwaite, P. (2011) Integrating health and social care in Torbay. Improving care for Mrs Smith [https://www.kingsfund.org.uk/insight-and-analysis/reports/integrating-health-social-care-torbay; accessed 3 June 2024].

Thistlethwaite, J. (2012) Interprofessional education: a review of context, learning and the research agenda, *Medical Education*, 46(1): 58–70.

Thompson, M., Hendry, A. and Mead, E. (2021) Three horizons of integrating health and social care in Scotland, in V.E. Amelung, K.V. Stein, N. Goodwin, E. Suter, E. Nolte and R. Balicer (eds) *Handbook Integrated Care* (2nd edn.). Switzerland: Springer Publishing.

TransForm (Transnational Form on Integrated Community Care) (2021a) ICC Approaches & Case Studies. Foundry Vancouver Granville. Poster and Workshop presentation. Available at: [https://transform-integratedcommunitycare.com/casestudy/foundry-vancouver-granville/; accessed 8 July 2024].

TransForm (Transnational Form on Integrated Community Care) (2021b) ICC Approaches & Case Studies. Foundry North Shore. Poster and Workshop presentation. [https://transform-integratedcommunitycare.com/casestudy/foundry-north-shore/; accessed 8 July 2024].

Tsiachristas, A. (2016) Financial incentives to stimulate integration of care, *International Journal of Integrated Care*, 16(4).

Vrijhoef, H.J., de Belvis, A.G., la Calle, M.D., de Sabata, M.S., Hauck, B., Montante, S. et al. (2017) IT-supported integrated care pathways for diabetes: a compilation and review of good practices, *International Journal of Care Coordination*, 20(1–2): 26–40.

West, M.A. and Lyubovnikova, J. (2012) Real teams or pseudo teams? The changing landscape needs a better map, *Industrial and Organizational Psychology*, 5(1): 25–28.

World Health Organization (2016) Global strategy on human resources for health: workforce 2030. Geneva: World Health Organization.

World Health Organization (2019) WHO global report on traditional and complementary medicine 2019. Geneva: World Health Organization.

World Health Organization (2024) Services organization and integration. [https://www.who.int/teams/integrated-health-services/clinical-services-and-systems/service-organizations-and-integration#:~:text=Integrated%20services%20are%20health%20services,within%20and%20beyond%20the%20health; accessed 3 May 2024].

Zonneveld, N., Driessen, N., Stüssgen, R.A. and Minkman, M.M. (2018) Values of integrated care: a systematic review, *International Journal of Integrated Care*, 18(4).

Mental health

Dr Sarah-Jane Fenton and Dr Sarah Carr

Introduction

Ultimately, there is no health without mental health

(World Health Organization, 2022: vi)

Mental health is an integral part of overall health and is a universal human right. Nearly a billion people around the world live with a diagnosable mental disorder, yet despite this, mental health systems and services globally remain fragile with the estimated treatment gap for severe mental health conditions standing at 90 per cent (World Health Organization, 2022). For children and young people, while 200 years ago childhood mortality accounted for nearly half of all deaths, today this has fallen to 3.9 per cent due to medical research, policy and governance, industry and changes within society (World Economic Forum, 2020). Contemporary data indicates that mental health now outstrips child mortality as the leading global cause of disability and poor outcomes for young people accounting for 45 per cent of the disease burden of those aged 10–24 years (World Economic Forum, 2020).

The sheer numbers requiring support across the life course means that the management and delivery of mental health services for all ages is highly complex and requires health systems to work and integrate with multiple sectors. Often there are fewer services in areas with higher levels of need, and there are widespread issues relating to equality of access to care. This is particularly acute in low- and middle- income countries (LMICs), where it is estimated that 75 per cent of people receive no treatment for mental disorders (Evans-Lacko et al., 2018).

This chapter focuses on understanding the scale of the challenge for contemporary management of healthcare systems of mental health, through drawing on learning from how the current mental health service delivery has been informed and shaped by its development and history. This contextual history is important as it has intergenerational effects on the way people perceive and receive treatment, and patterns of engagement in contemporary systems. The aim is to help you to develop an understanding of how social determinants impact upon and influence mental health before thinking about what this might mean for system development and management of mental health services. In starting with how or why people become unwell, we hope to ground thinking about system and process in *lived experience* and the reality of living with mental illness. The chapter develops an interest in understanding what 'good' looks like and for whom, as it turns to discussing how to measure success in mental health services and systems, before closing with a discussion about what the future might hold for mental health care management.

So, there's a growing realisation that people don't simply have needs that have to be met; they have assets (experience, skills and expertise) which can improve services.

(Coldham, 2012)

Definitions

Defining terms within mental health and illness depends on both the context (i.e. how the terms are understood within a particular health system and by those working in that system), and the way in which the individual experiencing mental distress understands their experience (i.e. their lived reality). Definitions within mental health are often contested and they vary between contexts, stakeholders within a system, cultures, and inter-generationally.

Not having a shared language or understanding can cause distress (Padmanathan et al., 2019). Language is powerful, it can be used to exacerbate or reduce stigma. For example, as Neilsen writes when reflecting on the need for us to move from a historically framed way of speaking about *committing suicide* (stemming from a time when suicide was deemed a crime) to talking about *people who die by suicide*, 'everyday expressions may carry connotations we have not considered and speak to ideas we don't condone' (Nielsen, 2016). The importance of changing the use of language relating to suicide and self-harm in the UK and why it matters is one example, but there are many ways in which language is used in relation to talking about mental health that reproduce stigma. As healthcare managers, be mindful about language and inclusivity as you build mental health care services and systems.

In this chapter, we do not seek to give final or certain 'definitions' but we will outline the concepts we are using (see Box 16.1) to help you to explore in your own context how and why language is used and in what ways, either as an inclusive tool to engage people with services or as a way to exclude people from narratives (including their own). These have been written by Dr Carr through integrating understanding from lived experience, academic or policy literature. We recognize that these may have different interpretations in different cultural contexts.

Box 16.1   An outline of key concepts

Well-being usually refers to a positive state either at an individual level or for whole societies. As a concept it is used to describe quality of life and is linked to thriving, having meaning or purpose, and it recognizes the interdependence of physical and mental health. Well-being is usually determined by environmental, social and economic conditions.

Mental health is a state of psychological and emotional well-being or an absence of mental illness.

Mental illness refers to a mental health problem that affects an individual's mood, thinking, feelings or behaviour and is diagnosed by a psychiatrist according to standard biomedical criteria (i.e. the Diagnostic and Statistical Manual [DSM] 5.)

Mental distress is a broad term that encompasses the emotional, psychological and social aspects of mental health problems as opposed to biomedical understandings.

Patient is a term commonly used by healthcare services that stresses the medical relationship with services and is usually associated with hospital settings.

Service user broadly describes people who use mental health services.

Survivor is a term often used by mental health activists who assert that some psychiatric treatment can be experienced as damaging, arguing that they have survived the psychiatric system, as well as a mental health crisis.

Lived experience and experiential knowledge is the knowledge that comes from having first-hand, personal (lived) experience of something. Lived experience in mental health can include experience of mental health problems themselves, experiences linked to healthcare settings or services and experience of stigma, discrimination and/or marginalization that may negatively affect mental health. It is also possible for those who care for relatives or friends with mental health problems to have their own lived experience and understanding of mental health problems through their caring relationship with a relative or friend.

The social determinants of mental health

The World Health Organization defines social determinants as: 'conditions in which people are born, grow, live, work and age, and people's access to power, money and resources' arguing that these are influenced by money, power and resources at global, national and local levels in ways that 'impact health outcomes and drive widening health inequities within and across countries' (World Health Organization, 2024a: vii). The aetiology (the origins or causes of disease) of mental illness are, like many physical health conditions, influenced by the social circumstances in which individuals live (see Chapter 4, Public health and global inequalities).

The role of epidemiology in mental health

Mental health epidemiological studies of the distribution and determinants of diseases in human populations have sought to understand how prevalent mental illness is in the general population, who develops mental illness, when, where and why. It is large studies at population level that help us to understand how social factors play a role in the aetiology of mental distress and mental disorder (Ford, 2008; Wiens et al., 2020). Such studies are essential to help global service planning (Baxter et al., 2013) and help us establish the link between social stressors and distribution of mental health outcomes across different population groups, showing that certain population subgroups are at higher risk of developing mental disorders because they are exposed to social, environmental or economic circumstances that place them at a disadvantage across the life-course (Allen et al., 2014).

The role of the social environment in mental health

Understanding how mental health and illness is impacted by the social environment is complex because there are so many factors that can affect mental well-being. For example, poverty, poor housing, trauma, unemployment, exposure to discrimination on grounds of race, gender, sexual orientation, disability and other characteristics or identities – all of these can shape the likelihood of developing mental illness (Kirkbride et al., 2024). You will notice that these influences are likely to be unfairly distributed across different population groups (see also Chapter 4, Public health and global inequalities). There are also factors linked to climate change, migration, conflict and political violence that are interwoven into our understanding of the disproportionate vulnerability of populations for developing poor mental health (see also Chapter 12, Climate change and sustainability). A useful policy framework to consider when trying to understand how to prioritize action is that of the Sustainable Development Goals (SDGs) as these recognize the interrelationships between poverty and other deprivations and identify priorities for improving health, education, reducing inequality, tackling climate change and increasing economic growth (United Nations, 2015).

From a healthcare system perspective, studies that help us identify where there are equity issues around becoming unwell ensure that we can further understand why these issues might be compounded by or reproduced in mental health systems. Mental health inequity exists not only in relation to the conditions in which people are living that might make them unwell, but also in relation to access to care, to engagement in care and in the outcomes of care (i.e. higher morbidity and mortality) (Ngui et al., 2010). There is an interaction effect between stigma and discrimination in relation to physical or mental health and resultant disability.

Mental health, disability and stigma

The evolving rights-based dialogue on mental health and disability promoted by global bodies like the United Nations (UN), reflects a broader trend towards recognizing the rights of people with mental health problems within disability legislation. It acknowledges the limitations of medical models that predominantly frame mental health problems as individual medical problems and overlooks societal influences and barriers to social inclusion that people face (Beresford and Carr, 2018). In terms of rights and recognition, the use of 'psychosocial disability' is gaining traction, especially within international frameworks like the UN Convention on the Rights of Persons with Disabilities (UNCRPD) (UN General Assembly, 2006). Many people with mental health problems, especially activists in the Global South, identify as having a 'psychosocial disability' and are forming alliances under this banner within the UN framework. They prefer the term 'disability' over 'patient' or 'service user' as it better acknowledges societal discrimination and supports personal identity recovery, distancing from the medical connotations associated with traditional psychiatric labels (Davar and Ravindran, 2015). Advocates argue that this terminology better captures the social and psychological dimensions of living with mental health problems and encompasses the broader impacts of stigma and societal discrimination (Minkowitz, 2015).

Stigma happens when a characteristic or trait that a person identifies as having leads to them being viewed negatively by others. Mental health stigma occurs when a person is viewed in a negative way because of their mental illness or psychiatric diagnosis (Hazell et al., 2022). This can happen in a variety of ways. Stigma can lead to the social shunning of individuals with mental health problems, particularly those with a schizophrenia label (Angermeyer and Dietrich, 2006). The pervasive stigma attached to mental illness can severely restrict the lives of those with mental health problems, further damaging their mental health and sense of self, reducing chances of meaningful occupation and relationships, and increasing social isolation (Thornicroft, 2006). Individuals can also experience self-stigma where they internalize social prejudice and feel ashamed of their mental ill health (Corrigan and Watson, 2002).

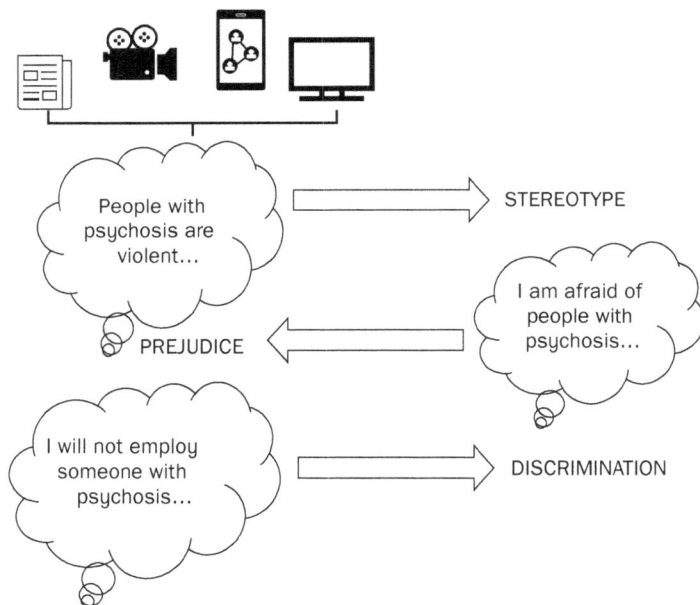

Figure 16.1 Example of how stigma forms, operates and is perpetuated resulting in active discrimination against individuals

Stigma often leads to discrimination, which is the process by which people with mental health problems are excluded or treated unfairly based on prejudice. This type of discrimination can happen in mental health services, affecting the quality of care (Henderson and Thornicroft, 2009). Figure 16.1 illustrates our view as to how stigma can form: people receive information (i.e. via the media, but also communities and/or societies) that generates or reinforces stereotypes about mental health; this is then internalized, resulting in prejudicial attitudes and behaviours that perpetuate stigma and create active discrimination against individuals. Stigma operates as a barrier to seeking mental health care (World Economic Forum, 2020), as a barrier to accessing employment and to functional recovery (Killackey and Alvarez-Jimenez, 2019), and as a barrier to gaining employment (Brohan and Thornicroft, 2010).

Learning activity 16.1

For this reflective activity, take 10 minutes to consider the following question based on your country context and mental health care settings: What do you think mental health care providers need to be mindful of in designing or delivering services given this identified stigma?
Useful prompt questions for your reflections include:

- How is mental health portrayed in the media or understood by the general public in your country context?
- What stereotypes can you identify about mental health in your country context, for example, what slang words or expressions do people use to describe people with poor mental health?
- What is it about mental health that is stigmatized?
- When you think about stigma or marginalized groups – what are the actual human behaviours, feelings, characteristics that are being categorized as 'deviant' and are therefore stigmatized in your context?

The architecture of mental health services and systems

A useful way to frame your understanding is to start by thinking about the people a system is meant to support. Integrating a focus on how the social determinants affect illness, how stigma and discrimination affect people's mental health and how disability relates to mental health is crucial for understanding the context in which services are delivered and how best to adapt those services to reach those most in need of them. However, in mental health holding a dual understanding of both the contemporary issues alongside historical context is particularly important as in most high-income countries (HICs), the history of mental health service delivery is one of oppression, incarceration and segregation, resulting in significant public fear and mistrust of mental health services and those who use them (Fernando, 2012).

The history of service provision and patient activism

During the nineteenth century mental health care management in most industrialized countries was driven by policies promoting the segregation and containment of those characterized as deviant or economically burdensome (Rogers and Pilgrim, 2014). By the mid-twentieth century, public concern about wrongful detainment and abuse of patients was increasing and psychopharmacological treatment was advancing (Turner, 2004). In the UK, in response to these mounting pressures, the Mental Health Act 1959 'set a direction for mental health services away from inpatient and towards outpatient and community care which enjoyed support across the political spectrum' (Glasby et al., 2021: 100). So 'deinstitutionalization' policies saw the gradual closure of old asylums and an ongoing move towards community-based mental health care.

Across Europe, America, Australia and other HIC contexts, the progress of deinstitutionalization happened at varying rates and with different models of care being introduced internationally (Garattini et al., 2023). These were shaped by local contexts, existing availability of community services, differing healthcare financing and structures and resulted in very different model adoption internationally (Garattini et al., 2023).

As deinstitutionalization policies progressed in the mid- to late-twentieth century, psychiatric patient's rights groups began to emerge across the UK, US, Canada, Australia and New Zealand. As with other movements during that era, much of the activism and campaigning focused on civil rights. For example, in the UK, the Mental Patients' Union (MPU) was founded in 1973 by a group of day hospital patients in London and one of its key aims was to 'oppose psychiatric oppression' (Rose, 2018). In the context of community-based mental health care, groups explored alternatives to psychiatry, and advocated for legal reform, citizenship, welfare, housing and employment rights (Sayce, 2015). As a result, patients and service users established themselves as key stakeholders in mental health service and system management. This is reflected in the UNCRPD, which states that service user and disabled people's organizations must have a role in setting disability strategies and policies, including those relating to mental health (OHCHR, 2010).

Understanding the historical shaping of services and the legacy of institutions, including patient and service user responses to this form of care provision, is integral to understanding enduring concerns often cited by patients (including outpatients) about 'being locked up' or 'never getting out' of the mental health system – these are intergenerationally transmitted through families to children and young people and they are shaped by our history (Fenton, 2016). While the inherited narrative is one about being detained within or trapped by services, the reality for most young people seeking access to healthcare in HIC health systems is that they cannot get into services in the first place due to lack of provision. This means there is a counter-narrative to this historical one of advocacy to *get into* services rather than advocacy to *get out* of them (Fenton, 2016). In many contexts globally, there are places where there is no mental health provision for young people to access at all, and limited services for adults.

Contemporary service organization

Contemporary services in HIC contexts are often divided between hospital (acute support) and community (long-term support) settings. That division is then usually affected by the age of individuals accessing services, so specialists are divided into those who work with children and young people or those who work with adults or older adults. This division broadly mirrors professional training pathways. Care is delivered across a spectrum of well-being and usually includes a focus on health promotion and prevention, as well as a focus on treatment of severe mental illness (SMI) in both acute health and community settings (see Figure 16.2).

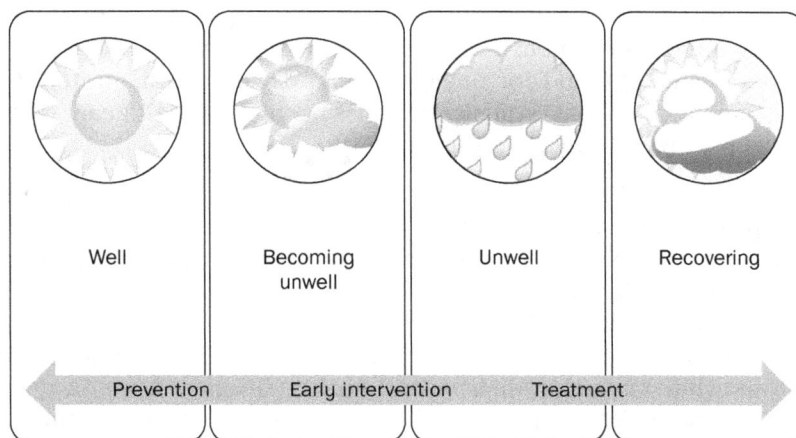

Figure 16.2 Treatment in relation to the spectrum of mental health

As we have seen, deinstitutionalization resulted in the need for the strategic management of complex mental health service systems, where community-based social support is as necessary as clinical interventions and inpatient care. In LMICs, workforce, capacity and resource issues also mean that services are often organized around multidisciplinary teams (MDTs).

Mental health care in high-income and lower-income countries differs from other forms of healthcare because it is highly multisectoral and interdisciplinary, and demands management that ensures integration, multi-agency and multidisciplinary working, and continuity of care for those with SMI (Rukundo et al., 2020). Multidisciplinary community mental health teams can include psychiatrists, psychologists, social workers, mental health nurses, occupational therapists, peer support workers and others. Ongoing higher level strategic difficulties of integration, resourcing and joint working can negatively affect the way some multidisciplinary teams function, and ultimately affect service user experience and quality of life (Rees et al., 2004).

In many European states and countries such as India, mental health care also operates within distinctive legal frameworks relating to involuntary detention and treatment of those who are very unwell (Georgieva et al., 2012). In this context, the provision and effective management of local community-based crisis prevention and early intervention services will reduce the likelihood of hospitalization (Bone et al., 2019). Complexity around legislation and practice also relates to how mental capacity is assessed (Furgalska, 2023), and the bidirectional relationship between mental health and human rights (Mahdanian et al., 2023). One key challenge is health and social care integration, because those living with mental health problems in the community have diverse social as well as clinical needs and this requires a holistic approach (see also Chapter 15, Integrated care). For example, socially oriented community support can have a preventative function, reducing the likelihood of a person having a mental health crisis that requires hospitalization (de Jong et al., 2016). The mental health service landscape is therefore a complex one, with the private, voluntary and community sector providing a significant amount of community-based care in many places, including social support, education, meaningful occupation, criminal justice, accommodation, welfare advice and so on. This service structure is vital for keeping people well and living in the community, and for timely hospital discharge. Integrated, coherent and system-wide management and investment strategies for mental health care that account for the needs of local populations are crucial (Carr, 2019).

Originating with mental health service users and their organizations, peer support and the recovery approach have influenced how mental health care and support is conceived, offered and managed. The concept of recovery was set to have major implications as an organizing principle for the design and management of mental health systems and provision of services (Anthony, 1993). During the late 1980s activists called for a radical reorientation of mental health services and systems towards supporting individuals to have meaningful and fulfilling lives while managing their mental health (Deegan, 1988). In this context the term 'recovery' does not refer to a process of clinical recovery or 'cure' from mental illness, but instead refers to the recovery of a life and an identity following a mental health crisis, focusing on the social and personal aspects of living with mental illness rather than privileging diagnosis and medication (Slade et al., 2014). The key processes of connectedness, hope and optimism about the future, identity, meaning in life and empowerment are crucial for shaping recovery-oriented approaches in mental health care (Leamy et al., 2011).

Mental health recovery means supporting people with mental health problems using approaches to support and personal mental health management that is determined and led by individuals themselves, working with practitioners and/or peer support workers (Thomas et al., 2019; WHO and Quality Rights, 2021). Peer support in mental health is a process where individuals with lived experience of mental health problems offer support and guidance to those experiencing poor mental health or recovering from a mental health crisis. This support is built on shared personal experiences and empathy, distinguishing it from traditional mental health care provided by practitioners. Peer support is now integrated into many modern mental health services and systems and has a role in improving clinical outcomes, enhancing personal empowerment, increasing treatment adherence and providing social support that is often lacking in traditional mental health care settings (Repper and Carter, 2011 ; Gillard et al., 2013). Integrating peer support into mental health systems means providing services that value lived experience as a source of expertise (Watson, 2019).

There is an important role for public health promotion of good mental health and wellbeing in mental health systems, and an increasing interest in prevention of SMI through early intervention and providing easier access to services before conditions become severe or enduring in a way that is debilitating and impairs engagement in functional and occupational activities. To explore this, we will take one Global North (see Box 16.2) and one Global South (see Box 16.3) case study both focusing on children and young people (as this is often the least developed part of international service infrastructure), in order to highlight how service provision requires a multisectoral approach and strong engagement at community level (World Health Organization, 2022, 2023).

Box 16.2 Case study – service organization change in England for children and young people

Mental health specialist services have long been referred to in the UK as the 'Cinderella services' (Glasby et al., 2021) within the health system, meaning they are poorly funded. Within this, children and young people's services have historically been significantly underfunded. However, rising prevalence rates and a change in emphasis to look at prevention and early intervention in youth mental health have meant there is a shift in both what is funded, and how the funding is distributed. We are going to take the Transforming children and young people's mental health provision: a green paper (Department of Health and Department for Education, 2017) as a case study. We will use this case study to understand what (policy and funding), where (in schools), and how (through new teams) this has changed service delivery in England.

Under the proposals set out in the Green Paper the Trailblazer programme launched in 2018 led by the Department of Health and Social Care, the Department for Education and NHS England and Improvement. It funded the creation of mental health support teams (MHSTs) and trained a new workforce of Education Mental Health Practitioners (EMHPs) to work directly in educational settings. These MHSTs had three core functions:

1   To provide direct support to children and young people with mild to moderate mental health problems to support educational settings.
2   To introduce or develop a whole school or college approach to mental health and well-being.
3   To advise staff in educational settings and liaise with external specialist services to help children and young people get the right support and stay in education.

Early evaluation findings of this programme found that schools and colleges welcomed: the funding for additional capacity to provide in-house mental health support; the programme's focus on prevention and early intervention; and that education settings reported positive effects from participating in the programme, including staff feeling more confident talking to children and young people about mental health issues, being able to access advice about mental health issues more easily, and having quicker access to support for children and young people with some mental health problems (Ellins et al., 2023). Despite this initial early progress, the evaluation also highlighted areas for future focus and improvement, including the finding that not all young people were benefiting from this investment. The evaluation highlighted how some identified groups of young people were at risk of falling between gaps in provision. These groups included young people whose mental health problems were neither 'mild to moderate', nor were they judged serious or urgent enough to meet the threshold for specialist National Health Service (NHS) help; or young people who had special educational needs, were neurodiverse, or whose mental health problems were related to traumatic circumstance, social determinants or life events, such as domestic violence or poverty.

These teams have continued to roll out across England, taking these early findings on board and now have over 400 mental health support teams across the country, representing a significant investment in the children and young people's mental health workforce and a shift in the location and model of service delivery for mild to moderate mental health need.

Further information: A summary of the early evaluation of the first 25 Trailblazer sites in the UK can be found on YouTube: https://youtu.be/4SazpCpBYKo?si=DivxOL SGKbShZxDa Or you can read a blog about this work here: https://theconversation. com/more-mental-health-support-in-schools-makes-sense-but-some-children-may-fall-through-gaps-225741

In the England case study example (Box 16.2), you can observe an explicit interest in building workforce and capacity for intervening early in life and early in illness (mild to moderate) to try to prevent SMI from developing. This is a significant shift in approach from a treatment in response to illness system, to one that seeks both to respond to and prevent illness. This shift has required reimagining the location of services (i.e. from health to education settings), as well as reconsidering the workforce involved in delivering or supporting the delivery of services.

When thinking about mental health service delivery in LMIC contexts, there are also considerations about the workforce that delivers services, the geographical reach of those services and the infrastructure available to support service delivery and resourcing. We will see some of these in our second case study example of service architecture in Colombia (see Box 16.3).

Box 16.3 Case study – service architecture in Colombia for children and young people

Colombia has had one of the longest internal armed conflicts with one of the highest number of victims (internally displaced persons, killed, disappeared) in the world (Londoño et al., 2012). Conflict is a key social determinant for health (Bornemisza et al., 2010), consequently this has shaped the social and environmental context and impacted youth mental health and development (Weber et al., 2024). Research mapping the provision of services to children and young people (Fenton et al., 2024) has found that:

- There is an unequal distribution of mental health care services across the country with most mental health care services in populous regions or capital cities.
- Accordingly, the number of mental health professionals (psychiatry and psychology) is limited in urban areas and there are almost none in rural and remote areas of the country.

- While there was a low prevalence of youth mental health problems in Colombia (4.5 per cent of individuals aged 12–17 years had mental illness and 5.4 per cent of young adults 18–24 years), the research indicated higher prevalence where there were fewer services, and it is expected that prevalence has increased in the last few years and will continue to do so.
- There were no specific child-only services registered nationally; however, provision may take place in adult settings. The number of children-only services is limited and usually it is not possible to identify beds only for children.
- Suicide was the second cause of violent and injury-after-violence related death for individuals aged 12–25.
- Triangulation of the data showed an association between lower numbers of professionals and higher rates of suicide in those areas. Suicide rates in Colombia are likely to be underestimated and thus association should be read carefully.

Further information: If you would like further information, then retrieve this open access article by Fenton et al. (2024) to see if it helps to prompt your thinking: *Macro level system mapping of the provision of mental health services to young people living in a conflict context in Colombia.* You can find it here: https://doi.org/10.1186/s12913-024-10602-2

Learning activity 16.2

For this reflective activity, take 10 minutes and use either or both examples in boxes 16.2 and 16.3 to help you to think about your country or context:

- What are the issues in relation to where services are delivered or not in the context of geography and sustainability of provision?
- By whom are services delivered and what workforce issues do you have in relation to need?
- For what ages are services currently provided?

Management in mental health systems

Given the scale of unmet need, mental health systems – however fragile – need to rapidly adapt to work in partnership with other sectors and draw professional expertise from education, social work, youth work and community organizations or non-governmental organizations (NGOs), and communities themselves, among others. Services will need to consider how best to reach rural or remote communities through digital or community-based interventions, and will need to engage in raising awareness where services are available (Kayiteshonga et al., 2022). There is also a need to address comorbidity and multimorbidity within health systems.

Research highlights the association between SMI and multimorbidity, with people with SMI having higher prevalence of physical health conditions, meaning services will need to adopt a multidisciplinary approach to improve outcomes (Pizzol et al., 2023).

International organizations, such as the World Health Organization (WHO), suggest that the foundations for changing mental health systems and services require three types of political commitment – expressed, institutional and budgetary – in order to progress mental health agendas (World Health Organization, 2022). While there may be political commitment expressed through policy, strategy or even legislation, budgetary resource pressures exist everywhere. It is interesting for us to consider this *institutional* element, and what it is that local leaders and service managers in mental health systems globally are likely grappling with.

In terms of pressures, there are three key issues we see affecting service delivery: rising need or demand for services (World Economic Forum, 2020; World Health Organization, 2022); lack of appropriate human resources (Qureshi et al., 2021; World Health Organization, 2022); and implementation challenges around integrating multisector services with existing mental health infrastructure (Qureshi et al., 2021; World Health Organization, 2022). While these pressures shape the broader context in which services are being delivered, at the institutional level there are other considerations that are helpful for healthcare managers to reflect on when working and we have included some of these below.

Involving mental health service users and patients

Mental health service user and patient involvement is a key feature of contemporary mental health management and should occur throughout the system, from policy and research to service development and delivery (Qureshi et al., 2021; World Health Organization, 2023). Service user-led organizations and peer support initiatives form an important part of the mental health service and support landscape, while activist groups campaign for more fundamental systemic reforms to tackle the discrimination, injustice and poverty that affect mental health (Rose et al., 2011). Experiential knowledge, that is knowledge that comes from lived experience, is becoming recognized as a legitimate form of evidence, influencing research, evaluation, policy and training. At the individual level, service users are expected to have choice and control over their care and support and share treatment decisions with practitioners. In the UK, patient governors have been appointed at NHS mental health trusts (MacDonald et al., 2015) and the English health and social care regulator employs inspectors who are 'experts by experience' (Richardson et al., 2019). Similarly, the Australian National Mental Health Commission engages those with lived experience in high-level service planning, governance and safety and quality assurance activities (Australian National Mental Health Commission , 2024).

Tackling racism in mental health

One of the most persistent drivers of inequity in services and inequality in relation to mental health outcomes is racism, which studies in the UK and US demonstrate impacts both access to treatment and treatment efficacy (Nazroo et al., 2020; Castro-Ramirez et al., 2021).

We need to consider therefore how racism might operate alongside structural stigma and discrimination, impacting treatment pathways and contributing to mental health disparities (Acker et al., 2023; Kapadia, 2023). As healthcare mental health service managers, tackling institutional rather than just individual racism and improving clinical processes is central to improving outcomes (Bhui et al., 2021).

Learning activity 16.3

We are going to take the UK as a case study for this learning activity. Below are some statistics taken from research about mental health in ethnic minority communities in the UK. As you will see from these statistics there are inequalities identified in the way in which black and minority groups are supported in mental health care.

- A study by Edbrooke-Childs and Palatay (2019) of nearly 15,000 young people who accessed mental health services found that those from minority ethnic backgrounds were more likely to be referred to mental health services through routes such as youth justice or social services, than they were through primary care health services.
- This echoed findings in adult mental health care that demonstrated that 'Black patients had more complex pathways to specialist care, with some evidence of ethnic variations in primary care assessments' (Bhui et al., 2018: 105).
- Data from NHS England showed that a disproportionate number of people from Black, Asian and minority ethnic communities were detained under the Mental Health Act (involuntarily admitted to hospital). The rates showed that Black or Black British people were over four times more likely to be detained involuntarily in hospital than White groups. Data also showed that this trend continued outside hospital settings in the community, with Community Treatment Orders for Black or Black British groups being over 10 times those of White groups. NHS England data further showed that Black people are more than four times more likely to be the subject of 'restrictive interventions' such as being restrained or held in isolation while admitted to hospital (NHS England, 2021).

Activity:

Drawing on your understanding of social determinants that influence mental health, how stigma operates and the effects of discrimination, reflect on these findings highlighting inequalities in mental health treatment and answer the following three questions:

1 What do you think the implications of these findings are for providers of mental health care?
2 Think about the country where you are living or working – do you have similar or different patterns or is this data unavailable?

Continued

Learning activity 16.3   *Continued*

3   What strategies are already in place or could be put in place by a health manager in your country to monitor and identify trends such as these and to implement changes in order reduce such inequalities in mental health care?

Tip: If you are finding these difficult to answer, have a look at this open access article by Nazroo et al., 2020 to see if it helps to prompt your thinking: *'Where next for understanding race/ethnic inequalities in severe mental illness? Structural, interpersonal and institutional racism'.* You can find it here: https://doi.org/10.1111/1467-9566.13001

Measuring mental health services and systems

Understanding what 'good' looks like in mental health services and systems, defining successful outcomes, establishing what works and how to improve the quality of care, are all particularly important in mental health, given the historical context of these services. In HICs, the most commonly used tools to understand and inform quality of care alongside clinical outcomes are: a combination of asking patients to report their experiences; a risk management system that monitors adverse events; and formal complaints processes. Increasingly, in the UK measures of success include patient-reported outcome measures (PROMs) and patient-reported experience measures (PREMs). Usually in the form of questionnaires, PROMs ask patients to rate their healthcare activities – these ask about symptoms, well-being and quality of life (so are about the patients themselves), whereas PREMs ask about their personal experience of services. Recent work exploring the adoption of PROMs and PREMs in mental health in Europe has called for international harmonization of these measures (de Bienassis et al., 2021).

It is important to obtain reliable, authentic patient feedback in mental health to inform and improve the quality of care. Alongside formal measures of outcome (PROMs) and experience (PREMS), often a range of other feedback is gathered to try to understand how services are doing. There are significant challenges in not just gathering but also analysing and using patient experience data. This was underlined by a study examining how patient experience data was used to improve the quality of inpatient care in NHS England (Weich et al., 2020). The study showed that around a quarter (22 per cent) of services were struggling to collect feedback on patients' experiences of inpatient care routinely, nearly half (51 per cent) were collecting feedback but unable to use this to improve the quality of care, and only around quarter (27 per cent) were able to collect, analyse and use patient experience data in inpatient settings to support change (Weich et al., 2020). Collecting data therefore cannot be an end in itself and as healthcare managers, the challenge remains to see how to authentically engage with feedback and how to analyse and use it to implement change and improve service delivery.

Learning activity 16.4

Care Opinion operates in the UK, Ireland and Australia. The organization is funded mainly through subscriptions from health and care organizations. They host a website where members of the public can share their opinions and stories about their care, and whereby they can receive a response from health organizations' patient experience teams. The websites host publicly available self-reports from patients or carers about their own/their loved one's experiences of mental health care.

Activity:

1   Type 'mental health' into the Care Opinion search function in either the UK, Ireland or Australia site. Pick one positive and one negative review from the publicly available options. We recognize that people have different lived experience of poor mental health themselves or for caring for others. If you find an excerpt you come across triggering or upsetting, then find another one to work with instead.
2   Having chosen a positive and a negative review, read these and list what aspects of care or services you think contributed first to the positive and second to the negative reviews.
3   Reflect on the items you have listed – what do they tell us are priorities for patients and or carers, and how might you want to take these priorities into account when planning care and treatment service delivery?

The future of mental health management

To reduce inequalities and ensure care quality in mental health, healthcare managers should remain aware of future trends and upcoming innovations. The evidence that should inform decisions is constantly evolving, with goals being determined by multiple stakeholders with an interest in mental health care, including those with lived experience. Goals include increasing the number of new and improved supports, treatments and interventions, improving choice and reducing health inequalities (Wykes et al., 2023).

In relation to these goals, artificial intelligence (AI), data-driven technology and digital mental health interventions are rapidly developing, but there are serious questions about human rights, ethics and social impacts (Mantelero, 2022). In mental health this applies to many areas, such as patient monitoring and coercion, privacy, algorithmic decision-making, data quality, bias and transparency (Carr, 2020; Bossewitch et al., 2022). Healthcare managers need to recognize the various implications of introducing AI and digital innovations in mental health.

The international psychiatric global mental health movement seeks to reduce gaps in treatment and 'global burden' or mental illness (Cooper, 2016). Priorities seek to reduce treatment gaps through initiatives, such as the mental health gap action programme (mhGAP) launched by the WHO in 2008 (World Health Organization, 2024b). However, critics assert that mental health interventions and policy and planning strategies in LMICs are often influenced at national and local level by Western biomedical models to the detriment of holistic, indigenous approaches and context specific strategies (Whitley, 2015; Bayetti et al., 2023). The need to consider intersectional experiences and contexts is also relevant for countries with increasingly diverse populations where culturally appropriate support (including that provided by communities themselves) must also be integral to future mental health systems development (Gopalkrishnan, 2018).

Present and future mental health support should be safe, effective, equitable, inclusive and meet the diverse needs of various ethnic, cultural and socioeconomic groups across the life course. To achieve this, it is necessary for healthcare managers to fully engage with those with lived experience, their communities and their organizations.

Conclusion

To be successful, healthcare managers need to understand the challenges and complexities associated with mental health, account for social and economic impacts, respond to social as well as clinical support needs for recovery, be guided by the voices of lived experience and operate within a human rights framework. As with all who are responsible for mental health services and systems, healthcare managers should consider and combat the effects of social and structural discrimination and stigma within and beyond those services and systems. Integrating the expertise of those with lived experience is crucial for creating anti-discriminatory cultures and for understanding the quality and impact of services and support. By using collaborative approaches, including multisectoral working, healthcare managers can meet contemporary challenges, intervening at early stages to prevent people becoming more unwell, supporting people living with mental illness and those who are close to them and to promoting good mental health and equitable access to support for all.

Learning resources

World Health Organization World mental health report: transforming mental health for all. Geneva: World Health Organization; 2022. Licence: CC BY-NC-SA 3.0 IGO: This report draws together the latest available evidence and global good practice to explore why and where change is needed and how it can be achieved. The report highlights the importance of voicing lived experience and outlines the need for strengthening systems of care for mental health [https://iris.who.int/bitstream/handle/10665/356119/9789240049338-eng.pdf?sequence=1].

World Economic Forum (WEF) 2020, A Global Framework for Youth Mental Health: Investing in Future Mental Capital for Individuals, Communities and Economies: The global framework for youth mental health was developed using a combination of evidence reviews and consultations with young people, families, clinicians, economists, policymakers and others from North and South America, Asia, Europe, Australia, New Zealand and Africa. The framework is based on eight key principles that underpin an approach to youth mental health: 1. Rapid, easy and affordable access, 2. Youth-specific care; 3. Awareness, engagement and integration; 4. Early intervention; 5. Youth partnership; 6. Family engagement and support; 7. Continuous improvement; 8. Prevention [https://www.weforum.org/publications/a-global-framework-for-youth-mental-health-db3a7364df/].

Early evaluation of the Children and Young People's Mental Health Trailblazer programme: a rapid mixed-methods study. NIHR: This report is of an early evaluation the Children and Young People's Mental Health Trailblazer programme in England, which was a national programme that funded the creation of mental health support teams (MHSTs) working in schools and further education colleges. The aim of the programme was to improve early intervention and access to support and promote good mental health and well-being for all children and young people. This report offers early insights into the impact of the proposals set out in the Transforming children and young people's mental health provision: a green paper. (Ellins, J. et al., 2023) [https://doi.org/10.3310/hsdr-tr-130818].

Institutional racism in mental health care. BMJ 334, 649–650: This editorial piece comments on the findings of the Healthcare Commission report of the 'Count me in' one-day census of National Health Service hospitals, private mental health hospitals and learning disability units. The paper defines institutional racism as the collective failure of an organization to provide an appropriate and professional service to people because of their colour, culture or ethnic origin. This can be seen or detected in processes, attitudes and behaviour that amount to discrimination through unwitting prejudice, ignorance, thoughtlessness and racist stereotyping, which disadvantages people in ethnic minority groups. (McKenzie, K. and Bhui, K., 2007) [https://doi.org/10.1136/bmj.39163.395972.80].

United Nations Human Rights Office of the High Commissioner (2019) A/HRC/41/34 - Right of everyone to the enjoyment of the highest attainable standard of physical and mental health - Report of the Special Rapporteur on the right of everyone to the enjoyment of the highest attainable standard of physical and mental health: This is the final report of the Special Rapporteur, Dainius Pūras, on the right of everyone to the enjoyment of the highest attainable standard of physical and mental health to the UN General Assembly. He argues that *'good mental health and well-being cannot be defined by the absence of a mental health condition, but must be defined instead by the social, psychosocial, political, economic and physical environment that enables individuals and populations to live a life of dignity, with full enjoyment of their rights and in the equitable pursuit of their potential'*. The report highlights the need for creating and sustaining environments that integrate rights-based approaches to mental health [https://www.ohchr.org/en/documents/thematic-reports/ahrc4134-right-everyone-enjoyment-highest-attainable-standard-physical].

Continued

Learning resources *Continued*

Lived Experience Leadership Digital Library: This online library is a National Mental Health Consumer and Carer Forum and National Primary Health Network Mental Health Lived Experience Engagement Network project that is supported by Mental Health Australia. It provides free access to resources on all aspects of lived experience involvement and leadership in mental health, including the lived experience workforce and co-design and co-production of services and support. The resources encompass full-text articles and reports, along with podcasts, websites and videos. [https://livedexperiencedigitallibrary.org.au/].

Practical Guide: Progressing transformative co-production in mental health. Bath: NDTi: This guide outlines some practical steps for co-producing mental health services and support with those who have lived experience. It offers practice lessons from real-life examples in the UK National Health Service and includes a link to a checklist of key questions to guide mental health co-production processes. (Carr, S. and Patel, M., 2016) [https://www.ndti.org.uk/assets/files/MH_Coproduction_guide.pdf].

Together for Mental Health (2019) Service User Involvement in the delivery of mental health services. London: Together for Mental Health: Produced by the UK mental health charity Together, this briefing gives a comprehensive overview of how to effectively involve and integrate service users/those with lived experience in mental policymaking, service development and delivery and commissioning. It is illustrated by case examples from the UK and presents a spectrum of involvement for organizations to assess their position and progress [https://www.together-uk.org/wp-content/uploads/2019/08/Service-User-Involvement-briefing.pdf].

References

Acker, J., Aghaee, S., Mujahid, M., Deardorff, J. and Kubo, A. (2023) Structural racism and adolescent mental health disparities in northern California, *JAMA Network Open*, 6, e2329825. https://doi.org/10.1001/jamanetworkopen.2023.29825.

Allen, J., Balfour, R., Bell, R. and Marmot, M. (2014) Social determinants of mental health, *International Review of Psychiatry*, 26: 392–407. https://doi.org/10.3109/09540261.2014.928270.

Angermeyer, M.C. and Dietrich, S. (2006) Public beliefs about and attitudes towards people with mental illness: a review of population studies, *Acta Psychiatrica Scandinavica*, 113: 163–179. https://doi.org/10.1111/j.1600-0447.2005.00699.x.

Anthony, W.A. (1993) Recovery from mental illness: the guiding vision of the mental health service system in the 1990s, *Psychosocial Rehabilitation Journal*, 16: 11–23. https://doi.org/10.1037/h0095655.

Australian National Mental Health Commission (2024) Mental Health Safety and Quality Engagement Guide. [https://www.mentalhealthcommission.gov.au/lived-experience/consumer-and-carers/safety-and-quality-engagement-guidelines/mental-health-safety-and-quality-engagement-guide; accessed 21 June 2024].

Baxter, A.J., Patton, G., Scott, K.M., Degenhardt, L. and Whiteford, H.A. (2013) Global epidemiology of mental disorders: what are we missing?, *PLOS ONE*, 8, e65514. https://doi.org/10.1371/journal.pone.0065514.

Bayetti, C., Bakhshi, P., Davar, B., Khemka, G.C., Kothari, P., Kumar, M., et al. (2023) Critical reflections on the concept and impact of 'scaling up' in Global Mental Health, *Transcultural Psychiatry*, 60: 602–609. https://doi.org/10.1177/13634615231183928.

Beresford, P. and Carr, S. (eds) (2018) *Social Policy First Hand: An International Introduction to Participatory Social Welfare*. Bristol: Policy Press.

Bhui, K., Dein, S. and Pope, C. (2021) Clinical ethnography in severe mental illness: a clinical method to tackle social determinants and structural racism in personalised care, *BJPsych Open*, 7, e78. https://doi.org/10.1192/bjo.2021.38.

Bhui, K., Stansfeld, S., Hull, S., Priebe, S., Mole, F. and Feder, G. (2018) Ethnic variations in pathways to and use of specialist mental health services in the UK: systematic review, *The British Journal of Psychiatry*, 182: 105–116. https://doi.org/10.1192/bjp.182.2.105.

Bone, J.K., McCloud, T., Scott, H.R., Machin, K., Markham, S., Persaud, K., et al. (2019) Psychosocial interventions to reduce compulsory psychiatric admissions: a rapid evidence synthesis, *EClinicalMedicine*, 10: 58–67. https://doi.org/10.1016/j.eclinm.2019.03.017.

Bornemisza, O., Ranson, M.K., Poletti, T.M. and Sondorp, E. (2010) Promoting health equity in conflict-affected fragile states, *Social Science and Medicine*, 70: 80–88. https://doi.org/10.1016/j.socscimed.2009.09.032.

Bossewitch, J., Brown, L.X.Z., Gooding, P.M., Harris, L., Horton, J., Katterl, S., et al. (2022) Digital futures in mind: reflecting on technological experiments in mental health & crisis support, *SSRN*. https://doi.org/10.2139/ssrn.4215994.

Brohan, E. and Thornicroft, G. (2010) Stigma and discrimination of mental health problems: workplace implications, *Occupational Medicine*, 60: 414–415. https://doi.org/10.1093/occmed/kqq048.

Carr, S. (2020) 'AI gone mental': engagement and ethics in data-driven technology for mental health, *Journal of Mental Health*, 29(2): 1–6. https://doi.org/10.1080/09638237.2020.1714011.

Carr, S. (2019) Mapping a complex landscape: a literature review of English mental health care and support, 2014–2017. Health Services Management Centre. [https://www.birmingham.ac.uk/Documents/college-social-sciences/social-policy/HSMC/publications/2019/mapping-a-complex-landscape.pdf; accessed 21 June 2024].

Castro-Ramirez, F., Al-Suwaidi, M., Garcia, P., Rankin, O., Ricard, J.R. and Nock, M.K. (2021) Racism and poverty are barriers to the treatment of youth mental health concerns, *Journal of Clinical Child & Adolescent Psychology*, 50: 534–546. https://doi.org/10.1080/15374416.2021.1941058

Coldham, T. (2012) Co-production: why Scie is giving a bigger voice to service users and carers. *The Guardian,* 26 June.

Cooper, S. (2016) Global mental health and its critics: moving beyond the impasse, *Critical Public Health*, 26: 355–358. https://doi.org/10.1080/09581596.2016.1161730.

Corrigan, P.W. and Watson, A.C. (2002) Understanding the impact of stigma on people with mental illness, *World Psychiatry*, 1: 16–20.

Davar, B.V. and Ravindran, T.K.S. (2015) *Gendering Mental Health: Knowledges, Identities, and Institutions*. Oxford: Oxford University Press.

de Bienassis, K., Kristensen, S., Hewlett, E., Roe, D., Mainz, J. and Klazinga, N. (2021) Patient-reported indicators in mental health care: towards international standards among members of the OECD, *International Journal for Quality in Health Care*, 34: ii7–ii12. https://doi.org/10.1093/intqhc/mzab020.

de Jong, M.H., Kamperman, A.M., Oorschot, M., Priebe, S., Bramer, W., van de Sande, R., et al. (2016) Interventions to reduce compulsory psychiatric admissions: a systematic review and meta-analysis, *JAMA Psychiatry*, 73: 657–664. https://doi.org/10.1001/jamapsychiatry.2016.0501.

Deegan, P.E. (1988) Recovery: the lived experience of rehabilitation, *Psychosocial Rehabilitation Journal*, 11: 11–19. https://doi.org/10.1037/h0099565.

Department of Health, Department for Education (2017) Transforming Children and Young People' Mental Health Provision: A Green Paper. [https://www.gov.uk/government/consultations/transforming-children-and-young-peoples-mental-health-provision-a-green-paper; accessed 21 Jun 2024].

Edbrooke-Childs, J. and Patalay, P. (2019) Ethnic differences in referral routes to youth mental health services, *Journal of the American Academy of Child Psychiatry*, 58: 368–375. e1. https://doi.org/10.1016/j.jaac.2018.07.906.

Ellins, J., Hocking, L., Al-Haboubi, M., Newbould, J., Fenton, S.-J., Daniel, K., et al. (2023) Early evaluation of the Children and Young People's Mental Health Trailblazer programme: a rapid mixed-methods study, *Health and Social Care Delivery Research*, 11: 1–137. https://doi.org/10.3310/XQWU4117.

Evans-Lacko, S., Aguilar-Gaxiola, S., Al-Hamzawi, A., Alonso, J., Benjet, C., Bruffaerts, R., et al. (2018) Socio-economic variations in the mental health treatment gap for people with anxiety, mood, and substance use disorders: results from the WHO World Mental Health (WMH) surveys, *Psychological Medicine*, 48: 1560–1571. https://doi.org/10.1017/S0033291717003336.

Fenton, S.-J. (2016) Mental health service delivery for adolescents and young people: a comparative study between Australia and the UK (E-thesis). University of Birmingham & University of Melbourne, Birmingham, UK.

Fenton, S.-J., Gutiérrez, J.R.R., Pinilla-Roncancio, M., Casas, G., Carranza, F., Weber, S., et al. (2024) Macro level system mapping of the provision of mental health services to young people living in a conflict context in Colombia, *BMC Health Services Research*, 24: 138. https://doi.org/10.1186/s12913-024-10602-2.

Fernando, S. (2012) Race and culture issues in mental health and some thoughts on ethnic identity, *Counselling Psychology Quarterly*, 25: 113–123. https://doi.org/10.1080/09515070.2012.674299.

Ford, T. (2008) Practitioner review: how can epidemiology help us plan and deliver effective child and adolescent mental health services?, *Journal of Child Psychology and Psychiatry*, 49: 900–914. https://doi.org/10.1111/j.1469-7610.2008.01927.x

Furgalska, M. (2023) 'Informed consent is a bit of a joke to me': lived experiences of insight, coercion, and capabilities in mental health care settings, *International Journal of Law in Context*, 1–19. https://doi.org/10.1017/S1744552323000174.

Garattini, L., Barbato, A., D'Avanzo, B. and Nobili, A. (2023) Including mental health care in a model of European health system, *Epidemiology and Psychiatric Sciences*, 32, e12. https://doi.org/10.1017/S2045796023000057.

Georgieva, I., Mulder, C.L. and Wierdsma, A. (2012) Patients' preference and experiences of forced medication and seclusion, *Psychiatric Quarterly*, 83: 1–13. http://dx.doi.org/10.1007/s11126-011-9178-y.

Gillard, S.G., Edwards, C., Gibson, S.L., Owen, K. and Wright, C. (2013) Introducing peer worker roles into UK mental health service teams: a qualitative analysis of the organisational benefits and challenges, *BMC Health Services Research*, 13, 188. https://doi.org/10.1186/1472-6963-13-188.

Glasby, J., Tew, J. and Fenton, S.-J. (2021) UK mental health policy and practice, in G. Ikkos and N. Bouras (eds) *Mind, State and Society: Social History of Psychiatry and Mental Health in Britain 1960–2010*. Cambridge: Cambridge University Press. https://doi.org/10.1017/9781911623793.012.

Gopalkrishnan, N. (2018) Cultural diversity and mental health: considerations for policy and practice, *Frontiers in Public Health*, 6: 179. https://doi.org/10.3389/fpubh.2018.00179.

Hazell, C.M., Berry, C., Bogen-Johnston, L. and Banerjee, M. (2022) Creating a hierarchy of mental health stigma: testing the effect of psychiatric diagnosis on stigma, *BJPsych Open*, 8, e174. https://doi.org/10.1192/bjo.2022.578.

Henderson, C. and Thornicroft, G. (2009) Stigma and discrimination in mental illness: Time to Change, *The Lancet*, 373: 1928–1930. https://doi.org/10.1016/S0140-6736(09)61046-1.

Kapadia, D. (2023) Stigma, mental illness & ethnicity: time to centre racism and structural stigma, *Sociology of Health and Illness*, 45: 855–871. https://doi.org/10.1111/1467-9566.13615.

Kayiteshonga, Y., Sezibera, V., Mugabo, L. and Iyamuremye, J.D. (2022) Prevalence of mental disorders, associated co-morbidities, health care knowledge and service utilization in Rwanda – towards a blueprint for promoting mental health care services in low- and middle-income countries?, *BMC Public Health*, 22: 1858. https://doi.org/10.1186/s12889-022-14165-x.

Killackey, E. and Alvarez-Jimenez, M. (2019) Psychosocial interventions for youth mental health, in L.B. Hickie and P.D. McGorry (eds) *Clinical Staging in Psychiatry: Making Diagnosis Work for Research and Treatment*. Cambridge: Cambridge University Press. https://doi.org/10.1017/9781139839518.012.

Kirkbride, J.B., Anglin, D.M., Colman, I., Dykxhoorn, J., Jones, P.B., Patalay, P., et al. (2024) The social determinants of mental health and disorder: evidence, prevention and recommendations, *World Psychiatry*, 23: 58–90. https://doi.org/10.1002/wps.21160.

Leamy, M., Bird, V., Le Boutillier, C., Williams, J. and Slade, M. (2011) Conceptual framework for personal recovery in mental health: systematic review and narrative synthesis, *The British Journal of Psychiatry: The Journal of Mental Science*, 199: 445–452. https://doi.org/10.1192/bjp.bp.110.083733.

Londoño, A., Romero, P. and Casas, G. (2012) The association between armed conflict, violence and mental health: a cross sectional study comparing two populations in Cundinamarca department, Colombia, *Conflict and Health*, 6, 12. https://doi.org/10.1186/1752-1505-6-12.

MacDonald, D., Barnes, M., Crawford, M., Omeni, E., Wilson, A. and Rose, D. (2015) Service user governors in mental health foundation trusts: accountability or business as usual?, *Health Expectations an International Journal of Public Participation in Health Care and Health Policy*, 18: 2892–2902. https://doi.org/10.1111/hex.12274.

Mahdanian, A.A., Laporta, M., Drew Bold, N., Funk, M. and Puras, D. (2023) Human rights in mental healthcare: a review of current global situation, *International Review of Psychiatry*, 35: 150–162. https://doi.org/10.1080/09540261.2022.2027348.

Mantelero, A. (2022) Beyond Data: Human Rights, Ethical and Social Impact Assessment in AI, Information Technology and Law Series. The Hague: T.M.C. Asser Press. https://doi.org/10.1007/978-94-6265-531-7.

Minkowitz, T. (2015) Advancing the rights of users and survivors of psychiatry using the UN Convention on the Rights of Persons with Disabilities, in S. Helen, A. Jill and B. Sapey (eds) *Madness, Distress and the Politics of Disablement*. Bristol: Policy Press.

Nazroo, J.Y., Bhui, K.S. and Rhodes, J. (2020) Where next for understanding race/ethnic inequalities in severe mental illness? Structural, interpersonal and institutional racism, *Sociology of Health and Illness*, 42: 262–276. https://doi.org/10.1111/1467-9566.13001.

Ngui, E.M., Khasakhala, L., Ndetei, D. and Roberts, L.W. (2010) Mental disorders, health inequalities and ethics: a global perspective, *International Review of Psychiatry*, 22: 235–244. https://doi.org/10.3109/09540261.2010.485273.

NHS England (2021) Mental Health Act Statistics, Annual Figures - 2020-21 [WWW Document]. NHS Engl. Digit. [https://digital.nhs.uk/data-and-information/publications/statistical/mental-health-act-statistics-annual-figures/2020-21-annual-figures; accessed 30 April 2024].

Nielsen, E. (2016) Mind your 'C's and 'S's: The Language of Self-harm and Suicide (and why it matters). *Institute of Mental Health Blog*, Nottingham. [https://imhblog.wordpress.com/2016/01/22/emma-nielsen-mind-your-cs-and-ss-the-language-of-self-harm-and-suicide-and-why-it-matters/; accessed 29 April 2024].

OHCHR (2010) Professional Training Series no. 17: Monitoring the Convention on the Rights of Persons with Disabilities: Guidance for Human Rights Monitors, HR/P/PT/17. [https://www.ohchr.org/sites/default/files/Documents/Publications/Disabilities_training_17EN.pdf; accessed 21 June 2024].

Padmanathan, P., Biddle, L., Hall, K., Scowcroft, E., Nielsen, E. and Knipe, D. (2019) Language use and suicide: an online cross-sectional survey, *PLOS ONE*, 14, e0217473. https://doi.org/10.1371/journal.pone.0217473.

Pizzol, D., Trott, M., Butler, L., Barnett, Y., Ford, T., Neufeld, S.A., et al. (2023) Relationship between severe mental illness and physical multimorbidity: a meta-analysis and call for action, *BMJ Mental Health*, 26. https://doi.org/10.1136/bmjment-2023-300870.

Qureshi, O., Endale, T., Ryan, G., Miguel-Esponda, G., Iyer, S.N., Eaton, J., et al. (2021) Barriers and drivers to service delivery in global mental health projects, *International Journal of Mental Health Systems*, 15, 14. https://doi.org/10.1186/s13033-020-00427-x.

Rees, G., Huby, G., McDade, L. and McKechnie, L. (2004) Joint working in community mental health teams: implementation of an integrated care pathway, *Health and Social Care in the Community*, 12: 527–536. https://doi.org/10.1111/j.1365-2524.2004.00523.x.

Repper, J. and Carter, T. (2011) A review of the literature on peer support in mental health services, *Journal of Mental Health*, 20: 392–411. https://doi.org/10.3109/09638237.2011.583947.

Richardson, E., Walshe, K., Boyd, A., Roberts, J., Wenzel, L., Robertson, R., et al. (2019) User involvement in regulation: a qualitative study of service user involvement in Care Quality Commission inspections of health and social care providers in England, *Health Expectations an International Journal of Public Participation in Health Care and Health Policy*, 22: 245–253. https://doi.org/10.1111/hex.12849.

Rogers, A. and Pilgrim, D. (2014) *A Sociology of Mental Health and Illness* (5th edn.). Maidenhead: McGraw-Hill Education.

Rose, D., Willis, R., Brohan, E., Sartorius, N., Villares, C., Wahlbeck, K., et al. (2011) Reported stigma and discrimination by people with a diagnosis of schizophrenia, *Epidemiology and Psychiatric Sciences*, 20: 193–204. https://doi.org/10.1017/s2045796011000254.

Rose, N. (2018) *Our Psychiatric Future*. Medford, MA: John Wiley & Sons.

Rukundo, G.Z., Nalugya, J., Otim, P. and Hall, A. (2020) A collaborative approach to the development of multi-disciplinary teams and services for child and adolescent mental health in Uganda, *Frontiers in Psychiatry*, 11. https://doi.org/10.3389/fpsyt.2020.579417.

Sayce, L. (2015) *From Psychiatric Patient to Citizen Revisited*. London: Bloomsbury.

Slade, M., Amering, M., Farkas, M., Hamilton, B., O'Hagan, M., Panther, G., et al. (2014) Uses and abuses of recovery: implementing recovery-oriented practices in mental health systems, *World Psychiatry*, 13: 12–20. https://doi.org/10.1002/wps.20084.

Thomas, E.C., Zisman-Ilani, Y. and Salzer, M.S. (2019) Self-determination and choice in mental health: qualitative insights from a study of self-directed care, *Psychiatric Services*, 70: 801–807. https://doi.org/10.1176/appi.ps.201800544.

Thornicroft, G. (2006) *Shunned: Discrimination Against People with Mental Illness*. Oxford: Oxford University Press.

Turner, T. (2004) The history of deinstitutionalization and reinstitutionalization, *Psychiatry, Community Psychiatry*, 3, 9: 1–4. https://doi.org/10.1383/psyt.3.9.1.50257.

UN General Assembly (2006) UN General Assembly, Convention on the Rights of Persons with Disabilities (CRPD): resolution / adopted by the General Assembly, A/RES/61/106 [https://www.un.org/en/development/desa/population/migration/generalassembly/docs/globalcompact/A_RES_61_106.pdf; accessed 21 June 2024].

United Nations (2015) The 17 Sustainable Development Goals [WWW Document]. U.N. Sustainable Development Goals. [https://sdgs.un.org/goals; accessed 30 April 2024].

Watson, E. (2019) The mechanisms underpinning peer support: a literature review, *Journal of Mental Health*, 28: 677–688. https://doi.org/10.1080/09638237.2017.1417559.

Weber, S., Carranza, F., Rengifo, J.R., Romero, C., Arrieta, S., Martínez, K., et al. (2024) Mapping mental health care services for children and youth population in Colombia's Pacific: potential for boundary spanning between community and formal services, *International Journal of Mental Health Systems*, 18, 9. https://doi.org/10.1186/s13033-024-00626-w.

Weich, S., Fenton, S.-J., Staniszewska, S., Canaway, A., Crepaz-Keay, D., Larkin, M., et al. (2020) Using patient experience data to support improvements in inpatient mental health care: the EURIPIDES multimethod study, *Health and Social Care Delivery Research*, 8, 21. https://doi.org/10.3310/hsdr08210.

Whitley, R. (2015) Global Mental Health: concepts, conflicts and controversies, *Epidemiology and Psychiatric Sciences*, 24: 285–291. https://doi.org/10.1017/S2045796015000451.

WHO and Quality Rights (2021) Peer support mental health services: Promoting person-centred and rights-based approaches. [https://www.who.int/publications/i/item/9789240025783; accessed 9 January 2025].

Wiens, K., Bhattarai, A., Pedram, P., Dores, A., Williams, J., Bulloch, A., et al. (2020) A growing need for youth mental health services in Canada: examining trends in youth mental health from 2011 to 2018, *Epidemiology and Psychiatric Sciences*, 29, e115. https://doi.org/10.1017/S2045796020000281.

World Economic Forum (WEF) (2020) A Global Framework for Youth Mental Health: Investing in Future Mental Capital for Individuals, Communities and Economies. [https://www.weforum.org/publications/a-global-framework-for-youth-mental-health-db3a7364df/; accessed 21 June 2024].

World Health Organization (WHO) (2022) World mental health report: transforming mental health for all. [https://www.who.int/publications/i/item/9789240049338; accessed 9 January 2025].

World Health Organization (WHO) (2023) Global mapping report on multisectoral actions to strengthen the prevention and control of noncommunicable diseases and mental health conditions: experiences from around the world. [https://www.who.int/publications/i/item/9789240074255; accessed 21 June 2024].

World Health Organization (WHO) (2024a) Operational framework for monitoring social determinants of health equity. [https://www.who.int/publications/i/item/9789240088320; accessed 21 June 2024].

World Health Organization (2024b) WHO EMRO Mental health gap action programme [WWW Document]. World Health Organ. - Reg. Off. East. Mediterr. [www.emro.who.int/mnh/mental-health-gap-action-programme/index.html; accessed 4 March 2025].

Wykes, T., Bell, A., Carr, S., Coldham, T., Gilbody, S., Hotopf, M., et al. (2023) Shared goals for mental health research: what, why and when for the 2020s, *Journal of Mental Health*, 32: 997–1005. https://doi.org/10.1080/09638237.2021.1898552.

Adult social care

Emily Burn and Catherine Needham

Introduction and overview

Adult social care is a term for the provision of services to support people with age-related frailty, disability or mental health conditions. In the international context it is often called long-term care, to distinguish it from services provided as part of health systems, although in the UK the term social care is used. Both long-term care and social care usually refer to services to assist people with the so-called Activities of Daily Living (e.g. washing, dressing, preparing food) or the Independent Activities of Daily Living (such as shopping and cleaning (NHS England, 2023). In this chapter we use the term adult social care, which has been the preferred term in the UK in recent decades, eclipsing earlier terms, such as social services and community care. As our focus is on adults, we do not include childcare or support for disabled children in our scope.

In many advanced democracies, the welfare states that were set up in the twentieth century made some provision for supporting people through old age and disability. However, population ageing and improved longevity for disabled people have increased the demand for social care services way beyond that envisaged by welfare state designers. Demand for long-term mental health support has also increased across many nations and it is widely recognized that services need to be expanded to meet this demand (World Health Organization, 2022). Doing so generates a range of challenges, including where the resources will come from to pay for social care and how to develop a large and suitably trained workforce.

It is also increasingly recognized that reducing social care to a functional account of basic needs (sometimes summarized as 'up, washed and dressed') is no longer adequate to meet people's expectations of what makes a good life. Social care campaigners have begun to apply a wider lens of well-being to care services and to consider the extent that people can aspire to 'have a life not a service' (Think Local Act Personal, 2018). Strengths-based or assets-based approaches focus on asking people what they enjoy and are good at, rather than on what they need or cannot do. We discuss more about this later in the chapter.

What is social care and why is it different from health?

Social care encompasses 'a wide range of activities to help people who are older or living with disability or physical or mental illness live independently and stay well and safe' (The King's Fund, 2023). For many people, social care will be provided in their own home or in residential care facilities and will also include support to access community activities. Many countries have established legal frameworks setting out long-term care provision. For example, Singapore passed the CareShield Life and Long-Term Care Act in 2019, which made provisions for a long-term care insurance scheme (CareShield Life, n.d.). The Social Support Act 2015 in the Netherlands established local authorities' duty to provide support for people in their homes (Government of the Netherlands, 2016). In England the legal framework for social care is set out in the Care Act 2014 (Care Act, 2014), which clarifies who is entitled to state-funded care services, how care should be provided and paid for and how it will be regulated.

The broad parameters of social care are similar across many countries in providing assistance to those who require additional support through age-related frailty, disability or mental health conditions. However, it is important to acknowledge that there are country differences in the expectations of who holds responsibility to provide this care. Razavi (2007) developed the concept of the 'care diamond' to distinguish between family, state, market and community to highlight the contribution that each makes to care (see Figure 17.1). In some countries, there is a greater expectation that the family will provide care to older and disabled people; in other countries it is assumed that this role will mainly be undertaken by the state or by the market (i.e. private companies).

Although we need to be wary of misleading generalizations, the literature on 'welfare regimes' and in particular 'care regimes' highlights regional or national patterns in care provision. For example, Theobald and Luppi (2018) note that Italy has had a strong emphasis on family care, Sweden has had a strong emphasis on publicly provided care, and Germany has a mix of private care and family care. However, in all of these countries, patterns are changing (e.g. an increase in the use of for-profit care services) and new models of care are emerging (e.g. the growth of live-in care in Italy and Germany).

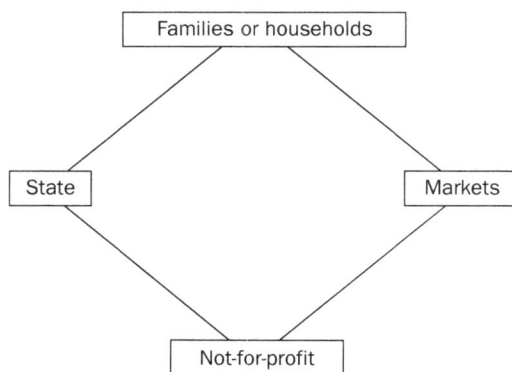

Figure 17.1 The Care Diamond
Source: Adapted from Razavi (2007: 21)

Even in countries with high levels of state and market involvement in social care, the majority of social care continues to be provided by the family. The European Care Strategy (European Commission, 2022: 16) noted that, 'the value of hours of long-term care provided by informal carers is estimated to be around 2.5% of EU GDP higher than the public expenditure on long-term care.' Most adults will be involved in care at some stage in their life. Data from the UK shows that between 1991 and 2018, two thirds of adults have been an unpaid carer for a family member or friend who was sick, disabled or who required support in old age. Women were particularly likely to be providing intense rates of care for another adult (over 50 hours a week). By the age of 46, half of women had been a carer. Half of men had been a carer by the age of 57 (Zhang et al., 2019).

The structure and scope of the paid care workforce differs between countries. In many countries there is a distinction between nursing, which is done by members of a registered profession, who are relatively well trained and renumerated, and social care, which is done by a low-paid and poorly trained workforce. These roles include care workers in residential homes or working to support people in their homes, community support and outreach workers and roles contributing to the running of facilities, such as cleaners and chefs. There are concerns about the recruitment and retention of the social care workforce (Bottery and Mallorie, 2024). Some countries have registration of care workers – e.g. Ireland, Wales and Scotland – but even then there are exceptions (for example, personal assistants are not registered) and there is often a 'grey economy' in care work where tasks like cleaning overlap with care. The rise of live-in care work by migrant workers in parts of Europe has raised concerns about the low visibility and absence of protections for this workforce. In the UK, there are new concerns about the rise of 'modern slavery' in care work (Booth, 2024).

Social care governance

There are differences between countries in how social care is organized and by whom. In some countries it is the responsibility of national government, whereas in others it is a local government jurisdiction. In the UK social care sits with local government, although national government plays a key role in determining funding and regulation. In the Nordic countries (Denmark, Finland, Iceland, Norway and Sweden), it has historically been the role of local government to control care services, along with health. In Australia, disabled and elder care was historically a responsibility of the six states rather than the federal government, with no local government involvement. Since 2016, the federal government in Australia has taken increasing control of disability services through the creation of the National Disability Insurance Scheme (National Disability Insurance Scheme, 2024).

Increasingly, the functioning of long-term care systems has received attention from international organizations looking to influence and support states to improve the provision of formal services and unpaid care. International organizations can draw attention to an issue and encourage action, although they are limited in their ability to compel state action. For example, the International Labour Organization (ILO) report *Care work and care jobs for the future of decent work* (Addati et al., 2018) explores the quality of care work, as well as the ways that unpaid work is recognized. Previous work from the ILO (Sheil-Adlung, 2015) has considered the difficulty meeting growing demand for long-term care services across 46 countries. UN Women (2017) discuss gender imbalances in care work and wider implications of this on women's lives.

The European Commission's (2022) European Care Strategy identified shared challenges for long-term care across member states. These included ensuring the timely access of affordable and high-quality, long-term care services at a time of rising demand, concerns about workforce sustainability and supporting unpaid carers. Member states are encouraged to take action to secure the supply and quality of services, as well as improving conditions for the workforce and the availability of support for unpaid carers. The European Commission requests that member states submit an annual plan detailing progress and work to strengthen data collection and demand forecasting. Daly (2023: 6) critiques the European Care Strategy as a continuation of the status quo, which 'spells a continuing reliance' on unpaid care with little emphasis on additional funding.

Learning activity 17.1 Assessing local social care provision

Write two to three brief sentences defining social care and its contribution to society in the context of your country's health and care system.

Note in bullet point form the different types of social care services in your area and identify which client groups these services are intended to support.

Drawing on your overview of local social care services, make an assessment of how they help local health services to meet their goals, or not. Building on this, set out how local health services affect the ways in which social care services function.

Changing approaches to social care

In many countries, support for older and disabled people was designed at a time when life expectancy was much lower than it is now, and when people were less likely to live into old age with a range of long-term health conditions. For those who did need additional support, this would come from families or long-stay hospitals or asylums. These residential facilities were often not much different from the workhouses and prisons that were built alongside them. Critiques of these 'total institutions' (Goffman, 1968) – which often housed the 'socially unacceptable' (e.g. unmarried mothers) as well as disabled people – emerged from the 1960s. High-profile scandals in many nations about abuse and neglect further undermined their respectability (Hide, 2021). Many countries have moved away from residential facilities for all but a small minority of people.

New approaches were also driven by fiscal pressures and the need for reform of post-Second World War systems, which did not anticipate large numbers of people drawing on social care. The acute illnesses that in the 1950s and 1960s tended to end lives not long after retirement have been replaced by chronic conditions, which people live with rather than die from (Crimmins, 2015). Life expectancies in the Global North (defined broadly as members of the Organisation for Economic Co-operation and Development) have advanced to 80 years (OECD, 2024), although averages mask wide differences based on social class and country. Disabled people also have a much higher life expectancy than in the past, creating new challenges around ageing with a disability. However, it should be borne in mind that ongoing health inequalities means that people with severe mental illness and people with learning disabilities have a shorter average life expectancy than the general population (Heslop et al., 2021; Office for Health Improvement and Disparities 2023). The increased prevalence of dementia has placed a particular strain on care services, given that people may live for several years with high levels of care needs.

Pressures for new approaches to social care have come not only from demographic changes, but also from disability rights movements, which have drawn attention to the primacy of independent living, human rights and dignity. From the 1980s there was increased concern about the tendency of the welfare state to police and discipline people, rather than to support them to flourish (Dukelow and Kennett, 2018). People living in institutions campaigned under the slogan of 'independent living'. Disability rights campaigns led to landmark legislation, such as the UK's Disability Discrimination Act 1995 and the US Americans with Disabilities Act passed in 1990. These acts created new duties on public bodies to make spaces accessible for disabled people.

Person-centred approaches for people with learning disabilities were also becoming influential from the 1980s, supporting the rights of people to live independently where possible. Within mental health services, the survivor movement challenged dominant psychiatric accounts of illness. Underpinning all of these approaches was the social model of disability, in which people were recognized to be disabled by society rather than by an impairment (Oliver, 2013). Under the banner of choice and control, people campaigned for greater independence and for individualized payments to make their own care purchases rather than having services provided by the state.

With greater attention paid to dignity, choice and control has come an understanding that where possible people would like to 'age in place'. For many people this will involve remaining in their home rather than moving to an institution. Home adaptations and the growth in domiciliary care services are designed to support people in their preferred place of living for as long as possible. This means that residential care facilities are increasingly seen as places of last resort for the final few months of life, rather than places for long-term stay. However, it is important to note that there is still a big variability between countries in the extent of care provision in residential facilities versus care at home, and that this is often a reflection of societal norms and preferences. In 2019 in Portugal, 35 per cent of long-term care recipients aged 65 and over received care at home, whereas this figure stands at 81 per cent of long-term care recipients over 65 in Spain (OECD, 2021). Some countries continue to invest heavily in new care homes, whereas others are decommissioning care homes and investing in other models.

Collective models of social care promoting co-living are seen to be a potential way to address social isolation and loneliness (for example, see Social Care Institute for Excellence, n.d.).

Ageing in place has come with an awareness that 'place' may not be a large family home that no longer meets the needs of residents. For example, there has been a growth in extra care facilities, in which people are able to rent or buy an apartment with options to step up or step down the care that is needed. In Australia and New Zealand, retirement villages are purpose-built housing developments that offer a range of services and accommodation options (Saville-Smith et al., 2019; Travers et al., 2022). There have been experiments with inter-generational housing to promote mixing between older and younger generations, fostering a sense of community and belonging (see Prasad (2019) for examples in Denmark and the Netherlands). In the UK, Shared Lives (2024) is a model where people who require support are matched with an approved carer, who includes the individual in their family and community life through either sharing a home or through regular visits. New Zealand has piloted a similar Home Share model (Office for Seniors, 2022).

Learning activity 17.2 Changing models of social care services

Create a table to identify and compare the different models of care available for frail older people in health and social care services where you live.

Have the underlying principles informing these models of health and social care services changed over time? Write a brief paragraph summarizing these changes and the reasons for them.

Opportunities and challenges facing the social care sector

A key challenge for social care is how to ensure that support is high quality and safe, while at the same time being person-centred and enabling wider well-being goals. Most formal care services will be inspected and regulated, which generates data about the models of care that are most likely to be high quality. Excessive levels of profit extraction, particularly in large care chains, have been raised as a concern in many countries, for example, the UK (Horton, 2022), Finland (Hoppania et al., 2024), Ireland (Mercille, 2024) and Canada (Brown, 2022).

Hedge fund investment in care chains has led to some complex ownership models, with care providers becoming subsidiaries of offshore companies and capital assets being sold on and leased back. In Belgium, a number of nursing homes owned by the French care home provider, Orpea, closed due to financial difficulties (The Brussels Times, 2023). When the Four Seasons care chain went into administration in the UK in 2019, local government staff reported difficulty in being able to work out who owned the care home (Jarrett, 2019; Rowland, 2019).

Quality concerns are not exclusive to the private sector of course. Abuse, neglect and poor-quality care may be a result of the culture of closed institutions, which are set apart from the rest of society, as much as related to the model of ownership. For example, in recent years there have been public scandals about abuse in care homes in Canada (Pederson et al., 2020),

Australia (Mercer, 2018), France (Acco and Mandia, 2022), and the UK (Buchanon, 2024) and we cannot assume that any country is immune from services that cause mistreatment and harm. A culture of transparency and openness is usually considered the best way to minimize these risks, which embeds equality and human rights to deliver care with dignity (Care Quality Commission, 2022).

Box 17.1   Case study – Royal Commission, Australia

Following concerns about abuse and substandard care in Australia, the government established a Royal Commission in 2018 to look into the quality and safety of care and support services for older people. Care services for older people often take place outside of the awareness of the local community. The Royal Commission's (2021) final report notes that building and maintaining social connections is an important component of high-quality care and that services should encourage and promote links with the local community. The Commission also recommended placing greater emphasis on the voices of people drawing on care and support, noting that the regulator should establish appropriate routes for people to report their experiences of care services throughout the year. The regulator should also ensure that they speak to at least 20 per cent of people drawing on care, or carers, when inspecting a service. In closed institutions, substandard care is less likely to be observed or reported. Incorporating mechanisms that hear the experiences of people accessing care and support is one way to address this.

One response to poor quality and unsafe care is to tighten up regulation. A review of quality assurance practices by the European Commission (Zigante and King, 2019) notes that regulation of social care is usually administered by a national body; however, other decentralized or arms-length bodies may monitor compliance. For example, in Sweden, providers are accredited by the regulator and the local district establishes local standards (Zigante and King, 2019: 27–28).

Improving quality in social care

Expected levels of service quality are set in regulation standards and differ from country to country. Standards can focus on governance, staffing levels or the suitability of premises or equipment. Regulation has also begun to incorporate standards focused on assessing outcomes for people who draw on care services.

In England, the Care Quality Commission (CQC) inspects both care and health services and issues quality ratings for care providers. Almost 80 per cent of regulated adult social care services in England were rated good in 2022/23 and 16 per cent were rated as 'requires improvement' (Care Quality Commission, 2023). Since 2024, local authorities have been assessed against how well they commission social care services. Regulators have a dual role in inspecting care as well as supporting care provision improvement.

There are concerns, however, about whether the inspection model is really effective at spotting and responding to and improving poor-quality care. This can be seen in the case of Whorlton Hall, a specialist hospital for people with learning disabilities and autism in County Durham in North East England. A BBC investigative documentary in 2019 found care workers were abusive to patients (The Health Foundation, 2019). An independent review of the CQC's actions to regulate Whorlton Hall between 2015–2019 found that the inspection process had not uncovered patient abuse. The review made a series of recommendations to improve identifying abuse (Murphy, 2020).

Disability campaigners have argued that a more effective mechanism to keep people safe from abuse is to increase consumer power in the sector. This is often done through financial mechanisms that enable people to purchase their own care rather than relying on state services. In many countries – including the UK, the USA, Canada, Japan, Australia, France and Germany – care services can be purchased via cash transfers to individuals or their families. The idea is that people have the best sense of what types of support they need and whether it is of a high quality. If it isn't, then they can move their money to a different provider. The signals here are more immediate and effective than when it requires a regulator to spot low quality care, report it to a state commissioner and then make changes through a contractual process.

Box 17.2   Case study – social care in Germany

In Germany, people drawing on care can choose to receive a care allowance that can be used to organize support that meets the individual's needs. Funded by long-term care insurance, the amount of care allowance is graduated according to an individual's assessed care need (Federal Ministry for Family Affairs, Senior Citizens, Women and Youth, n.d.). Social care policy in Germany has aimed to strengthen informal care and to support people to stay in their own homes (European Commission, 2021). Individuals are free to use their care allowance and may pass it on to acknowledge the people who have provided support (Federal Ministry for Family Affairs, Senior Citizens, Women and Youth, n.d.). People cared for by family members or friends are visited twice a year by care professionals to discuss concerns and pass on advice (Handbook Germany, n.d.).

However, it is important to note that there are barriers to effective consumer power in social care – which is often a 'distress purchase' made at a time of crisis with little prior experience of what constitutes good care. Just as there are limits to how much regulation can assure good care, so too there are limits to the extent that individuals and families can be smart customers in a care context.

Given the limits to consumer sovereignty, another approach is to involve people with lived experience in the design and delivery of social care, as co-producers. Co-production brings together practitioners and people using care services to jointly design and deliver support. It shifts the focus from doing things *to* and *for* people to doing things with them:

> This is not about consultation or participation – except in the broadest sense. The point is not to consult more, or involve people more in decisions; it is to encourage them to use the human skills and experience they have to help deliver public or voluntary services
>
> (Stephens et al., 2008: 10–11)

In England, co-production is promoted through the Care Act 2014, which requires partnership between practitioners and people using services. It is an alternative to the gatekeeping approach whereby social workers and other professionals ration access to services. There is an emphasis on power sharing, relationships and mutual respect for knowledge and expertise. It has also been a key principle in social care reform in Scotland (Feeley, 2021), Wales (Welsh Government, 2019) and Northern Ireland (Kelly and Kennedy, 2017) – and outside the UK (for example, in Norway (Tingvold and Olsvold, 2023)).

The greater involvement of people with lived experience has contributed to a reframing of what is meant by social care. Rather than seeing care as a package of supports to be purchased in chunks of time by the state or the individual, it can be seen as a set of tools to support people in more flexible ways. An influential account of social care by the social movement Social Care Future summarizes the aspiration as: 'We all want to live in the place we call home with the people and things that we love, in communities where we look out for one another, doing the things that matter to us' (Social Care Future, 2024).

Strengths-based approaches in social care

Achieving this vision involves a reframing of the process of care assessment away from needs and towards strengths-based approaches and asset-based approaches. This approach recognizes that people are often embedded in reciprocal caring relationships, in which they give support to others, as well as requiring support themselves. People may also have skills and capabilities they can develop in ways that support their own development and contribute to community well-being. In this approach, it is also important to raise what people care about and what helps them to feel good. For example, strengths-based assessments should have a whole life focus and consider significant life events and the skills someone has accrued (see Box 17.3). Thinking about someone's wider support networks can also highlight what is important to them.

Box 17.3   An example of a strengths-based approach to social care

Improving Adult Care Together (IMPACT) is a UK centre for implementing evidence in adult social care. IMPACTAgewell® is based in Northern Ireland. Older people referred to the project are met in their homes by IMPACTAgewell® Officers who work with the individual to identify options that could improve their well-being. With their consent, the individual is introduced to community groups providing support. Key professionals are brought together in locality hub meetings to share information and learning about the local population's needs.

See https://impact.bham.ac.uk/wp-content/uploads/2023/12/Asset-Based-Approaches-report.pdf for further information.

Elements of a strengths-based approach (adapted from IMPACT, 2023)

- **Link workers who can connect people to local organizations and community activities.** Link workers should build relationships within the local community, professionals and the voluntary sector.
- **An adequate range of accessible community activities.** Activities should cater for a range of needs and interests. There is appropriate support for individuals connecting with community activities.
- **Resources should be continually updated.** Awareness of community activities should be kept up to date and developed with communities and local agencies.
- **Referrals should be efficient.** Appropriate digital resources and data systems should support connections between individuals and link workers.

There has been a lot of optimism about the scope for these ways of working to improve social care. Approaches such as social prescribing and local area coordination have been based on these and have shown positive evaluations at the individual level (Morton et al., 2015; Lunt et al., 2021). However, a scoping review of the evidence of strengths-based approaches in social work and social care highlighted a number of issues. It was difficult to clearly define such approaches, which tend to be defined by what they *are not* (Caiels et al., 2021). There were also concerns that they could magnify inequalities, benefitting people who already have strong networks and good support, or could overly emphasize self-help and resilience. The approach also continues to clash with legal eligibility criteria, which are based on need (Caiels et al., 2021).

Technology and innovation

Another route to doing social care differently is through the judicious use of new technology (see Box 17.4). Within England, Whitfield and Hamblin (2022) find a strong pro-technology rhetoric from the Department of Health and Social Care but a tendency for 'pilotitis' (the tendency to continuously introduce small-scale projects without progressing to full implementation) and a lack of engagement with key practical questions (e.g. the implications for pendant alarms with the upcoming analogue switch off) and ethical issues (e.g. the lack of data security with consumer devices, such as the Amazon Echo) (Whitfield and Hamblin, 2022).

In countries that are further advanced with care tech than the UK, such as Japan, studies have found a similar techno-optimism. Wright's (2023) ethnographic work looking at the use of care robots in Japanese care homes, found that the devices were more expensive and required more human labour to maintain the devices, compared to traditional care. He called for more rather than less commitment to the essential humanness of care and relationships, looking at how this can be supported rather than replaced.

Studies looking at the establishment of artificial intelligence-based technologies in social care found a number of implementation difficulties relating to resource management, training and acceptance of the new technology (Litchfield et al., 2023). This study has informed guidance for commissioners on introducing technology to social care services (Glasby et al., 2023). A framework developed by Greenhalgh et al. (2017) considers the factors that inform the non-adoption, abandonment, scale-up, spread and sustainability of technology-based health and social care programmes.

Box 17.4   Different interventions included in the term 'care technology'

- technologies to assist (e.g. devices to assist with walking or lifting);
- technologies used to monitor (e.g. telecare devices such as trackers and sensors);
- technologies to organize and record care (e.g. digital care records or care worker check in systems);
- technologies used to collect and analyse data (e.g. integrated records across health and social care); and
- technologies used to connect (such as smartphones and iPads, and apps, such as Zoom and FaceTime).

(Adapted from Whitfield and Hamblin, 2022).

Learning activity 17.3 Technology and social care

Write a paragraph on how technology is used within your service.

- What are the barriers and enablers that have facilitated or obstructed the use of technology? Have concerns around ethics and data sharing and data protection prevented the introduction of new forms of technology?
- What are the advantages and disadvantages of introducing new technology into social care services?
- What might be done to maximize the advantages and mitigate the disadvantages?

The interface between social care and health

Integrated care brings social care and health together to provide joined-up services that place the individual at the centre of provision. Integration recognizes the mutual dependencies between social care and health – neither could function without the other. In many countries there are challenges in drawing a sharp line between health and care services. For people with dementia, for example, it can be hard to distinguish between the health needs of this condition and the social care needs that it creates. Humphries (2022: p. 7) describes how a bath would be funded differently in the UK depending on whether it was a bath for 'health' or 'care' reasons. Exley et al. (2024) also note that this has been a challenge in the Netherlands. The difficulty of drawing this distinction, particularly for older people close to the end of life who have both health and care needs and may be frequently in hospital or residential care, has led to decades of attempts to bring the two systems closer together.

Integration can take on different forms. In England the creation of integrated care systems has given a statutory basis for integration and there is optimism that these organizations will be able to make a step change that was lacking in earlier iterations (Charles, 2022). In the United States, accountable care organizations, the inspiration for integrated care systems in England, bring together providers across a geographic area to coordinate care to facilitate integrated service delivery (Shortell et al., 2014). Reforms introduced in Italy in 2022 aim to develop integrated services closer to local communities (Cinelli and Fattore, 2024).

Exley et al.'s (2024) study looking at integration in the Netherlands, Italy and Scotland, highlights the common impetus in many countries to bring health and care closer together. They also note that the pandemic accelerated this agenda, as it highlighted the ways that integrated services grounded in positive relationships between stakeholders and a culture of openness had brought partners together, facilitating a faster response to COVID-19.

Reed et al.'s (2021) discussion of integration across the four countries in the United Kingdom notes that integration has had a limited impact on outcomes and that health continues to dominate resource allocation. There is a pattern in many nations of integrated structures for health and social care being introduced with great fanfare, only later to be shelved or superseded. In part this reflects the difficulty of bringing together two distinct organizational forms, with different funding mechanisms.

Although it is too soon to say whether the current structures of integration in the UK will deliver the required transformation, it is notable that concerned voices continue to express the same issues as in previous eras: the continued over-focus on hospital issues, such as discharge, the lack of investment in prevention or the lack of parity of esteem (Integration of Primary and Community Care Committee, 2023). In the Netherlands, a decentralized, bottom-up approach is taken, which has made gradual progress towards integration (Nies et al., 2021). However, barriers to integration remain, such as fragmented financing arrangements and monitoring systems which favour acute healthcare (Exley et al., 2024). Given continued complexity, managers need to navigate the ever-present and dynamic tensions between health and social care.

Learning Activity 17.4 Integrating social care and health

Construct a table of the advantages and disadvantages of integrating social care and health services, both at the level of service delivery, and at the funding and organizational level.

What might make it hard for healthcare managers to work effectively with social care managers within a service focused on integration, and how might such barriers be overcome?

Where next for social care?

All countries will continue to need to address the issues of population ageing and that people will live longer with multiple health conditions. While life expectancy has increased, there has been relatively little change in healthy life expectancy, or the amount of time that someone can expect to live in good health (GOV.UK, 2023). In the UK and elsewhere it will be important to build further the public profile of social care as part of mobilizing political pressure for greater investment.

There are clear economic benefits from investing in social care (Future Social Care Coalition, 2023), however, public discussions about care should also focus on the wider social benefits that come from bolstering social support and care. Countries that have reformed their care funding arrangements in recent years – such as Germany and Japan (see Box 17.5) – have been able to reframe discussions to focus on the positives of social care as 'mutual support' and a key part of the national infrastructure (Curry, 2024).

Box 17.5   Social care policy reform in Japan and Germany

Both Japan and Germany have reformed social care funding. Both reforms introduced a social care insurance system to provide access to a minimum level of care to the population (Curry et al., 2018, 2019).

In Germany, risk is pooled, and people contribute insurance premiums set at a national level. Only a basic level of service provision is funded, and people are expected to make further contributions to the cost of their care. Eligibility to access funded care and support is established by a national framework and providers cannot charge people different rates for care. The reforms have contributed to a strong social care market; however, there are concerns about the level of profits drawn by some providers.

In Japan, the care insurance system is funded using a mix of insurance contributions, taxation and personal contributions, with people paying into the care system from the age of 40. Service provision is viewed to be reasonably generous; however, there are mechanisms to control demand. The social care system is reviewed by the national government every 3 years. Reviews offer the chance to control demand and expenditure on services by adjusting the amount that people are expected to contribute to the costs of their care. While the reforms are viewed to be a success, an ageing population and workforce shortages are a continual challenge for the system.

The very significant contribution that unpaid carers make to society frequently goes unrecognized (Petrillo and Bennett, 2023) and by not supporting unpaid carers there is a risk that care is hidden in the private sphere of the family. This is often to the detriment of women, who are more likely to give up work to provide care. Attempts to stabilize the social care workforce in the Global North have frequently relied on migration. However, this can have a destabilizing effect on the social care workforce in other countries. The contribution of migrant workers to the care system needs to be valued, but this is too often missing from migration policies (Mooten, 2021).

In the UK, there are two clearly articulated directions of travel in social care reform. The first is more integration, further dissolving the boundaries between health and social care through initiatives, such as integrated care systems. The second – and somewhat contradictory – impetus is towards a National Care Service (NCS), which would give care a separate structure and status akin to that of the NHS. Plans for an NCS are at different stages in different parts of the UK, from draft legislation in Scotland (Scottish Government, n.d.) and government proposals in Wales (Welsh Government, 2022) to more nascent think tank ideas in England (Fabian Society, 2023). Each of these variants of the NCS proposes a different structure, which will have distinct implications for social care services. However, there is a shared aim to promote consistency of access of quality services.

In the UK, as in many other countries, attempts to reform social care have been seen as politically risky (due to the implications for higher taxation) and many people still find it difficult to get timely access to good-quality care services. Social care remains a pressing policy issue and continued efforts need to be made with people who draw on care and support to generate new approaches. Other countries that have advanced social care reform may be a source of learning for those such as the UK who have yet to make sufficient progress. Thinking about how reforms to social care can be reframed from negative accounts of deficit to more positive stories of facilitating support and community cohesion may offer a way to proceed (Curry, 2024).

The challenges for managers

So, what does this mean for managers of health and social care? Whether health and care systems are formally integrated or not at a national or regional level, being a manager in health or care requires an understanding of the interconnectedness of these care and service domains. Working towards understanding the touchpoints between social care and other local public service systems will help managers to understand how people engage with these services and can be supported most effectively. Some of these points of contact between systems may be obvious and others more hidden. It is well known that people can be stuck in hospital for longer than they need if there are delays in putting in place the social care services that they will need to support them at home. However, it is important also to be aware of other intersections – for example, how pressures on unpaid carers can increase their susceptibility to a range of stress-related health conditions affecting their well-being and ability to provide appropriate support.

Health and social care operate as complex adaptive systems (Plsek and Greenhalgh, 2001) where different parts are dependent on one another in ways that are hard to control or even predict. Making a change in one area will have wider effects on other parts of the system. For example, a change in the eligibility criteria used to assess access to local authority support may lead to additional strain for the voluntary, community and social enterprise sector. Furthermore, there may be tensions between changes initiated by national policy and changes pursued at a regional or local level. Managers must be adept at managing uncertainty within the health and social care systems as it will often be difficult to control or anticipate the outcomes from any changes.

There are a number of workforce challenges that come from this complex system. Managers may be overseeing services with complex delivery chains where parts of the service are delivered by the for-profit or non-profit sectors. Here, the role of a manager is to oversee commissioning teams, and work closely with regulatory and quality assurance bodies, to ensure effective service delivery. There are also issues in ensuring sufficiency of provision in a sector that has struggled to meet rising demand. Workforce shortages are a particular issue in rural areas or where there is plenty of alternative employment with better pay and conditions. Managers have to work within organizations to create a narrative around the value of social care as a career to attract the sorts of high-calibre and committed workers that the sector needs.

Excellent relational skills and interacting and connecting with others within and across public services can provide vital intelligence about how different parts of the system function. Part of this influence requires being able to decipher and develop a wider story of what is going on in the social care system. Skills in data analysis will facilitate this. Many organizations now have data dashboards to improve intelligence about their local communities, but managers do not always have the data analysis skills to make best use of these. Managers should reflect on their skill set and seek opportunities to address any knowledge gaps (see Box 17.6). Similarly, organizations should consider their suite of training opportunities to ensure managers can develop their skills. Lack of data sharing between health and care organizations also continues to be a barrier to effective interventions.

Box 17.6   The 21st Century Public Servant

The 21st Century Public Servant is a framework developed at the University of Birmingham that sets out the skills, roles and values required to be an effective leader and manager in public services. First developed in 2014, it identified 10 characteristics of effective leaders. These included an awareness of place and scale (what needs to happen at the neighbourhood, at the town/city or regional level), and a commitment to working co-productively with citizens (Needham and Mangan, 2014). Following a turbulent decade of a global pandemic and pressures on public service expenditure, the work was updated (Needham et al., 2024). This new research highlighted that the 'easy' work of public services has been automated or outsourced, and that much of what public service managers deal with now has high levels of complexity. They need to be multi-lingual in working across organizations, providing allyship for excluded voices, deploying data effectively and prioritizing self-care to avoid burnout.

Managers also need the skills to facilitate co-production and co-design with the local community, working in partnership to harness knowledge about what works when it comes to service delivery. Activism from disabled people, older people and people with mental health conditions was prompted by a history of marginalization and stigmatization. Overcoming this legacy requires humility in acknowledging people as experts in their own lives, and an ability to build trust with communities who are cynical about engagement. Much of this engagement and co-production work may be done by frontline staff rather than by managers themselves, and it can be challenging, time intensive and expensive. Managers need to build a strong narrative within teams about why this work is crucial to ensure that health and care services promote equity and human rights as well as better service outcomes.

Learning Activity 17.5 Skills required by health managers

Note in bullet point form the skills that are needed by health managers to work effectively within the social care system. How do these differ from their core skills, if at all?

Write a brief paragraph on the benefits of co-producing health and social care services with the local community, using an example of a specific service. What skills do managers need to co-produce services effectively?

Conclusion

Social care is a high-profile area that intersects closely with, yet is distinct from, health systems. While 'care' is organizationally separate from 'cure' in many countries, these continue to be closely interlinked for people who – by virtue of their complex needs – may not distinguish between health and social care. Thinking about how decisions made in health services affect social care and vice versa can help develop deeper understanding of how the two systems interact with one another. Managers need to be skilled to traverse and work within these two systems, understanding how decisions that they make can have wider implications on people's experience of care and the outcomes they achieve.

Across the globe, social care systems are struggling to meet rising demand and maintain service quality. Managers will always be in a vital intermediary position, negotiating the demands of national, regional and local policy and the realities of frontline service delivery. It is all too easy to get overwhelmed by the complexity of social care, characterizing it as a 'problem' that is too complicated to resolve. To counter this sense of gloom, there are areas of hope. Arguably, there is increasing international recognition of the importance of social care for people's lives and wider social cohesion. This has been achieved in no small part by the work of self-advocacy groups campaigning to get their story heard.

Ambitions for social care services are rightly growing; however, the challenge will be how to achieve this vision. Learning from people who draw on support and unpaid carers about what works is a starting point. Understanding how other nations have reformed their social care system and the impact of this on people's experience of services is another avenue to pursue, although social care models may not be transferable depending on a nation's governance structures and cultural context. These actions offer a foundation on which to make the changes needed for a sustainable social care system that emphasizes people's desire for 'a life not a service'.

Learning resources

Organisation for Economic Co-operation and Development (OECD): A membership organization that encourages collaboration to promote economic growth. The OECD holds data on membership states' social care workforce and services and allows for some international comparisons [https://www.oecd-ilibrary.org/social-issues-migration-health/data/oecd-health-statistics/long-term-care-resources-and-utilisation-edition-2022_a11247fc-en].

Eurocarers: A European network of organizations with an interest in unpaid care. This network advocates for unpaid carers, undertaking research and policy work. Eurocarers provides country profiles of the social care system, with a particular interest in unpaid care [https://eurocarers.org/country-profiles/].

European Care Strategy: Presented by the European Commission, it aims to support member states to develop 'high-quality, affordable and accessible care services with better working conditions and work-life balance for carers'. The strategy covers both early childhood education and care (ECEC) and social care [https://ec.europa.eu/social/main.jsp?langId=en&catId=89&furtherNews=yes&newsId=10382#navItem-relatedDocuments].

Continued

Learning resources *Continued*

The European Commission: Has produced a series of profiles on member states' social care systems [https://op.europa.eu/en/publication-detail/-/publication/b39728e3-cd83-11eb-ac72-01aa75ed71a1].

The King's Fund: Works to understand trends, challenges and opportunities in health and social care. Their annual Social care 360 review provides an overview of adult social care trends in England and analysis of a range of data sets [https://www.kingsfund.org.uk/insight-and-analysis/long-reads/social-care-360].

International Journal of Care and Caring: This academic journal has published a special issue that has a number of open access articles exploring experiences and perceptions of unpaid care of older people across countries in Southern Africa, highlighting a range of perspectives on unpaid care [https://bristoluniversitypressdigital.com/view/journals/ijcc/7/2/ijcc.7.issue-2.xml].

Social Care Future: A movement that draws attention to the improvements needed in social care, so that people can live the life that is meaningful to them. Social Care Future wants to reframe how we think about social care, encouraging support for a positive social care future [https://socialcarefuture.org.uk/].

The Nuffield Trust: Aims to improve health and care policy. There are regular blogs and reports on social care [https://www.nuffieldtrust.org.uk/topics/social-care].

The Centre for Care: An Economic and Social Research Council Research Centre that works to develop understanding of care. The Centre produces regular commentaries discussing key issues in care and the latest research findings [https://centreforcare.ac.uk/commentary/].

Social Care Institute for Excellence (SCIE): Works towards the improvement of social care by sharing evidence of what works in practice. Resources are themed, including a section on integrated care and strengths-based approaches [https://www.scie.org.uk/care-themes/].

Improving Adult Care Together (IMPACT): A centre that works to implement evidence on adult social care to facilitate improvements to services and support cultural change [https://impact.bham.ac.uk/].

References

Acco, A. and Mandia, D. (2022) French police raid nursing home group Orpea amid probe over malpractice. Reuters [https://www.reuters.com/business/frances-orpea-reduce-its-international-activities-2022-11-15/; accessed 24 February 2024].

Addati, L., Cattaneo, U., Esquivel, V. and Valarino, I. (2018) Care work and care jobs for the future of decent work. International Labour Organization [http://www.ilo.org/global/publications/books/WCMS_633135/lang--en/index.htm; accessed 24 February 2024].

Booth, R. (2024) Modern slavery in social care surging since visa rules eased, *The Guardian*, 21 January [https://www.theguardian.com/society/2024/jan/21/modern-slavery-in-social-care-surging-since-visa-rules-eased; accessed 24 February 2024].

Bottery, S. and Mallorie, S. (2024) Social Care 360: Workforce and Carers. The King's Fund [https://www.kingsfund.org.uk/insight-and-analysis/long-reads/social-care-360-workforce-carers; accessed 14 May 2024].

Brown, J. (2022) The financialization of senior's housing in Canada. Canada Human Rights Commission [https://www.homelesshub.ca/sites/default/files/attachments/Brown-The-Financialization-of-Seniors-Housing-ofha-en.pdf; accessed 14 May 2024].

Buchanan, M. (2024) Sutton: Three jailed for abusing care home residents with learning disabilities. BBC News [https://www.bbc.com/news/uk-england-london-67884252; accessed 24 February 2024].

Caiels, J., Milne, A. and Beadle-Brown, J. (2021) Strengths-based approaches in social work and social care: reviewing the evidence, *Journal of Long-Term Care*: 401–422. DOI: 10.31389/jltc.102.

Care Act 2014 (2014) [https://www.legislation.gov.uk/ukpga/2014/23/contents; accessed 10 December 2024].

CareShield Life (n.d.) CareShield Life and Long-Term Care Act [https://www.careshieldlife.gov.sg/careshield-life/careshield-life-and-long-term-care-act.html; accessed 14 May 2024].

Care Quality Commission (2022) How CQC identifies and responds to closed cultures [https://www.cqc.org.uk/guidance-providers/all-services/how-cqc-identifies-responds-closed-cultures; accessed 14 May 2024].

Care Quality Commission (2023) Appendix: CQC ratings charts [https://www.cqc.org.uk/publications/major-report/state-care/2022-2023/ratings-charts; accessed 8 March 2024].

Charles, A. (2022) Integrated care systems explained. The King's Fund [https://www.kingsfund.org.uk/insight-and-analysis/long-reads/integrated-care-systems-explained; accessed 8 March 2024].

Cinelli, G. and Fattore, G. (2024) The 2022 community-based integrated care reform in Italy: from desiderata to implementation, *Health Policy*, 139:104943. DOI: 10.1016/j.healthpol.2023.104943.

Crimmins, E.M. (2015) Lifespan and healthspan: past, present, and promise, *The Gerontologist*, 55(6): 901–911. DOI: 10.1093/geront/gnv130.

Curry, N. (2024) Shifting the narrative: building public support for social care reform. Nuffield Trust [https://www.nuffieldtrust.org.uk/news-item/shifting-the-narrative-building-public-support-for-social-care-reform; accessed 26 February 2024].

Curry, N., Castle-Clarke, S. and Hemmings, N. (2018) What can England learn from the long-term care system in Japan? Nuffield Trust [https://www.nuffieldtrust.org.uk/sites/default/files/2018-05/1525856899_learning-from-japan-final.pdf; accessed 14 May 2024].

Curry, N., Schlepper, L. and Hemmings, N. (2019) What can England learn from the long-term care system in Germany? Nuffield Trust [https://www.nuffieldtrust.org.uk/research/what-can-england-learn-from-the-long-term-care-system-in-germany; accessed 14 May 2024].

Daly, M. (2023) Long-term care as a policy issue for the European Union and United Nations organisations, *International Journal of Care and Caring*, Early View. DOI: 10.1332/239788221X16887213701095.

Dukelow, F. and Kennett, P. (2018) Discipline, debt and coercive commodification: post-crisis neoliberalism and the welfare state in Ireland, the UK and the USA, *Critical Social Policy*, 38(3): 482–504. DOI: 10.1177/0261018318762727.

European Commission (2021) Long-term care report. Trends, challenges and opportunities in an ageing society. Vol. 2: Country profiles [https://ec.europa.eu/social/BlobServlet?docId =24080&langId=en; accessed 29 May 2024].

European Commission (2022) European Care Strategy [https://eur-lex.europa.eu/legal-content/EN/TXT/?uri=CELEX%3A52022DC0440; accessed 24 February 2024].

Exley, J., Glover, R., McCarey, M., Reed, S., Ahmed, A., Vrijhoef, H., et al. (2024) Governing integrated health and social care: an analysis of experiences in three European countries, *International Journal of Integrated Care*, 24(1):9. DOI: 10.5334/ijic.7610.

Fabian Society (2023) Support guaranteed: the roadmap to a national care service [https:// fabians.org.uk/wp-content/uploads/2023/06/Fabians-Support-Guaranteed-Report-WEB. pdf; accessed 26 February 2024].

Federal Ministry for Family Affairs, Senior Citizens, Women and Youth (n.d.) Assistance for people in need of longterm care [https://www.serviceportal-zuhause-im-alter.de/english/ programmes/funding/longterm-care.html; accessed 14 May 2024].

Feeley, D. (2021) Independent Review of Adult Social Care in Scotland [https://www.gov. scot/binaries/content/documents/govscot/publications/independent-report/2021/02/ independent-review-adult-social-care-scotland/documents/independent-review-adult-care-scotland/independent-review-adult-care-scotland/govscot%3Adocument/independent-review-adult-care-scotland.pdf; accessed 29 May 2024].

Future Social Care Coalition (2023) Carenomics: unlocking the economic power of care [https://futuresocialcarecoalition.org/wp-content/uploads/2023/09/FSCC-Carenomics-2. pdf; accessed 26 February 2024].

Glasby, J., Litchfield, I., Parkinson, S., Hocking, L. and Tanner, D. (2023) If I knew then what I know now... A short guide to introducing new technology in adult social care [https:// www.birmingham.ac.uk/documents/college-social-sciences/social-policy/brace/ai-and-social-care-booklet-final-digital-accessible.pdf; accessed 14 May 2023].

Goffman, E. (1968) *Asylums: Essays on the Social Situation of Mental Patients and Other Inmates. New impression edition.* London: Penguin Books Ltd.

Government of the Netherlands (2016) Social Support Act (Wmo 2015) – Care and support at home. Ministerie van Algemene Zaken [https://www.government.nl/topics/care-and-support-at-home/social-support-act-wmo; accessed 14 May 2024].

GOV.UK (2023) Understanding the drivers of healthy life expectancy [https://www.gov. uk/government/publications/understanding-the-drivers-of-healthy-life-expectancy/ understanding-the-drivers-of-healthy-life-expectancy-report; accessed 14 May 2024].

Greenhalgh, T., Wherton, J., Papoutsi, C., Lynch, J., Hughes, G., A'Court, C., et al. (2017) Beyond adoption: a new framework for theorizing and evaluating nonadoption, abandonment, and challenges to the scale-up, spread, and sustainability of health and care technologies, *Journal of Medical Internet Research*, 19(11):e367. (DOI: 10.2196/ jmir.8775).

Handbook Germany (n.d.) Home care [https://handbookgermany.de/en/home-care; accessed 14 May 2024].

Heslop, P., Byrne, V., Calkin, R., Pollard, J., Sullivan, B., Daly, P., et al. (2021) The Learning Disabilities Mortality Review (LeDeR) Programme Annual Report 2020 [https://leder.nhs.uk/images/annual_reports/LeDeR-bristol-annual-report-2020.pdf; accessed 10 December 2024].

Hide, L. (2021) Mental hospitals, social exclusion and public scandals, in G. Ikkos and N. Bouras (eds) *Mind, State and Society: Social History of Psychiatry and Mental Health in Britain 1960–2010*. Cambridge: Cambridge University Press. DOI: 10.1017/9781911623793.009.

Hoppania, H-K., Karsio, O., Näre, L., Vaittinen, T. and Zechner, M. (2024) Financialization of eldercare in a nordic welfare state, *Journal of Social Policy*, 53(1):26–44. DOI: 10.1017/S0047279422000137.

Horton, A. (2022) Financialization and non-disposable women: real estate, debt and labour in UK care homes, *Journals Environment and Planning A: Economy and Space*, 54(1):144–159. DOI: 10.1177/0308518X19862580.

Humphries, R. (2022) *Ending the Social Care Crisis: A New Road to Reform*. Bristol: Policy Press.

IMPACT (2023) How to embed asset-based approaches in health and social care: Integration across public and community sectors [https://impact.bham.ac.uk/wp-content/uploads/2023/12/Asset-Based-Approaches-report.pdf; accessed 14 May 2024].

Integration of Primary and Community Care Committee (2023) Patients at the centre: Integrating primary and community care. Report of Session 2023–24. House of Lords. [https://committees.parliament.uk/publications/42610/documents/211770/default/; accessed 8 March 2024].

Jarrett, T. (2019) Four Seasons Health Care Group – financial difficulties and safeguards for clients. Briefing paper number 8004. House of Commons Library [https://researchbriefings.files.parliament.uk/documents/CBP-8004/CBP-8004.pdf; accessed 23 February 2024].

Kelly, D. and Kennedy, J. (2017) Power to people [https://www.health-ni.gov.uk/sites/default/files/publications/health/power-to-people-full-report.PDF; accessed 29 May 2024].

Litchfield, I., Glasby, J., Parkinson, S., Hocking, L., Tanner, D., Roe, B., et al. (2023) 'Trying to find people to fit the tech...': A qualitative exploration of the lessons learnt introducing artificial intelligence-based technology into English social care, *Health & Social Care in the Community*, 2023(9174873). DOI: 10.1155/2023/9174873.

Lunt, N., Bainbridge, L. and Rippon, S. (2021) Strengths, assets and place – The emergence of local area coordination initiatives in England and Wales, *Journal of Social Work*, 21(5):1041–1064. DOI: 10.1177/1468017320918174.

Mercer, P. (2018) Australia's elder abuse scandal 'beyond belief', BBC News [https://www.bbc.com/news/world-australia-45543804; accessed 24 February 2024].

Mercille, J. (2024) European long-term care marketisation: a political economy framework, *Social Policy & Administration*, [Online.] DOI: 10.1111/spol.13013.

Mooten, N. (2021) Racism, discrimination and migrant workers in Canada: Evidence from the literature [https://www.canada.ca/content/dam/ircc/documents/pdf/english/corporate/reports-statistics/research/racism/r8-2020-racism-eng.pdf; accessed 8 March 2024].

Morton, L., Ferguson, M. and Baty, F. (2015) Improving wellbeing and self-efficacy by social prescription, *Public Health*, 129(3):286–9. DOI: 10.1016/j.puhe.2014.12.011.

Murphy, G. (2020) CQC inspections and regulation of Whorlton Hall: second independent report. Care Quality Commission [https://www.cqc.org.uk/sites/default/files/20201215_glynis-murphy-review_second-report.pdf; accessed 24 February 2024].

National Disability Insurance Scheme (2024) What is the NDIS? [https://www.ndis.gov.au/understanding/what-ndis; accessed 14 May 2024].

Needham, C. and Mangan, C. (2014) The 21st Century Public Servant [https://21stcenturypublicservant.wordpress.com/wp-content/uploads/2014/09/21-century-report-281014.pdf; accessed 29 May 2024].

Needham, C., Mangan, C., McKenna, D. and Lowther, J. (2024) The 21st Century Public Servant [https://21stcenturypublicservant.wordpress.com/wp-content/uploads/2024/11/full-report-revisiting-the-21st-century-public-servant.pdf; accessed 30 September 2024].

NHS England (2023) Health Survey for England, 2021 part 2 [https://digital.nhs.uk/data-and-information/publications/statistical/health-survey-for-england/2021-part-2/social-care; accessed 10 December 2024].

Nies, H., Stekelenburg, D., Minkman, M. and Huijsman, R. (2021) A decade of lessons learned from integration strategies in the Netherlands, *International Journal of Integrated Care*, 21(4):15. DOI: 10.5334/ijic.5703.

OECD (2021) Health at a Glance 2021: OECD Indicators. OECD. https://doi.org/10.1787/ae3016b9-en.

OECD (2024) Life expectancy at birth (indicator) [http://data.oecd.org/healthstat/life-expectancy-at-birth.htm; accessed 24 February 2024].

Office for Health Improvement and Disparities (2023) Research and analysis. Premature mortality in adults with severe mental illness (SMI) [https://www.gov.uk/government/publications/premature-mortality-in-adults-with-severe-mental-illness/premature-mortality-in-adults-with-severe-mental-illness-smi; accessed 29 May 2024].

Office for Seniors (2022) Homeshare: An option to facilitate older homeowners to age in place report [https://officeforseniors.govt.nz/assets/Homeshare-an-option-to-facilitate-older-homeowners-to-age-in-place-report.pdf; accessed 26 February 2024].

Oliver, M. (2013) The social model of disability: thirty years on, *Disability & Society*, 28(7): 1024–1026. DOI: 10.1080/09687599.2013.818773.

Pedersen, K., Mancini, M., Common, D. and Wolfe-Wylie, W. (2020) 85% of Ontario nursing homes break the law repeatedly with almost no consequences, data analysis shows. CBC [https://www.cbc.ca/news/marketplace/nursing-homes-abuse-ontario-seniors-laws-1.5770889; accessed 24 February 2024].

Petrillo, M. and Bennett, M. (2023) Valuing Carers 2021: England and Wales [https://centreforcare.ac.uk/wp-content/uploads/2023/05/Valuing_Carers_WEB2.pdf; accessed 29 May 2024].

Plsek, P. E. and Greenhalgh, T. (2001) The challenge of complexity in health care, *The BMJ*, 323: 625–8. DOI: 10.1136/bmj.323.7313.625.

Prasad, G. (2019) Supported independent living: Communal and intergenerational living in the Netherlands and Denmark [https://www.housinglin.org.uk/_assets/Resources/Housing/OtherOrganisation/Supported-Independent-Living-Communal-and-intergenerational-living-in-the-Netherlands-and-Denmark.pdf; accessed 14 May 2024].

Razavi, S. (2007) The political and social economy of care in a development context: Conceptual issues, research questions and policy options. United Nations Research Institute for

Social Development [https://cdn.unrisd.org/assets/library/papers/pdf-files/razavi-paper.pdf; accessed 23 February 2024].

Reed, S., Oung, C., Davies, J., Dayan, M. and Scobie, S. (2021) Integrating health and social care: A comparison of policy and progress across the four countries of the UK. Nuffield Trust [https://www.nuffieldtrust.org.uk/sites/default/files/2021-12/integrated-care-web.pdf; accessed 8 March 2024].

Rowland, D. (2019) Corporate care home collapse and 'light touch' regulation: a repeating cycle of failure, *British Politics and Policy at LSE*, 8 May [https://blogs.lse.ac.uk/politicsandpolicy/corporate-care-homes/; accessed 24 February 2024].

Royal Commission: Aged Care Quality and Safety (2021) Final Report [https://www.royalcommission.gov.au/aged-care/final-report; accessed 16 May 2024].

Saville-Smith, K., James, B. and Bawden, M. (2019) Provision of residential care and occupation right agreements by retirement village operators [https://assets.retirement.govt.nz/public/Uploads/Monitoring-and-Reports/56439919cd/Interface-Retirement-Villages-Aged-Care-Findings-Report-Final-22-June.pdf; accessed 14 May 2024].

Scheil-Adlung, X. (2015) Long-term care protection for older persons: A review of coverage deficits in 46 countries. Working Paper No. 50. International Labour Organization. [https://www.ilo.org/public/libdoc/ilo/2015/115B09_148_engl.pdf; accessed 24 February 2024].

Scottish Government (n.d.) National Care Service [http://www.gov.scot/collections/national-care-service/; accessed 26 February 2024).

Shared Lives (2024) Shared Lives Plus. Homepage [https://sharedlivesplus.org.uk/; accessed 29 May 2024].

Shortell, S., Addicott, R., Walsh, N. and Ham, C. (2014) Accountable care organisations in the United States and England. Testing, evaluating and learning what works. The King's Fund. [https://assets.kingsfund.org.uk/f/256914/x/74b750cdcd/accountable_care_organisations_us_and_england_2014.pdf; accessed 29 May 2024].

Social Care Future (2024) Living good lives in the place we call home - An outline programme for the next government [https://socialcarefuture.org.uk/noticeboard/living-good-lives-in-the-place-we-call-home-an-outline-programme-for-the-next-government/; accessed 8 March 2024].

Social Care Institute for Excellence (n.d.) Alternative models of housing with care and support [https://www.scie.org.uk/housing/role-of-housing/promising-practice/models/alternative-model/; accessed 29 May 2024].

Stephens, L., Ryan-Collins, J. and Boyle, D. (2008) Co-production: A manifesto for growing the core economy, New Economics Foundation [https://neweconomics.org/uploads/files/5abec531b2a775dc8d_qjm6bqzpt.pdf; accessed 6 March 2024].

The Brussels Times (2023) Ten care homes across Belgium to close over financial difficulties, *The Brussels Times* Newsroom, 17 February [https://www.brusselstimes.com/373847/ten-care-homes-across-belgium-to-be-closed-over-financial-difficulties; accessed 29 May 2024].

The Health Foundation (2019) Whorlton Hall abuse scandal. Policy navigator [https://navigator.health.org.uk/theme/whorlton-hall-abuse-scandal; accessed 24 February 2024].

The King's Fund (2023) Key facts and figures about adult social care [https://www.kingsfund.org.uk/insight-and-analysis/data-and-charts/key-facts-figures-adult-social-care; accessed 24 February 2024].

Theobald, H. and Luppi, M. (2018) Elderly care in changing societies: concurrences in divergent care regimes – a comparison of Germany, Sweden and Italy, *Current Sociology*, 66(4): 629–642. DOI: 10.1177/0011392118765232.

Think Local Act Personal (2018) TLAP 'I' statements from Making It Real 2018 Local Government Association [http://www.local.gov.uk/our-support/partners-care-and-health/care-and-health-improvement/autistic-and-learning-disabilities/learning-disabilities/better-lives/tlap-i-statements-making-it-real-2018; accessed 3 January 2024].

Tingvold L. and Olsvold N. (2023) Configurations of care work: fragile partnerships in the co-production of long-term care services, *Societies*, 13(11): 234. DOI: 10.3390/soc13110234.

Travers, M., Liu, E., Cook, P., Osborne, C., Jacobs, K., Aminpour, F., et al. (2022) Business models, consumer experiences and regulation of retirement villages [http://www.ahuri.edu.au/research/final-reports/392; accessed 14 May 2024].

UN Women (2017) Long-term care for older people: A new global gender priority. Policy brief no. 9 [https://www.unwomen.org/sites/default/files/Headquarters/Attachments/Sections/Library/Publications/2017/UN-Women-Policy-Brief-09-Long-term-care-for-older-people-en.pdf; accessed 24 February 2024].

Welsh Government (2019) Social Services and Well-being (Wales) Act 2014: Code of practice in relation to the performance and improvement of social services [https://gov.wales/sites/default/files/consultations/2019-05/code-of-practice.pdf; accessed 29 May 2024].

Welsh Government (2022) Towards a national care and support service for Wales [https://www.gov.wales/establishing-national-care-and-support-service; accessed 26 February 2024].

Whitfield, G. and Hamblin, K. (2022) Technology in social care: spotlight on the English policy landscape, 2019–2022. Centre for Care Working Paper 1 [https://centreforcare.ac.uk/wp-content/uploads/2022/12/Technology-in-social-care-report-Dec-2022_FINAL.pdf; accessed 24 February 2024].

World Health Organization (2022) World mental health report: Transforming mental health for all. [https://iris.who.int/bitstream/handle/10665/356119/9789240049338-eng.pdf?sequence=1; accessed 14 May 2024].

Wright, J. (2023) *Robots Won't Save Japan: An Ethnography of Eldercare Automation*. Ithaca, New York: ILR Press.

Zhang, Y., Bennett, M.R. and Yeandle, S. (2019) Will I Care? The likelihood of being a carer in adult life. Carers UK [https://www.carersuk.org/reports/will-i-care-the-likelihood-of-being-a-carer-in-adult-life/; accessed 24 February 2024].

Zigante, V. and King, D. (2019) Quality assurance practices in long-term care in Europe: emerging evidence on care market management. European Commission [https://data.europa.eu/doi/10.2767/167648; accessed 24 February 2024].

Informatics for healthcare systems

Paul Taylor

Introduction

Health informatics is the study of how information and information technology can be applied to improve the effectiveness of healthcare services. This chapter looks at the key challenges in health informatics from the perspective of a healthcare manager. It considers how information is created, stored, analysed and applied in looking after patients and managing organizations. Some of the different kinds of systems used in healthcare organizations are described and some of the technical challenges identified. The promise and challenges affecting the adoption of new technologies are described.

The information cycle

The key aim in informatics is to improve our capacity to use data. This is partly about being better able to record and access data about the patients we are treating, and partly about learning from it to improve the treatments and services we offer future patients. In informatics we often talk about the data cycle, about how data are (1) stored and retrieved (2) analysed and interpreted and (3) used to drive improvements. We can use this three-arc cycle to look at the use of data at different levels: within a clinical service; in the management of individual patients; within a healthcare organization, such as an NHS trust or GP practice; and across the whole of a comprehensive system, such as the NHS.

Use of data in the management of individual patients

Consider the example of a patient who reads in her newspaper about the risks of osteoporosis in her age group and decides to visit her GP and ask advice. The GP will need to assess the risk of osteoporosis in this patient based on information about her history and exposure to key risk factors. Traditionally this would have been a subjective assessment of the woman's risk, but now it could be based on a quantitative calculation using an online calculator (Schini et al., 2024). The GP can then compare the risk with guidelines and, if appropriate, order a test, for example, a DEXA scan to measure the patient's bone density.

This scenario involves two complex computations: the risk calculator and the DEXA scan. The risk calculation involves an equation that was derived from an analysis of data on risk factors and outcomes from a large population of patients. A DEXA scan exploits the fact that the proportion of X-rays absorbed by a given tissue type is a function of the energy of X-rays. Hence, if we can assume a simple mix of tissue types, a comparison of X-rays taken at two different energies allows an estimate of the proportion of bone in each cross-section, and hence a quantitative measure of bone health. These applications are good examples of 'high tech' medicine, but computer systems would also be used in the booking of the appointments and the transmission of the test results. One of the key lessons of health informatics is that the computerization of simple administrative systems is often harder to achieve than the programming of apparently more sophisticated analytical tools. These applications can also lead to a greater transformation in patient experience and outcomes (see Box 18.1).

Box 18.1   Case study – using AI in breast cancer screening

In 2016 Geoffrey Hinton, probably the most influential researcher in artificial intelligence (AI) of the last 30 years, suggested it was no longer worth training radiologists, since within 5 years AI would be able to interpret medical images. He now admits that he was wrong. Although 531 of the 692 AI systems that had been approved by the US Food and Drug Administration (FDA) for medical use by October 2023 were for applications in radiology, www.radworking.com, a US job board for the specialty, was listing 470 vacancies for physician roles in spring 2024.

It is not that progress in AI has been slower than Hinton expected, but that it has proved difficult for innovators and entrepreneurs to identify viable business models for the application of AI to radiology, pass the necessary regulatory hurdles and bring products to market. One challenge is that, in the UK, regulations governing the use of ionizing radiation require that radiology exams are reviewed by a qualified professional, which makes it hard for an AI tool to deliver cost-savings.

One approach has been to build tools that identify those chest X-rays that contain cancer and select a proportion to be fast-tracked for further investigation (e.g. CT scans) without the need for human interpretation (Tam et al., 2021). This potentially speeds up the diagnostic process since the CT scan can be scheduled before the patient has left the hospital, so it offers a clinical benefit, but a marginal one in terms of mortality and not an obvious cost saving. Another is to identify a proportion of chest X-rays that do not contain cancer, and which do not need to be reviewed at the hospital, although the current regulatory constraints mean that these will still be reviewed, perhaps by radiologists employed elsewhere, which again limits the cost saving that can be generated (Dyer et al., 2021).

Kheiron Medical has taken a different approach, building software to identify cancer on mammograms. These images are traditionally reviewed by two human film readers; since individual readers spot different abnormalities, additional reviews can increase sensitivity and improve cost-effectiveness. Replacing one of the readers will generate savings so long as the algorithm can match human performance. A recent retrospective study using 10 years' worth of data showed that replacing one of the human readers with Kheiron Medical's tool would have detected approximately the same number of cancers while recalling fewer women. Since the tool referred more women for arbitration (the process of resolving differences in interpretation between readers) the workload would have been reduced by between 30 per cent and 44 per cent rather than halved, but the scope for savings should be sufficient to build a business case (Sharma et al., 2021).

Use of data in running a healthcare service

Running a clinic or service efficiently is partly about ensuring that the service can meet demand. The better we can predict demand, the easier it is to ensure the required capacity is available. Demand for beds can be predicted from an assessment of the number of people currently in the hospital combined with an estimate of the number of people likely to require admission and the number likely to be discharged. The estimate of likely admissions will be based on what time of year it is, what day of the week it is and other information. Researchers are increasingly looking at how we can improve our estimates of demand based on fine-grained information about patients, for example, estimating how likely it is that a patient currently in the Accident and Emergency department will need to be admitted (King et al., 2022).

Decisions about how much capacity to provide require an assessment of the likely demand as well as the costs of spare capacity and the consequences of failing to meet demand. The mathematics of queuing theory, which is the study of systems where the service users arrive at variable rates and impose variable demands on the system, can help understand how systems behave in different situations. A good rule of thumb is that once the amount of spare capacity falls below 15 per cent, then the likelihood that the service will be overwhelmed rapidly increases (Proudlove, 2020).

Use of data across a healthcare system

It is increasingly easy to collect, analyse and disseminate data, with the result that senior managers sometimes describe themselves as drowning in data. What, then, is the really important data when it comes to running a national service like the NHS? One key distinction is between measures of process and measures of outcome. Clearly measures of outcome are of greater intrinsic interest since the clinical outcomes of a stay in hospital are the real reason for the hospital visit. A distinction is sometimes made between two classes of measures of outcome, those in which the outcome is assessed by the physician, which would be the traditional approach, and those in which it is assessed by the patient. In England, patient reported outcome measures (PROMs) have been recorded since 2009 for a range of surgical procedures, driven by government policy, as a way for the public to compare providers' performance (Kyte et al., 2016).

Relying on measures of outcome is problematic. One unambiguous and unignorable outcome is mortality, but this has the flaw, when it comes to assessing quality of care, of being relatively rare. Worse, when it does occur it is often inevitable, and it is only avoidable deaths that can serve as a measure of how well or poorly a hospital is performing. Nevertheless, there has been a great deal of attention paid to the use of adjusted mortality as a way of detecting failing hospitals (Taylor, 2013). Measures of process have less intrinsic interest than measures of outcome but may provide a more direct assessment of what is happening. In England, key measures of process (percentage of patients waiting for more than four hours in the A&E department, percentage of patients waiting 18 weeks for treatment) are used to assess performance and have, at times, assumed sufficient importance for some to claim that clinical priorities are distorted to meet targets (Mason et al., 2012).

Whether we are looking at the care of individual patients, the running of clinical services or the management of the healthcare system as a whole, there are challenges in how we improve the recording of data, how we turn data into knowledge and how we improve access to knowledge. In the next three sections we review each of these.

Learning activity 18.1

Reflect on a challenge that you face as a manager, on a difficult decision that you have to make in allocating resources within your organization. What information is available to you to help make this decision?

Now think about how that information is collected. Is there a possibility that the data might be biased in some way? Is there some systematic effect whereby in certain circumstances data might not be collected or could be entered erroneously?

What practical steps could you take to improve the accuracy and completeness of the data on which you rely?

Improving the recording of data

A key goal for research in health informatics has been to support the development of electronic healthcare records that store information acquired by clinicians, as explained shortly. Increasingly the recording of patient data also involves the acquisition of data directly from patients, as described in the final part of this section.

The development of electronic health records

The computerization of clinical systems means that medical data is increasingly stored digitally in electronic health records (EHRs). This has benefits that relate to the physical disadvantages of paper. However, simply replacing paper storage with some form of electronic storage is not adequate to achieve the important benefits that can accrue from making the data computable. For this we need to be able to extract the essential meaning from the record of each clinical encounter in a form that allows us to aggregate information across episodes, throughout populations and in different organizations. This, inevitably, requires imposing some kind of discipline on how information is recorded, constraining the clinician who previously was able to use free text to record whatever seemed relevant or important in any way that allowed the efficient transfer of information between colleagues. There are two ways in which this happens: one is to impose a structure on how data is recorded, in effect forcing the clinician to use some kind of form or template; the other is to restrict the clinician to using some set of standard terms These are discussed in the next two sections.

Standards and interoperability; technical challenges in integrating systems

A large and complex hospital will contain many, possibly hundreds, of different computer systems that need to be able to exchange information if the hospital is to function efficiently. Increasingly, patients with serious conditions are cared for under collaborative arrangements, which means that the requirement for interoperability extends to systems in different hospitals and other care organizations. A precondition of this interoperability is standardization. For systems to work together, the implementors have to agree to define, at some level, how information is represented, so that it is mutually intelligible. The agreement and emergence of standards is a universal problem in a digital economy, and a complex one that requires a degree of cooperation between organizations that are commercial competitors.

In the healthcare IT sector, there has been a multiplicity of attempts to define standards to allow the better integration of healthcare systems. Some of these have been highly successful. DICOM®, for example, is the standard for medical imaging (Pianykh, 2012). It defines an image format, just as a JPG does, but also a messaging standard that allows different image acquisition and display devices in a radiology department to work together seamlessly. HL7 FHIR defines a messaging standard for the exchange of information, such as test results, but also billing information (Bender and Sartipi, 2013). There are other standards that allow for the exchange of medical documents with a degree of structure (HL7 Clinical Document Architecture, IHE Cross Enterprise Document Sharing or XDS).

Increasingly, hospitals are finding that the best way to ensure that the systems used by the different departments within the organization work efficiently together is to buy a comprehensive system that will meet or almost meet all of their requirements. These systems are incredibly expensive and their implementation in a trust requires top to bottom organizational change and has often proved traumatic; after the Addenbrookes NHS Trust in Cambridge implemented Epic, the Care Quality Commission found that services were so disrupted the trust was placed in special measures. Another difficulty is that the UK market for such systems has become dominated by a very small number of US suppliers, with Epic being predominant.

A more ambitious approach to securing interoperability has been to define a language and a set of open-source tools that allow clinicians to share definitions of the kind of information required for a particular clinical application. The openEHR initiative allows for the definition of what are known as archetypes, structured descriptions of the data fields and the data types that would be expected to be recorded as part of, for example, a blood pressure measurement (Heard and Beale, n.d.).

Controlled clinical terminologies

There are a variety of controlled clinical terminologies in use, with different applications. The two most important ones for most readers of this book will be the International Classification of Diseases (ICD) and the Systematics Nomenclature of Medicine or SNOMED. ICD is sponsored by the World Health Organization and provides a structured list of diagnosis codes, each with a succinct definition and an explicit list of inclusion and exclusion criteria for all diagnoses, grouped into a small set of broad categories known as chapters. ICD predates the world of computers and has an important history as an aid to statisticians attempting to standardize the recording of diseases, and especially of causes of death. SNOMED, in contrast, is very much the child of the computer age and was developed to provide a complete terminology covering everything that might be recorded on the computer record. It has a more flexible organization than ICD, terms are grouped into multiple hierarchies and although, in theory, each term is defined using an underlying logic, in practice both the meaning of the terms and the organization of the terminology is confusing. SNOMED is a vast and contentious undertaking which, despite widespread international support, has not become a ubiquitous standard (Spackman et al., 1997).

Personal health data

Traditionally, research in health informatics has focused on the systems used by clinicians to record data about their patients. Increasingly, however, patients and members of the public have access to other systems for recording information relevant to their health. This is in part due to the growing market for consumer products, such as Fitbits and exercise bands, and in part due to the increasing viability of patient self-testing in the monitoring of long-term conditions, such as diabetes and hypertension.

There is also a trend towards personal health records. In many countries there is a multiplicity of health providers and patients may contract with a variety of organizations; in such an environment it can make sense for the patient to contract with an appropriate service provider to host an integrated record that is controlled by the patient: a personal health record. The primary market for such services is the US, and the rationale is weaker in a setting such as the UK where most healthcare is provided by the NHS. Nevertheless, patients increasingly expect access to their records and that those records should have features of personal health records, allowing them to upload data about their health, for example.

Turning data into knowledge

This section deals with how we analyse data to obtain new insights. A complete account would deal with every aspect of medical research, including clinical trials and epidemiological surveys. So construed, the topic is too vast to be dealt with in a chapter like this. Instead, this section focuses on two approaches to the analysis of data that are commonly used in health informatics and are directly applicable in health service management, and raise some important issues that affect how data are used to generate new information. Issues around the use of patient data for research are considered in Box 18.2.

Box 18.2   Case study – linked data sets

Patient data is a valuable resource. A variety of NHS and government bodies mandate the collection of data for administrative and other purposes. Other organizations, including universities and private companies, compete to get the best possible data for their research. The result is a complex arrangement of dataflows (Zhang et al., 2023). Much research in healthcare is now carried out using very large collections of linked data. These can be enormously valuable, especially if the datasets are large and combine information about patients' exposure to risk factors with information about their later health outcomes, for example, if they link GP records with hospital records. One such dataset is Clinical Practice Research Datalink or CPRD. It will supply data, for a substantial fee, to researchers whose proposals must pass a strict test of scientific merit as well as reaching appropriate ethical standards. Commercial organizations can apply but will only be considered if their research is deemed to be in the public interest. CPRD holds GP records for more than 20 million patients, from more than 800 GP practices in the UK. The data, which is uploaded automatically from the IT systems used by participating GPs, includes everything these GPs record about their patients: diagnoses, hospital referrals, prescriptions, vaccinations, test results, whether they smoke, how much they drink. All this information is added to the database without the patient's consent. That may seem at odds with a patient's rights. The legal and ethical justification is not based on the value of the resource or the science it enables, but on the idea that since the data is anonymized, the patient no longer has any rights over it.

This is a problem because, if the data is rich enough, patients can often be identified even after the most obvious identifying labels have been removed. In 2011 you could buy anonymized data on all 648,384 hospitalizations in Washington State. A privacy researcher was able to find 81 news stories published in the state that year containing the word 'hospitalization'. In 35 of them a single individual whose record featured in the hospital data could be confidently identified as the person named in a news report. In ten of these cases there were references in the hospital data to potentially sensitive information not revealed in the news story (Sweeney, 2013).

In practice, the only way to protect privacy and confidentiality is to ensure that these collections are only made available to approved researchers in controlled environments. This is awkward because it means that people have to trust that researchers will treat the data with respect, but the general public knows much less about research than it does about, say, healthcare, and confidence is easily lost. At the time of writing the NHS is awarding the contract for a federated data platform, which would support mainly operational rather than research uses, to Palantir, a controversial company; this has led privacy campaigners to urge that patients should exercise their right to have their data removed from the system.

Risk prediction

One obvious example of how we turn data into knowledge is when we use data to generate a rule or an equation that we can use to predict outcomes in the future (see Box 18.3). A well-known technique for this is regression, which is used to derive an equation from a set of data points for which we have values for the dependent variable (the thing we are trying to predict) and values for the independent variable (the thing we are using to do the predicting). If there are multiple 'predictor variables', the approach is called multiple regression. If the output is a binary classification (e.g. high-risk patient or not), the approach involves multiple logistic regression. The term logistic refers to the use of the logit function, a mathematical manoeuvre that allows us to adapt the world of probabilities (which lie between the bounds of 0 and 1) to the maths of regression (where numbers can range up and down to infinities).

One application that has received a consistent level of attention is predicting hospital admissions, specifically, looking at the readmission of patients who were admitted as emergencies (Kansagara et al., 2011). The most obvious goal of this research is to identify patients who would benefit most from 'care transition interventions', that is to say who could receive some additional care after discharge which, if sufficiently well-targeted and sufficiently effective, could improve patients' health and well-being and generate savings for the system by preventing future hospital admissions. The aim of this kind of mathematical analysis applied to healthcare is often to devise a new test that will identify a subgroup for whom some intervention will prove cost-effective. The approach is often to take a set of historical data and divide it into two sets: the training set and the test set. Each set must include a set of 'input variables' and at least one 'output' or 'outcome variable'. Essentially the task is to use the training set to explore the influence that the input variables have on the outcome to derive a prediction rule and then to test the prediction rule by applying it to the input variables in the test set and seeing if the outcome generated matches the outcome recorded in the data.

Box 18.3   Case study – mathematical modelling and the pandemic response

On 12 March 2020, the UK government announced that although other countries had locked down, due to the COVID-19 pandemic, the UK would not. But things quickly changed. Schools were closed on 18 March, pubs and restaurants on the 20th. A lockdown was announced on the 23rd. The changes were forced by a combination of empirical evidence of how the disease had already taken hold and by mathematical modelling, including a model developed by a team at the London School of Hygiene and Tropical Medicine (LSHTM) (Davies et al., 2020).

You can build a simple mathematical model of an epidemic in a spreadsheet, using three columns to represent the Susceptible, the Infectious and the Recovered (SIR) (see Figure 18.1). The number of people moved from the Susceptible to the Infectious group each day is the average number of contacts each individual has, multiplied by both

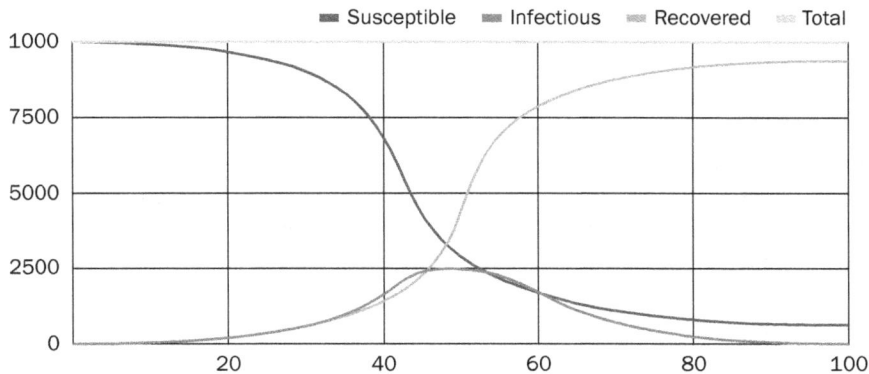

Figure 18.1 A mathematical model of an epidemic showing how the proportions of individuals that are susceptible, infectious or recovered change over time

the likelihood that a contact is with an infectious person and the likelihood that such contacts will lead to infection. The number moved from Infectious to Recovered is the number of infectious individuals multiplied by the average rate of recovery.

The graph above starts with 9999 susceptible people and one infectious person (Taylor, 2020). The number of contacts per person per day is 13 and the probability of a contact resulting in disease transmission is 3 per cent. Fifteen per cent of the infectious population recover each day. Dividing the product of the first two numbers by the third gives R0, the expected number of transmissions from a single case, 13 x 3 ÷ 15, or 2.6. When everyone is susceptible, each infectious person will infect, on average, 2.6 others, leading to an exponential increase until the supply of non-infectious people begins to run out. The model used by the LSHTM is superficially similar to this simple model. Susceptible people pass through a latent phase between becoming infected and being infectious, and then either have a mild subclinical version of the disease, or a more serious illness with both a preclinical phase and a clinical phase requiring a stay in hospital.

In the absence of treatments or vaccines only one of the parameters in an SIR model – the average number of contacts per person per day – can be manipulated to alter the course of a pandemic. In the LSHTM model the average number of contacts was calculated for every five-year age band in each county, by combining data on the proportion of people in each age band with survey data. The model predicted that, if nothing were done to mitigate the effects of the epidemic in the UK, 85 per cent of the population would be infected, there would be 24 million clinical cases and 370,000 deaths. At its peak, 220,000 ICU beds would be required. In February 2020 there were 4122 adult ICU beds open in England. The effects of different policies – school closures, social distancing, shielding of the elderly and self-isolation of symptomatic individuals, and of combinations of them – were simulated by adjusting the average number of contacts. The most effective single strategy, shielding the elderly, still resulted in 220,000 deaths and a need for 120,000 ICU beds.

Statistical process control

Often, we use statistics to test a hypothesis about two sets of measurements, for example, between two kinds of hospitals, one employing a particular technique that is not favoured in the others. The conventional approach to analysing such data is to see it as a test of a 'null hypothesis', which, in this case, would be that there is no difference between the two sets of measurements. If the null hypothesis is true then the data from the two groups are treated as coming from the same distribution, they should cluster around a single mean; if not then we would expect to see two distributions, perhaps overlapping but with a separation between the means. Analysis of the variation in the data can reveal the likelihood that the null hypothesis is false.

But what if we are not running a trial and we do not have a hypothesis that we wish to test? What if we are simply trying to analyse the variation to see what, if anything, needs to be done to improve quality or maintain patient safety? One approach, known as statistical process control (SPC), is to attempt to distinguish 'common cause' from 'special cause' variation (Benneyan et al., 2003). The idea is to measure the variation within a sample and identify cases where the variation seems sufficiently extreme to warrant attention. To test for 'special cause variation' we must first decide what proportion of the distribution counts as extreme, how far along either extremity to set the threshold so that a data point lying beyond the threshold is said to be 'special cause variation' and therefore worthy of investigation. We generally measure variation in units known as standard deviations. In SPC, the threshold on variation is conventionally set at three standard deviations from the mean. At this threshold 0.27 per cent of plotted data can be expected to fall in the extremities. Hence a typical plot, which might contain 30 or so points, will very rarely contain a point in the extremity, unless it is there because the data item at that point is not part of the same distribution as the other items, i.e. it reflects some 'special cause variation'.

The basic analytical tool in SPC is a graphical device called the control chart. The technique is commonly used to look for fluctuations in measurements taken of a process at different points in time. The measurements are plotted, with the measured value on the y-axis and time point of the measurement on the x-axis. The quality of the process is assessed by looking for special cause variation. The task can be made easier by superimposing on the plot a solid line to indicate the mean and dotted lines at three standard deviations above and below the mean, these two thresholds are referred to in SPC as the upper and lower control limits (see Figure 18.2).

SPC was developed in the 1920s and first used to study processes in manufacturing. SPC has now been applied by a variety of agencies and teams with an interest in quality to a range of problems in healthcare, including, controversially, looking for GPs or GP practices with unusually high death rates. British GP Harold Shipman was convicted of murdering 15 of his elderly patients but is believed to have killed many more, perhaps as many as 250 (Smith, 2004). It seems unbelievable that murder on such a scale could go undetected. (Mohammed et al., 2001) argue that Shipman did stray outside SPC control limits derived from the district where he worked with their analysis suggesting 'special cause variation' in 1993, 1995, 1996, 1997 and 1998. The difficulty in using SPC as a kind of screening test, however, is that since there are 9,000 practices in England, every year 45 would be in the top 0.5 per cent of the distribution and would come under investigation.

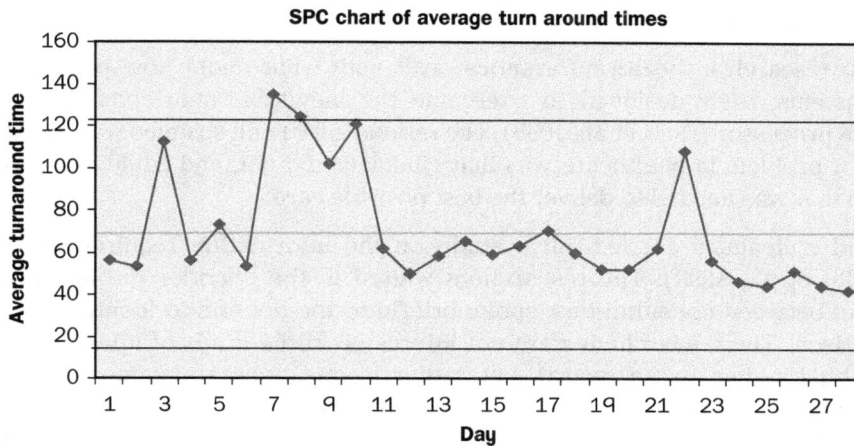

Figure 18.2 A control chart showing mean turnaround times for pathology tests over a 28-day period (Taylor, 2006). The data show the spread of the points around a mean, drawn in grey. The dark horizontal lines indicate the upper and lower control lines. Two data points, days 7 and 8, are above the upper control limit and suggest special cause variation.

Learning activity 18.2

Consider a measure that is collected repeatedly in your organization, something that is measured every day, or every week or every month. How is this information used? Could it be used to assess whether initiatives aimed at improving services are having an effect? Or could the measure be used to monitor a critical process and identify potential problems at an early stage?

It is worth thinking about what comparisons are being made. It is often the case that a current number is simply compared, informally, to a previous number, one that was obtained last month or last year. Have a look at the material on the SPC – multiple chart tool available here [https://www.england.nhs.uk/statistical-process-control-multiple-chart-tool/] and consider whether SPC is an appropriate technique for looking at variation over time.

Applying insights to drive improvements

The third arc in the data cycle, after the recording and analysis of patient data, deals with how the results of the analysis can be applied to improve the delivery of healthcare. Improved access to information can be used to drive improvements in clinical outcomes through improved clinical decision-making, improved management decision-making and better health behaviour.

Improving clinical decision-making

Much early research in health informatics dealt with what might now be called decision support systems, tools designed to overcome the inevitable shortcomings of a human information processor (Hunt et al., 1998). The rationale for such systems was the assumption that a major problem in healthcare was that clinicians did not, and could not, retain all the knowledge that was needed to deliver the best possible care.

Ely and colleagues carried out a study on the information requirements of family doctors (Ely et al., 1999). The researchers waited in the corridor during consultations and then, in between consultations, spoke briefly to the doctors to identify the questions that had arisen. The researchers were not interested in the kinds of question that can be answered by looking at the record, but rather in questions about medical knowledge: 'what is the name of this kind of rash?', 'what is the right dose for this drug?' The doctors generated 1101 questions during the study, an average of 0.32 questions per patient. Of these, 702 (64 per cent) were not pursued. Doctors said that they might later seek answers to 123 of these questions. For a further 148 they said that on reflection they were confident that they knew enough to take the right decision, which leaves 431 questions that were never going to be answered.

One of the most revealing findings of the study was that the mean time spent pursuing an answer was 118 seconds and the median time was 60 seconds. Unless the answer can be found in less than two minutes, the question will simply never be pursued. To be effective, decision support systems need to be able to provide clinicians with information in real time, or near real time. One way of doing this is to ensure that the systems are integrated into the systems that support the rest of clinical work. Decision support systems have been shown to be effective where evidence-based clinical guidelines have been computerized and incorporated into, for example, the systems that clinicians use to record patient histories, make referrals or order tests.

Improving management decision-making

Most business organizations, including healthcare providers, rely on computer systems for the storage and analysis of data. Simple relational database management systems, commonplace since the 1970s, have evolved. Data warehouse systems, central repositories of data integrated from different sources, are now used to allow a form of enterprise-level analysis known as business intelligence. This term, in use since the 1990s, is associated with technologies such as data marts (a subset of a data warehouses focused on a single functional area), online analytical processing or OLAP and the use of scorecards and dashboards to visualize performance metrics. Recent years have seen dramatic changes in the market for health IT products in the United States, through the Affordable Care Act (ACA) and the Health Information Technology for Economic and Clinical Health Act, a component of the 2009 economic stimulus package. The result is that data and analytical tools are now expected to play a role in the transformation of American healthcare into a more efficient, value-driven system, one in which incentives are more in line with patient health (Davidson, 2015).

The question of how best to visualize complex information is increasingly urgent as the functionality of information systems advances, enabling more users to interact with data and explore it in an open-ended way. In many industries, managers have for years had access to near real-time reports tailored to their needs. Healthcare, in contrast, has typically relied on centralized production of reports which are a) historical and b) standardized for all recipients. A typical interface for a contemporary business intelligence system would include an interactive 'dashboard' providing customizable graphical displays of key metrics, historical trends and reference benchmarks. These are now standard in healthcare too. The health informatics literature includes some studies demonstrating that patients and clinicians make better decisions when data are provided to them in a clear and easily interpreted visual language. The impact on management decision-making is of less interest to researchers but likely to be equally important: clear and unambiguous visual displays improve the speed and reliability of decision-making (Koopman et al., 2011).

Improving health behaviour

Increasingly in health informatics, the goal is to improve a patient's health not by improving the clinician's performance or the efficiency of the health service but by intervening directly in the patient's own life. In fact, it may not be appropriate to talk of a 'patient' at all because initiatives are increasingly aimed at improving population health. The hope is that applications delivered via smartphones or tablets can have a significant effect on health behaviour. There are now a great many apps aimed at, for example, supporting smoking cessation, improving diet and encouraging exercise. The most obvious target for these applications, from the point of view of the health service, is to improve patient self-management of long-term conditions, such as diabetes, which account for a huge and growing proportion of health service spending. The potential market for such applications is huge and the hype around them has been considerable; evidence of benefit is more limited (Milne-Ives et al., 2020).

Learning activity 18.3

Think of a clinical team or service that you are familiar with. What is its mission? Think for a moment about the role of the team, about what it should be trying to accomplish, from the perspective of the wider organization.

Now think about how it is assessed, about the key performance indicators on which it is judged. Are these the right ones, or are the factors that affect performance on these indicators outside the team's control?

Could its performance be measured better, focusing on measures relevant to the mission you identified. What data would help a manager identify performance problems in the service?

Conclusion: future challenges in health informatics

Artificial intelligence

Research into artificial intelligence (AI) dates to the 1950s but the trajectory of the research shifted dramatically in 2012 when graphical processing units or GPUs, powerful chips originally designed for gaming consoles, began to be used to program neural networks. A further breakthrough came in 2017 with the invention of the 'transformer', a neural network architecture that provided an incredibly efficient way of analysing large volumes of structured data. This has enabled the creation of what are known as 'foundation models': general purpose AI programs trained on vast amounts of data. The best-known foundation models are probably OpenAI's GPT models, which power ChatGPT. These models are trained on trillions of bytes of data, at phenomenal expense (it is estimated that training GPT4 cost around $300 million) (Taylor, 2024).

Researchers have already begun to assess the potential of these foundation models to help with administrative tasks, such as the generation of discharge summaries (Ellershaw et al., 2024). The current state of the art seems too unreliable for more safety-critical tasks, and it is hard to see how technology built on top of a generic foundation model could gain approval as a medical device, given the regulatory constraints that would impose on the manufacturers of the underpinning models. There are also concerns with bias and fairness, given that the material such tools are trained on is likely to reflect existing societal biases (see Box 18.4). An alternative approach is to train bespoke medical foundation models. Retfound, for example, was trained on 1.6 million retinal images and can support tasks in the interpretation of such images, including, potentially, predicting the development of non-ophthalmic diseases, such as Parkinson's Disease (Zhou et al., 2023).

Box 18.4   Case study – bias and fairness in AI

Research in AI has seen astonishing success and associated hype since graphical processing units were first repurposed to program neural networks in 2012. This growth has also seen increased attention on the potential harms of AI. Since the technology uses data to train its algorithms, if there are problems with the data there will be problems with the algorithms. This is especially worrying with AI because the algorithms tend to be opaque, and biases may not be apparent. It has been shown, for example, that algorithms for the detection of skin lesions perform poorly on darker skin tones since these are under-represented in the training data (Daneshjou et al., 2022).

Algorithms can also be biased because of poor decisions about what kind of data to focus on in training. A commonly used algorithm for identifying patients who might benefit from an intervention to prevent subsequent hospital admission is optimized to reduce healthcare costs. That is how it was designed. This, however, has the consequence that the algorithm is less likely to recommend the intervention for Black patients, since, on average, less is spent in caring for them and therefore there is less scope for saving money later by spending more on early interventions. The researchers who identified the bias estimated that if the algorithm was calibrated according to health needs rather than potential cost savings (using the number and severity of chronic illnesses, rather than costs incurred, as the measure of need) twice as many Black patients would be recommended for the intervention (Obermeyer et al., 2019).

The problems get more complicated in applications that are built on top of 'foundation models', large AI programs, such as OpenAI's GPT models, which are trained on vast amounts of data scraped from the web that will inevitably contain undesirable associations and negative stereotypes. Language models represent words in what are termed 'embedding spaces', statistical models derived from analyses of how words are used. Imagine if we analysed a corpus of millions of sentences containing, say, 10,000 different words and used the cells of a spreadsheet to count how often pairs of words appeared together. There might be a row for 'red' and a column for 'car': the cell at their intersection would show how often they co-occurred. Since a spreadsheet is in effect a matrix and any matrix can be expressed as the product of two smaller matrices, it is mathematically possible to find a more compact representation, one with a row for each word but only, say, a hundred columns, each containing a number that summarizes something about the way the word is used in conjunction with other words. The sequence of numbers in a row can be seen as a set of co-ordinates determining the position of the word in a conceptual space – the embedding space – within which words with similar meanings will be found close together. One approach to mitigating bias in language models is to train an algorithm to predict a set of protected attributes from a word embedding, and then, in effect, remove the information the prediction uses from the data. This would ensure, for example, that any association between the word 'surgeon' and the characteristic 'male' or between the word 'nurse' and the characteristic 'female' is removed (Zhang et al., 2018).

Cybersecurity

The focus in this chapter has been on the potential of information technology to improve outcomes in healthcare. It is, however, increasingly important also to be aware of the risks. The Tracking Healthcare Ransomware Events and Traits (THREAT) database identified 374 ransomware attacks on US healthcare organizations between January 2016 and December 2021 (Neprash et al., 2022). One of the most high-profile attacks in the UK, the 2017 WannaCry attack, led to a £5.9 million reduction in NHS activity (Ghafur et al., 2019). Healthcare organizations are a common target for ransomware attacks. They typically rely on a complex mix of computer systems, which are often poorly maintained and both continuity of provision and confidentiality of data are paramount. Defences against such attacks are partly a matter of designing systems that can prevent such attacks, partly a matter of training staff, especially to detect 'phishing' emails, but also about putting in place backup and recovery plans (known as business continuity and disaster recovery or BC/DR plans).

The risks grow more and more complicated as the range of internet-enabled devices in healthcare becomes greater and more diverse. Many of the implanted devices, such as pacemakers, given to patients are accessible remotely. It is important that the security policy of a trust and the training of its staff cover not just the systems within the trust, but also the external systems, and devices, used to deliver care to patients (Straw et al., 2024).

Learning activity 18.4

One of the concerns that some people have with AI is that it will enable widespread automation and lead to wholesale unemployment. In practice, the impact of new technologies on jobs is complicated. One useful analysis of the impact of technology and AI on the future of healthcare work suggests that it will be tasks rather than jobs that are automated (Moulds and Horton, 2023).

Moulds and Horton (2023) suggest that the tasks performed in a role can be divided into four categories based on two binary classifications: tasks that computers will be able to do better vs tasks that humans will be able to do better; and tasks that we will be happy to delegate to computers vs tasks that we will want still to be done by humans, but possibly with computer support.

Consider one or more roles in your organization and think about the different tasks performed in each role.

- Which of these tasks do you think will be tractable for computers in the near future?
- Which of these tasks do you think it will be acceptable to delegate to a computer?

Learning resources

The Lancet Digital Health: A high impact UK journal that is open access, so there is no paywall. Its focus is on academic research so some of the work described here will be some years from practical implementation, but articles on the evaluation of commercial systems and on issues of ethics and policy will also appear [https://www.thelancet.com/journals/landig/home].

American Medical Informatics Association (AMIA): The largest and most prestigious professional body in health informatics. It runs a major journal and conference and a number of campaigns, including major initiatives in education. The website also hosts a blog, as well as carrying information about health informatics meetings and events [https://www.amia.org/].

Digital Health: A UK-focused website with news and comment on issues in health informatics; it carries advertising, and the job adverts are a good way to look at the range of roles that health informatics specialists fulfil. The site also hosts a network for chief information officers to exchange ideas [https://www.digitalhealth.net/].

Journal of Medical Internet Research (JMIR): One the more successful open access journals; it focuses on applications of health informatics that support the consumers of healthcare rather than those that are more aimed at the practitioners of healthcare. This field is sometimes called consumer health informatics, ehealth or mhealth [http://www.jmir.org/].

References

Bender, D. and Sartipi, K. (2013) HL7 FHIR: an Agile and RESTful approach to healthcare information exchange, in Proceedings of the 26th IEEE International Symposium on Computer-Based Medical Systems, *Institute of Electrical and Electronics Engineers (IEEE)*, pp. 326–331.

Benneyan, J.C., Lloyd, R.C. and Plsek, P.E. (2003) Statistical process control as a tool for research and healthcare improvement, *BMJ Quality & Safety*, 12(6): 458–464.

Daneshjou, R., Vodrahalli, K., Novoa, R.A., Jenkins, M., Liang, W., Rotemberg, V., et al. (2022) Disparities in dermatology AI performance on a diverse, curated clinical image set, *Science Advances*, 8(32), p. eabq6147.

Davidson, A.J. (2015) Creating value: unifying silos into public health business intelligence, *eGEMs*, 2(4): 1172.

Davies, N.G., Kucharski, J.J., Eggo, R.M., Gimma, A. and Edmunds, J.W. (2020) Effects of non-pharmaceutical interventions on COVID-19 cases, deaths, and demand for hospital services in the UK: a modelling study, *The Lancet. Public Health*, 5(7): e375–e385.

Dyer, T., Dillard, L., Harrison, M., Naunton Morgan, T., Tappouni, R., Mailk, Q., et al. (2021) Diagnosis of normal chest radiographs using an autonomous deep-learning algorithm, *Clinical Radiology*, 76(6): 473.e9-473.e15.

Ellershaw, S., Tomlinson, C., Burton, O., Frost, T., Hanrahan, J.G., Khan, D.Z., et al. (2024) Automated Generation of Hospital Discharge Summaries Using Clinical Guidelines and Large Language Models. [https://openreview.net/pdf?id=1kDJJPppRG; accessed 24 June 2024].

Ely, J.W., Osheroff, J.A., Ebell, M.H., Bergus, G.R., Levy, B.T., Chambliss, M.L. and Evans, E.R. (1999) Analysis of questions asked by family doctors regarding patient care, *BMJ*, 319(7206): 358–361.

Ghafur, S., Kristensen, S., Honeyford, K., Martin, G., Darzi A. and Aylin P. (2019) A retrospective impact analysis of the WannaCry cyberattack on the NHS, *NPJ Digital Medicine*, 2: 98.

Heard, S. and Beale, T. (n.d.) openEHR. [https://openehr.org/; accessed 27 May 2024].

Hunt, D.L., Haynes, B.R., Hanna, S.E. and Smith, K. (1998) Effects of computer-based clinical decision support systems on physician performance and patient outcomes: a systematic review, *JAMA: The Journal of the American Medical Association*, 280(15): 1339–1346.

Kansagara, D., Englander, H., Salanitro, A., Kagen, D., Theobald, C., Freeman, M. et al. (2011) Risk prediction models for hospital readmission: a systematic review, *Journal of the American Medical Association*, 306(15): 1688–1698.

King, Z., Farrington, J., Utley, M., Kung, E., Elkhodair, S., Harris., S., et al. (2022) Machine learning for real-time aggregated prediction of hospital admission for emergency patients, *NPJ Digital Medicine*, 5(1): 104.

Koopman, R.J., Kochendorfer, K.M., Moore, J.L., Mehr, D.R., Wakefield, D.S., Yadamsuren, B. et al. (2011) A diabetes dashboard and physician efficiency and accuracy in accessing data needed for high-quality diabetes care, *Annals of Family Medicine*, 9(5): 398–405.

Kyte, D., Cockwell, P., Lencioni, M., Skrybant, M., von Hildebrand, M., Price, G., et al. (2016) Reflections on the national patient-reported outcome measures (PROMs) programme: where do we go from here?, *Journal of the Royal Society of Medicine*, 109(12): 441–445.

Mason, S., Weber, E.J., Coster, J., Freeman, J. and Locker, T. (2012) Time patients spend in the emergency department: England's 4-hour rule – a case of hitting the target but missing the point?, *Annals of Emergency Medicine*, 59: 341–349.

Milne-Ives, M. Lam, C., De Cock, C., Van Velthoven, M.H. and Meinert, E. (2020) Mobile apps for health behavior change in physical activity, diet, drug and alcohol use, and mental health: systematic review, *JMIR mHealth and uHealth*, 8(3): e17046.

Mohammed, M.A., Cheng, K., Rouse, A. and Marshall, T. (2001) Bristol, Shipman, and clinical governance: Shewhart's forgotten lessons, *The Lancet*, 357(9254): 463–467.

Moulds, A. and Horton, T. (2023) What do technology and AI mean for the future of work in health care?, *The Health Foundation*. [https://www.health.org.uk/publications/long-reads/what-do-technology-and-ai-mean-for-the-future-of-work-in-health-care; accessed 20 June 2024].

Neprash, H.T., McGlave, C.C., Cross, D.A., Virnig, B.A., Puskarich, M.A., Huling, J.D., et al. (2022) Trends in ransomware attacks on US hospitals, clinics, and other health care delivery organizations, 2016–2021, *JAMA Health Forum*, 3(12): p. e224873.

Obermeyer, Z., Powers, B., Vogeli, C. and Mullainathan, S. (2019) Dissecting racial bias in an algorithm used to manage the health of populations, *Science*, 366(6464): 447–453.

Pianykh, O.S. (2012) *Digital Imaging and Communications in Medicine (DICOM)*. Berlin Heidelberg: Springer.

Proudlove, N.C. (2020) The 85% bed occupancy fallacy: the use, misuse and insights of queuing theory, *Health Services Management Research*, 33(3): 110–121.

Schini, M. et al. (2024) An overview of the use of the fracture risk assessment tool (FRAX) in osteoporosis, *Journal of Endocrinological Investigation*, 47(3): 501–511.

Sharma, N., Ng, A.Y., Jonathan, J.J., Khara, G., Ambrozay, E., Austin, C.C., et al. (2021) Retrospective large-scale evaluation of an AI system as an independent reader for double reading in breast cancer screening, bioRxiv. doi: 10.1101/2021.02.26.21252537.

Smith, D.J. (2004) The Shipman Inquiry. Chairman Dame Janet Smith. Third Report. Death Certification and Investigation of Deaths by Coroners. Manchester: The Shipman Inquiry, 2003.

Spackman, K.A., Campbell, K.E. and Côté, R.A. (1997) SNOMED RT: a reference terminology for health care, *Proceedings AMIA Annual Fall Symposium*, 1997: pp. 640–644.

Straw, I., Dobbin, J., Luna-Reaver, D. and Tanczer, L. (2024) Simulation-based research for digital health pathologies: a multi-site mixed-methods study, *Digital Health*, 10, 20552076241247940.

Sweeney, L. (2013) Matching Known Patients to Health Records in Washington State Data, arXiv [cs.CY]. [http://arxiv.org/abs/1307.1370; accessed 19 December 2024].

Tam, M.D.B.S., Dyer, T., Dissez, G., Naunton Morgan, T., Hughes, M., Illes, J., Rasalingham, R. and Rasalingham, S. (2021) Augmenting lung cancer diagnosis on chest radiographs: positioning artificial intelligence to improve radiologist performance, *Clinical Radiology*, 76(8): 607–614.

Taylor, P. (2006) *From Patient Data to Medical Knowledge*. Blackwell Publishing Ltd. [https://onlinelibrary.wiley.com/doi/book/10.1002/9780470994702].

Taylor, P. (2013) Standardized mortality ratios, *International Journal of Epidemiology*, 42(6): 1882–1890.

Taylor, P. (2020) Susceptible, infectious, recovered, *London Review of Books*, 42(9): 7 May. [https://www.lrb.co.uk/the-paper/v42/n09/paul-taylor/susceptible-infectious-recovered; accessed 19 December 2024].

Taylor, P. (2024) Llamas, pizzas, mandolins: AI doomerism, *London Review of Books*. [https://www.lrb.co.uk/the-paper/v46/n06/paul-taylor/llamas-pizzas-mandolins; accessed 24 June 2024].

Zhang, B.H., Lemoine, B. and Mitchell, M. (2018) Mitigating Unwanted Biases with Adversarial Learning, in Proceedings of the 2018 AAAI/ACM Conference on AI, Ethics, and Society. New York, NY, USA: Association for Computing Machinery (AIES '18), pp. 335–340.

Zhang, J., Morley, J., Gallifant, J., Oddy, C., Teo, T.T., Ashrafian, H.,et al. (2023) Mapping and evaluating national data flows: transparency, privacy, and guiding infrastructural transformation, *The Lancet. Digital Health*, 5(10): e737–e748.

Zhou, Y., Chia M.A., Wagner, S.K., Ayhan, M.S., Williamson, D.J., Struyven, R.R., et al. (2023) A foundation model for generalizable disease detection from retinal images, *Nature*, 622(7981): 156–163.

Healthcare innovation

Robert J. Romanelli and Sonja Marjanovic

Introduction

Healthcare innovation is concerned with making the health system work better in areas of quality, safety, patient experience, efficiency, effectiveness and value for money (Marjanovic et al., 2020a; Jones et al., 2021). In general, innovation tends to refer to developing and/or implementing new products, technologies or services or applying existing products, technologies or services in new ways (Marjanovic et al., 2020a).

Healthcare innovations can involve medicines, therapies, diagnostics, devices, digital health technologies or new service models for delivering care, such as remote care pathways and integrated care models. While healthcare innovations are often high-tech, this is not universally true. The misconception that innovation is necessarily high-tech or science-intensive can act as a barrier to healthcare staff engaging with it, even when they have meaningful contributions to make.

Innovation can be supply or demand driven. In terms of the supply-side impetus, innovation can be initiated in response to scientific or technological advances that create new opportunities for further research and development (R&D). For example, without scientific and technological advances in artificial intelligence (AI), the development of AI-based diagnostic imaging innovations for cancer would not be possible (Joy Mathew et al., 2020). Similarly, advances in research into neurodegeneration have made possible recent progress in developing treatments for early-onset Alzheimer's disease that may help slow down cognitive decline (Alzheimer's Society, 2020). The impetus to innovate can also arise from an identified unmet health need or, in other words, be demand-driven. For example, the public health challenge of delivering care in the first waves of the COVID-19 pandemic accelerated the focus on technology-enabled remote monitoring innovations to support evolving demands for health service delivery (Greenhalgh et al., 2020; Green et al., 2022). Supply- and demand-side stimuli for innovation need not be mutually exclusive. Unmet needs (i.e. demand) can trigger investments in R&D that can lead to scientific advances (i.e. supply). An example of this is an increased focus on innovation to address the growing problem of antimicrobial resistance (Anderson et al., 2023).

Regardless of where the stimulus for innovation comes from, the ability to achieve the intended impact will depend on how well the supply of innovations aligns with areas of unmet needs and on the willingness and ability of health systems to afford innovations and implement them successfully.

Healthcare staff can adopt innovations that have been developed externally (e.g. innovations developed by organizations in other countries, or in other locations in the same country). Alternatively, healthcare staff can also be directly involved in developing innovations, for example, through participation in R&D, such as in clinical trials. The agents of innovation range from individuals in academic and research institutes to industry actors, such as small- and medium-sized enterprises (SMEs), large biopharmaceutical companies and health-technology companies, as well as clinical entrepreneurs from healthcare delivery organizations. Most often, innovation occurs through collaboration between diverse actors.

Against this backdrop, the aim of this chapter is to provide an evidence-based overview of key practical considerations related to developing and implementing innovations. In this chapter, we use the term implementation to broadly refer to adoption, scale and spread of innovations, where adoption is defined as the initial implementation of an innovation, scale is defined as increasing levels of implementation in the setting where it is adopted, and spread is defined as the adoption of innovation in additional settings

The chapter is targeted at leaders and managers in healthcare delivery organizations who are interested in understanding healthcare innovation and embedding innovation into the culture and practice of service delivery. The chapter aims to support these leaders and managers to become more familiar with the concept of healthcare innovation and, thereby, more comfortable with understanding how innovations can be used to make meaningful changes for the benefit of healthcare providers and patients.

The innovation pathway

Who funds innovation?

Funding for innovation can come from a variety of sources. For example, academic and research institutions often achieve scientific advances through basic, translational and clinical research with financial support from government departments, charities or industries, such as in the case of pharmaceutical-funded clinical trials. SMEs, such as biotechnology firms, can raise funding from public sector support schemes, as well as more commonly from private business angels and venture capitalists, particularly for high-risk and high-reward R&D.

Large firms, such as biopharmaceutical companies, are usually shareholder controlled and invest to secure a financial return for shareholders. If we look at the financial ecosystem for medicines R&D globally, approximately two thirds of funding comes from biopharmaceutical companies, just over one-quarter comes from public sector and not-for-profit funders and the remaining 10 per cent from venture capitalists (Kalindjian et al., 2022). However, the relative contribution of financial investment in terms of amounts invested is not necessarily indicative of its relative importance. Without public and not-for-profit investments, there would not be sufficient contributions into the innovation pipeline for private sector investors to take up (Schot and Steinmueller, 2018). For example, the discovery of novel drug targets is often identified through basic and translational research conducted in academic settings but generates opportunities for private industry to develop and commercialize innovative products aimed at these targets.

In general, the funding landscape for developing innovations is more mature than that for financing implementation, spread and scale efforts (Marjanovic et al., 2020b), as we discuss in the Healthcare innovation in practice section. In publicly funded health systems, like the National Health Service (NHS) in the United Kingdom (UK), funding for adopting innovations will generally come from national or regional organizations involved with financing health services and/or specialized funding programmes for testing innovations in the NHS.

The stages of research and development

All innovations initially go through early-stage R&D (e.g. basic and translational research) and, subsequently, late-stage R&D (e.g. clinical trials and other types of testing), which are pre-requisites for the development of new drugs, vaccines, devices, diagnostics, digital health technologies and service models (Figure 19.1). To illustrate, early-stage R&D for drugs and vaccines involves target selection, lead optimization and pre-clinical testing. Late-stage R&D involves clinical trials in patients. Phase I trials are conducted to determine the safety, including safe dosage of a drug, and to identify side effects/adverse events. They generally involve a small number of participants, either healthy volunteers or people with the condition the drug is meant to treat. Phase II trials are conducted to assess the efficacy of a drug and to further evaluate safety, including potential side effects/adverse events. They tend to involve a larger number of participants (compared to phase I trials) and specially include those with the condition that the drug is meant to treat. Phase III trials involve a larger number of participants (than phase I or II trials) and are used to confirm the efficacy of a drug in comparison to usual care or an alternative treatment and to further monitor side effects/adverse events. All three are needed for drugs or therapies to be approved by regulators for use.

Early-stage R&D for digital health technologies often involves proof of market, proof of concept, design/prototyping (i.e. coming up with an early model) and alpha testing (i.e. early stage testing in a controlled environment), whereas late-stage R&D involves what is known as beta testing (i.e. to obtain feedback from a real-world use environment) (Marjanovic et al., 2020b). Service model innovations, as part of their early-stage R&D, undergo concept design, piloting and testing, followed by service prototype development and further testing during their late-stage R&D.

Commercialization

Innovators often seek to protect the intellectual property (IP) of their innovations, which can include patents, copyright or trademarks. Innovators need to apply for IP protection through

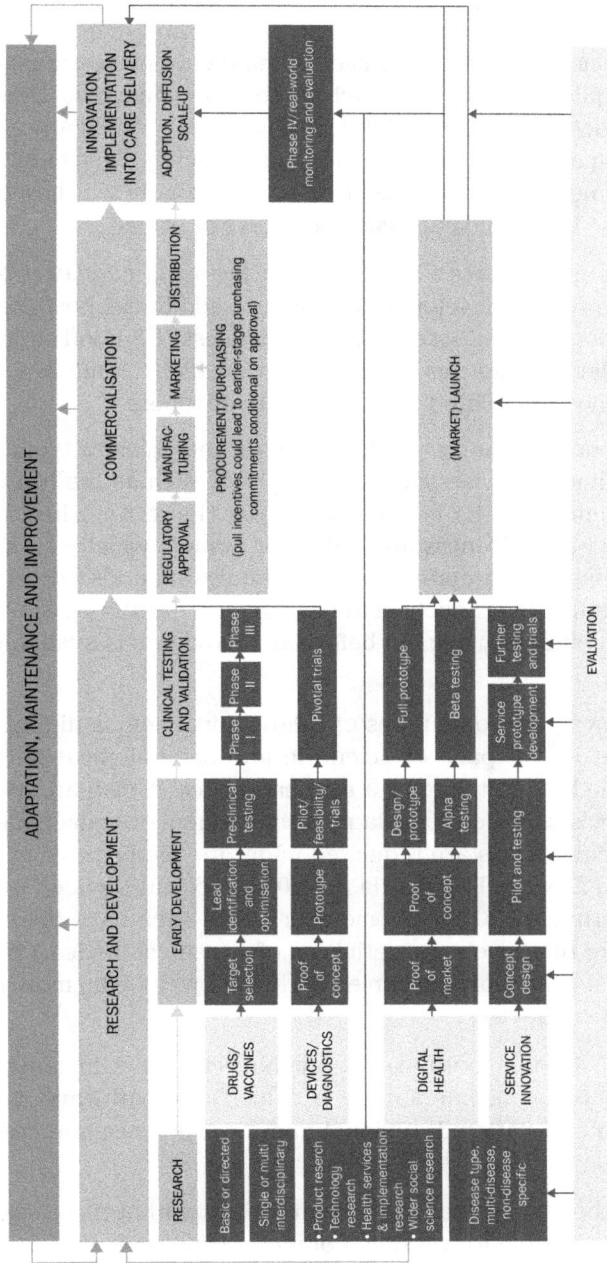

Figure 19.1 Healthcare innovation pathway
Source: Adapted from Marjanovic et al. (2020b).

institutions, such as the UK IP Office or to IP offices in other geographies where they need their product to be protected, such as the United States Patent and Trademark Office or the European Union (EU) IP Office.

Innovative products, such as drugs, vaccines, devices and diagnostics, require regulatory review before they can be licensed for use by healthcare professionals and/or patients. National or regional regulatory agencies, such as the Medicines and Healthcare products Regulatory Agency (MHRA) in the UK and the EU's European Medicines Agency (EMA) are responsible for reviewing and approving products for licencing. They determine if a product is safe and efficacious and/or effective based on studies conducted during early- and late-stage R&D, such as phase I/II/III clinical trials in the case of drugs.

Regulatory agencies may approve a product for licensing or may provide conditional approval, requiring the product developers to conduct additional post-licensing studies to evaluate real-world and longer-term safety and effectiveness (US Food and Drug Administration (FDA), 2018). Regulatory agencies can also later decide to remove a product from the market based on emerging data related to safety or effectiveness.

Depending on the country context, products and technologies can undergo an appraisal by a national health technology assessment (HTA) body, such as the National Institute for Health and Care Excellence (NICE) in England or the Haute Autorité de Santé (HAS) in France, to determine cost-effectiveness and value for money, which can influence a health system's willingness to pay for an innovation. HTA bodies may also determine how a new product compares to alternative products in the existing care pathway. HTA typically occurs after regulatory approval and licensing but before an innovation is available for distribution and use.

The regulatory pathway for some types of innovation, such as digital health technologies, is evolving in light of the pace of scientific and technological developments. Such products may be classified as 'software as a medical device' if they are used by healthcare professionals to make decisions about the diagnosis, treatment or management of health conditions. In the UK, medical devices are regulated under the Medicines and Medical Devices Act 2021 and the Medical Devices Regulation Act 2002 (Medical Device Coordination Group (MDCG), 2019; UK Government, 2002). EU member states each have their own policies for the regulation of software that meets the definition of a medical device. Other digital health technologies are designed to support consumer health and well-being more broadly and thus are not classified as medical devices.

Innovations can have different pathways to reaching end users, including healthcare professionals, patients or public consumers more widely. These pathways will depend on the nature of the innovation and national, regional and local policies and commissioning and procurement processes.

Health systems and healthcare delivery organizations within these systems often have established functions responsible for product commissioning and procurement. Some products and services are procured via specialized commissioning at the national level (e.g. NHS England), whereas others may be procured at the regional (e.g. integrated care board or primary care networks) or local (e.g. hospital trusts) levels. NHS Supply Chain provides lists of available products and is also a source of competitive landscape intelligence for innovators considering new product or technology development efforts (Lillie et al., 2023; Health Innovation Network, n.d.).

Innovation implementation into care delivery

Once licensed, or more generally approved for use, some innovations quickly move to wide-scale adoption, spread and scale. One example of this is the cholesterol-lowering drug class of statins (O'Keeffe et al., 2016). Other innovations however, such as electronic medical records have taken much longer to embed and there are still challenges to interoperability between different systems and care providers (Sheikh et al., 2014). Innovations can also sometimes appear to be deceptively simple, but their adoption, spread and scale can be riddled with challenges. For example, remote blood pressure monitoring devices may not ideally accommodate people of all weights and ages and the health workforce may struggle to engage with the volume of data coming from monitoring devices, unless these data are conveyed in a user-friendly matter. Digital health innovations, more broadly, may face challenges related to public trust in data security and a general apprehension regarding surveillance.

In addition, what is suitable for implementation in one setting may not necessarily be appropriate for others. Certain healthcare innovations, such as drugs and vaccines, may be restricted in terms of how they are used and by whom and, thus, have limited or no scope for adaptation. Other innovations, such as new service delivery models, can (and at times must) be adapted before they can be adopted, scaled up or spread. For adaptation to be successful, a balance needs to be found between adherence (or fidelity) to the original innovation's key features essential to its effectiveness, and pragmatic and monitored changes that allow the innovation to be more successful in specific contexts and for certain end-users (Bopp et al., 2013). As discussed further in the section titled 'Healthcare innovation in practice' in this chapter, various factors related to the innovation itself, and to the wider context in which is it being implemented (such as workforce capacity and skills, available information and incentives) can impact adoption, spread and scale (Marjanovic et al., 2020b; Papoutsi et al., 2024).

Who is involved in innovation?

We previously noted that innovations can come from varied sources and involve multiple actors across the public, private and not-for-profit sector (Kalindjian et al., 2022). For example, many of the products developed through R&D in biotechnology or pharmaceutical companies are seeded by basic and translational research discoveries made in academia. Industry may run a clinical trial programme for a promising new drug, but the trial is conducted, and participants are often recruited, from within healthcare delivery organizations. Individuals within healthcare delivery organizations can themselves be a source of innovation, for example, through clinical entrepreneurship.

On the implementation side, decisions about what innovations are needed and if and how they are adopted, spread and scaled up involve those who hold commissioning and procurement budgets at national, regional/local and organizational levels. These decisions should be informed by frontline staff, and by evidence on patient experience and outcomes. Frontline staff are often responsible for the implementation of new products, technologies and services and, thus, are integral in determining not only what is needed but also how innovations could be successfully adapted to a local context.

Theoretical and disciplinary perspectives on healthcare innovation

Science, technology and innovation studies perspectives

Historically, much of the science, technology and innovation literature on innovation (across different sectors) adopted an industrial strategy perspective and focused on research and innovation as vehicles for economic competitiveness and growth (Schot and Steinmueller, 2018). Over time, organizational science, business management and health service scholars have increasingly contributed to the theory and evidence base on healthcare innovation.

Early perspectives assumed a linear process in which investing in research and research infrastructure would lead to innovation and result in competition and economic growth (Bush, 1945; Kuznets, 1973; Schot and Steinmueller, 2018). Gradually, perspectives that better recognized the complexity of innovation emerged, most notably *national, regional and sectoral innovation systems* (Nelson, 1993; Etzkowitz and Leydesdorff, 2002; Orsenigo and Malerba, 2002; Freeman, 2008; Consoli and Mina, 2008; Edquist and Hommen, 2008; Lundvall, 2010) and *sociotechnical systems* perspectives on innovation (Geels and Schot, 2007; Fuenfschilling and Truffer, 2014; Broerse and Grin, 2019). These schools of thought recognized that innovation systems take shape, change and adapt as a result of interactions between various individuals, organizations, networks, institutions, ideas and opportunities, capabilities, values, behaviours, regulations, policies, socioeconomic, political and cultural contexts (Marjanovic et al., 2020a). In these perspectives, innovation is recognized as emergent and non-deterministic (Consoli and Mina, 2008).

In the *national, regional and sectoral innovation systems* schools of thought, innovation results from interconnected activity across a 'triple helix' of government, industry and research at universities/research institutes (Etzkowitz and Leyesdorff, 2002). In the literature on health innovation systems specifically, this has since been expanded to highlight the importance of those involved in clinical service delivery, with healthcare providers (and to a degree patients via input into practitioner–patient interactions) having key roles in the exchange of knowledge and information with the scientific research community (Consoli and Mina, 2008). This fourth dimension of 'society' was later termed as the 'quadruple helix' in innovation systems thinking (Carayannis and Campbell, 2009). More recently, a new perspective – that of transformative change – further emphasized issues of sustainable and more inclusive societies as key drivers of innovation and places even greater focus on end users (Schot and Steinmueller, 2018).

Within *sociotechnical systems thinking, the multilevel perspective on sociotechnical transitions* is particularly helpful in understanding innovation system evolution and change. It focuses on the adaptive and iterative nature of innovation, with systems 'transitioning' from incumbent to new forms, over time, through co-evolving interactions between technical

Table 19.1 Key implications of innovation systems and sociotechnical perspectives for decision-making about innovation

Key practical implications	Explanation
Decisions about if and how to support innovation development need to consider the fit of product and context	Innovation achieves desired impact (or not), as a result of interactions between the physical properties of 'the product' and the context in which it will be developed and used (e.g. socioeconomic, scientific and technological, cultural, political, legal, policy and regulatory)
Innovation can be orchestrated to a degree 'top-down' by system leaders	Innovation systems thinking accommodates for emergence to a degree, but focuses on the ability to manage, govern, coordinate and orchestrate innovation at national, regional or sectoral levels. This gives rise to the possibility of system level change and transformation being driven by national level actors and their orchestration (i.e. in a more top-down fashion).
Innovation can also be driven by 'bottom-up' efforts	Sociotechnical regimes perspectives see change and transformation being driven through the experience and results of experiments happening in niches gradually impacting on the wider system. This gives scope for bottom-up, individual and organizationally driven experimentation and innovation, including grassroots efforts, impacting on system level transformation and change.

and social aspects of the innovating system. Deeply rooted structures in an innovation system (i.e. sociotechnical regimes) consist of formal rules and informal practices, relationships and behaviours that remain relatively stable and/or only incrementally evolve when there is strong alignment between social and technical aspects of a system. When technical aspects (e.g. science and technological advances) and/or societal needs (e.g. unmet health needs) shift, the regime will begin to change. This can start in protected spaces for innovation (termed as 'niches') that might have particularly enabling conditions, such as good access to funding, enabled leadership or permissive regulation (Geels and Schot, 2007; Geels, 2011; Broerse and Grin, 2019). Processes, conditions and outcomes from individual or interconnected niches can, over time, scale, spread and lead to a new sociotechnical regime.

Table 19.1 summarizes how the science, technology and innovation literature brings practical value to decision-makers who may invest in or make policy decisions about supporting innovation.

Health services and implementation sciences perspectives

While the science, technology and innovation literature has emphasized the developmental aspect of innovations, particularly in the context of complex production-consumption systems, the health services and implementation sciences literature, the broader social sciences literature and the complexity sciences literature have emphasized adoption, scale and spread of innovations.

Several frameworks have shaped our understanding of the key requirements for the implementation of innovations within health systems. Next, we discuss three influential frameworks: the Implementation Outcomes Framework (IOF), the Consolidated Framework for Implementation Research (CFIR) and the non-adoption, abandonment and challenges to scale-up, spread and sustainability (NASSS) framework.

The IOF was developed to advance the concept of measuring the implementation of an intervention (e.g. new treatments, practices or services), with the view that successful implementation is a necessary pre-condition for the intervention to bring about desired changes in clinical or service outcomes (Proctor et al., 2011). The IOF was largely derived from a pre-existing framework designed to measure the impact of an intervention (called the Reach, Effectiveness, Adoption, Implementation and Maintenance (RE-AIM) framework) (Glasgow et al., 1999), as well as from Everett M. Rogers' seminal text, *Diffusion of Innovations* (Rogers, 1962), and a conceptual model for moving innovations into practice (Simpson and Flynn, 2007). The IOF is composed of eight domains related to the success of implementation: appropriateness; feasibility; acceptability; implementation costs; adoption; penetration; fidelity; and sustainability. These domains have practical value for decision-makers who are considering if a specific innovation should be adopted – often in comparison to potential alternatives – and the potential for the innovation to be scaled up and spread.

The CFIR framework considers innovations in terms of 'what works, where and why across multiple contexts', and brings into play a wider range of considerations (Damschroder et al., 2009: 1). The CFIR is derived from at least 19 published theoretical frameworks for implementation research and is composed of five core domains: intervention characteristics; outer setting; inner setting; individual characteristics; and the process of implementation. Each domain is composed of multiple constructs, which are considered to interact to influence successful implementation. The CFIR is of practical value for decision-makers, as it underscores the importance of the setting (and different levels and features of the setting) when considering how to successfully adopt, scale up and spread.

More recently, the NASSS framework was developed to 'help predict and evaluate the success of a technology-supported health or social care program' (Greenhalgh et al., 2017, 2017: 1). The NASSS is composed of seven domains that need to be considered when making decisions related to implementing innovations. These domains relate to characteristics of: the condition (i.e. health condition, illness, sociocultural factors); technology; value proposition (i.e. supply side value for the innovation developer and demand-side value for users); adopters (e.g. staff, patients, carers); organization(s) (e.g. capacity to innovate, readiness); wider system (e.g. policy, regulatory, professional, interorganizational context); and embedding and adapting over time. NASSS embraces the complexity of health innovation, emergence and uncertainty. Each of the domains that NASSS considers can have varied levels of complexity (i.e. simple, complex or complicated), which can impact adoption, spread and scale up efforts. While NASSS and CFIR share certain features, NASSS is rooted in considerations for technology-based innovations, especially (including digital health innovations which are increasingly prominent); although, it can also be used to inform implementation of non-technology-based innovations (Papoutsi et al., 2024). NASSS has recently gained attention in informing scale and spread, as well as sustainability, flagging the need to adapt over time, ostensibly in response to continual technological or other contextual advances (Papoutsi et al., 2024).

Table 19.2 Key implications of health services and implementation science perspectives for decision-making about innovation (IOF, CFIR and NASSS)

Key practical implications	Explanation
***Alignment* of the nature of an innovation with its adoption context is essential for successful implementation**	The IOF flags criteria for a good fit of an innovation with its implementation context (e.g. appropriateness; feasibility; acceptability and implementation costs) and differentiates between perceived and actual fit. The CFIR considers a host of contextual factors related to individual characteristics (e.g. leaders, implementation teams), the 'inner setting' (e.g. structural, relational, resource and cultural characteristics in a unit or organization) and 'outer setting' (e.g. policies, attitudes, conditions, financial resources and other external conditions local, regional and national levels). NASSS considers the nature of the intervention (e.g. technology) and adoption context (e.g. adopting individuals, organizations, wider system) and the value proposition for both suppliers and adopters.
Decisions about whether and how to adopt an innovation need to consider the *complexity* of both the innovation and its adoption context	NASSS puts emphasis on levels of complexity (simple, complicated, complex) of the innovation, the health condition it is targeting and the different domains of the adoption context. The levels of complexity will have a role in the nature of resources, structures and processes that need to be mobilized to support effective implementation and impact.
When spreading and scaling innovations, a *balance between fidelity and adaptability* is required	For innovations to have maximal impact they should have the potential for adaptation without loss of requisite fidelity. NASSS emphasizes adaptation over time as key to embedding innovation, spread and scale (e.g. in light of changing technological developments and changing contexts, uncertainty and emergence, as well as the need for organizational resilience). CFIR emphasizes adaptability of both the intervention and of implementation processes in light of learning and evaluation. IOF places emphasis on intervention fidelity.

Table 19.2 summarizes how health services and implementation science perspectives, and the IOF, CFIR and NASSS frameworks in particular, bring practical value to decision-makers who are considering adoption, spread and scale up of innovation.

Healthcare innovation in practice

While innovation development and implementation have been well studied – and we have good theoretical understanding of what is required to be successful at both – innovation is challenging to put into practice.

First and foremost, innovations take time to develop and implement. There are many pieces to a complex puzzle that must come together and many influences on both the development/supply and implementation/demand side (as introduced in the discussion of theoretical and disciplinary perspectives in the section titled 'Theoretical and disciplinary perspectives on healthcare innovation' in this chapter), which need to be considered collectively to support an innovating health system.

In the UK, both researchers in this area and those involved with policy efforts have tried to unpack the challenges to innovation and identify ways to tackle them to support an innovative NHS. For example, the Accelerated Access Review (UK Government, 2016) provided recommendations to the NHS on how to improve patient access to innovative medical and health-related products. The recommendations aimed to tackle varied challenges, including those relating to identifying innovations of value, accelerating the development-to-adoption pathway into the NHS (including regulatory and payment hurdles) and obtaining evidence on real-world impact. Among others, recommendations included developing an enhanced horizon scanning process to identify innovations; setting up an Accelerated Access Pathway to align regulatory, reimbursement, evaluation and diffusions processes to bring innovations to patients more quickly; improving digital infrastructure to capture information on the use of innovation and outcomes; establishing incentives to support local uptake and spread; and establishing an Accelerated Access Partnership to help coordinate innovation activities across institutions.

The Nuffield Trust, an independent health charity and think tank in the UK, also published a report looking at the challenges to innovation and its adoption in the NHS (Castle-Clarke et al., 2017) outlining barriers related to: an approach to innovation that was overly supply-side and top-down driven (i.e. stemming from innovation developers and/or centralized planners), rather than demand-side and bottom-up (i.e. stemming from those who use or benefit from innovations); a reliance on evidence from randomized controlled trials, which are time and resource intensive; NHS cultures where 'looking for new solutions' is not integrated into the jobs of frontline staff; and a focus on adopting innovations that provide short-term cost savings, rather than longer-term gains in efficiency. The scale up and spread of innovations, which are key to maximizing clinical and population health benefits, have similar challenges (Papoutsi et al., 2024). As the Nuffield Trust report points out, there is little funding to support adaptation and spread across healthcare delivery organizations within the health system and there are behavioural and cultural barriers related to bringing in innovations developed from outside, and perceived threats to individual, professional judgement and autonomy (Castle-Clarke et al., 2017).

Learning activity 19.1

You are asked by senior leadership in your health system to advise them on deciding between purchasing one of two potential innovative technology platforms that are designed to help digitize patient flow through a hospital. The hospital leadership is hoping to implement technology that can help with efforts to ensure that patients get the most appropriate care while in hospital and that they are discharged in timely ways. The leadership is hoping that the technology can help with clinical decision support related to moving patients from the Accident & Emergency department into the correct hospital wards, in light of available bed space, and that can help with real-time data on patient vital signs to make decisions about care while in hospital, and with decisions about timely discharge and planning for subsequent care needs.

Reflecting on the health service and implementation science frameworks, IOF, CFIR and NASSS, what factors would you advise senior leadership to consider when deciding which of the two technology platform innovations to choose and why?

Consider also the challenges to innovation adoption discussed in this section.

- How might these challenges affect the implementation of the chosen innovation?
- Are there other challenges that you believe are particularly relevant?
- How might you address some of these challenges to create a culture that is more conducive to adopting, scaling and spreading the innovation that is ultimately selected?

Building on prior national and international studies of healthcare innovation and based on a substantial body of work conducted by the not-for-profit research institute RAND Europe and academic partners (including most recently a large-scale multi-year, mixed-methods NIHR-funded study on creating an innovating NHS) (Marjanovic et al., 2020b), there are a series of key influences on an innovating NHS that can affect both the development and implementation of innovation. These influences include: 1) funding and policy levers; 2) workforce: capacity, skills, leadership, motivations and accountabilities; 3) information and evidence, including regulation and HTA; 4) relationships and networks for collaboration and coordination; 5) physical and IT infrastructure; and 6) service user engagement and explicit consideration of inequalities (Figure 19.2).

Health system leaders and managers need to understand these influences, and why they can affect innovation efforts, in order to maximize the chances of creating and nurturing environments that enable innovation. This is essential for ensuring a good alignment (i.e. fit) between an innovation and its development context and/or its adoption environment, which is requisite for innovation adoption (as introduced in the section titled 'Theoretical and disciplinary perspectives on healthcare innovation'). We elaborate on each of these six categories of influences based on insights from prior work (Marjanovic et al., 2020b) and provide some examples of programmes that exist to address challenges associated with each. The examples are not exhaustive but illustrate some of the key efforts focused on the UK context, as the core focus of this chapter.

Funding and wider policy levers

Funding is a necessary but not a sufficient determinant of successful innovation development and implementation. Funding is needed to both feed R&D pipelines and to support adoption of innovation in care pathways. Public funding can be seen as a policy lever to help support innovation activity. While there are various funding mechanisms that support the development of innovations, there are limited mechanisms that support innovation adoption, including the

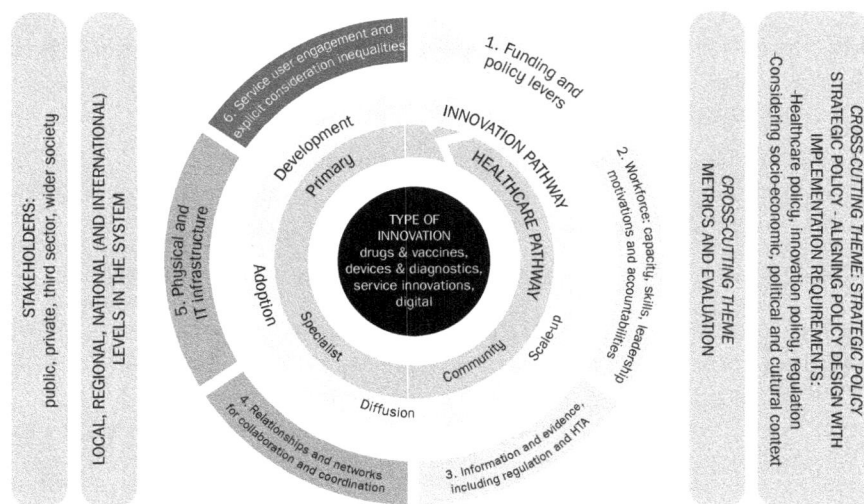

Figure 19.2 Key influences on the development and implementation of innovations
Source: Adapted from Marjanovic et al. (2020b).

adaptation of innovations for different settings. This creates a significant barrier to getting evidence-based innovations into the hands of healthcare professionals and patients. Some examples of practical support available in the UK that could help health system leaders and managers in pursuing innovation opportunities are illustrated in Box 19.1.

Wider policy levers, such as strategic policy documents, can also provide incentives and help innovators prioritize areas of innovation, as they can signal where there is likely to be more funding and wider support for innovative activity in the healthcare innovation ecosystem. For example, the NHS Long Term Plan highlights areas where healthcare improvements are needed and where innovation can play a role in improving quality, safety and efficiency of care services, such as in early cancer diagnosis, innovation in mental health and digital innovation (NHS England, n.d.). Similarly, budget announcements, such as the focus on NHS productivity in the 2024 Budget (Atkins, 2024), have signalled the need for considering how digital innovation can help achieve productivity gains.

Box 19.1 Examples of funding sources for research, innovation development and adoption in the UK

Funding that supports research and development – examples:

- **Medical Research Council**: Funder of basic and translational research for academic and other research institutes, centres and units in the UK.

- **National Institute of Health and Care Research (NIHR)**: Funder of clinical and applied research, including public health and service delivery research. Also has programmes of support that can evaluate different types of innovation (e.g. rapid evaluation centres for service innovations, real-world implementation evaluations).
- **Small Business Research Initiative (SBRI) for Healthcare**: Supports the development of new innovations by small businesses and/or partnerships with academics and the NHS, with the goal of aligning the demand for innovation with supply and promoting faster adoption and spread of products that solve the problems faced by the NHS. The funding programme also collaborates with NHS England in priority areas, such as cancer (**Innovation Open Calls**).
- Other sources of funding can be accessed from various research charities. Early-stage innovation funding can be accessed from business angels, venture capital and biopharma investment.
- Regional **health innovation networks (HINs)** can help make needed introductions to the investor community.
- **NHS AI Diagnostic Fund**: This programme provides funds to accelerate the deployment of promising AI imaging and decision support tools to help diagnose patients more quickly. A total of £21 million will be provided to 11 imaging networks, comprising 64 NHS Trusts across England.
- The **Artificial Intelligence (AI) Award** is an **NHS AI Lab** that supports the testing of various AI technologies at different stages of development, from early-stage testing to evaluating technologies in practice.

Many programmes (e.g. NIHR, SBRI Healthcare) can support efforts across the four UK nations, but devolved nations can also have additional funding programmes. For example, NHS Research Scotland and Health and Care Research Wales support high-quality research in Scotland and Wales respectively.

Funding that supports innovation testing and implementation – examples:

- **MedTech Funding Mandate**: This programme helps to point NHS organizations to diagnostic and other medical technologies that have been recommended by NICE and that payers need to secure funding arrangements for.
- Information on how to secure funding for innovation adoption in the NHS can be found through discussion with local commissioning bodies (e.g. Integrated Care Boards), specialized commissioners (e.g. NHS England) and via various **procurement frameworks**. Various other payment schemes may exist for specific types of innovations or in specific (e.g. pre-commercial procurement commitments, outcome-based commissioning models).

Workforce matters: capacity, skills and leadership, and motivations and accountabilities

Engaging with innovation requires a skilled and empowered workforce who can devote time to the process, within a supportive environment. Innovation opportunities often create new workforce demands. For example, the promise of new Alzheimer's disease drugs that slow down cognitive decline has significant implications on workforce capacity and skills within existing care pathways, including potentially the need for more neurologists and neurora-diologists to manage diagnosis and treatment and to monitor patients (Ulyte et al., 2024). Similarly, advances in cancer diagnosis, such as liquid biopsy tests, will require a critical mass of appropriately trained and skilled diagnostic laboratory workforce to collect, pre-pare, store and process blood samples, as well as a clinical workforce to analyse test results and make appropriate care decisions (Tsimberidou et al., 2023).

When health system leaders and managers are thinking about whether to engage wider staff within their organizations, either in developing or implementing innovation, it is impor-tant to consider the types of staff who need to engage and the training and skills required. This necessitates identifying ways to ensure staff have permission, time and headspace to engage with innovative activities. Given existing pressures on healthcare staff, it can be especially challenging to free up scarce time for individuals to identify issues and come up with innovative solutions. However, without protected time, it is difficult to embed innova-tion into practice.

There are some national programmes that can not only help 'buy out' time of busy clinical and non-clinical staff but also invest in developing skills to support innovation and entrepre-neurship (see Box 19.2). However, freeing up time can only go so far if staff are already too busy delivering frontline care. More efforts are needed to create a culture within the NHS to allow staff to experiment with innovative thinking and ways of doing things. Not everyone in the health system needs to be an innovator in terms of developing new products, technologies or service models, but at minimum staff should understand what impact innovation can have, why it matters and what evidence-based innovations are available to help improve service delivery. An international example of relevance would be the Swedish–French Accelerator 2.0, a 12-month programme that provides expert support in the form of mentoring, onsite and online training to help Swedish companies validate innovation solutions in precision health and their fit to the French market.

Embedding innovation into healthcare delivery organizations requires investing in a mix of technical and social skills. Technical skills might include the ability to identify and priori-tize innovation needs; horizon scan for available innovations; critical appraisal of evidence; intellectual property literacy; and the ability to adopt and adapt proven innovations. Social skills might include inspirational and inclusive leadership; managing and communicating risk; and networking and relationship management. It is not just up to health system leaders to support skills and capability building. Innovation developers/suppliers can also provide training support and guidance. In addition to having the requisite skills, individuals need to be motivated to innovate and have accountability. The mix of incentives and accountabili-ties needs careful consideration to mitigate against unintended consequences (e.g. tokenistic innovation roles or tick box actions).

Box 19.2   Examples of initiatives to support a workforce engaged with innovation in the UK

- **Clinical Entrepreneurs Programme**: A workforce development programme for clinical and non-clinical NHS staff, launched in 2016. The programme aims to provide commercial skills, knowledge and experience to individuals who wish to successfully develop and spread innovative solutions to benefit patients, staff and the wider NHS.
- **NHS England Genomics Education**: Provides genomics education, training and experience for the NHS healthcare workforce through Health Education England.
- **NHS Innovation Accelerator programme and fellowships** to support individuals to help develop skills and build networks to enable adoption of innovation in the NHS.
- **NIHR Academic Clinical Medicine Fellowships** to support clinicians in developing research skills.

Information and evidence, including regulation and HTA

Health system leaders and managers need to understand various types of information and evidence, to support an innovating health system and staff involved with innovation activity. For example, innovators developing novel solutions need information on the issues facing health systems and how innovations can help; information on funding schemes to support R&D; how to protect IP; and how to navigate the regulatory landscape. Staff in healthcare delivery organizations, who are responsible for implementing innovations, need information related to the types of innovations available and the evidence to support their safety, efficacy and cost-effectiveness and how the innovation can fit within existing care pathways. They also need information on how to adopt innovations and adapt them to their specific contexts, as well as information on how to de-implement products or services that are being replaced by an innovation. Patients and the public also require information to enable them to contribute to identifying unmet needs, to participate in trials and to be aware of what innovations they can access.

It is important to ensure that information and evidence is widely communicated within the health system and across the healthcare innovation ecosystem to build trust in the value of proven innovations. As innovation landscapes change, key resources such as HTA assessments and clinical guidelines also need to be kept up to date.

Box 19.3 provides examples of organizations in the UK that can help with access to information and evidence to help NHS leaders and managers support their staff in navigating innovation pathways. Key international examples include the EMA, an agency of the EU in charge of evaluating pharmaceutical products and providing centralized market authorization for member states, and the FDA, which is responsible for market authorization across the 50 US states.

**Box 19.3   Examples of programmes related to information
and evidence in the UK**

- **Medicines and Healthcare products Regulatory Agency (MHRA)**: An executive agency of the Department of Health and Social Care (DHSC) that is responsible for ensuring that medicines and medical devices work as intended and have an acceptable safety profile.
- **National Institute for Health and Care Excellence (NICE)**: An executive non-department of the DSHC that publishes guidance on the use of health technologies, including new and existing medicines, treatment and procedures. NICE also conducts health technology assessment (HTA) to determine the cost-effectiveness of a health innovation, which can impact on whether and how much the NHS will pay. NICE has an advisory service (NICE Advice), which can help innovators prepare for an HTA and can also help them understand how to engage with NHS payers and commissioners.
- **NHS Innovation Service**: This service aims to help individuals and companies at various stages of the innovation pathway, providing access to coordinated support and guidance from organizations with the right expertise, from arriving at an idea to developing an innovation, generating evidence needed for regulation and HTA to information about commissioning and adoption.
- Other sources of information of relevance for innovators can be accessed from technology transfer offices, knowledge transfer networks and regional organizations, such as **HINs**.

Relationships and networks

There are many initiatives that focus, to varying degrees, on enabling collaborations or coordinating innovation activities, some of which are nationally coordinated but locally run. The effective function of a networked healthcare innovation ecosystem depends on clear roles and responsibilities, minimizing unnecessary duplication of effort and coordination both within and between regions. There are a myriad of things that can get in the way of effective coordination, such as lack of awareness of what initiatives and programmes exist, the 'politics of ownership', short-term relationships and churn in lines of authority and siloed working. Effective and well-coordinated collaboration requires understanding the pathway through which innovations are developed and implemented, and considering how an innovation may relate to (i.e. fit with, complement) other solutions being explored to improve healthcare. This includes appreciating and being able to navigate the complexity of an innovation and of its implementation context (an important aspect that is highlighted in conceptual frameworks such as NASSS, as discussed previously).

Box 19.4 provides some examples of the types of organizations that help with collaboration and coordination of R&D activities in the health system in the UK. These organizations can also be a helpful point of contact for NHS staff wishing to explore collaborative R&D. A key international example includes Horizon Europe, a funding programme (2021–2027) for research and innovation across the EU, with the goal of fostering collaboration across member states.

Box 19.4 Examples of programmes related to relationships and networking

- **Applied Research Collaboration (ARC)**: The NICE research funds 15 ARCs across England to support applied health and care research and research on implementation of health and care evidence into clinical practice. Each ARC represents a partnership between NHS providers, universities, charities, local authorities, HINs and other organizations to increase the rate at which research findings are implemented into practice.
- **The Health Innovation Network**: This network, formerly known as the Academic Health Sciences Network, was established in 2013 to help the adoption and spread of innovation to improve health outcomes and generate economic growth. The network connects the NHS, academic organizations, local authorities and charities and provides support to generate a pipeline of evidence-based innovations and the adoption and spread of proven innovations across England.
- Innovators can reach out to various other networked research translation and innovation organizations to explore shared interests and complementarities and to access information. These include **NIHR Biomedical Research Centres**, **Academic Health Science Centres** and quality improvement networks like the **Q community**.
- Other key points of contact in regions across the country (e.g. **integrated care systems**, **primary care networks**) can help point innovators from the NHS to organizations and individuals who can offer various types of advice and support.
- Scotland has a range of innovation offerings, including the **NHS Health Innovation South East Scotland,** which is a 'test bed' for innovative solutions to health and social challenges, **NHS West of Scotland Innovation Hub**, provides end-to-end support from innovation conception to procurement and the **Digital Health & Care Innovation Centre**, which supports collaborations to co-design digital health and care solutions

---

Physical and IT infrastructure

Innovation raises new requirements for well-functioning facilities, equipment and data/IT infrastructure. For example, advances in technologies for cancer diagnosis, such as liquid biopsy platforms and multianalyte tests, lead to new capacities required in genomic testing laboratories. Advances in the field of dementia drugs could lead to increased diagnosis rates and impact on needed infrastructure in terms of imaging scanner capacity. Advances in AI lead to increased data management capacity needs, data processing and analytics infrastructure. Yet health systems, like the NHS, still face challenges related to basic facilities, including issues with physical infrastructure, bed capacity shortages and struggling to ensure that EMRs are well-functioning and interoperable. Given this, programmes are needed not only to support development of high-tech innovations but also to support innovation that addresses physical and data/IT infrastructure (see Box 19.5).

Box 19.5 Examples of sources of information about capital and infrastructure funding in the UK

- **UKRI Research Capital Investment Fund** supports the sustainability of research by contributing to replacement of premises or infrastructure, improved use of space and increasing sharing and use of research equipment.
- **The Department of Health and Social Care capital investment budget** can support NHS estates, facilities and equipment.

Service user engagement and explicit consideration of inequalities

Services users have key roles to play in helping identify innovation needs, informing the design of new products, technologies and service models to make sure they are user-friendly and fit for purpose. Further, service users can make significant contributions by participating in research, such as in clinical trials or serving as members of public advisory boards. However, there are many challenges to engaging service users, as well as other stakeholders, including carers and the public, in R&D activities. These challenges relate to limited knowledge of how to engage these stakeholders effectively and how to manage time and other resource constraints, as well as limited awareness among the public about potential opportunities.

Health system leaders and managers need to raise awareness about R&D activities taking place in their organizations and why it is relevant for service users, carers and the public, as well as about opportunities for participating or contributing to these activities. These individuals also need to be trained and prepared for engaging effectively. In addition to patient participation panels in NHS organizations or in specific disease-focused research charities, there are numerous sources of support for patient involvement and engagement in research and innovation in the UK. Some examples are presented in Box 19.6. Some international examples include the Patient Engagement Resource Centre (PERC), a European resource for patient engagement in research, and the Patient-Centered Outcomes Research Institute (PCORI), a not-for-profit organization in the US that funds research on outcomes that matter to patients and to help them make better-informed healthcare decisions.

Innovation can also have an important role to play in helping to tackle health inequalities among marginalized or vulnerable groups, for example, through solutions that can improve access, outcomes or patient experience, or by developing more tailored or personalized diagnostics, treatments and other interventions that prevent or reduce their morbidity and mortality. However, innovation is a human activity and, as such, is prone to reflect human biases. This affects not only what gets developed but also if, where and how innovations are implemented. Thus, innovation can have unintended consequences that create or exacerbate inequalities (Weiss et al., 2018). The key to mitigating these untoward consequences is to involve diverse patients and the wider public in decision-making activities across the innovation pathway, ranging from helping to identify unmet needs and neglected areas to evaluating the impacts of innovations on different communities, especially those who have been historically marginalized. While these populations can be particularly difficult to engage, there are organizations that specialize in this (see Box 19.6).

Box 19.6   Service user engagement and involvement with research and innovation

- **Patient Entrepreneurs Programme**: The NHS Clinical Entrepreneurs Programme is piloting a 12-month programme that started in March 2024, to support patients or carers who are working on healthcare innovations to improve patient care.
- **Core20PLUS5**: An approach developed by the NHS to inform action to reduce healthcare inequalities among the most deprived 20 per cent of the national population, especially among ethnic minority communities, people with a learning disability, people with multiple long-term health conditions, and other groups with protected characteristics, across five clinical areas of focus: maternity, severe mental illness, chronic respiratory disease, early cancer diagnosis and hypertension case-finding/lipid management.
- **National Voices**: A coalition of health and social care charities in England to incorporate the voice of people with lived experiences to influence changes in health and social care at the national and local levels.
- **People Street**: An organization that helps tackle inequalities and brings public perspectives to research and innovation efforts, mobilizing lived experience of individuals and communities to help with service design, research and wider decision-making.
- Numerous medical research charities have patient panels who can engage a lay perspective in research and innovation activities. Charites can also provide an intermediary voice for service users, but the engagement of charity staff should not substitute for efforts to engage service users and/or carers directly.

Learning activity 19.2

You are approached by a clinician in your organization who has an idea for a new diagnostic algorithm that combines two routinely used blood tests to diagnosis a rare disease. She has piloted the approach on a small group of her own patients in a research

Continued

Learning activity 19.2 *Continued*

study, with approval from the Health Research Authority (HRA) and believes that this novel algorithm could provide a quicker and more accurate diagnosis, potentially avoiding the need for other more expensive tests. But she is unsure about how to further develop the innovation.

- How could your organization support this clinician in developing her idea into an innovative diagnostic offer?
- What other departments and professional groups in your organization should be brought into discussions around how to take this forward?
- Which stakeholders outside your organization would you advise her to connect with?
- Where might she seek advice on how to develop the evidence base for the innovation?
- What factors other than the scientific performance/diagnostic accuracy should she consider in taking product development forward?

Examples of innovation in practice: navigating the innovation journey

In this section, we provide three real-world innovation case vignettes to bring to life some of the learning discussed earlier in this chapter, illustrating how innovations have entered the NHS and how barriers to adoption can be overcome. For these vignettes (Marjanovic et al., 2020b), we selected a:

1 Digital innovation: cognitive behavioural therapy (CBT) for insomnia provided via a digital health technology (i.e. software app) (Box 19.7).
2 Service model innovation: a new diagnostic cascade pathway for Familial Hypercho-lesterolemia (FH) (Box 19.8).
3 Low-tech innovation: blood donation chair (Box 19.9).

These cases represent distinct types of innovations and a range of enablers that influence their adoption.

Box 19.7   Sleepio: a digital health technology approach to treating insomnia

Millions of people globally suffer from insomnia, ranging from difficulty falling asleep, staying asleep, or experiencing poor quality sleep. Approximately 10 per cent of the UK population is estimated to suffer from the condition (Hafner et al., 2023). Sleepio is a software app that aims to help people overcome insomnia and improve sleep quality through CBT. Sleepio was developed by Big Health, a UK-based company.

Sleepio first entered into NHS use in 2013 after it was listed on the NHS Health Apps Library, a now discontinued effort to make it easier for patients to find NHS-endorsed health apps and programmes. In 2014, an Improving Access to Psychological Therapies (IAPT) service in Manchester helped establish a pilot in which Sleepio was provided for free to the IAPT service, in return for outcomes evidence generation for the company. Following a successful pilot, the IAPT service decided to commission Sleepio and the results helped with efforts to introduce Sleepio into other services in the North West and North of England. In 2015, one of the founders of Big Health became a fellow of a national programme that focused on helping support adoption of innovation in the NHS (the NHS Innovation Accelerator programme) and through this experience established relationships with various individuals and organizations that helped with the route to market (e.g. commissioning groups, NHS staff). However, most of the commissioning was done at local level, which created challenges for scale and spread. Some collaborative commissioning partnerships helped spread the service in London (e.g. The Health London Partnership) but access to the app through the NHS was to some extent a 'postcode lottery'. The absence of robust cost and health economics impact analysis also created barriers to widescale adoption. However, since the time of conducting this case study, the evidence base, including on health economics, has grown. In 2022, following an evaluation in the Thames Valley region of England, NICE recommended Sleepio for treating insomnia symptoms in primary care (Sampson et al., 2022). While some localities in the UK offer it for free, enabling a degree of spread, it is still not widely available free of charge, throughout the NHS (Sampson et al., 2022; Atenstaedt, 2023).

While Sleepio's entry into the UK market was slow, a series of enabling conditions as well as innovator and early adopter efforts made entry into the NHS possible. First, insomnia is a condition with a high societal burden with a **clear demand** for innovation, especially in light of the potential of digital interventions to enable people to access care in the comfort of their own home and to reduce demand pressures on face-to-face services. Second, the lived experience of insomnia by one of the founders was a **motivation for developing** Sleepio. The innovation also **fit within existing care pathways** (i.e. it was a complement to existing services, rather than a major disruptor), which helped create a receptive environment. Third, developing Sleepio entailed a **stakeholder-inclusive process that involved patients and healthcare professionals** in both designing the digital delivery of CBT and, in testing it, to help maximize the chances of relevant and user-centric content. Stakeholder engagement also facilitated **adaptation and improvement** over time. A **robust evidence base** on the clinical effectiveness of Sleepio, from randomized controlled trials and a NICE medtech innovation briefing, helped establish trust in this innovation and its quality among service-users, clinicians and commissioners. The company's participation in national initiatives, such as the NHS Innovation Accelerator fellowship programme, facilitated the establishment of **relationships and networks** that could help support uptake, alongside other personal networking efforts and word-of-mouth recommendations. The innovators behind Sleepio also helped with **support and training for healthcare providers** with its adoption.

Box 19.8   Cascade model for genetic testing of familial hypercholesterolemia: an example of a diagnostic service innovation

Familial hypercholesterolemia (FH) is a genetic condition that causes increased cholesterol levels from birth and, if left untreated, increases the risk of cardiovascular disease (CVD). Although FH is not a common condition, affecting only 1 in 250 people, there is a 50 per cent chance that a parent with FH will pass the condition on to their children. Cascade testing is a way of identifying relatives of individuals with FH and testing them for the gene mutation associated with the condition, which if identified can help promote timely treatment.

Cascade testing for FH first began in the Netherlands in 1994 and was shown to be effective in detecting individuals at risk. Genetic testing of FH in the UK first started at Great Ormond Street Hospital (GOSH) in 1997. In 2003, the UK government announced a two-year pilot programme to assess feasibility and cost-effectiveness of cascade testing in five centres in England. The promising results of the pilots led to guidance from NICE in 2008 (National Institute For Health And Care Excellence, 2019), recommending that genetic testing should be offered to individuals suspected to have FH and cascade testing should be pursued as a cost-effective means to identify relatives of people with FH who may also have the condition (guidance last updated in 2019). However, initial roll out across the UK was slow, in part due to challenges with clear commissioning routes. FH and cascade testing did not fall into specialized national commissioning routes, meaning the need to negotiate with local clinical commissioning groups (CCGs), many of whom did not see it as a priority. A lack of champions for the service and associated workforce demands for cascade testing (especially on nurse time) presented further barriers to uptake and spread. In 2010 the British Heart Foundation (BHF), in partnership with NHS Wales and the Welsh Assembly Government, funded an FH service in Wales. At the time, cascade testing in England was only being carried out in a few locations, largely where pilot studies had been run and staff had been able to continue securing funding for the services. However, FH gradually grew in importance and visibility in health policy and, in 2013, the Department of Health (now Department of Health and Social Care) developed a wider CVD outcomes strategy, which set out the needs to develop and spread good practice in relation to FH and CVD more broadly. Following the success of the Welsh trial, the BHF also started funding nurses in England (via CCGs) to provide cascade testing, but with agreements that bound CCGs to take steps to commission the service longer term, if the pilots were successful. By 2018, services had spread to approximately one-third of England (although with adaptation and variation in implementation models to fit local pathways, populations and settings) (National Institute For Health And Care Excellence, 2018). Wider developments with genomics testing services in the NHS, in addition to reductions in the costs of gene sequencing, further helped support service rollout; however, at the time of the case study development, there were efforts underway to help support wider scale spread of the service.

The initial adoption and spread of the FH cascade testing in the NHS was enabled **by information and evidence** of effectiveness and impact from use in other contexts (the Netherlands), as well as evidence of **cost-effectiveness**. **Funding** from not-for-profit organizations (BHF and HEART UK) helped pay for the needed software that supported nurses and aided the process of establishing familial pedigrees (PASS Clinical), facilitating the introduction of FH services in the UK. **Reduction in costs** of genetic testing, as well as **policy emphasis** on personalized medicine and interest in this space helped support commissioning.

Box 19.9   NHS Blood donor chair – an example of a low-tech innovation

NHS Blood and Transplant (NHSBT) is responsible for managing blood donation across England. NHSBT identified problems associated with blood donation that related to poor patient experience and process disruption due to donor fainting, which could occur up to 300 times per day in England. This was linked to old systems for blood collection and the nature of chairs used for blood donation. An innovative NHS Blood Donor Chair was developed in response to these issues and resulted in a product that was easier to clean and transport.

NHSBT first did research to identify the types of chairs available globally but did not identify any that they felt met NHS needs. They also developed a business case to understand the value for money that an improved chair could lead to. They then engaged in a procurement process and developed a tender in collaboration with the NHS National Innovation Centre (NIC), an organization that existed at the time to help support innovation in the NHS. The tender focused on the design of an improved blood donation chair and was informed by a consultation with blood collection teams and blood donors. Following a rigorous process of shortlisting companies, who had responded to the tender and provided design prototypes, two companies spent many months working with NHS staff and blood donors to advance a prototype and to test it. Following testing in 20 different locations involving over 200 blood donations, the Renfrew Group was awarded the contract to manufacture the new chair. The NHSBT was given intellectual property rights and are the only client of the chairs, purchasing them for rollout across England (at the time of conducting this case study). The innovative blood donor chair was awarded the 'Procurement Initiative of the Year' at the annual Health Service Journal awards in 2011.

Several enablers helped with product entry into the NHS. **Using established system networks** (e.g. the NHS National Innovation Centre, which existed at the time) helped broker contacts and helped establish relationships between stakeholders in NHS Blood and Transplant (NHSBT), innovators and NHS, clinical staff and blood donors. In turn, the **engagement of diverse stakeholders** helped inform the product design and

user-friendly specifications. A **pre-commercial procurement agreement guaranteed a viable commercial market** for innovators acting as an incentive for product development. The existence of a **centralized buyer** (NHSBT) supported adoption and spread across the NHS. There were also no significant technical or training barriers as the **product fitted within existing staff competencies and clinical pathways.**

The case examples presented illustrate the varied processes and influences involved in developing and adopting innovation, as discussed in as discussed in the section titled 'Healthcare innovation in practice'. Across the case examples, we observe many shared forces at play. In particular, these relate to the importance of efforts to establish and nurture appropriate relationships and networks between diverse stakeholders, the need to ensure appropriately skilled NHS staff and a good fit between an innovation and its adoption context (both the immediate implementation environment and sometimes wider policy landscape). The examples highlight the importance of establishing a robust evidence base for conveying value for money and supporting financing and procurement decisions, but also point to the need to navigate complexities in the NHS landscape, for example, as they relate to decentralized versus centralized procurement for different types of innovations. Enabling innovation to progress through a pathway – from development to adoption and spread – takes time and effort, and knowing how to create receptive conditions and capabilities is key to maximizing the chances of success.

Learning activity 19.3

Based on the case vignettes, reflect on an innovation that may have been developed or adopted in your organization or department.

- Was this innovation a new product, technology or service model, or was it using an existing product, technology or service model in a new way?
- Was it developed by you or one of your colleagues or was it developed elsewhere?
- If it was developed elsewhere, how well did you or your colleagues accept it?
- How did your organization develop or identify this innovation?
- What were the enablers that influenced if and how the innovation was developed and/or adopted?
- What enablers could influence how the innovation could be scaled up or spread?

Conclusions

This chapter has described why innovation matters, what influences the ability of health systems to be innovative and how leaders and managers in NHS organizations can attempt to embed innovation into health services. It has also provided some examples of the types of practical support available in the health system in the UK and some international examples. The chapter has outlined some theoretical and disciplinary perspectives on innovation to help readers familiarize themselves with how innovation has been studied across the pathway from development through to implementation.

Of course, innovation is not a magic bullet to address all the challenges facing health systems, and innovations can have disruptive and even negative consequences. Health system leaders and managers should consider where and how innovation can sit within broader efforts to transform care pathways and support efficient and effective care delivery and new ways of working.

For innovation to be sustainable, scalable and to spread also requires coordination between local and national efforts and priorities. Health system managers and leaders are key in mobilizing coordinated efforts, as well as in supporting cultures that rely on evidence-informed decisions and can help overcome obstacles like siloed thinking or the 'not invented here' syndrome. Ultimately, what matters is what works.

Learning resources

The NHS Innovation Service: The NHS Innovation service provides information, guidance and advice for innovators on the steps they need to take at different stages of the innovation pathway. It offers free advice and a free review for innovators to establish what their needs are and connect them with organizations that can help. It also has information on funding opportunities [https://innovation.nhs.uk/].

HINs: HINs can support innovators with innovations at various stages of development. There are 15 HINs in different parts of the country. HINs can support with guidance on the value proposition and evidence base related to an innovation, with efforts to create a proof of concept or innovation prototype, with various types of evaluation activities (e.g. impact modelling, health economics) and with information that can help innovators navigate the NHS. HINs can also broker contacts with health and care system experts and help with innovation adoption efforts

[https://thehealthinnovationnetwork.co.uk/how-we-can-help-you/support-for-innovators/].

NHS Clinical Entrepreneurs Programme: This programme provides training and support for clinical and non-clinical NHS staff and wider healthcare professionals interested in healthcare innovation. It aims to equip individuals with the knowledge, experience and commercial skills needed to develop and spread innovations. This is embedded in a wider ethos of supporting innovation, with a view to helping address the challenges facing the NHS. It is a free workforce development programme offering training, mentoring and networking opportunities [https://nhscep.com/].

Continued

Learning resources *Continued*

NHS Innovation Accelerator (NIA): This is a fellowship programme to support health and care staff to develop innovation skills, as well as to support the adoption and spread of innovation. The aim is to help accelerate innovation, help innovators grow their business and help improve patient experience and outcomes through support for innovation adoption [https://nhsaccelerator.com/].

National Institute of Health and Care Research (NIHR): NIHR funds diverse types of applied and clinical research and evaluation to improve health and well-being, as well as to support economic growth. It has research funding opportunities across various funding programmes [https://www.nihr.ac.uk/research-funding/funding-programmes].

Small Business Research Initiative (SBRI) Healthcare: SBRI Healthcare provides funding to support innovation development by small businesses and partnerships with academics and the NHS, in order to help solve the problems faced by the NHS [https://sbrihealthcare.co.uk/].

The Medicines and Healthcare products Regulatory Agency (MHRA): As the executive agency responsible for ensuring that medicines and medical devices work as intended and have an acceptable safety profile, the MHRA provides information for innovators on regulatory requirements innovations need to meet, as well as other useful information related to market authorizations and product approvals

[https://www.gov.uk/government/organisations/medicines-and-healthcare-products-regulatory-agency].

NICE Advice service: A source of scientific and strategic information and advice for health tech and pharmaceutical companies in particular, to help them in their innovation efforts and to support engagement with the NHS and access. It brings together and builds on prior NICE services, such as the Office for Market Access and NICE Scientific Advice. Although targeted mainly at industry, it provides useful information of relevance also for innovators in the NHS [https://www.nice.org.uk/about/what-we-do/life-sciences/nice-advice-service].

References

Alzheimer's Society (2020) Three promising drugs for treating Alzheimer's disease bring fresh hope. [Online]. [https://www.alzheimers.org.uk/blog/three-promising-drugs-for-treating-alzheimers-disease-bring-fresh-hope; accessed 28 March 2024].

Anderson, M., Panteli, D., Van Kessel, R., Ljungqvist, G., Colombo, F. and Mossialos, E. (2023) Challenges and opportunities for incentivising antibiotic research and development in Europe, *The Lancet Regional Health – Europe*, 33, 100705.

Atenstaedt, R. (2023) Should the Sleepio programme be available free of charge across the whole of the UK?, *Public Health in Practice*, (Oxf), 6, 100408.

Atkins, V. (2024) The 2024 Budget and NHS productivity [Online]. [https://www.gov.uk/government/speeches/the-2024-budget-and-nhs-productivity; accessed 28 March 2024].

Bopp, M., Saunders, R.P. and Lattimore, D. (2013) The tug-of-war: fidelity versus adaptation throughout the health promotion program life cycle, *Journal of Primary Prevention*, 34: 193–207.

Broerse, J. and Grin, J. (2019) *Toward Sustainable Transitions in Healthcare Systems*. (1st edn.). Abingdon: Routledge.

Bush, V. (1945) Science, the endless frontier: A report to the president on a program for postwar scientific research. Office of Scientific Research and Development (US). Reprinted in July 1960. Washingon, DC: National Science Foundation.

Carayannis, E. and Campbell, D. (2009) 'Mode 3' and 'Quadruple Helix': Toward a 21st century fractal innovation ecosystem, *International Journal of Technology Management*, 46.

Castle-Clarke, S., Edwards, N. and Buckingham, H. (2017) Falling short: Why the NHS is still struggling to make the most of new innovations [Online]. [https://www.nuffieldtrust.org.uk/research/falling-short-why-the-nhs-is-still-struggling-to-make-the-most-of-new-innovations#:~:text=6.,System%20barriers%20play%20a%20significant%20role,adapt%20are%20obvious%20cultural%20problems; accessed 28 March 2024].

Consoli, D. and Mina, A. (2008) An evolutionary perspective on health innovation systems, *Journal of Evolutionary Economics*, 19: 297–319.

Damschroder, L.J., Aron, D.C., Keith, R.E., Kirsh, S.R., Alexander, J.A. and Lowery, J.C. (2009) Fostering implementation of health services research findings into practice: a consolidated framework for advancing implementation science, *Implementation Science*, 4, 50.

Edquist, C. and Hommen, L. (2008) *Small Country Innovation Systems: Globalization, Change and Policy in Asia and Europe*. Cheltenham: Edward Elgar Publishing.

Etzkowitz, H. and Leydesdorff, L. (eds) (2002) *Universities and the Global Knowledge Economy: A Triple Helix of University-Industry-Government Relations*. Boston, MD Cengage Learning.

Freeman, C. (2008) *Systems of Innovation*. Cheltenham: Edward Elgar Publishing.

Fuenfschilling, L. and Truffer, B. (2014) The structuration of socio-technical regimes— Conceptual foundations from institutional theory, *Research Policy*, 43: 772–791.

Geels, F. (2011) The multi-level perspective on sustainability transitions: responses to seven criticisms, *Environmental Innovation and Societal Transitions*, 1: 24–40.

Geels, F. and Schot, J. (2007) Typology of sociotechnical transition pathways, *Research Policy*, 36: 399–417.

Glasgow, R.E., Vogt, T.M. and Boles, S.M. (1999) Evaluating the public health impact of health promotion interventions: the RE-AIM framework, *American Journal of Public Health*, 89: 1322–7.

Green, M.A., Mckee, M. and Katikireddi, S.V. (2022) Remote general practitioner consultations during COVID-19, *The Lancet Digital Health*, 4: e7.

Greenhalgh, T., Koh, G.C.H. and Car, J. (2020) Covid-19: A remote assessment in primary care, *The BMJ*, 368, m1182.

Greenhalgh, T., Wherton, J., Papoutsi, C., Lynch, J., Hughes, G., A'Court, C., et al. (2017) Beyond adoption: a new framework for theorizing and evaluating nonadoption, abandonment, and challenges to the scale-up, spread, and sustainability of health and care technologies, *Journal of Medical Internet Research*, 19: e367.

Hafner, M., Romanelli, R.J., Yerushalmi, E. and Troxel, W.M. (2023) The societal and economic burden of insomnia in adults: An international study. Santa Monica, CA, RAND Corporation.

Health Innovation Network (n.d.) NHS procurement explained [Online]. Health Innovation Network. [https://thehealthinnovationnetwork.co.uk/how-we-can-help-you/support-for-innovators/nhs-procurement-explained/; accessed 28 March 2024].

Jones, B., Kwong, E. and Warburton, W. (2021) Quality improvement made simple. [Online]. [www.health.org.uk/publications/quality-improvement-made-simple; accessed 24 December 2024].

Joy Mathew, C., David, A.M. and Joy Mathew, C.M. (2020) Artificial intelligence and its future potential in lung cancer screening, *EXCLI Journal*, 19: 1552–1562.

Kalindjian, A., Ralph, L., Middleton, S., Parkinson, S., Phillips, W.D., Romanelli, R.J., et al. (2022) The financial ecosystem of pharmaceutical R&D. An evidence base to inform further dialogue. [Online]. [https://www.rand.org/pubs/external_publications/EP68954.html; accessed 24 December 2024].

Kuznets, S. (1973) Modern economic growth: Findings and reflections, *The American Economic Review*, 63: 247–258.

Lillie, W., Ruth, R. and Charkitte, W. (2023) What is commissioning and how is it changing? [Online]. The King's Fund. [https://www.kingsfund.org.uk/insight-and-analysis/long-reads/what-commissioning-and-how-it-changing; accessed 24 December 2024].

Lundvall, B.-Å. (2010) *National Systems of Innovation: Toward a Theory of Innovation and Interactive Learning*. London: Anthem Press.

Marjanovic, S., Altenhofer, M., Hocking, L., Chataway, J. and Ling, T. (2020a) Innovating for improved healthcare: Sociotechnical and innovation systems perspectives and lessons from the NHS. *Science and Public Policy*, 47: 283–297.

Marjanovic, S., Altenhofer, M., Hocking, L., Morgan Jones, M., Parks, S., Ghiga, I., et al. (2020b) Innovating for improved healthcare: Policy and practice for a thriving NHS. Santa Monica, CA, RAND Corporation.

Medical Device Coordination Group (MDCG) (2019) Guidance on Qualification and Classification of Software in Regulation (EU) 2017/745-MDR and Regulation (EU) 2017/746-IVDR European Commission.

National Institute for Health and Care Excellence (NICE) (2018) Familial hypercholesterolaemia: Implementing a systems approach to detection and management. [Online]. [https://assets.publishing.service.gov.uk/media/5b646bbced915d37793abcda/familial_hypercholesterolaemia_implementation_guide.pdf; accessed 24 December 2024].

National Institute for Health and Care Excellence (NICE) (2019) Guideline: Familial hypercholesterolaemia: identification and management. [Online]. [https://www.nice.org.uk/guidance/cg71; accessed 24 December 2024].

Nelson, R.R. (1993) *National Innovation Systems. A Comparative Analysis*. Oxford: Oxford University Press.

NHS England (n.d.) NHS Long Term Plan. [Online]. [https://www.longtermplan.nhs.uk/; accessed 28 March 2024].

O'Keeffe, A.G., Nazareth, I. and Petersen, I. (2016) Time trends in the prescription of statins for the primary prevention of cardiovascular disease in the United Kingdom: a cohort study using The Health Improvement Network primary care data, *Journal of Clinical Epidemiology*, 8: 123–132.

Orsenigo, L. and Malerba, F. (2002) Innovation and market structure in the dynamics of the pharmaceutical industry and biotechnology: towards a history-friendly model, *Industrial and Corporate Change*, 11: 667–703.

Papoutsi, C., Greenhalgh, T. and Marjanovic, S. (2024) Approaches to spread, scale-up, and sustainability. [Online]. [https://www.cambridge.org/core/books/approaches-to-spread-scaleup-and-sustainability/B2A69BE3D579E3BDB5922340CE23D617; accessed 28 March 2024].

Proctor, E., Silmere, H., Raghavan, R., Hovmand, P., Aarons, G., Bunger, A., et al. (2011) Outcomes for implementation research: conceptual distinctions, measurement challenges, and research agenda, *Administration and Policy in Mental Health and Mental Health Services Research*, 38: 65–76.

Rogers, E.M. (1962) *Diffusion of Innovations*. New York: The Free Press.

Sampson, C., Bell, E., Cole, A., Miller, C.B., Marriott, T., Williams, M., et al. (2022) Digital cognitive behavioural therapy for insomnia and primary care costs in England: an interrupted time series analysis, *BJGP Open*, 6, BJGPO.2021.0146.

Schot, J. and Steinmueller, W.E. (2018) Three frames for innovation policy: R&D, systems of innovation and transformative change, *Research Policy*, 47: 1554–1567.

Sheikh, A., Jha, A., Cresswell, K., Greaves, F. and Bates, D.W. (2014) Adoption of electronic health records in UK hospitals: lessons from the USA, *The Lancet*, 384: 8–9.

Simpson, D.D. and Flynn, P.M. (2007) Moving innovations into treatment: a stage-based approach to program change, *Journal of Substance Use and Addiction Treatment*, 33: 111–120.

Tsimberidou, A.M., Kahle, M., Vo, H.H., Baysal, M.A., Johnson, A. and Meric-Bernstam, F. (2023) Molecular tumour boards — current and future considerations for precision oncology, *Nature Reviews Clinical Oncology*, 20: 843–863.

UK Government (2002) The Medical Devices Regulation [Online]. [https://www.legislation.gov.uk/uksi/2002/618/contents/made; accessed 28 March 2024].

UK Government (2016) Accelerated Access Review: final report. Review of innovative medicines and medical technologies. Wellcome Trust.

Ulyte, A., Moriarty, S. and Marjanovic, S. (2024) Preparing for the potential rollout of new Alzheimer's drugs: Towards a policy, research, and innovation agenda. [Online]. [https://www.rand.org/pubs/commentary/2024/01/preparing-for-the-potential-roll-out-of-new-alzheimers.html; accessed 28 March 2024].

US Food and Drug Administration (FDA) (2018) The drug development process: Step 3: Clinical Research [Online]. [https://www.fda.gov/patients/drug-development-process/step-3-clinical-research; accessed 28 March 2024].

Weiss, D., Rydland, H.T., Øversveen, E., Jensen, M.R., Solhaug, S. and Krokstad, S. (2018) Innovative technologies and social inequalities in health: a scoping review of the literature, *PLOS ONE*, 13: e0195447.

The healthcare workforce

Billy Palmer

Introduction

For any healthcare system, its workforce is both the largest single cost but also the greatest asset. There has been a growing recognition of the importance of healthcare staff, but all health systems are still facing some degree of challenge around supporting a sustainable workforce. The nature of the workforce challenge means it is both a very local issue – this distribution of staff between services is crucial to ensure that all patients can receive appropriate care – and a very global issue, given the huge amount of international migration of healthcare workers.

Government, employers, unions and patients all have perspectives on the nature of workforce challenges and the often-noisy debate on this does not always result in either an accurate diagnosis of the staffing problems or correct prescription on what to do about them. So, despite substantial endeavours to improve healthcare workforce planning, it continues to often fall short and be criticized (Anderson et al., 2021).

As we discuss in this chapter, the demand for healthcare staff is growing, but it is also important to note that their role is changing too. In part, this is because of the changing patterns of illness with, for example, an increase in chronic conditions likely requiring a more ongoing, monitoring staff role. There has also been a growing emphasis on person-centred care, which has changed the way healthcare professionals need to engage with patients. Similarly, the increasing recognition of the importance of overall well-being, prevention and of the social determinants of health means healthcare workers are having to consider and promote a wider set of health factors and treatments or programmes (Dahlgren and Whitehead, 1991).

It would also be remiss not to recognize how fundamentally the COVID-19 pandemic affected the workforce, including the dramatic change in working conditions and workload that many faced. Inevitably, this led to increased rates of burnout among the health workforce and this has had knock-on consequences, with there being recognized implications in terms of a negative impact on quality and safety of care, engagement, productivity, absenteeism and turnover (Smallwood et al., 2023).

In this chapter we look at the healthcare workforce which, put simply, covers 'all individuals whose job it is to protect and improve the health of their communities' (World Health Organization, 2006). The chapter begins with an overview of the size of the workforce in different countries, before covering the key trends and differences in the inflows and outflows of countries' healthcare workforce, including training, migration and retention. The chapter also looks at pay and employment models, as well as highlighting some key considerations around trying to ensure that there is the right balance of professions within the workforce and between different areas. The focus of the chapter is on healthcare workforce and so not directly on the social care workforce, although there are implications for the latter, including in the discussions on sources of recruitment and destination of leavers of nurses, healthcare assistants and other healthcare staff.

Size of the global healthcare workforce

In the region of 65 million people worked in healthcare in 2020 (World Health Organization, 2022). These staff are the single most important resource for any health services and, moreover, the healthcare workforce also accounts for a material proportion of the overall labour market within a country. Across developed countries, on average around one in ten jobs are within the health and social care sector, although this differs with over one in five in the labour market working within health and social care in Norway, whereas in Mexico it is less than one in 30 (OECD, 2023a).

Within these overall workforce numbers, there are a range of different professions. Norway, Switzerland and Finland have high numbers of practising nurses (all at nearly one practising nurse per 50 residents) whereas Latvia, Greece, Poland, Hungary, Israel and Mexico have fewer than a third of this level (at fewer than one per 170 residents). There is similar variation in relative staffing for practising doctors – with a two-fold difference between Austria (one per 182) and Korea (one per 391) – and in total hospital employment, with the latter particularly high in Switzerland and the United Kingdom (Figure 20.1).

The range of jobs within health services is vast – covering professionally qualified clinical staff, their clinical support staff, administrative and estates staff and managers. In English hospital and community services there are, for example, 323 different job roles from accountant to applied psychologist and from receptionist to radiographer. These staff also work across a huge array of services, from ambulance and emergency departments to allergy clinics and from tropical medicine to transport services (NHS Digital, 2023). This huge diversity creates challenges for healthcare managers who must consider how to deploy, support and remunerate staff fairly and effectively.

The growing number of healthcare workers

Across developed economies, total numbers in employment rose by a tenth in the decade to 2021, but the increase in health and social care employment – at 24 per cent – far outstripped

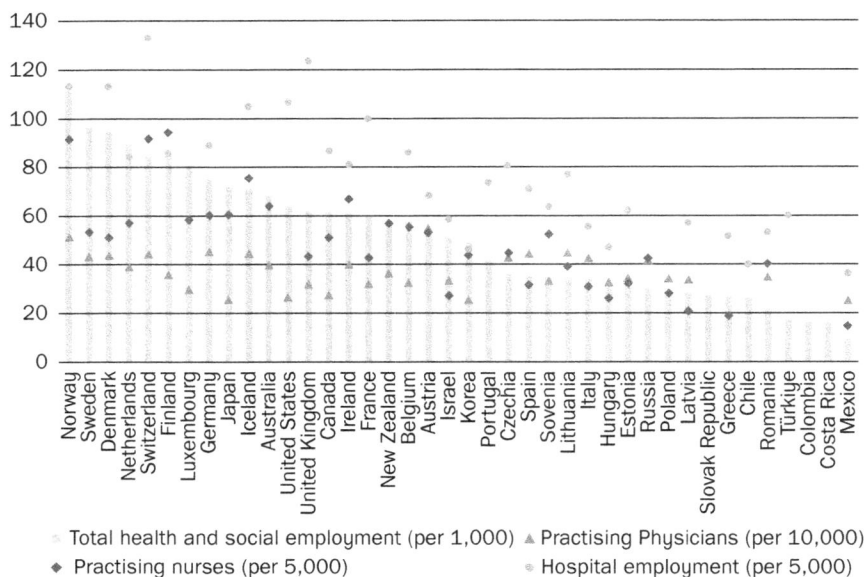

Figure 20.1 Size of health workforce relative to the population
Source: Analysis of Organisation for Economic Co-operation and Development (OECD) data (OECD, n.d.).

this level (OECD, 2023a). More starkly still, the global health workforce was reported to have increased by 29 per cent between 2016 and 2020 (World Health Organization, 2022). This increase was accelerated further during the pandemic. In some nations and professions, the increase is enormous – in the 8 years to 2018 the number of practising nurses in China and India both doubled (to 4 million and 2 million respectively), with a further increase of 1 million nurses in China in the subsequent 3 years to 2021. The largest relative increase has likely been in Indonesia which had 2.7 times more practising nurses in 2020 than 2015 (OECD, 2023b).

Yet there is a general consensus that many more healthcare staff are needed. In part, this is to address existing shortages, technological changes requiring a different skill mix and – in some countries at least – treating ageing populations with more complex care needs. As such, many countries, including the USA, Canada and England, have all predicted vast increases in health sector jobs over the next decade or so (Government of Canada, 2021; U.S. Bureau of Labor Statistics, 2023; NHS England, 2023a). Moreover, the World Health Organization (WHO) have estimated that 18 million more health workers are needed to achieve universal healthcare by 2030 in low- and lower-middle income countries (World Health Organization, n.d.).

Managing the supply of healthcare workers

Workforce planning is the process of analysing and forecasting the supply of, and demand for, workers in order to assess shortfalls and determine what interventions need to be put in place to ensure that there are 'the right people – with the right skills in the right places at the right time – to fulfil… the strategic objectives' (National Institute of Health, Office of Management,

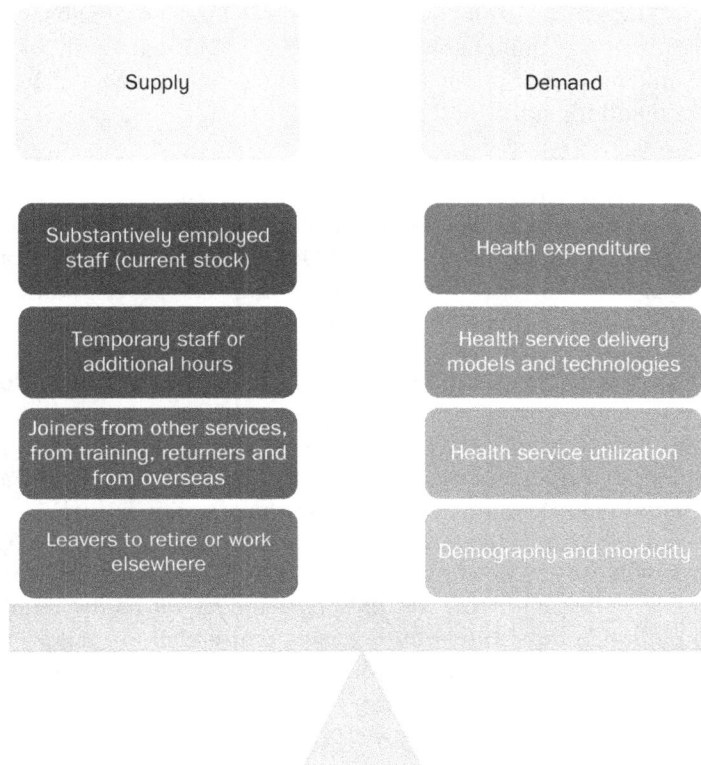

Figure 20.2 Key considerations in workforce planning
Notes: The factors are not intended to be a comprehensive list.
Source: Adapted from Ono et al. (2013).

n.d.). On the supply side, this involves estimating current staffing levels and projecting likely inflows and outflows. On the demand side, planning involves predicting how changes in the size and needs of the population, and in how services are designed and used, will impact on the likely number of staff needed to deliver the intended level of care (Figure 20.2).

Workforce planning is typically the responsibility of each country's respective ministry of health. That said, international organizations, such as WHO, European Commission, World Bank and OECD, as well as national and individual bodies, are involved, particularly around projecting workforce shortages. There is variation in the resource dedicated to workforce planning, with some countries, such as Australia and England, having dedicated, substantially funded health workforce planning agencies to improve data and modelling approaches while in other countries such planning is under-resourced (Ono et al., 2013).

Workforce planning – given the uncertainties in both the demand for and supply of staff – represents a formidable challenge (Ono et al., 2013). It requires long-term planning – to assess future demand and ensure that there are sufficient training places for medical, nursing and other clinical students to meet it – but also has to be agile to short-term shocks. The NHS in England in particular saw demand for nurses rapidly rise as a result of a hospital quality scandal (relating to Mid-Staffordshire NHS Foundation Trust) and subsequent inquiry and development of safe staffing guidelines (Francis, 2013; National Audit Office, 2016). More recently, the pandemic proved another example – with global reach – of how unforeseeable events can affect demand for staff.

Many countries are hindered by a lack of reliable, timely data and information. For example, countries often do not even have a grip of the current workforce shortages, including in Chile, where a shortage has been indirectly measured by comparing doctor-to-population ratio to a single country (Spain) and time point (2008) (Ono et al., 2013; Parzonka et al., 2023). As workforce models become more complex and comprehensive, additional assumptions have to be made with some proving difficult, including:

- the trend in productivity – output per worker – which has a direct influence on balancing the supply and demand for care. Where workforce models do try to account for productivity, some countries have assumed productivity gains – previously in Australia and Canada (Ono et al., 2013) and now in England (NHS England, 2023a), while previous planning in Belgium assumed a gradual decline in working time per doctor although they recognized the assumption was arbitrary and fragile (Ono et al., 2013).
- reconciling estimates of demand for care with assumptions on healthcare expenditure available to employ staff. Not only is this difficult as the number of staff that can be employed is determined by levels of pay which are not wholly predictable, but in the countries that have considered healthcare expenditure – such as previous modelling in England and Norway – the results are quite different to when only assessments of patient demand are factored in (Ono et al., 2013).

Training

While many – but not all – countries are seeking a more sustainable domestic pipeline of homegrown clinicians to meet demand, the approaches differ. In the last decade, many countries have increased the number of medical graduates by half or even higher (more than doubling in Latvia, Turkey and Bulgaria, for example). While the vast majority have seen substantial increases in graduate numbers, a few countries have seen numbers plateau, including the UK in the 2010s, Norway, Korea and Austria. However, some countries have bold ambitions with, for example, England recently having announced large increases in future training numbers, including medical school intakes expected to double by 2031 (NHS England, 2023a).

The supply of homegrown clinicians is not just an artifact of the number of training places but also affected by levels of attrition during training and participation in clinical services on graduation (see Box 20.1). Many countries have identified this training pipeline as being leaky and adopted various initiatives to shore it up. A relatively common policy is to offer free or heavily subsidized education in exchange for subsequently working in publicly funded health care services. The tie-in arrangements range in restrictiveness with, for example, Malaysia offering medical school scholarships in return for a 10-year commitment (for a typical 5-year course), whereas in Wales in return for covering tuition costs and a bursary for living costs, students must commit to working in their NHS for 2 years. Other policies include using pre-registration paid employment as a bridge between training and fully qualified employment, as in Ireland and Australia (Palmer et al., 2023).

Box 20.1   Case studies – turning off the taps on training numbers

There is typically an assumption that with the rising demand for healthcare, so too will the education infrastructure need to provide more domestically trained clinicians. However, this is not always the case and the reasons vary. For example, in Korea – where in order to become a midwife one must receive a year-long education in a hospital that provides a midwifery programme – due to the sudden decrease in birth rate, the childbirth numbers in many university hospitals fell and, as a result, midwifery programmes had to be shut down. By 2004, midwifery student numbers had fallen to just a quarter of the level in 1991 (Lee, 2006). Subsequently, the number of practising midwives in Korea fell by a quarter from 1,331 in 2007 to 1,009 in 2015.

Meanwhile, in England, the numbers starting nurse training fell fairly consistently from 2006 to around 2013 (Beech et al., 2019). At the time, the number of training places was being constrained by a ring-fenced budget for education and training. The government's response was to shift funding of tuition fees to students and thus remove what it considered was the cap on numbers caused by the limited national budget available to otherwise fund tuition fees. In the event, there was no immediate increase in training, though numbers did increase around 2020–22 but, worryingly, have fallen away considerably over the last 2 years.

In other clinical professions – particularly medicine – there has been a reluctance to change training numbers; a nationally commissioned UK analysis in 2014 predicted an 80 per cent oversupply of infectious disease consultants and 30 per cent undersupply of old age psychiatric consultants and yet training places commissioned for these two specialties remained unchanged for the subsequent year (National Audit Office, 2016). In part, this may have been due to the importance of doctors in training in providing services, so, by reducing training places, services might become unsustainable in the short term. Curious workforce planning decisions around training numbers in England are as old as the NHS itself with, for example, a powerful committee in 1955 determining that there was a risk of training too many doctors and recommending reducing student intakes moving forward (Palmer, 2022); in the event the number of hospital doctors doubled between 1949 and 1970.

Learning activity 20.1

- Consider all the types of organizations and stakeholders – including your own, if relevant – that play a role in education, including clinical placements during courses.
- Create a table for the trade-offs facing these organizations by outlining the challenges (including costs) and opportunities for increasing clinical training places for each of these.

Table 20.1 Countries with significant proportion of doctors who were foreign-trained

Country	Proportion of foreign-trained (2022 or latest available)	Largest single source country
Israel	58%	Russia (5,300)
Norway	42%	Poland (2,700)
New Zealand	42%	UK (3,200)
Ireland	40%	Pakistan (2,400)
Switzerland	38%	Germany (7,800)
Australia	32%	UK (6,600)
UK	32%	India (19,000)
Sweden	30%	Poland (1,300)

Note: Includes countries with available information and at least 25 per cent foreign-trained doctors in latest year of data.

Source: OECD (n.d.).

International migration

There is a large variation between countries in their reliance on foreign-trained clinicians. In 2022 or the latest year available, foreign-trained doctors accounted for over a quarter of the workforce in a number of countries (Table 20.1), although for some of these countries a significant proportion of foreign-trained doctors were actually native-born (see case study). There is typically lower reliance on foreign-trained nurses, although in New Zealand they account for nearly a third (31%) and in Ireland a half (49%) of nurses (OECD, n.d.).

First approved by member states in 2010, the WHO Global Code of Practice on the International Recruitment of Health Personnel – while being voluntary – aims to promote ethical practice with the primary aim of avoiding active recruitment from countries with already pressing workforce challenges (World Health Organization, 2010). A study using data to 2018 looking at migration of clinicians to countries in the European region, identified apparent declines in the numbers of nurses trained in developing countries but practising overseas, which might suggest increased adherence to the Code's principles on ethical recruitment. The increase in doctors recruited from overseas was explained as being driven by arrivals from countries experiencing conflict and volatility (Williams et al., 2020). Recently there has been concern, including in England, about the increase in recruitment from so called 'red list' countries (those from which active recruitment should be avoided); however, it is difficult to determine the extent to which this is passive (i.e. not active) recruitment or in contravention of the Code (Church, 2023).

A country's reliance on overseas recruitment may make them vulnerable given increased competition both from the native country and elsewhere for the same pool of staff (see Box 20.2). As highlighted earlier, most countries are rapidly increasing their clinical workforce, which means it might be less certain that opportunities to easily recruit from overseas will be available.

Box 20.2   Case study – outsourced training

One aspect of overseas recruitment that has – to date – been under-appreciated is the use of overseas medical schools to train your native-born students. Training is expensive – in England the cost to the taxpayer may be broadly in the region of £500,000 to train a consultant doctor, once you account for the cost of postgraduate training as well as undergraduate courses (and this does not include the costs of training those that do not complete the training or choose to work elsewhere) (Jones, 2024). It can also place a burden on services.

Even though there are few countries with readily available data on the proportion of their doctors who were foreign-trained but native-born, the variation is staggering. In Australia and England, these foreign-trained but native-born doctors represent around 1 in 250 of their workforces, whereas in Norway it is closer to 1 in 4 (23 per cent), and in Israel is it almost a third (30 per cent).

There are also called 'offshore medical schools' that are primarily aimed at foreign students wishing to practice medicine in their country of origin (Mclean and Charles, 2018). These are typically aimed at American and Canadian citizens and often located in the Caribbean basin but with examples too in Mexico and Australia. The curricula of these medical schools are based on that of the health systems to which they advertise.

An extreme case is Luxembourg – a very wealthy country in Europe – which does not train any doctors at all. Admittedly, it is not a large country (population of 640,000 in 2021) but that is still almost twice the size of, say, Iceland, which trains its own doctors.

Learning activity 20.2

- Speak to those involved in international recruitment – including the migrant clinical workforce – in your organization (or a nearby / related employer, if necessary) about personal and organizational motivations and experiences. Document the key ethical and practical implications of international recruitment.
- Outline what you consider could be the main challenges around offshore medical schools, including educational standards, clinical placements, financial, reputation and cultural. For each challenge, consider how national and local organizations of the destination countries of the graduates could mitigate any risk.

Retention

Efforts to reduce the rate of staff leaving are not just about sustaining numbers. They can also benefit patients by retaining valuable skills and experience in the health service and wider services from reduced disruption due to turnover and the need to recruit more staff to fill staffing gaps. Data from the UK suggest that for doctors leaving the register, wanting to live or practise overseas and retirement were the main reasons (General Medical Council, 2023). For nurses in the UK, the top three main reasons for leaving were retirement, physical or mental health, and burnout or exhaustion (Nursing and Midwifery Council, May 2023).

With many countries seeing an ageing workforce, attention is turning to how to get them to continue to contribute to delivery of healthcare or education in older life. There is substantial variation from country to country in the proportion of older clinicians, although this data alone does not tell us the nature of the problem. For example, the UK has a very small proportion (14%) of doctors aged 55 or over, which could either suggest there is little scope for improvement (as there are fewer doctors reaching possible retirement age) or, to the contrary, that there is huge scope for improvement (as it could suggest very high leaver rates among older doctors). The reverse could be argued for Italy, which has a very high proportion of doctors aged 55 or over (55%).

In most if not all countries, on a wider societal level, issues around retirement and ageing workforce are an important policy topic (Department for Work and Pensions, 2010). In healthcare specifically, many systems have sought to improve retention of their older workforce. Recent initiatives in England have focused on, for example, retirement conversations, flexible working and opportunities to work while still taking your pension (NHS England, 2023b).

Health service policymakers have to manage a huge array of levers to affect changes in retention – pay is one but so too are work environment, discrimination, flexibility, autonomy, training and staffing levels, to list to a few (Bimpong et al., 2020). Moreover, policymakers also need to keep up with the changing career behaviours and expectations of subsequent 'generations' of clinicians. England, for instance, has seen a doubling of doctors pausing their training, often taking up temporary non-training roles, for example, and a doubling of doctors leaving altogether, after their initial period of postgraduate training, including to work abroad (Palmer et al., 2023). Similarly, while in 2009 only 20 per cent of pensions awarded in England to family doctors (general practitioners (GPs)) were taken ahead of normal retirement age; by 2017 that had reached 52 per cent (Review Body on Doctors' and Dentists' Remuneration, 2023). However, there have been some promising initiatives to show that retention rates are amenable (see Box 20.3).

Box 20.3   Case study – Retention Direct Support Programme in England

The Retention Direct Support Programme was launched in 2017 to improve retention among nurses working in England's NHS hospitals. While data, guidance and liaison officers (to help form and execute plans) were provided to support individual employers, the bespoke plans were developed locally. As well as this delegated approach to development of the strategy, it is also interesting (and perhaps unusual) that employers were not given a numeric target to meet and the Programme has no other direct goals.

The action plans developed locally varied, although themes around development and education, increased flexibility and career progression were fairly common. The phased rollout meant that researchers were able to more clearly investigate the impact of the Programme and a subsequent independent evaluation appears to show significant success, with nurse turnover rates falling by 4 per cent, decreased exits from the public hospital sector down by 5 per cent, and even an apparent improvement in patient outcomes, with some evidence for a reduction in patient mortality.

The lessons are perhaps wider than just for retention, as they provide weight to the argument that a model in which information is provided to managers of multi-unit organizations, who trade off coordinating decisions across units and adapt them to local conditions, has scope for success.

Source: adapted from Moscelli et al. (2023).

The health of staff is also an important consideration both as a moral obligation of the employer but also in terms of the effect on workforce capacity. While, of course, health issues may manifest differently from country to country, figures from England lay bare the potential scale of the sickness absence issues. The reported data suggest some 27 million reported sick days across 2022, equating to around an average of 75,000 full-time equivalent staff and, if anything, this will be a substantial underestimate due to under-recording of incidences. Around a quarter (6 million days) were recorded for staff being sick due to mental health and well-being related reasons, with absences related to anxiety, stress, depression and other psychiatric illnesses having increased substantially over the last few years (Palmer and Rolewicz, 2023).

Sickness absences are important, in the longer term, for retention. Recent analysis highlighted that absences for both physical and mental health reasons are strongly associated with increased likelihood of leaving the NHS acute sector. For example, an NHS consultant missing 3 days of work for mental health reasons is 58 per cent more likely to leave 3 months later compared to those that have not had absences (Kelly et al., 2022).

Learning activity 20.3

- Discuss career expectations and motivations with some early career clinicians in your organization (or a nearby / related employer, if necessary).
- Reflect on their responses – how might any identified changes in behaviours have implications for your organization and the healthcare service more widely?

Pay, rewards and employment models

Healthcare workers – and specialist (consultant) doctors in particular – can be employed on various contractual models. In particular, some are self-employed, whereas others are salaried employees. In addition, whereas some are substantive employees, others are contracted on a temporary basis either through in-house temporary staffing bank, a collective staffing bank (i.e. run across multiple employers) or through an agency. In addition, other staff working in healthcare settings may be employed by an outsourcing company and, further, some staff are essentially employed by another body from the organization they work for (in England this includes doctors in training who are employed at a regional level and an increasing number of the workforce in general practice who are employed by pan-practice primary care networks). This could have huge significance when, for example, it comes to the organizations where these staff work, trying to promote fairness or introduce a comprehensive change to terms or conditions.

The employment model will, to a degree, influence the level of pay. However, there are wider differences in the pay-setting processes in different countries. In some countries the salaries of specialists are usually negotiated individually between the specialist and hospitals (e.g. USA and Sweden), in other countries associations of physicians and associations of hospitals collectively negotiate salary scales and increases (e.g. Canada, France, Germany), while in some the salary scale is fixed by the government department (e.g. England, albeit with a pay review body that makes recommendations). The length of time between negotiations also varies, with this being irregular in some countries but, for example, every 4 years in Canada (Quentin et al., 2018). There are also differences in the arrangements for arbitration and the role that national governments play. In some instances, wider employment factors are prioritized in contract negotiations with, for example, the Canadian province of British Columbia prioritizing minimum nurse to patient ratios (Hutchings, in progress).

There are many ways to compare earnings between countries, including by adjusting for exchange rates or in relation to the costs of goods (purchasing power) or average earnings in that country, and none are perfect. However, notwithstanding that note of caution, there are substantial differences in levels of pay between countries. For example, salaried specialists' salaries vary from 1.4 times the average wage in Poland to 4.7 times in Hungary and self-employed specialists' salaries vary from 3.2 times the average wage in Switzerland to 6.8 times in Korea (Figure 20.3).

As individuals' satisfaction with pay is determined by assessments of both the absolute and relative level (Valet, 2023), it is important too to consider how different staffing groups' salaries differ within the same country. In Korea, England, Ireland and Germany the average salaried specialist earnings are at least three times higher than that for nurses whereas the disparity is half this (1.5 times) in Poland and Costa Rica (OECD, n.d.).

Learning activity 20.4

- Select three or four clinical staff groups and collate the available information on their pay range in your organization and across different providers and settings.
- Speak to your HR department about the mechanisms they have locally to determine pay, including any recruitment and retention premia, and how effective these are.

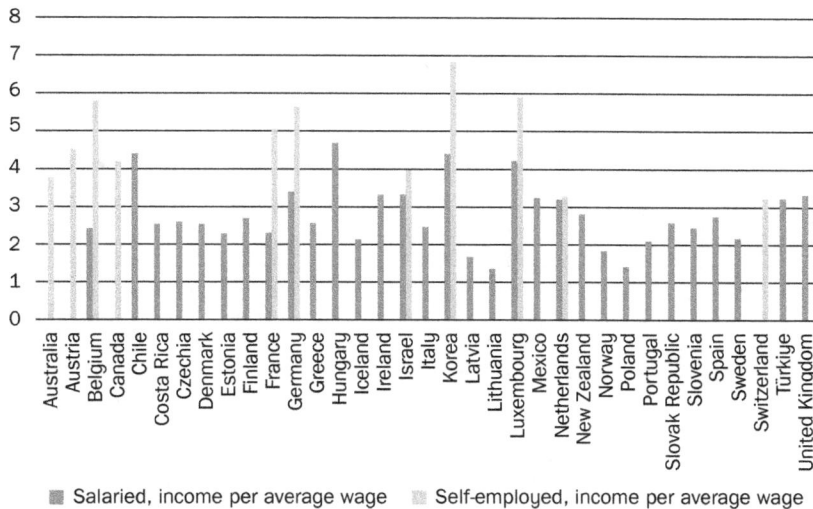

Figure 20.3 Remuneration of specialist medical practitioners relative to average earnings, 2022 (or nearest year)
Source: Analysis of OECD data (OECD, n.d.).

Rebalancing the mix of professions

Introducing new or a different balance of staff to a service has the potential to meet changing needs of patients, improve cost-effectiveness, keep up with increased demand for care and potentially unlock the potential of technological or medical advancements, but such changes are not a guarantee of improvements in care or costs; in fact, if changes in the balance of staff or introduction of new roles is poorly implemented then care and costs can be compromised. In particular, there are challenges around designing the role, education, training, supervision, public awareness, acceptance by other professions and developing career pathways.

As well as rebalancing the split of established roles, such as doctors and nurses, there are various emerging roles. These can be broadly categorized as: advanced (e.g. advanced clinical practitioners or nurse practitioners), assistance (e.g. nurse or physician associates), new (e.g. mental health peer support workers or health and well-being coaches), extended (e.g. health visitors) and new training roles (e.g. new apprenticeship careers).

As ever, international comparison on workforce data needs to be treated with a degree of caution, but the available data do appear to reveal differences in the use of certain professions, including doctors and nurses. These two professions account for little more than two-thirds of hospital staff in the United States (34 per cent), Canada (35 per cent) and UK (37 per cent) compared to nearly two-thirds in Italy (63 per cent) and almost three-quarters (72 per cent) in Austria (Figure 20.4) (OECD, n.d.). Drilling down to more specific staff groups and, in particular, emerging roles, reveals even more stark differences with, for example, an estimated 120,000 physician associates (who perform various medical tasks under the supervision of a doctor) across the United States as of mid-2020 compared to 2,000 across the United Kingdom and 30 across Australia (Hooker and Berkowitz, 2020).

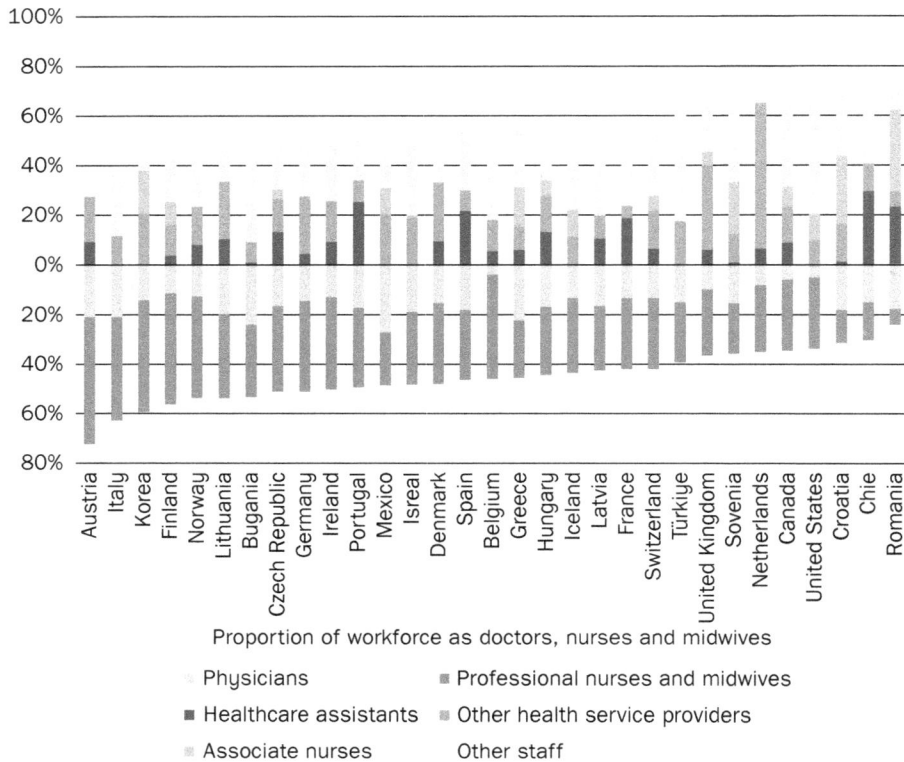

Figure 20.4 Breakdown of staff employed in hospitals, by profession grouping
Source: Analysis of OECD data (OECD, n.d.).

In some cases, the changing balance of staff has been gradual, whereas in others it has been rapid and dramatic. In 2019, NHS England and the doctors' professional association (the British Medical Association (BMA)) published a five-year framework to implement the then system-wide strategy (BMA and NHS England, 2019), which called for 20,000 more staff (excluding GPs) working in primary care by 2023/24. On top of this, the incoming government committed to recruiting an additional 6,000 more primary care staff. In the event, the government exceeded this ambition, with 29,000 added even a year in advance (by March 2023). While in some respect this is welcome, the scale of the skill-mix change is dramatic; the ratio of fully qualified, permanent family doctors (GPs) to other clinicians has fallen from 1:1 to 1:2 in 8 years. This has obvious implications on capacity for supervision, for example. The phenomenon also raises questions about whether the salary reimbursement is appropriately balanced with, specifically, many of these additional staff groups effectively being provided free of direct salary costs to the individual family surgeries (general practice), unlike, for example, the cost of salaried GPs where the entire cost is borne by the surgery. Similar arguments have been levelled at whether the high levels of postgraduate salary reimbursement for doctors in postgraduate training could incentivize a skill-mix that is not optimal in the long-term (Beech et al., 2019).

A key consideration when it comes to clinical staff and, in particular, the introduction of new professions, is regulation. Regulation can take many forms with, at the most formal end, statutory regulation, whereby you cannot describe yourself as a regulated health-care professional without appropriate registration to a professional body. Where there is no formal regulation, greater responsibilities fall on individuals (including the need to be aware of their own limitations and scope of practice) and employers (including providing assurance of appropriate qualifications). Many different approaches to regulation are used internationally, even across staff with similar scopes of practice. For example, a cross-country comparison of 11 countries, with similar scopes of practice for advanced nurse practitioners, found nine had – at that time – specific regulations in place (including Australia, Canada, the Netherlands, New Zealand and the US) while Finland and England did not (Maier and Aiken, 2016). While regulation can have benefits in terms of protecting the public and even advancing a profession, it is also important to recognize a trade-off: it is often costly and complex to introduce and results in some degree of additional burden on staff (Palmer et al., 2023).

There are different approaches to the challenge of providing assurance around the competence of healthcare leaders. In France, individuals aspiring to be hospital or assistant hospital directors must undertake a specific programme lasting 2 years, with requirements around previous experience and a formal examination to train entry. The training has three aspects: cultural, human and technical (École des Hautes Etudes en Sante Publique, n.d.). However, the situation across the channel in England, is somewhat different. Since 2015, all executive and non-executive director posts (or equivalent) have been required to meet the requirements of the *fit and proper persons regulations*, which include they are 'of good character' and have not been responsible for or contributed to any serious misconduct or mismanagement in the course of conducting regulated activity (NHS Providers, n.d.). Subsequent reviews have made various recommendations (Figure 20.5), but the competence of NHS managers remains a topic of political and public debate (Booth, 2023).

Learning activity 20.5

- Ascertain the stated policy intentions around changing the mix of professions in your country.
- Create a table of what you consider to be the key challenges in meeting these intentions and who you believe holds primary responsibility for mitigating any risks, including at national, regional and local levels.

Distribution within health services

Typically, countries have a disproportionately high number of doctors in their capital city and fewer doctors relative to the size of the population in remote areas; however, this varies considerably between nations. At the extreme, in Lithuania's remote areas the physician

The NHS leadership review (Rose review), 2015	Kark Review of the fit and proper person test, 2019	The Messenger Review of NHS leadership, 2022
• Require senior managers to attend accredited courses for a qualification • Set, teach and embed core management compentencies and associated expected behaviours at each management level • Establish a mechanism for providing ongoing career suport for all those in a management role	• Develop competencies for directors • A central database of director's qualifications, training and appraisals • Expand the definition of serious misconduct	• Consistent management standards delivered through accredited training • A simplified, standard appraisal system for the NHS • Targeted interventions on collaborative leadership and organisational values

Figure 20.5 Some key findings from independent reviews of NHS leadership in England
Source: Adapted from Rose Review (Rose, 2015), Kark Review (Kark and Russell, 2019), Messenger Review (Messenger and Pollard, 2022).

density is half that of metropolitan areas, whereas in Japan there are more doctors relative to the number of people in remote compared to metropolitan areas (OECD, 2023a). For nurses and midwives, the geographic distribution is – for Europe at least – the opposite, with higher numbers, relative to size of the population, in more sparsely populated areas (Winkelmann et al., 2020).

It is not always clear how undesirable the variation is – some differences in doctors relative to the size of the population may just be due to availability of other staff groups or different care models – but many governments have tried to rebalance the geographical variation. France, Czech Republic and England have all, for example, introduced financial incentives for GPs to work in underserved areas. In Australia, tuition fees for medical courses are part-paid in return for commitment to work in eligible regional, remote or rural areas for 3 years after completion of training. Similarly, there are student loan forgiveness schemes for working in underserved or remote areas for doctors, nurses, midwives and physician associates in the United States and for family doctors and nurses in Canada (Palmer et al. 2023).

As well as addressing geographical variation, countries have also sought to address specific shortages in particular services, settings and specialties. For instance, many countries have sought to respond to concerns about shortages in the number of general practitioners. Policies have included increasing the proportion of medical training places allocated to general practice, with England, the Netherlands, France and Canada all, for instance, committing to having somewhere in the region of 40–50 per cent of training places dedicated to family medicine (OECD, 2023a).

Learning activity 20.6

- Speaking to colleagues from HR and clinical services, outline the key enablers and barriers to rebalancing the geographical workforce imbalances.
- Reflect on how your context differs from elsewhere in your country, and internationally too, and draw out which settings and services face most similar challenges to your own organization.

Conclusion

Workforce planning and management is a hugely complex task. Health systems should use intelligent workforce planning approaches to make best estimates on the number of training places across the different professions needed to meet future workforce needs. They can also ensure that there are appropriate processes in place to set pay and conditions to promote sufficient levels of recruitment and retention. However, healthcare leaders also need to recognize that even the best-laid plans will often go awry, perhaps because of funding changes, changing government workforce targets or changes in the global market for these valuable clinicians. And so, leaders need both long- and short-term levers to ensure that there are the right staff, in the right place, at the right time.

Action has been patchy; some countries have been bold in trying to address some distinct issues, but these efforts have neither been exhaustive, in terms of seeking to address all issues, nor comprehensive, in terms of all health systems engaging with the issue. Moreover, where action has been taken there has been a disappointing lack of published evaluation to help understand the impact, any unintended consequences and implications for translating to different settings and services. This gap in evidence is hard to accept given the consequences of workforce shortages.

Learning resources

Organisation for Economic Co-operation and Development (OECD): Equipping Health Workers with the Right Skills provides a comparative overview of practices in 16 countries to anticipate future skills needs in the health workforce, and of how such information is used by policymakers and social partners to foster better alignment with labour market needs [https://www.oecd.org/health/equipping-health-workers-with-the-right-skills-9b83282e-en.htm].

World Health Organization (WHO): Published Global strategy on human resources for health: Workforce 2030 that intended to address, in an integrated way, all aspects

Continued

Learning resources *Continued*

ranging from planning, education, management, retention, incentives, linkages with the social service workforce, so they can inform more incisive, multi-sectoral action, based on new evidence and best practices [https://iris.who.int/bitstream/handle/10665/250368/9789241511131-eng.pdf].

Health Systems and Policy Monitor (HSPM): Website provides up-to-date information on health systems, as well as policy reform for most EU countries including on workforce issues [www.hspm.org].

European Commission – Health Workforce: Website provides information and resources and details of events about the EU healthcare workforce [https://health.ec.europa.eu/health-workforce_en].

Organisation for Economic Co-operation and Development (OECD) statistics portal: Provides a range of measures around various countries' workforces, including numbers of graduates and currently practising clinicians and remuneration levels [https://stats.oecd.org/].

NHS England: Published the **NHS Long Term Workforce Plan** in 2023. It includes details of its workforce modelling and sections on training, retaining and reforming the workforce [https://www.england.nhs.uk/long-read/nhs-long-term-workforce-plan-2/].

NHS Pay Review body (and equivalent for doctors and dentists): Their reports include a huge array of data on the workforce in the UK [https://www.gov.uk/government/organisations/nhs-pay-review-body].

References

Anderson, M., O'Neill, C., Macleod Clark, J., Street, A., Woods, M., Johnston-Webber, C., et al. (2021) Securing a sustainable and fit-for-purpose UK health and care workforce, *The Lancet*, 397(10288).

Beech, J., Bottery, S., Charlesworth, A., Evans, H., Gershlick, B., Hemmings, N., et al. (2019) Closing the gap: key areas for action on the health and care workforce. London: Nuffield Trust, Health Foundation, The King's Fund.

Bimpong, K.A.A., Khan, A., Slight, R., Tolley, C.L. and Slight, S.P. (2020) Relationship between labour force satisfaction, wages and retention within the UK National Health Service: a systematic review of the literature, *BMJ Open*, 10(7): e034919.

BMA and NHS England (2019) Investment and evolution. A five-year framework for GP contract reform to implement The NHS Long Term Plan. [https://www.england.nhs.uk/publication/gp-contract-five-year-framework/; accessed 9 January 2025].

Booth, R. (2023) Labour vows to make NHS managers accountable after Lucy Letby failings. *The Guardian* [Online] [https://www.theguardian.com/society/2023/aug/28/

labour-vows-to-make-nhs-managers-accountable-after-lucy-letby-failings; accessed 14 March 2024].

Church, E. (2023) NMC register grows but concern over 'red list' recruitment. [Online] [https://www.nursingtimes.net/news/workforce/nmc-register-grows-but-concern-over-red-list-recruitment-30-11-2023/; accessed 15 March 2024].

Dahlgren, G. and Whitehead, M. (1991) Policies and strategies to promote social equity in health. Background document to WHO Strategy paper for Europe. Institute for Futures Studies, Arbetsrapport.

Department for Work and Pensions (2010) A comparative review of international approaches to mandatory retirement. [Online] [https://assets.publishing.service.gov.uk/media/5a7acf33ed915d670dd7eb6f/674summ.pdf; accessed 14 March 2024].

École des Hautes Etudes en Sante Publique (n.d.) Health Care Institution Management Program. [Online] [https://www.ehesp.fr/en/programs/civil-service-executive-degree-programs/health-care-institution-management-program/; accessed 14 March 2024].

Francis, R. (2013) Report of the Mid Staffordshire NHS Foundation Trust Public Inquiry. The Mid Staffordshire NHS Foundation Trust Public Inquiry. [https://www.gov.uk/government/publications/report-of-the-mid-staffordshire-nhs-foundation-trust-public-inquiry; accessed 14 March 2024].

General Medical Council (2023) The state of medical education and practice in the UK. Workforce report 2023. London: GMC.

Government of Canada (2021) Industrial projections (2022–2031), Canadian Occupational Projection System (COPS). [Online] [https://occupations.esdc.gc.ca/sppc-cops/l.3bd.2t.1ilshtml@-eng.jsp?lid=27&fid=1&lang=en; accessed 15 March 2024].

Hooker, R. and Berkowitz, O. (2020) A global census of physician assistants and physician associates, *Journal of the American Academy of PAs*, 33(12): 43–45.

Hutchings, R. (in progress) *How Do other countries determine pay for healthcare staff?* London: Nuffield Trust.

Jones, K., Weatherly, H., Birch, S., Castelli, A., Chalkley, M., Dargan, A., et al. (2024) Unit costs of health and social care 2023 manual. Technical report. Personal Social Services Research Unit (University of Kent) & Centre for Health Economics (University of York).

Kark, T. and Russell, J. (2019) A review of the Fit and Proper Person Test. Department of Health and Social Care. [https://assets.publishing.service.gov.uk/media/5c937b7e40f0b633f5bfd89c/kark-review-on-the-fit-and-proper-persons-test.pdf; accessed 15 February 2025].

Kelly, E., Stoye, G. and Warner, M. (2022) *Factors associated with staff retention in the NHS acute sector*. London: The Institute for Fiscal Studies.

Lee, K.H. (2006) Nurse-midwifery education through graduate programs to provide a sufficient number of high quality nurse-midwives, *Journal of Educational Evaluation for Health Professions*, 3(5).

Maier, C.B. and Aiken, L.H. (2016) Task shifting from physicians to nurses in primary care in 39 countries: a cross-country comparative study, *European Journal of Public Health*, 26(6): 927–934.

Mclean, S. and Charles, D. (2018) A global value chain analysis of offshore medical universities in the Caribbean. *Studies and Perspectives*. United Nations.

Messenger, G. and Pollard, L. (2022) Leadership for a collaborative and inclusive future. Department of Health and Social Care.

Moscelli, G., Sayli, M., Blanden, J., Mello, M., Castro-Pires, H. and Bojke, C. (2023) Non-monetary interventions, workforce retention and hospital quality: evidence from the English NHS. University of York.

National Audit Office (2016) Managing the supply of NHS clinical staff in England. HC 736. Session 2015-16.

National Institute of Health, Office of Management (n.d.) Workforce Planning. [Online] [https://hr.nih.gov/workforce/workforce-planning#:~:text=Workforce%20Planning%20is%20the%20process,to%20fulfill%20its%20mandate%20and; accessed 1 January 2024].

NHS Digital (2023) HCHS staff in NHS trusts and core orgs March 2023: area of work, job role tables. [Online] [https://digital.nhs.uk/data-and-information/publications/statistical/nhs-workforce-statistics/march-2023; accessed 15 January 2025].

NHS England (2023a) NHS long term workforce plan. [Online] [https://www.england.nhs.uk/publication/nhs-long-term-workforce-plan/; accessed 14 March 2024].

NHS England (2023b) Retaining doctors in late stage career guidance. [Online] [https://www.england.nhs.uk/long-read/retaining-doctors-in-late-stage-career/; accessed 14 March 2024].

NHS Providers (n.d.) Fit and proper persons regulations in the NHS. [Online] [https://nhsproviders.org/fit-and-proper-persons-regulations-in-the-nhs/the-fit-and-proper-persons-regulations; accessed 14 March 2024].

Nursing and Midwifery Council (2023) NMC register leavers survey. May 2023. [https://www.nmc.org.uk/globalassets/sitedocuments/data-reports/may-2023/annual-data-report-leavers-survey-2023.pdf; accessed 9 January 2025].

OECD (2023a) Health at a glance 2023: OECD indicators. [Online] https://doi.org/10.1787/7a7afb35-en.

OECD (2023b) Statistics. Health resources: Nurses. [Online] [https://stats.oecd.org/Index.aspx?ThemeTreeId=9; accessed 2 January 2023].

OECD (n.d.) Statistics. [Online] [https://stats.oecd.org/#; accessed 9 January 2024].

Ono, T., Lafortune, G. and Schoenstein M. (2013) Health workforce planning in OECD countries: a review of 26 projection models from 18 countries. OECD Health Working Paper No. 62. Paris: Organisation for Economic Co-operation and Development.

Palmer, W. (2022) Doing right when you are wrong: perspectives on workforce planning in the NHS in uncertain times. [Online] [https://www.nuffieldtrust.org.uk/news-item/doing-right-when-you-are-wrong-perspectives-on-workforce-planning-in-the-nhs-in-uncertain-times; accessed 15 March 2024].

Palmer, W. and Rolewicz, L. (2023) All is not well: Sickness absence in the NHS in England. [Online] [https://www.nuffieldtrust.org.uk/resource/all-is-not-well-sickness-absence-in-the-nhs-in-england; accessed 14 March 2024].

Palmer, W., Julian, S. and Vaughan, L. (2023) Independent report on the regulation of advanced practice in nursing and midwifery. London: Nuffield Trust.

Palmer, W., Rolewicz, L. and Dodsworth, E. (2023) Waste not, want not; strategies to improve the supply of clinical staff to the NHS. London: Nuffield Trust.

Parzonka, K., Ndayishimiye, C. and Domagala, A. (2023) Methods and tools used to estimate the shortages of medical staff in European countries—scoping review, *International Journal of Environmental Research and Public Health*, 20(2945).

Quentin, W., Geissler, A., Wittenbecher, F., Ballinger, G., Berenson, R., Bloor, K., et al. (2018) Paying hospital specialists: experiences and lessons from eight high-income countries, *Health Policy*, 122(5): 472–484.

Review Body on Doctors' and Dentists' Remuneration (2023) Fifty-first report 2023. London: Office of Manpower Economics.

Rose, Lord (2015) Better leadership for tomorrow: NHS leadership review. Department of Health and Social Care.

Smallwood, N., Mismark, M. and Willis, K. (2023) Burn-out in the health workforce during the COVID-19 pandemic: opportunities for workplace and leadership approaches to improve well-being. *BMJ Leader*, 7(3):178–181. doi: 10.1136/leader-2022-000687.

U.S. Bureau of Labor Statistics (2023) Occupational employment projections, 2022-32. [Online] [https://www.bls.gov/emp/; accessed 15 March 2024].

Valet, P. (2023) Perceptions of pay satisfaction and pay justice: two sides of the same coin?, *Social Indicators Research*, 166: 157–173.

Williams, G., Jacob, G., Rakovac, I., Scotter, C. and Wismar, M. (2020) Health professional mobility in the WHO European Region and the WHO Global Code of Practice: data from the joint OECD/EUROSTAT/WHO-Europe questionnaire, *European Journal of Public Health*, 30 (Suppl 4): iv5–iv11.

Winkelmann, J., Muench, U. and Maier, C. (2020) Time trends in the regional distribution of physicians, nurses and midwives in Europe, *BMC Health Services Research*, 20(937).

World Health Organization (2006) The world health report 2006: working together for health. Geneva: World Health Organization. [Online] [https://www.who.int/publications/i/item/9241563176; accessed 2 January 2024].

World Health Organization (2010) WHO global code of practice on the international recruitment of health personnel. 20 May. [https://www.who.int/publications/i/item/who-global-code-of-practice-on-the-international-recruitment-of-health-personnel; accessed 9 January 2025].

World Health Organization (2022) Global strategy on human resources for health: workforce 2030: Reporting at Seventy-fifth World Health Assembly. [Online] [https://www.who.int/news/item/02-06-2022-global-strategy-on-human-resources-for-health--workforce-2030; accessed 2 January 2024].

World Health Organization (n.d.) Health workforce. [Online] [https://www.who.int/data/gho/data/themes/health-workforce; accessed 2 January 2024].

Service user perspectives, experiences and involvement

Jo Ellins and Tina Coldham

Introduction

At some point in our lives, we will all use health services. Our experiences may be great or not so good, but either way there is much that we can learn about how to design and deliver services so that they are responsive to the needs of people who use them. In this chapter, we introduce, explore and perhaps even demystify the world of involvement in healthcare. While policymakers, managers and professionals may debate the purpose of involvement and the best way to do it, the reality is that we all play a role in our health-care, whether we recognize it or not. This spans from decisions we make about whether and where to seek help when a new symptom emerges, through to the various activities that people undertake, often on a daily basis, to manage life with a long-term health condi-tion or conditions.

The real issue is how to ensure that people can participate in ways that are positive, meaningful and beneficial, and what this means for service users, health professionals and the relationships between them. In addressing this issue, we have sought to blend insights from theoretical and research literature with practical tools and learning, and a selection of international case study examples. Attention is paid both to involvement practices and the wider organizational contexts in which such practices are situated, and the ways in which these contexts can both enable and constrain successful partnership working.

Definitions

Before we embark, it is important to acknowledge that there is a great deal of terminol-ogy used in this area, and this is often ambiguous and frequently contested. Traditionally, people receiving healthcare services were referred to as 'patients' but, with its connotations of passivity and dependence, this language feels rather at odds with the modern view of individuals as active participants in their health and care (Neuberger, 1999). There are many other terms available, such as service user, client, consumer, customer and survivor (often, but not exclusively, used by people who have experienced mental health difficulties). All of these have their proponents and their critics, and none has been universally accepted. The term 'carer' is also problematic. It means different things to different people; implies a burden that can devalue the person that is being cared for; and is a term that many people who provide care neither recognize nor associate with (Molyneaux et al., 2011).

There is no easy answer to this terminological problem but, wherever possible, people should be allowed to choose for themselves how they are defined in order to avoid the use of terms that are considered inappropriate, insensitive or offensive. A key principle is to use 'people-first' language, which places the person before the illness or disability (Crocker and Smith, 2019). This would mean, for example, referring to 'people who have diabetes' rather than 'diabetics'.

The same issues arise when thinking about 'involvement'. When an activity captures the imagination of others, it often grows its own language, rules and principles, and codes of conduct. People argue over all of this, endeavouring to come to a place of agreement and understanding of what 'good' looks like. It is so with involvement. Ironically, this can take valuable energy away from 'getting on with it'. Involvement is a vast area of work, and is growing in its understanding and also complexity. People seek to make sense of this through definitions, but it is challenging.

Broadly, involvement refers to an activity that is 'carried out "with" or "by" members of the public rather than "to", "about" or "for" them' (INVOLVE, 2012: 6). Sometimes this activity is referred to as engagement, participation or co-production, and views differ about whether these terms are inter-changeable or mean different things (Jerofke-Owen et al., 2023). There is huge variation in when and how terms are used, even within the same context. For example, in England, the term involvement is widely used across healthcare policy and practice. However, where the focus is on working with the public at a neighbourhood or local area level, this is often described as 'community engagement'. In primary care, such activities are referred to as 'patient participation'. None of this is wrong, but the lack of shared agreement about what key terms mean – both within and across different countries and health systems – can be confusing. Rather than getting tied up in semantic knots, we would encourage you to choose a term that best fits your context and focus on reaching a shared understanding of roles, responsibilities and expectations.

Why involving people and communities matters

Given that service user and community involvement is now widely promoted in many health systems internationally, there is still a surprising degree of uncertainty about what 'involvement' actually means and why it is important (McCoy et al., 2019). A useful place to start is with the different ways in which the value of, and need for, involvement are justified. These rationales are diverse and reflect differing moral, ideological and practical commitments. They are also important because they underpin and frame how we think about the goals of involvement, who should be involved and how, and what counts as success. Broadly, there are four main justifications put forward, two of which focus on the involvement process, with the remaining two concerned about its outcomes (McCoy et al., 2019). The process-oriented justifications see involvement as intrinsically important, a good thing in itself, whereas the outcome-oriented justifications value involvement because of what it can achieve. Of course, these different rationales and the evaluation criteria that they give rise to are not mutually exclusive, may be combined, and frequently overlap in policy and practice.

The first of these justifications offers a rights-based perspective. With its roots in the disability and mental health survivor movements, it holds that involving people in the services they use respects, and promotes, their right to autonomy and self-determination (Soresi et al., 2011). This is captured by the phrase 'nothing about us, without us', adopted and promoted by the disabled people's movement, and related calls for healthcare services and professionals to see and value 'the person in the patient' (Fenney et al., 2022). Involvement is also justified in terms of collective rights and ideals, specifically those relating to democracy and visions of a good society. In connecting individual citizens to the decisions that affect their lives, involvement has the potential to increase public accountability, transparency and good governance. Sometimes, this is framed as a much-needed counterweight to declining trust in governing and public institutions (Stoker, 2006).

Alternatively, involvement is promoted in instrumentalist terms as a means by which to improve service experiences, quality of care and health outcomes. On this view, services will be more appropriate and responsive to users' needs when those users are involved in their design, delivery and improvement. There is a growing body of evidence that involvement can improve care experiences and outcomes, although success appears to depend on wider contextual factors related to, for example, timing, resourcing and leadership (Bombard et al., 2018). Relatedly, and increasingly so, involvement is justified with reference to economic benefits. Some studies have shown that individuals who are more knowledgeable and confident in their ability to manage their healthcare are more judicious in their use of health services, have better outcomes and incur lower costs (Hibbard et al., 2013). This has drawn attention to the potential efficiency savings that can be made by encouraging people to be more effective 'self-managers', alongside which the promotion of independence and self-reliance have become key goals of health policy in many countries.

We would, however, urge caution in seeing involvement in purely economic terms. If involvement is approached as a way to contain or even reduce costs, strategies can become narrowly focused on shifting the burden of care onto individuals (and their friends and families), overlooking other important goals, such as improving care quality and upholding the right to self-determination (Kidd, 2014). Moreover, people's access to the skills, resources and networks of support that enable them to participate effectively in their health and care varies considerably (Nieminen et al., 2008; Janamian et al., 2022). If insufficient attention is given to *equipping* people to become more effective self-managers, the risk is that some will thrive, while others are left feeling abandoned. This has the potential to increase existing health inequalities or even create new ones (McDonald, 2014).

Learning activity 21.1

Select an example of involvement from your own organization or country, and examine it in relation to the following questions:

- Can you identify the rationale underpinning this involvement: is it process-oriented; outcomes-oriented; are both rationales evident; or is reason for involvement unclear?
- In what ways might the underpinning rationale have shaped decisions about purpose and goals, who is involved, how and when?
- If the rationale is outcomes-oriented, are the desired goals of involvement realistic and achievable?
- What would you have done differently if you had been leading this involvement?

What do we mean by involvement?

Efforts to define 'involvement' are longstanding and ongoing, and there are more than 60 frameworks for understanding service user involvement in health research alone (Greenhalgh et al., 2019). One of the earliest frameworks developed remains the most influential and widely used. Sherry Arnstein (1969) understood involvement in terms of the distribution of power between citizens and public officials. This was represented using the image of a ladder, with eight levels of participation ranked according to the increasing degree of control that the public has over decisions and resources (Figure 21.1). Implicit in Arnstein's model is a normative assumption that citizens should be aiming to climb the ladder, away from bottom rungs of 'manipulation' and 'placation', to full 'citizen control' at the top. This is reflected in the description of the activities forming the lower rungs of the ladder as 'non-participation' and 'tokenism'.

Notwithstanding the enduring influence of Arnstein's work, the ladder model is not without its shortcomings (Tritter and McAllum, 2006). Above all, it assumes that the involvement methods higher up the ladder are inherently better than those lower down, irrespective of how appropriately or successfully they are used. While we share the view that a commitment to share power is essential if tokenism is to be avoided, the 'best approach' to involvement should be determined by the particular circumstances in each case and will be shaped by a number of considerations including the time, skills and resources available, and any wider (e.g. political or regulatory) constraints on decisions to be taken. Arguably, consultation that is carried out with a genuine commitment to listen and learn is far preferable to poorly conceived and disorganized partnership working. We also disagree with Arnstein's categorization of information as 'tokenism'. As we discuss in more detail shortly, high-quality information builds knowledge and understanding and is, therefore, fundamental to empowerment. However, informing people of a decision already made does not allow for active involvement. The model also fails to consider the breadth and diversity of participation. Is citizen power

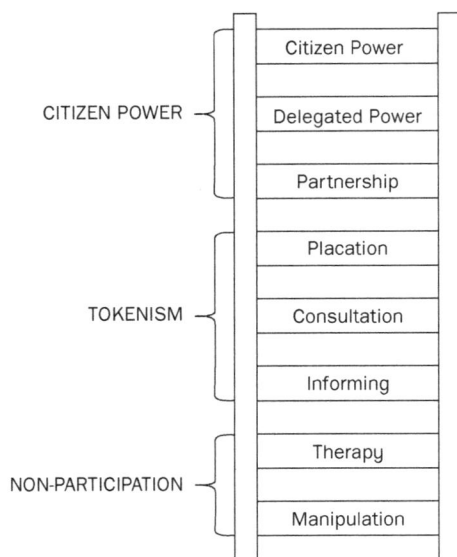

Figure 21.1 Arnstein's Ladder of Participation

the ultimate goal, if, in reality, this might mean a small number of people making decisions on behalf of others, whose views and interests they may neither understand nor share?

A common characteristic of several of the conceptual frameworks that followed Arnstein (e.g. Charles and DeMaio, 1993; Carman et al., 2013) is that they distinguish between involvement at different levels across the healthcare system (Box 21.1).

Box 21.1   Levels of involvement

- **Micro**: people's involvement in their own treatment, care and support
- **Meso**: service user and community involvement in planning, delivering and improving services in their area.
- **Macro**: public involvement in strategic decisions about healthcare services and policy at a system or national level.

Although the practices and processes at these levels may look different, and some of the skills required for effective partnership working may also be different, there are also important similarities – above all, that clear communication and a focus on building trust and constructive relationships are critical to success. A further distinction can be made between involvement activities in terms of the extent of power-sharing with service users, communities and/or the public. In community or public consultations, decision-making power

Table 21.1 Different levels and types of involvement

	Consultation	Collaboration	Co-production or shared leadership
Micro	Patient-reported outcome measures (PROMs) to assess the impact of surgery or treatment from the service user perspective	Service users are asked about their expectations and support needs when a care plan is developed	Treatment or care decisions are made together by service users and professionals using a shared decision-making approach
Meso	Organizations survey service users about their care experiences	Service users sit on governance, steering or advisory groups	Service users co-lead quality improvement initiatives
Macro	Public engagement activities are held to inform healthcare priorities or policy development	Members of the public are involved in setting priorities for national bodies funding healthcare research	National programmes of work are jointly led with patient charities or service user groups

still resides with the consulting body or organization. A degree of power-sharing occurs where service users or community members collaborate in decision-making processes and, at the other end of the spectrum, is full power-sharing in the form of co-production or shared leadership approaches.

Table 21.1 provides examples of consultation, collaborations and co-production/shared leadership at each of the three levels of the healthcare systems described above.

The term people- or person-centred care is widely used across health systems internationally to describe the relationships and approaches that comprise involvement at the micro level. The Australian Commission on Safety and Quality in Health Care describes a person-centred approach as one that:

> Treats each person respectfully as an individual human being, and not just as a condition... It involves seeking out and understanding what is important to the patient, their families, carers and support people, fostering trust and establishing mutual respect. It also means working together to share decisions and plan care
>
> Australian Commission on Safety and Quality in Health Care (n.d.)

As this definition captures, person-centred care includes both principles (e.g. care is compassionate and tailored to people's individual needs) and specific activities (e.g. shared decision-making). It also emphasizes that good care is often a 'triadic' interaction, one in which the important role of family and friends – for example, in providing emotional, social and/or practical help – is recognized, valued, integrated and supported (Adams and Gardiner, 2005). This is sometimes referred to as the Triangle of Care (Martin, 2019). The aim is that all parties involved work together as a team, with mutual respect for the knowledge and skills that each person brings to the relationship.

Involving people in their own care and support

Internationally, research evidence and feedback from service users shows a fairly consistent picture about what matters most to people when using health services and what good care looks like. These priorities are summarized in Box 21.2.

Box 21.2   What matters most to people when using health services?

- Fast access to reliable healthcare advice.
- Effective treatment delivered by trusted professionals.
- Continuity of care and smooth transitions.
- Involvement and support for family and carers.
- Clear information, communication and support for self-care.
- Involvement in decisions and respect for preferences.
- Emotional support, empathy and respect.
- Attention to physical and environmental needs.

Source: The Picker Institute (https://picker.org/who-we-are/
the-picker-principles-of-person-centred-care/).

A key concept is that of patient empowerment, which is defined by the World Health Organization (WHO) (1998: 6) as, 'a process through which people gain greater control over decisions and actions affecting their health'. Internationally, there is growing recognition of the personal (and community) assets that people can draw on to promote their well-being, alongside which health systems are seeking to encourage and equip individuals to participate more actively in their health and care. Such efforts are closely aligned to strategies to improve the efficiency and financial sustainability of health services, in an era of increasing demand and spiralling costs. Empowerment is a relational process, meaning that it is developed in and through interpersonal relationships and the wider social environments in which these occur (Entwistle et al., 2010). This draws attention to the vital role that healthcare services and professionals must play in fostering interactions and environments that enable patients to be partners in their care. In the remainder of this section, we focus on three important ways in which this can be achieved.

Equipping patients with timely and helpful information

Good quality and timely information plays a crucial, and yet frequently under-appreciated, role in patient involvement. For people to participate confidently and effectively in their care, they need to understand their health and the factors that contribute to this; what services are available to support them and how to access and navigate these; what actions they can take to manage and live well with any health conditions they may have; what treatments or interventions may be offered and their potential benefits and risks; and what to do if there are problems in their care. Much of the information that service users receive is verbal, directly from healthcare professionals and staff, in the course of routine interactions. But less than half of what people are told during consultations is remembered afterwards (Kessels, 2003). Hence it is important that information-giving also includes printed or other materials that can be accessed and used at home, or in other settings, after the consultation.

Effective information is accessible, understandable, balanced, relevant and actionable. The reality, however, is that not all materials possess these characteristics. For example, studies that have assessed the quality of patient information frequently report that materials are written in a directive style, with patients characterized and addressed in passive terms, rather than as active participants in their care (e.g. Dixon-Woods, 2001; Coulter et al., 2006). Their purpose is typically to 'educate' patients to ensure compliance with medical treatments and instructions. Such materials are written from a professional perspective, tend to focus on biomedical processes and goals, and often fail to address the topics, issues and outcomes that matter most to service users.

A further consideration is about whether information is written and/or presented in a way that is comprehensible to those using it. The term health literacy refers to the confidence and skills that people have to access, understand, appraise and apply information to make decisions about their health and healthcare (Liu et al., 2020). This ranges from basic skills, such as reading and writing, through to being able to critically analyse and compare information from diverse sources. The latter advanced skills are becoming ever more important with the explosion of online and digital health information, and the increasing difficulty of assessing whether sources are reliable and can be trusted. An international study of more than 42,000 people in 17 European countries, carried out between 2019 and 2021, revealed the scale of the problem. This found that 44 per cent of respondents had low health literacy, with 33 per cent having skills that were categorized as 'problematic' and a further 13 per cent as 'inadequate' (HLS_{19} Consortium of the WHO Action Network M-POHL, 2021). This substantial variation in population health literacy does not appear to be routinely taken into account in information design. Studies have shown that many information materials are written at a reading level too high for people with low health literacy to understand. These findings have been reported for all major information sources including patient leaflets (Nash et al., 2023), medication labels (Pons et al., 2019), consent forms (Eltorai et al., 2015), discharge summaries (DeSai et al., 2021), and online health materials (Worrall et al., 2020).

The good news is that there is growing understanding of how to design information, so it is understandable to people with low health literacy. Simplifying language and avoiding use of complex medical terminology is widely recommended, as is using non-written forms of communication, such as diagrams, pictures and infographics (U.S. Department of Health and Human Services, 2010). Involving service users in developing and pilot testing new materials helps to ensure that content and presentation is accessible, appropriate and meets their information needs. In terms of verbal information, there is good evidence that 'teach back' techniques – where patients are asked to explain in their own words what a healthcare professional has just told them – increases the likelihood that information is understood and retained (Talevski et al., 2020).

Learning activity 21.2

Select a patient information resource either from your organization or one available on the internet. Assess the quality of this information resource by answering the following questions:

- Is the resource written in plain and user-friendly language? There are several free tools that you can use to help you make your assessment, including Microsoft Editor, Hemmingway Editor [https://hemingwayapp.com/] and Readable [https://readable.com/]
- Does the resource address readers as active participants in their care, or as passive recipients?
- Does it use specific presentation strategies to improve comprehension for readers with low health literacy?
- How can readers check the accuracy of the information – for example, are sources of evidence listed; are these sources up-to-date?
- Are there any details about how the resource was developed and what, if any, role service users had in this process?

Collaborative relationships with healthcare professionals

Notwithstanding recent advances in digital and remote services, the vast majority of healthcare remains an interpersonal experience, delivered through person-to-person interactions. It is unsurprising, then, that interpersonal qualities and skills are highly valued by service users and are at the core of their views of what makes a good healthcare provider. People value humanity, empathy, being listened to, being provided with information about their health conditions and treatment options, and being involved in decisions about their care (Grundnig et al., 2022). This is at odds with the traditional, paternalistic style of decision-making ('doctor knows best') that dominated healthcare for many decades. Instead, the healthcare professional's role should be to promote and facilitate patient (and, in many cases, family) participation: to work with, rather than do to.

While the goal is often described as a patient-professional partnership, which implies that decisions are fully shared by both parties, in reality people's preferences for involvement varies. There may be times when an individual may decline or feel unable to participate and want their healthcare provider to make decisions for them. Ultimately, what is important is that people have opportunities to share decisions and, when they choose to take up these opportunities, can readily access information and support to enable them to do so effectively. Involvement is not an all-or-nothing event; it is a matter of degrees. Even where a person would prefer a healthcare professional to make decisions for them, they may still want to understand their treatment options and have their views and priorities taken into account in the process. Additionally, it should not be assumed that certain groups lack the interest or ability to participate due to characteristics, such as age, education, race and ethnicity, gender identity or disability. No single demographic characteristic has been shown to reliably predict preferences or expectations for involvement (Keij et al., 2022).

Supporting people to practise effective self-management and self-care

As people with health conditions have come together and campaigned for better understanding in society, so they have experienced the value of collective action and peer support. While helping people to take control is a personal journey, it is profoundly political in trying to change the balance of power, often to the detriment of the individual. Policy shifts like 'care in the community' sought to close down asylums that separated out people with mental health problems from society (Jones et al., 2018). With this, though, there came a need for community provision to cater for people's needs. As some people gained a voice, they also started to help themselves, often in the absence of, or alongside, state provision.

Patient and user-led organizations have played an important role in promoting self-management, allied to calls for ways of working that recognize and harness people's personal strengths and assets. The goal is for people to claim more autonomy and control over their health and their life and place this aspect of their lives in perspective with work, family and other important facets of modern-day living. Organizations also debate and advocate for better interaction with health and care professionals so that they are not in charge all the time, and a person is not 'a victim' of their condition, but rather they work in partnership, valuing both the learnt and lived experience.

Self-help and self-management are also seen as valuable by healthcare services and policymakers and are increasingly presented as being vital for ensuring the long-term financial sustainability of health systems in the face of increased costs and demand. Thus, there are an ever-growing number of services that seek to support and enable self-management across many different health conditions and problems (see Box 21.3 for an example from the United States Veterans Health Administration).

Box 21.3   Veterans Affairs Whole Health Coaching Programme

The Veterans Health Administration provides care for more than 9 million veterans across the United States. Its Whole Health Coaching Programme aims to equip people to take more control of their health, focusing on self-care, skill building and support. Since 2012, more than 2,300 clinicians, staff, veterans and other have been trained in the coaching model. The Whole Health approach starts with the question 'What matters to you?'. Coaches use motivational interviewing and other person-centred communication approaches to support veterans to explore the links between their health and other aspects of their life and connect them with resources and opportunities to help them achieve their goals. This includes peer support and a range of complementary and integrative services, including yoga and meditation classes. An evaluation of the Programme reported significant improvements in mental health, stress and perceived health competence, and participants were highly satisfied with their coaching experience (Purcell et al., 2021).

Involving service users and communities in planning, delivering and improving services

The importance of involving users and communities in shaping healthcare services has grown significantly in recent decades. Indeed, alongside safety and clinical effectiveness, patient experience is now widely recognized as an integral component of healthcare quality. Internationally, it is common for healthcare organizations to have mechanisms in place for gathering feedback from people either during or after they have used their services; in some countries, such as England, this is a legal duty (National Health Service Act, 2006). In part, this move towards greater public involvement in health service planning, delivery and improvement has been driven by high-profile failures in service and clinical quality. This has exposed the risks of paternalism in healthcare and made clear that the only reliable way of understanding what people need and expect from health services is to ask them directly.

Looking at the many toolkits and guides available, it is easy to reach the conclusion that the key to success in involvement lies in picking the right method. Methods do matter, and it is important to select one that is well-suited to the particular context, purpose and resources available. But we know from a now sizeable evidence base that the same method can result in very different outcomes, and findings consistently show that it is not what involvement comprises, but how it is done, that makes the greatest difference (Dalton et al., 2015). There are numerous examples of what has been described as 'tokenistic' involvement (Ocloo and Matthews, 2016). What these examples share in common is that professional and system interests and power dominate decision-making, despite the rhetoric of partnership working. Arnstein (1969) rightly identified that genuine involvement means sharing power, so that everybody is heard and valued. If this does not happen, at best, involvement will have limited impact; at worst, it will undermine trust and create frustration, resentment and even disengagement.

In the UK, a set of standards for involvement in healthcare research were developed in 2019 by a partnership of professional and public representatives (National Institute for Health and Care Research, 2019). The standards were designed to provide a framework to support the planning of involvement activities and support learning, including identifying lessons learned where such activities failed to achieve expected outcomes. In Table 21.2, we have adapted these standards to describe what 'good' involvement in health services looks like.

Co-production

A concept that has gained increasing popularity in recent years is that of co-production. The term was coined in the 1970s by US economist Elinor Ostrom, as a way to understand the reciprocal relationship between the users and providers of public goods or services (including healthcare) (Ostrom, 1973). It challenges professionally led and needs-based approaches that see service users as passive recipients of treatment or care, their role limited to complying with decisions made by others on their behalf. Instead, co-production starts from the

Table 21.2 UK Public Involvement Standards

Standard	Questions to support planning and reflection
1: Inclusive opportunities Public involvement partnerships are accessible and include a range of people and groups, as informed by community and service needs.	• How is information about involvement opportunities shared, and does it appeal to different communities? • Are there fair and transparent processes for involving the public and do they reflect equality and diversity duties? • Is there choice and flexibility in opportunities offered to the public?
2: Working together Work together in a way that values all contributions, and that builds and sustains mutually respectful and productive relationships.	• Have all the potential different ways of working together been explored, and have these plans and activities been developed together? • Is there is a shared understanding of roles, responsibilities and expectations of public involvement? • Have individuals' influence, ideas and contributions' been recognized and addressed?
3: Support and learning Offer and promote support and learning opportunities that build confidence and skills for public involvement.	• Have specific resources been designated to support learning and development opportunities for everybody involved, both the public and staff? • Do the public know where to go for information and support about public involvement?
4: Governance Involve the public in management, regulation, leadership and decision-making.	• Are public voices heard, valued and respected in decision-making? • Is there visible and accountable responsibility for public involvement throughout the organization? • Are realistic resources (including money, staff, time) allocated for public involvement?
5: Communications Use plain language for well-timed and relevant communications, as part of involvement plans and activities.	• Are the needs of different people being met through inclusive and flexible communication methods? • Are processes in place to offer, gather, act on and share feedback with the public?
6: Impact Seek improvement by identifying and sharing the difference that public involvement makes to service planning, delivery and improvement.	• Are the public involved in deciding what the assessment of impact should focus on, and the approach to take? • Are there processes in place to help reflect on public involvement? • Are the changes, benefits and learning resulting from public involvement acted on?

principle that people have assets to contribute to personal and community well-being, and that harnessing these assets through collaborative ways of working can achieve better outcomes for all (Boyle and Harris, 2009). This extends well beyond the traditional focus in involvement on seeking public views about health services to encompass several forms of co-creation, including people with lived experience co-delivering services as peer support workers or peer mentors. Conversely, clinical and managerial leaders do not have all the answers to the challenges that health services face, implying a change of role from being a 'fixer' to that of a 'facilitator'.

There have been many efforts to define the guiding principles of co-production. The UK Social Care Institute for Excellence (SCIE) (2022), for example, contends that the principles of equality, diversity, accessibility and reciprocity (getting something back for putting something in) are critical to putting co-production into practice. Fundamentally, co-production depends on a shift in the balance of power between service professionals and managers, and the public. It is this commitment to true partnership working, not any particular method or goal, that sets co-production apart. Sharing power can only happen where there is mutual trust and respect, and so time needs to be invested in building relationships and breaking down traditional hierarchies. None of this is easy, and it can profoundly challenge managerial and professional norms. But it can also make a real difference, as can be seen in the quote below, from a peer mentor in a service that supports people facing multiple disadvantages:

> When I was a peer mentor […] it was a massive part of my recovery to actually see the impact I was having on somebody else, seeing that light turn on in their eyes sort of thing and getting them to engage with services when they hadn't done so previously
>
> (Woodall et al., 2019)

Involving the public in strategic decisions about healthcare services and policy

At the macro level, the purpose of involvement is to inform strategic decisions about what healthcare services are provided and how these are financed and organized, which can include participation in priority-setting processes or being consulted about major service changes or new policy directions. In highly centralized health systems these decisions are taken nationally while, in more decentralized systems, they are typically taken regionally or by individual provider organizations. At the macro level, considerations of equity in how involvement opportunities are offered and taken up are paramount given that decisions are being taken in 'the public interest' (Fredriksson et al., 2018). Strategic involvement can extend beyond service and policy considerations to include healthcare research. In England, for example, all of the funding committees of the NIHR have public members who are involved in reviewing and making decisions about funding applications.

Internationally, there are a growing number of patient charities and voluntary organizations that seek to represent and amplify the voice of service users, carers and specific interest groups in the policy process. This works particularly well in countries, such as the Netherlands, where there is a long history of involving 'social partners' – including voluntary sector and employer organizations, as well as trade unions – in democratic decision-making structures and processes. Some patient organizations in the Netherlands receive a subsidy from the Dutch government, which can help to legitimize and fund their influencing work (van de Bovenkamp et al., 2010). An alternative model of public involvement, from Germany, is presented in Box 21.4 below.

Box 21.4   Patient participation in the Federal Joint Committee in Germany

The Federal Joint Committee is the highest decision-making body in the German healthcare system. It issues binding directives, including making decisions about which services will be covered by statutory health insurance for around 70 million Germans. Representatives from leading national patient advocacy and self-help groups sit on the Committee. They can take part in discussions and submit petitions, but they are not entitled to vote on the directives. The involvement of patient groups has been reported to have enhanced transparency, and an awareness of and attention to service user perspectives in decision-making processes (Conklin et al., 2010).

User-led organizations have been influential in defining and promoting a social model of disability. This is a civil rights approach to disability; it proposes that, while someone has a physical impairment, they are disabled by attitudes, discrimination and inaccessible environments that prevent them from being a full part of society. Organizations, such as the Australian Federation of Disability Organisations [https://www.afdo.org.au/], have been vocal in drawing attention to how people with disabilities and who experience ill health, and mental illness in particular, have been silenced and excluded from decision-making. Rather than waiting for an invitation to 'be involved', they have sought to claim power for themselves in campaigning for their members and attempting to shape how services are created. Some user-led organizations have also become service providers, which presents an opportunity to put the social model of disability into practice through services that focus on promoting independence and peer support (Paxton et al., 2005).

Making person-centred care a reality

Healthcare providers are increasingly encouraged to work in partnership with people who use services, and design and deliver care in ways that align with their needs, circumstances and preferences. Yet feedback from, and research with, service users suggests that there is still some way to go to achieve truly person-centred healthcare, and barriers to involvement and user-driven quality improvement are widely reported (Harding et al., 2015). One response has been to focus on equipping service users with the resources and skills to participate more confidently in decisions about their healthcare. This can range from the provision of simple tools that prompt people to ask questions during clinical consultations to elicit important information (e.g. Ask Me 3: https://www.ihi.org/resources/tools/ask-me-3-good-questions-your-good-health), through to highly structured programmes that support people to develop the knowledge and skills to manage ongoing and long-term health conditions (e.g. The Chronic Disease Self-Management Programme for arthritis: https://www.cdc.gov/arthritis/programs/index.html). Such strategies can enable people to be more active participants in their care, but studies consistently show that the most effective approaches are tailored to people's individual capabilities, needs and preferences, and seek to address cultural, language, physical and other accessibility barriers (Alden et al., 2014; Taylor et al., 2014). In short, one size does not fit all.

There has also been increasing recognition of the skills, attitudes and behaviours that healthcare professionals need to work effectively in partnership with service users, and a growing emphasis on workforce training and development to underpin and drive progress towards person-centred care. As Coulter and Oldham (2016: 115) note, 'Working with patients in a more person-centred manner places new demands on health professionals. It requires excellent listening, communication and negotiation skills and the capacity to respond flexibly to people's individual needs'. In England, the bodies that oversee workforce development in health and care have produced an education and training framework for person-centred approaches, built around a core set of communication and relationship-building skills (Health Education England, Skills for Health and Skills for Care, 2017). This was developed with input from several key groups, including organizations representing people who use health and care services (see Box 21.5).

Box 21.5   Health Education England Education and Training Framework for Person-Centred Approaches

The framework describes nine core communication and relationship building behaviours that patients and carers would like to see in health and care professionals:

1   Introducing yourself; 'Hello my name is…'[1]
2   Really listening to me and hearing me.
3   Asking open questions to explore and understand me, my personal situation, and what matters to me and my community.
4   Acknowledging what I am doing already to manage, and reassuring me that what I am experiencing is understandable.
5   Not judging me.
6   Checking if there is something else I want to talk about.
7   Giving me the opportunity to be an equal partner in how we guide and continue our conversation.
8   Working with me and my carers in a way that means we can trust each other.
9   Sensitively giving me an idea of how long we have available for our conversation.

Source: Skills for Health, Skills for Care and Health Education England (2017) https://www.skillsforhealth.org.uk/wp-content/uploads/2021/01/Person-Centred-Approaches-Framework.pdf.

---

1   In England, Dr Kate Granger, a doctor and terminally ill cancer patient, led the #hellomynameis campaign. This raised awareness of the importance of healthcare professionals introducing themselves to patients, when delivering care to them. For more information, see https://www.hellomynameis.org.uk/.

Person-centred organizations

Efforts to equip people and professionals with knowledge and skills for partnership working are crucial, but alone are unlikely to fully bring about desired changes in practice. This is because, while involvement is ultimately about what happens in the interactions between individuals and groups, these interactions are both enabled and constrained by wider organizational, financial and political factors (Hower et al., 2019). This points to the need for a systemic approach to implementing person-centred care. Such an approach seeks to 'hard wire' into everyday ways of working a focus on what matters most to service users (and their families) by attending to multiple factors at the individual, team, organization and system levels (Ocloo et al., 2021).

What might this look like in practice? An answer to this question is proffered by Stephen Stirk and Helen Sanderson, who conducted detailed case study research to understand what makes a 'person-centred organization'. Stirk and Sanderson (2012: 11) define a person-centred organization as one that has 'people at its heart – both people it serves and people it employs'. Leaders and managers in these organizations apply the values of person-centredness (such as treating people with respect and compassion, listening to them and engaging them in decisions that matter) to staff and service users alike. Stirk and Sanderson draw attention to the importance of human resource and team-working processes and practices, arguing that the expectation that staff deliver the best possible services and experiences requires changes in how they are recruited, trained, organized, supervised and rewarded. Their work identified eight key characteristics that are the foundation of a person-centred organization (see Box 21.6).

Box 21.6   Eight characteristics of person-centred organizations

1 **Visionary leadership**: person-centred organizations have a clear vision and mission, with leaders who motivate, inspire and ensure that everything is aligned to deliver this.
2 **Shared values and beliefs**: everyone shares, can articulate and most importantly demonstrate the person-centred values of the organization.
3 **Outcomes for individuals**: everything is orientated to achieving the outcomes people who are supported want in their lives.
4 **Community focus**: both the people supported and the organization contribute to and feel part of their local community.
5 **Empowered and valued staff**: managers work with staff in a person-centred way, and staff are appreciated, valued and listened to.
6 **Individual and organizational learning**: person-centred organizations are continuously developing and improving. Learning takes place at all levels, and learning from people supported directly influences staff, team and organizational development.

7   **Working together:** starts with the people supported, in co-designing what they want their service to look like. Decision-making is as close to them as possible.

8   **Person-centred practices embedded throughout the organization**: the whole organization shares a common language and practices to deliver the other seven key elements. This is part of the DNA of the organization – person-centred practices are simply the way things get done.

Source: Adapted from Stirk and Sanderson (2012).

Stirk and Sanderson's work on person-centred organizations highlights the strong connection between how staff are managed and feel about their jobs, and outcomes for service users. Indeed, extensive research has demonstrated that, when healthcare staff feel valued, engaged and supported, this translates not only into more positive patient experiences, but also leads to higher quality of care, and lower rates of workforce turnover and sickness absences, adverse events, healthcare acquired infections and patient mortality (Braithwaite et al., 2017). These findings are neatly summed up by West and Dawson (2020: 20), who note that 'When we care for staff, they can fulfil their calling of providing outstanding professional care for patients'.

Learning activity 21.3

Looking at Stirk and Sanderson's eight characteristics, how person-centred would you say that your organization or team is? Which of the characteristics are most in need of improvement?

Devise an action plan detailing what steps your organization or team could take to become a more person-centred one. Before you do so, consider how you could involve service users and/or staff in this process.

Assessing involvement and its impact

Evaluation is a crucial, and yet often overlooked, part of any involvement process. Evaluation can fulfil several important purposes; it can:

• Generate learning and insights to improve the design and effectiveness of future involvement activities.
• Inform service user or public participants about what difference their contributions have made.
• Identify good practice and help build an evidence base about what works.

- Highlight the factors that help people to contribute and identify barriers to participating, to inform thinking about how best to support and enable effective partnership working.
- Assess the diversity (or not) of those taking part, and highlight which groups, experiences, interests and perspectives were not included.
- Provide evidence of the impact of involvement, which may be linked to a formal requirement to justify the funding and other resources invested.

There are many different kinds of question that evaluation can pose. An evaluation of the involvement process, for example, might explore how people were recruited to participate; whether the involvement approach chosen was appropriate and to what extent it supported meaningful and inclusive participation; and what support participants were offered and how useful this was perceived to be. Whereas an impact evaluation is interested in what difference the involvement made. Before this can be assessed, there must first be agreement about which outcomes to focus on, and how these will be assessed or measured. At the start of the chapter, we described four dominant rationales for involvement. Each of these is related to a different understanding of what counts as success (see Table 21.3).

Irrespective of the underpinning rationale, attention should always be paid to ensuring that opportunities and practices promote inclusivity and take account of structural and cultural factors that can limit involvement. Marginalized and minority groups, and those that experience discrimination and stigma, have long been under-represented in involvement processes. This includes people who are older (especially older adults living in institutional care

Table 21.3 Potential criteria for evaluating success in involvement

Involvement rationale	Example criteria for evaluating success
Rights-based	• People feel respected and listened to. • Efforts are made to understand and address power imbalances between staff/managers and service users. • The process is guided by values of equity, inclusivity and non-discrimination.
Democratic	• Decision-making processes are open and transparent. • The process fosters genuine dialogue and participants' views influence decisions taken. • The process increases trust and mutual understanding between participants and officials.
Instrumentalist	• Improvements in service appropriateness, accessibility and/or quality. • People report more positive experiences of using services and/or reduction in complaints. • Better service and health outcomes for under-served populations.
Economic	• More appropriate and/or efficient use of available resources. • Reductions in use of healthcare services, especially unscheduled and emergency care. • Increased use of preventive services (e.g. screening).

settings), who have learning and physical disabilities, are LGBTQ+, belong to an ethnic minority group and who live in poverty (Ocloo et al., 2021). Standard involvement methods – for example, acting as a service user representative on a governance body, taking part in a public consultation – are likely to be a key part of the explanation for this. These methods often presuppose a 'typical' participant who is able to freely give their time, understands formal and technical jargon, and has the confidence to question and challenge those in professional roles. The effect is to legitimize some groups and contributions, while de-legitimizing or even silencing others (Snow, 2022).

Efforts to increase equality, diversity and inclusion in involvement often focus on broadening the range of characteristics of those taking part. While this is crucial, it is equally important that involvement activities, and the spaces in which these take place, are accessible and inclusive, and that there is an explicit commitment to non-discrimination. This, ultimately, requires a rebalancing of power in partnership working. A useful framework to guide this is offered by Snow, who proposes that truly meaningful involvement should be: approachable, acceptable, available, appropriate and affordable (see Box 21.7).

Box 21.7   Five dimensions of accessible and inclusive involvement

Approachable: for example, are service users aware that opportunities for involvement exist and are relevant to them?

Acceptable: for example, have provisions been made to support the involvement of people with specific language and communication needs?

Available: for example, are the venues where activities are taking place accessible, both physically (e.g. to those with limited mobility) and psychologically (e.g. do they feel safe and familiar)?

Appropriate: for example, is there a fit between the involvement opportunity and participants' preferences, needs and values?

Affordable: for example, will any costs that participants might incur (e.g. transportation, time off work, childcare costs) be reimbursed?

Source: Snow (2022).

Conclusion

Our main aim in this chapter has been to offer a series of practical reflections about what works in involvement. These can be summarized as follows:

- Involvement is about 'working with' not 'doing to'. This cannot happen if managerial and clinical decision-makers are unwilling to challenge power inequities and embrace what can be learned from service users' experiential knowledge.

- Successful involvement is defined by the values and principles that underpin and guide it, not by any particular methods, tools or techniques. Fundamentally, success lies in building relationships and trust, and consideration of how this will be achieved should be prioritized in the planning of any involvement activity.
- Partnership working may come naturally to some, but many service users and professionals will need training and support to develop the communication and other skills that are required. The importance of timely and high-quality information in empowering people in their own healthcare cannot be underestimated.
- Marginalized and minority groups face a greater number of barriers to participating in healthcare, at all levels. If these barriers are not addressed through a commitment to accessible and inclusive involvement, there is a risk that existing inequalities will be reinforced, or even increased.
- Involvement is enabled and constrained by the physical and social environment in which it takes place. This calls for a systemic approach, with a crucial role for clinical and managerial leaders to identify and change the organizational factors and processes that can hamper partnership working.

All of the above point to the vital role that healthcare managers have in enabling meaningful, appropriately resourced and effective involvement, which happens in ways and spaces that are accessible and inclusive, and which makes a difference.

Learning resources

Australian Commission on Safety and Quality in Healthcare: Partnering with consumers: The Australian Commission on Safety and Quality in Healthcare is the national body for safety and quality in Australia, and partnering with consumers is a Commission priority. This website includes fact sheets, tools, e-learning modules, podcasts and vodcasts and links to further resources on key topics including person-centred care, health literacy and shared decision-making [https://www.safetyandquality.gov.au/our-work/partnering-consumers].

Health Improvement Scotland: Community Engagement: Health Improvement Scotland is the national health improvement organization for the NHS in Scotland. This website hosts a range of resources about engaging communities in shaping health and care services, including a toolkit of engagement methods that outlines each method's strengths and weaknesses and the resources required [https://www.hisengage.scot/].

Helen Sanderson Associates Person-Centred Approaches: Helen Sanderson Associates is an international team that provides support to organizations to become more person-centred. The website hosts information about several person-centred practices, including free tools and templates, videos and links to training opportunities [https://www.helensandersonassociates.com/person-centered-approaches/].

Continued

Learning resources   *Continued*

International Association of Patients Organizations (IAPO): A global network of more than 300 organizations in 71 countries, which supports and empowers patients across all disease areas. IAPO's key purpose is to promote patient-centred healthcare, advocating for change at national, regional and international levels [www.iapo.org.uk].

Social Care Institute for Excellence (SCIE) co-production training and resources: a UK agency promoting evidence-based and co-produced improvement in social care. This website includes guidance about what co-production is and how to do it, a report exploring the impact of co-production, practical resources and practice examples [https://www.scie.org.uk/co-production/].

UK Standards for Public Involvement: These standards were developed to improve the quality and consistency of public involvement in health and social care research, but they equally apply to and can be used as a framework for public involvement in service delivery and improvement. This website also includes guidance about how to apply the standards and case study examples [https://sites.google.com/nihr.ac.uk/pi-standards/home].

McMaster University Public Engagement in Health Policy Project: The Public Engagement in Health Policy Project aims to strengthen public engagement in health policymaking in Canada, through research, education and leadership opportunities. The website includes details of and outputs from the Project's different elements, including work on digital engagement, equity-centred engagement, black community-led engagement and deliberative approaches [https://www.engagementinhealthpolicy.ca/].

Patient Information Forum (PIF): UK-based organization providing guidance and support on developing patient information. The organization also runs an independent quality mark scheme for information materials. The website includes a host of materials and resources, and a service for peer-reviewing draft information materials [https://pifonline.org.uk/].

The Ottawa Hospital Research Institute Patient Decision Aids Inventory: The Ottawa Hospital Research Institute is the research arm of one of Canada's largest learning and research hospitals. A key area of their research is around patient decision aids, which help people to understand and be involved in decisions about their care. The website includes a database of hundreds of decision aids, organized by health topic, as well as a toolkit to support implementation of decision aids in clinical practice [https://decisionaid.ohri.ca/AZinvent.php].

References

Adams, T. and Gardiner, P. (2005) Communication and interaction within dementia care triads: developing a theory for relationship-centred care, *Dementia*, 4(2): 185–205.

Alden, D.L., Friend, J., Schapira, M. and Stiggelbout, A. (2014) Cultural targeting and tailoring of shared decision making technology: a theoretical framework for improving the effectiveness of patient decision aids in culturally diverse groups, *Social Science & Medicine*, Mar; 105: 1–8. doi: 10.1016/j.socscimed.2014.01.002. Epub 2014 Jan 15.

Arnstein, S. (1969) A ladder of citizen participation, *Journal of the American Institute of Planners*, 35(4): 216–224.

Australian Commission on Safety and Quality in Health Care (no date) 'Person-centred care' [https://www.safetyandquality.gov.au/our-work/partnering-consumers/person-centred-care; accessed 25 April 2024].

Bombard, Y., Baker, G.R., Orlando, E., Fancott, C., Bhatia, P., Casalino, S., et al. (2018) Engaging patients to improve quality of care: a systematic review, *Implementation Science*, 13: 98. doi: 10.1186/s13012-018-0784-z.

Boyle, D. and Harris, M. (2009) *The challenge of co-production. How equal partnerships between professionals and the public are crucial to improving public services.* London: NESTA.

Braithwaite, J., Herkes, J., Ludlow, K., Testa, L. and Lamprell, G. (2017) Association between organisational and workplace cultures, and patient outcomes: systematic review, *BMJ Open*, 8 Nov; 7(11): e017708. doi: 10.1136/bmjopen-2017-017708.

Carman, K.L., Dardess, P., Maurer, M., Sofaer, S., Adams, K., Bechtel, C., et al. (2013) Patient and family engagement: a framework for understanding the elements and developing interventions and policies, *Health Affairs* (Millwood), Feb; 32(2): 223–231. doi: 10.1377/hlthaff.2012.1133.

Charles, C. and DeMaio, S. (1993) Lay participation in health care decision making: a conceptual framework, *Journal of Health Politics, Policy and Law*, Winter; 18(4): 881–904. doi: 10.1215/03616878-18-4-881.

Conklin, A., Morris, Z. and Nolte, E. (2010) *Involving the public in healthcare policy. An update of the research evidence and proposed evaluation framework.* Cambridge: RAND Europe.

Coulter, A. and Oldham, J. (2016) Person-centred care: what is it and how do we get there?, *Future Hospital Journal*, Jun; 3(2): 114–116. doi: 10.7861/futurehosp.3-2-114.

Coulter, A., Ellins, J., Swain, D., Clarke, A., Heron, P., Rasul, F., et al. (2006) *Assessing the quality of information to support people in making decisions about their health and healthcare.* Oxford: Picker Institute Europe.

Crocker, A.F. and Smith S.N. (2019) Person-first language: are we practicing what we preach?, *Journal of Multidisciplinary Healthcare*, 8 Feb;12: 125–129. doi: 10.2147/JMDH.S140067.

Dalton, J., Chambers, D., Harden, M., Street, A., Parker, G. and Eastwood, A. (2015) Service user engagement in health service reconfiguration: a rapid evidence synthesis, *Journal of Health Services Research and Policy*, Jul; 21(3): 195–205. doi: 10.1177/1355819615623305. Epub 2015 Dec 20.

DeSai, C., Janowiak, K., Secheli, B., Phelps, E., McDonald, S., Reed, G., et al. (2021) Empowering patients: simplifying discharge instructions, *BMJ Open Quality*, 10: e001419. doi: 10.1136/bmjoq-2021-001419.

Dixon-Woods, M. (2001) Writing wrongs? An analysis of published discourses about the use of patient information leaflets, *Social Science & Medicine*, May; 52(9): 1417–1432. doi: 10.1016/s0277-9536(00)00247-1.

Eltorai, A.E., Naqvi, S.S., Ghanian, S., Eberson, C.P., Weiss, A.P., Born, C.T., et al. (2015) Readability of invasive procedure consent forms, *Clinical and Translational Science*, Dec; 8(6): 830–833. doi: 10.1111/cts.12364. Epub 2015 Dec 17.

Entwistle, V.A., Carter, S.M., Cribb, A. and McCaffery, K. (2010) Supporting patient autonomy: the importance of clinician-patient relationships, *Journal of General Internal Medicine*, Jul; 25(7): 741–745. doi: 10.1007/s11606-010-1292-2. Epub 2010 Mar 6.

Fenney, D., Wellings, D., Lennon, E. and Hadi, F. (2022) Towards a new partnership between disabled people and health and care services: getting our voices heard. [https://www.kingsfund.org.uk/insight-and-analysis/long-reads/new-partnership-disabled-people-health-care; accessed 25 April 2024].

Fredriksson, M., Eriksson, M. and Tritter, J. (2018) Who wants to be involved in health care decisions? Comparing preferences for individual and collective involvement in England and Sweden, *BMC Public Health*, 18: 18. doi: 10.1186/s12889-017-4534-y.

Greenhalgh, T., Hinton, L., Finlay, T., Macfarlane, A., Fahy, N., Clyde, B., et al. (2019) Frameworks for supporting patient and public involvement in research: systematic review and co-design pilot, *Health Expectations*, Aug; 22(4): 785–801. doi: 10.1111/hex.12888. Epub 2019 Apr 22.

Grundnig, J.S., Steiner-Hofbauer, V., Drexler, V. and Holzinger, A. (2022) You are exactly my type! The traits of a good doctor: a factor analysis study on public's perspectives, *BMC Health Services Research*, 22: 886. doi: 10.1186/s12913-022-08273-y.

Harding, E., Wait, S. and Scrutton, J. (2015) *The state of play in person-centred care: report summary. A pragmatic review of how person-centred care is defined, applied and measured.* London: The Health Policy Partnership.

Health Education England, Skills for Health and Skills for Care (2017) Person-Centred Approaches: Empowering people in their lives and communities to enable an upgrade in prevention, wellbeing, health, care and support. A core skills education and training framework. [www.skillsforhealth.org.uk/images/pdf/Person-Centred-Approaches-Framework.pdf; accessed 4 March 2025].

Hibbard, J.H., Greene, J. and Overton, V. (2013) Patients with lower activation associated with higher costs; delivery systems should know their patients' scores, *Health Affairs* (Millwood). Feb; 32(2): 216–222. doi: 10.1377/hlthaff.2012.1064.

The HLS$_{19}$ Consortium of the WHO Action Network M-POHL (2021) *International report on the methodology, results, and recommendations of the European Health Literacy Population Survey 2019-2021 (HLS$_{19}$) of M-POHL.* Vienna: Austrian National Public Health Institute.

Hower, K.I., Vennedey, V., Hillen, H.A., Kuntz, L., Stock, S., Pfaff, H., et al. (2019) Implementation of patient-centred care: which organisational determinants matter from decision maker's perspective? Results from a qualitative interview study across various health and social care organisations, *BMJ Open*, 1 Apr; 9(4): e027591. doi: 10.1136/bmjopen-2018-027591. Erratum in: *BMJ Open*. 27 Jun; 9(6): e027591corr1. PMID: 30940764; PMCID: PMC6500213.

INVOLVE (2012) *Briefing notes for researchers: involving the public in NHS, public health and social care research.* Eastleigh: INVOLVE.

Janamian, T., Greco, M., Cosgriff, D., Baker, L. and Dawda, P. (2022) Activating people to partner in health and self-care: use of the Patient Activation Measure, *Medical Journal of*

Australia, 6 Jun; 216(Suppl 10): S5–S8. doi: 10.5694/mja2.51535. PMID: 35665937; PMCID: PMC9328281.

Jerofke-Owen, T.A., Tobiano, G. and Eldh, A.C. (2023) Patient engagement, involvement, or participation — entrapping concepts in nurse–patient interactions: a critical discussion, *Nursing Inquiry*, 30: e12513. doi: 10.1111/nin.12513.

Jones, A., Hannigan, B., Coffey, M. and Simpson, A. (2018) Traditions of research in community mental health care planning and care coordination: a systematic meta-narrative review of the literature, *PLOS One*, 22 Jun; 13(6): e0198427. doi: 10.1371/journal.pone.0198427. PMID: 29933365; PMCID: PMC6014652.

Keij, S.M., de Boer, J.E., Stiggelbout, A.M., Bruine de Bruin, W., Peters, E., et al. (2022) How are patient-related characteristics associated with shared decision-making about treatment? A scoping review of quantitative studies, *BMJ Open*, 24 May; 12(5): e057293. doi: 10.1136/bmjopen-2021-057293.

Kessels, R.P. (2003) Patients' memory for medical information, *Journal of the Royal Society of Medicine*, May; 96(5): 219–222. doi: 10.1177/014107680309600504.

Kidd, L. (2014) Handing more control to patients could just be cost-cutting in disguise, *The Conversation* [https://theconversation.com/handing-more-control-to-patients-could-just-be-cost-cutting-in-disguise-34511; accessed 25 April 2024].

Liu, C., Wang, D., Liu, C., Jiang, J., Wang, X., Chen, H., et al. (2020) What is the meaning of health literacy? A systematic review and qualitative synthesis, *Family Medicine and Community Health*, May; 8(2): e000351. doi: 10.1136/fmch-2020-000351. PMID: 32414834; PMCID: PMC7239702.

Martin, K. (2019) The Triangle of Care. *Carers included: a guide to best practice in mental health care in Scotland*. Glasgow: Carers Trust Scotland.

McCoy, M.S., Warsh, J., Rand, L., Parker, M. and Sheehan, M. (2019) Patient and public involvement: two sides of the same coin or different coins altogether?, *Bioethics*, Jul; 33(6): 708–715. doi: 10.1111/bioe.12584. Epub 2019 Apr 8.

McDonald, C. (2014) Patients in control. Why people with long-term conditions must be empowered [https://ippr-org.files.svdcdn.com/production/Downloads/patients-in-control_Sept2014.pdf; accessed 25 April 2024].

Molyneaux, V., Butchard, S., Simpson, J. and Murray, C. (2011) Reconsidering the term 'carer': a critique of the universal adoption of the term 'carer', *Ageing and Society*, 31(3): 422–437. doi: 1017/S0144686X10001066.

Nash, E., Bickerstaff, M., Chetwynd, A.J., Hawcutt, D.B. and Oni, L. (2023) The readability of parent information leaflets in paediatric studies. *Pediatric Research*, 94: 1166–1171. doi: 10.1038/s41390-023-02608-z.

National Health Service Act (2006) London: The Stationery Office. [https://www.legislation.gov.uk/ukpga/2006/41/contents; accessed 25 April 2024].

National Institute for Health and Care Research (NIHR) (2019) UK standards for public involvement. [https://sites.google.com/nihr.ac.uk/pi-standards/home; accessed 25 April 2024].

Neuberger J. (1999) Do we need a new word for patients? Let's do away with 'patients', *The BMJ*, 26 Jun; 318(7200): 1756–1757. doi: 10.1136/bmj.318.7200.1756.

Nieminen, T., Martelin, T., Koskinen, S., Simpura, J., Alanen, E., Härkänen, T. et al. (2008) Measurement and socio-demographic variation of social capital in a large population-based survey, *Social Indicators Research*, 85: 405–423. doi: 10.1007/s11205-007-9102-x.

Ocloo, J. and Matthews, R. (2016) From tokenism to empowerment: progressing patient and public involvement in healthcare improvement, *BMJ Quality & Safety*, Aug; 25(8): 626–632. doi: 10.1136/bmjqs-2015-004839. Epub 2016 Mar 18.

Ocloo, J., Garfield, S., Franklin, B.D. and Dawson, S. (2021) Exploring the theory, barriers and enablers for patient and public involvement across health, social care and patient safety: a systematic review of reviews, *Health Research Policy and Systems*, 20 Jan; 1: 8. doi: 10.1186/s12961-020-00644-3.

Ostrom, E. (1973) *Community Organization and the Provision of Police Services*. Beverley Hills: SAGE.

Paxton, W., Pearce, N., Unwin, J. and Molyneux, P. (2005) *The voluntary sector delivering public services. Transfer or transformation?* York: Joseph Rowntree Foundation.

Pons, E.D.S., Moraes, C.G., Falavigna, M., Sirtori, L.R., da Cruz, F., Webster, G. et al. (2019) Users' preferences and perceptions of the comprehensibility and readability of medication labels, *PLOS One*, 22 Feb; 14(2): e0212173. doi: 10.1371/journal.pone.0212173.

Purcell, N., Zamora, K., Bertenthal, D., Abadjian, L., Tighe, J. and Seal, K.H. (2021) How VA Whole Health Coaching can impact veterans' health and quality of life: a mixed-methods pilot program evaluation, *Global Advances in Integrative Medicine and Health*, 5 Mar; 10: 2164956121998283. doi: 10.1177/2164956121998283.

Snow, M.E. (2022) Patient engagement in healthcare planning and evaluation: a call for social justice, *International Journal of Health Planning and Management*, Dec; 37(Suppl 1): 20–31. doi: 10.1002/hpm.3509. Epub 2022 May 28.

Social Care Institute for Excellence (SCIE) (2022) Co-production: what it is and how to do it. [https://www.scie.org.uk/co-production/what-how/; accessed 25 April 2024].

Soresi, S., Nota, L. and Wehmeyer, M.L. (2011) Community involvement in promoting inclusion, participation and self-determination, *International Journal of Inclusive Education*, 15(1): 15–28. doi: 10.1080/13603116.2010.496189.

Stirk, S. and Sanderson, H. (2012) *Creating Person-Centred Organisations*. London: Jessica Kingsley Publishers.

Stoker, G. (2006) *Why Politics Matters: Making Democracy Work*. Basingstoke: Palgrave Macmillan.

Talevski, J., Wong Shee, A., Rasmussen, B., Kemp, G. and Beauchamp, A. (2020) Teach-back: a systematic review of implementation and impacts, *PLOS One*, 14 Apr; 15(4): e0231350. doi: 10.1371/journal.pone.0231350.

Taylor, S.J.C., Pinnock, H., Epiphaniou, E., Pearce, G., Parke, H.L., Schwappach, A., et al. (2014) A rapid synthesis of the evidence on interventions supporting self-management for people with long-term conditions: PRISMS – Practical systematic Review of Self-Management Support for long-term conditions. Southampton (UK): *NIHR Journals Library*, Dec.

Tritter, J. and McCallum, A. (2006) The snakes and ladders of user involvement: moving beyond Arnstein, *Health Policy*, 76: 156–168.

U.S. Department of Health and Human Services, Office of Disease Prevention and Health Promotion (2010) Health literacy online: a guide to writing and designing easy-to-use health web sites [https://health.gov/healthliteracyonline/2010/Web_Guide_Health_Lit_Online.pdf; accessed 25 April 2024].

van de Bovenkamp, H.M., Trappenburg, M.J. and Grit, K.J. (2010) Patient participation in collective healthcare decision making: the Dutch model, *Health Expectations*, Mar; 13(1): 73–85. doi: 10.1111/j.1369-7625.2009.00567.x. Epub 2009 Aug 28.

West, M. and Dawson, J. (2012) NHS staff management and health service quality. [https://assets.publishing.service.gov.uk/media/5a7b92d040f0b62826a0473d/dh_129658.pdf; accessed 25 April 2024].

Woodall, J., Davison, E., Parnaby, J. and Hall, A-M. (2019) A meeting of minds: how co-production benefits people, professionals and organisations. Insights and inspiration from five strategic investments in England. [https://www.tnlcommunityfund.org.uk/media/A-Meeting-of-Minds_How-co-production-benefits-people-professionals-and-organisations.pdf?mtime=20190919092658&focal=none.; accessed 25 April 2024].

World Health Organization (WHO) (1998) *Health promotion glossary*. Geneva: World Health Organization.

Worrall, A.P., Connolly, M.J., O'Neill, A., O'Doherty, M., Thornton, K.P., McNally, C., et al. (2020) Readability of online COVID-19 health information: a comparison between four English speaking countries, *BMC Public Health*, 20: 1635. doi: 10.1186/s12889-020-09710-5.

Measuring and managing healthcare performance

Arne Wolters

Introduction

The management of healthcare performance increasingly relies on the use of data. Whether you are a nurse in a local healthcare system, a senior policymaker within a governmental department or a patient in the waiting room at your local primary care provider, chances are you are either looking at, collecting, generating or interpreting data about the healthcare system.

These data are used for delivery of day-to-day care to patients, but also commonly summarized in performance metrics, measures that are used as indicators of healthcare quality or performance. When performance metrics were first introduced in managing healthcare systems in the 1980s, most of the metrics were collected just for that purpose, to manage performance (Black, 1982). Over time, and with the increase of electronic health records (EHRs), these metrics are typically derived from data that are collected as part of routine healthcare provision.

In England, the National Health Service (NHS) reported that 90 per cent of NHS hospitals used EHRs (NHS England, 2023). These records are typically used for direct care purposes, but are increasingly feeding into performance metrics, and are also accessible to patients. In a 2018 survey by Zheng and Jiang (2022) in the United States, researchers found that 40 per cent of patients accessed their own EHR at least once in the previous 12 months. Technological advancements have also led to increased use of electronic patients records in developing countries, where a study by Akanbi et al. (2012) showed that 91 per cent of healthcare organizations surveyed in sub-Sahara Africa (predominantly HIV-related health centres) use open source healthcare software.

With this increase in the availability of data comes an increase in available metrics. Although this provides great opportunities for the increased use of data in performance management, it is important that performance metrics are carefully chosen to be relevant, of high quality, a true indicator of performance and easy to interpret. A risk that needs to be carefully managed is the plethora of metrics available causing a loss of focus on key metrics that matter, and overwhelming users with irrelevant information.

Although performance metrics are often simple in appearance, much goes on underneath the surface of even a simple metric. The way metrics are derived, collected and interpreted can make a big difference in our perception of the performance of a healthcare system. Take urgent and emergency care as an example. Patients that present at an emergency department can present with a wide range of conditions that all require immediate treatment. A common single measure of quality that is often used to assess performance of an emergency department is the time it takes to be seen. In the United Kingdom in particular, the key metric is the percentage of patients that have been admitted to hospital, transferred to another healthcare service or discharged from the emergency department within 4 hours of arrival. On the surface, this metric is easy enough to derive and interpret and would allow easy comparison between different hospitals; however, in practice it is not as straightforward. Some hospitals operate a large-scale consultant-led emergency department, treating a wide range of patients arriving themselves or by ambulance. Other hospitals only provide walk-in clinics or operate Urgent Care Centres, which serve a different case mix of patients and conditions. Some hospitals will provide a mix of both. This difference in services on offer will drastically impact the likely performance on a waiting time target, making it very difficult to draw conclusions from a seemingly straightforward metric.

In this chapter, we are taking a deep dive into some of the challenges, helping you as a healthcare manager to understand what performance metrics are, how they can be used (well) to manage performance, and consider some of the challenges, opportunities and pitfalls in devising your own metrics.

What are performance metrics?

As a patient follows a healthcare pathway a large volume of information is recorded in their EHR (or records, across different healthcare organizations). A simple care pathway will generate data including: scheduled date and time of a doctor's appointment, actual date and time of appointment, presenting complaint, results from diagnostic tests, medication prescribed, medication dispensed, date of a referral, scheduled date and time of a hospital appointment, actual date and time of appointment (or no show), further diagnostic testing, admittance to a hospital ward, ward transfers, any treatments provided in hospital, date and time of discharge, discharge location. Although a long list, this is just the tip of the iceberg of information recorded during any healthcare interaction.

In and of itself, information on a single patient does not make a metric. However, in addition to this patient pathway, consider the thousands of other patients that are seen and treated in a modern healthcare system every day. From this, you might derive metrics that are more interesting. For instance, the average waiting time for a consultation with a general practitioner (GP) at a local primary care provider. If you consider this information for a large number of patients every month, and then compare one month to the next, suddenly you are looking at a metric around the timeliness of care provided.

In addition to metrics on waiting times, common metrics may include volume of referrals, average length of stay in hospital, number of re-admissions to hospital within 30 days of discharge, rates of mortality or the rate of antibiotic prescribing.

What all these examples have in common is that a metric is usually an aggregate measure, over a large number of patients in a hospital or region, and typically over a certain amount of time. By aggregating information on individual patients, these metrics allow users to better understand what is happening in a healthcare system as a whole. These metrics can be indicative of the performance of a system, so-called performance metrics.

A single performance metric is not very informative in trying to understand the quality of care provided by a healthcare system, given there are so many different facets to good-quality care. At the beginning of the twenty-first century the Institute of Medicine (2001) identified six domains where improvement was required to make sure that healthcare systems provide good-quality care. These domains are still relevant today, and provide a good framework for a comprehensive set of performance metrics that can be indicative of the quality of care provided. These domains are summarized in Table 22.1.

Other frameworks or models can be used to consider a comprehensive set of performance metrics. For instance, Donabedian's framework (2005) that considers structure (characteristics of the care provider), process (characteristics of care delivery) and outcomes (effect of healthcare on individuals or a population) as three distinct domains that each can be measured.

Metrics as a proxy for actual performance

It is important to realize when working with performance metrics that these are often approximations of actual performance, an attempt at capturing something that really matters. As mentioned before, performance metrics are often derived from data that are already routinely collected as part of day-to-day care. This allows for the data collection burden to be minimized, as collecting an entirely separate metric would take valuable time away that clinicians can otherwise spend with patients. As a result, the metrics used to measure performance are typically proxies of actual performance.

Taking emergency departments as an example, good-quality care means that all patients receive timely and appropriate care, based on their actual need. Triaging the needs of patients is essential to ensure this, particularly if an emergency department is operating at or close to capacity. International standards on triage in emergency departments by Mackway-Jones et al. (2006) categorize patient need in five categories (or colours): immediate (red), critical (orange), urgent (yellow), standard (green) and non-emergency (blue). These categories each come with their own recommended maximum waiting time (from 0 to 240 minutes), although these may vary between countries. This triage often happens on the fly and may not be explicitly recorded in electronic systems.

A metric for good-quality of care in an emergency department may want to consider performance against the maximum recommended waiting time for each category. However, with the lack of consistent data collection, deriving this metric may be difficult or impossible. Instead, a common metric used measures the percentage of patients that are admitted, transferred or discharged within 4 hours after presenting at an emergency department. What

Table 22.1 Six domains of care quality that provide a good framework for a comprehensive set of performance metrics

Domain	Description	Example of metric
Safe	Measures that capture any harm to patients as a result of the care that is intended to help them. This can also include harm due to the delay of care provided.	Number of serious incidents; number of never events; % of patients receiving harm-free care.
Effective	Measures that capture the provision of evidence-based treatment and services to all those who could benefit, and refraining from providing these services to those who will not (avoiding underuse and overuse, respectively)	30-day re-admission rate; cancer survival rate.
Patient-centred	Measures that capture if care provided is respectful and responsive to individual patient preferences, needs and values and ensures that patients' values guide all clinical decisions.	Patient-reported outcome measures (PROMs); Patient-reported experience measures (PREMs).
Timely	Measures that capture waiting times and sometimes harmful delays for those who receive and provide care.	Average waiting time; 4-hour waiting time breaches at emergency departments; % of breaches of target referral to treatment time.
Efficient	Measures that capture waste, including waste of staff resources, equipment, supplies, ideas and energy.	% of outpatient appointments cancelled by hospital; % of 'did-not-attend' (DNA) for new outpatients; % of DNA for follow-up patients; theatre utilization.
Equitable	Measures that capture any variation in the quality of care provided to individuals because of personal characteristics. such as age, gender ethnicity, sexual orientation, religion, geographic location and socio-economic status.	Access to services by patient characteristics; Variation in PROMs/PREMs by patient characteristics.

Source: Adapted from Institute of Medicine (2001).

happens within those 4 hours, and after, is dependent on clinical judgement, essential for good-quality care, but not measured by the performance metric.

Trends over time

When looking at a performance metric, or proxy for performance, the question might arise 'What does good look like, what is a good level of performance?' For some metrics, this question might have a simple answer. For instance, one of the example metrics in Table 22.1 for safe care is the number of never events. This is the number of events that should never happen in a hospital, e.g. wrong site surgery. Clearly the metric should be as close as possible to zero, if not zero, to consider care provided as high quality.

For other metrics this is more complicated. Consider the average length of stay for patients on an inpatient ward. Of course, most patients would like to be able to be discharged to their home as soon as possible. However, patients should only be discharged when they are medically fit to be discharged. Overall, a shorter length of stay may be preferable, but if stays are too short, and patients are not sufficiently recovered, this may lead to re-admissions.

Looking at a performance metric at a single point in time will be of limited value. Judging a performance metric over time will provide much more insight (as illustrated in Box 22.1). Being able to judge whether performance metrics are staying constant with time, trending up, or trending down will give much better insights into the performance the metric tries to capture. Particularly where the metric is merely a proxy of the actual performance, the specific value of the metric may be almost irrelevant.

Box 22.1 The value of trends over time, and how to interpret them, considering average length of stay for inpatients in Germany

Figure 22.1 shows an example of a performance metric over time. In this case, the average number of days inpatients in Germany spend in hospital between admission and discharge. This figure shows the trend of this metric from 2010 to 2021. In this period, we see a downward trend in the average length of stay, starting at an average of 9.5 days in 2010, coming down as far as 8.7 days in 2020, with a slight subsequent increase to 8.8 days in 2021.

As explained above, looking at the value itself, makes it difficult to judge as to whether or not this metric reflects good performance. The number of 9.5 days in 2010 seems reasonable, but could be high or low, depending on context. This also shows that looking at a quantitative metric alone might not be sufficient to draw any conclusions. The value of monitoring performance metrics, and particularly changes in metrics, comes when you combine these with qualitative insights or other forms of intelligence.

What we can conclude from this trend is that in Germany average lengths of stay have been coming down, with the exception of the last year. A small uplift in 2021 could be the result of the impact of the global COVID-19 pandemic on hospital use, with a lot of delayed care from 2020. Whether or not the overall downward trend is appropriate, and reflective of improvement in quality of care, can only be determined with further information about the healthcare system. If concerted efforts have been made to improve patient care, and drive down the length of stay, you might conclude that this reduction in the metric is indicative of an improvement of the quality of care. If, on the other hand, the system has been under increased pressure, with increasing delays at emergency departments resulting in potential pressure to release patients more quickly from hospital, this might be an indication of a deterioration of the quality of care. If the re-admission rate following discharge does not increase over the same period, you might rule out this possible interpretation.

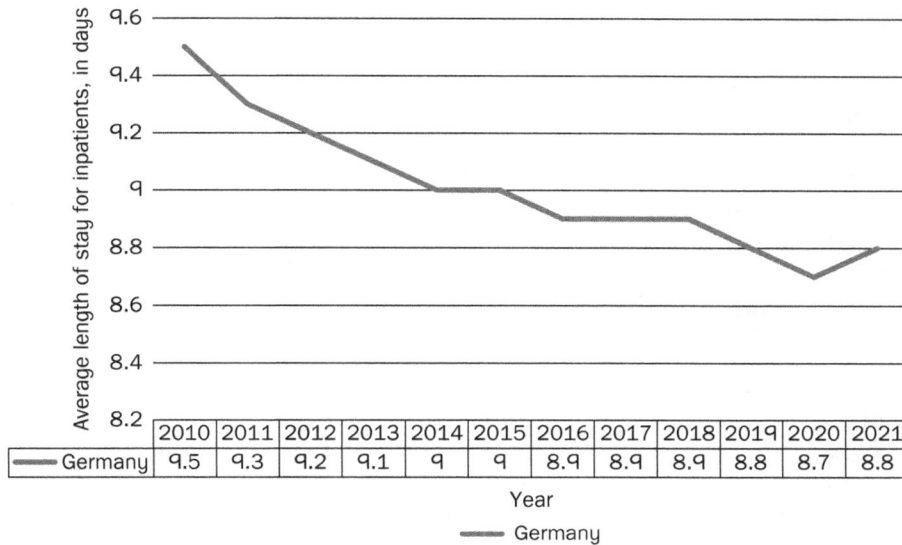

	2010	2011	2012	2013	2014	2015	2016	2017	2018	2019	2020	2021
Germany	9.5	9.3	9.2	9.1	9	9	8.9	8.9	8.9	8.8	8.7	8.8

Year

Germany

Figure 22.1 Average length of stay (in days) for inpatients in Germany, over time
Source: OECD (2024a).

Common challenges with performance metrics

When working with performance metrics, it is important to consider the quality of the metric itself. We already covered the fact that performance metrics are often a proxy for actual performance, but the proxy itself is typically derived from data. These data can have their own data quality issues, such as lack of precision, missing data, bias or changes over time.

Lack of precision

Most metrics are derived from routinely collected information, also called secondary data. That means that the data have not been collected for the purpose of measuring performance, but instead these data are re-used, and re-interpreted. It is important to consider the precision of data at the point of data collection, particularly if the person collecting the information is not aware of all of the uses of the data. Although it can be difficult to judge the level of precision of a performance metric, there are examples where you can clearly identify the lack of precision. The National Child Measurement Programme in England regularly collects information on weight of school-going pupils, among other measures. Weight is recorded in kilograms with one decimal point. By chance, you would expect 10 per cent of the weight measurements to be whole numbers; however, the national data shows this is the case in 16 per cent of pupils, with some local areas showing 30 per cent of recorded weight being a whole number (NHS England, 2018). This is a clear indication of the lack of precision in the data.

Missing data

Another common problem is missing data, or incomplete data. Sometimes relevant data has simply not been collected, or recorded correctly, resulting in missing data. It is important to consider what to do with missing data, particularly if the data are not missing at random.

If, say, information on one in every 100 doctors' appointments is missing, it may not affect trends in data. However, if the missing records are always for patients with diabetes, this can heavily impact the quality of a performance metric. When dealing with missing data it is also important to consider the difference between different types of missingness. For example, in ethnicity data a patient might not be asked about their ethnicity (missing), might prefer not to provide the information (not stated) or skip the question (not known). Similarly, it is important to distinguish between data that is missing from a dataset (typically recorded as NULL), and data with a valid value that is equal to zero (0). For instance, when deriving the average number of GP appointments in a year, patients who have zero appointments should be included in the average, whereas patients for whom the data is missing (NULL) are typically excluded from the analysis.

Bias

Both lack of precision and missingness can lead to bias in your data. But performance metrics can also be biased in other ways, and users should always be aware of this. This is a common problem in self-reported data or survey data, where respondents who are most likely to provide information may share common characteristics that are not representative of the population as a whole. But administrative data systems may also come with intrinsic biases. For instance, during the COVID-19 pandemic the United Kingdom introduced a contact tracing app to identify patients who may have been exposed to a carrier of the virus. Data shows that people with fewer formal qualifications were less likely to download the contract tracing app onto their smartphone (The Health Foundation, 2020). This not only biases the data but carries the risk that as a result people with fewer formal qualification would be less well-protected by the measures put in place to reduce the spread of the pandemic.

Changes over time

Although metrics can be used to detect changes in performance over time, the metric itself, or the data from which the metric is derived might change. Being aware of these changes, and potential breaks in trends of metrics over time, is essential. Particularly in healthcare data, even if a metric has not changed, the population served by a healthcare system may be changing. For example, recent trends in most healthcare systems in developed countries show an ageing population with increasingly complex needs (Chowdhury et al., 2023; World Health Organization, 2024). Patients admitted to hospital may present with more complex needs now than they did a decade ago. These changes in 'case mix' need to be addressed when considering trends in metrics over long periods of time.

How are performance metrics chosen[1]

With the increased availability of data due to digitization of the healthcare system and increased use of EHRs, metrics are more readily available than ever. This poses two important questions: who decided what performance metrics to use, and what for?

Different actors in a healthcare system will want to use performance metrics for different reasons. These reasons are summarized in Table 22.2.

---

1 This section draws on material included in the chapter on performance by Martin Bardsley in the 3rd edition of this book.

Table 22.2 Different users of performance metrics and their use purposes

Users	Purpose
Governments	Setting of national performance metrics, often accompanied by targets. These are used to monitor performance, promote accountability and drive policy change.
Regulators	Provide oversight of specific elements within the healthcare system, assessing of compliance with agreed standards, and surveil performance to identify poor practice requiring improvement.
Commissioners or purchasers of care	Monitor health outcomes in a local population to assess performance of a system or provider.
Providers of care – managers	Monitor and improve all aspects of quality of care provided to patients (including efficiency of the system).
Clinicians	Audit the performance of clinical teams against agreed standards, and drive improvement locally.
Patients and the public	Judge the quality of care provided in a local system, and influence political decisions. Patients may also use performance metrics to inform the choice of care provider.

Governments

Governments will be interested in a set of national performance metrics that will allow them to monitor performance. These performance metrics may be accompanied by policy-driven targets, in an attempt to improve performance (see next section). These national performance metrics are often made publicly available, promoting accountability of healthcare providers or local systems. These performance metrics tend to be high level, so they can be easily compared across different healthcare providers, local systems of different sub-populations. While most performance metrics are derived from routinely collected data, the government is in a position to mandate the collection of specific metrics.

Regulators

Regulators will have similar powers to governments in their ability to set certain national metrics. Their focus is typically on specific elements of the healthcare system where they assess performance for compliance with agreed standards and surveil performance across providers. Where regulators identify poor performance, or non-compliance with standards they will typically have powers to demand improvement in the quality of care given by healthcare providers. These powers will differ between countries, but can include public reporting, limiting the range of care services a provider can offer, close supervision by the regulator until significant improvements are made or in some cases financial penalties.

Commissioners or purchasers of care

Commissioners or purchasers of care typically use performance metrics to assess performance of providers in their local system. In addition to performance, they will be particularly interested in health outcomes for patients in their local system. This will help understand the need in the population and allow them to commission services that meet those needs. These metrics may be different from national metrics, as they can be tailored to the local population and their needs.

Healthcare providers and managers

Healthcare providers, and managers within those organizations, will typically monitor performance of their organization across a wide range of metrics. Metrics used can be very specific to the local provider/organization, and often have a strong focus on efficiency. Providers may want to maximize efficiency within their system while maintaining timely, safe and effective care for their patients. These metrics will also be used to support local improvement programmes.

Clinicians

Clinicians are responsible for the care provided to patients. They may use performance metrics to monitor the performance of clinical teams against agreed standards or to monitor local improvement programmes aimed at increasing the quality of care. While they may use high-level metrics to monitor overall trends, local improvement projects typically require specific metrics that may only exist within one provider or setting.

Patients and the public

Finally, patients and the public may use published performance metrics to judge the performance of local healthcare systems. Public access to metrics supports accountability for the healthcare system and providers to provide good-quality services, but it also allows patients and the public to influence political decisions related to healthcare (e.g. elections). Patients are increasingly given a choice of healthcare provider. Published metrics will help inform patients to make that choice. Although patients typically rely on metrics that are already published, they are increasingly given the opportunity to influence what metrics are collected by sharing what matters to them through involvement and engagement practices by decision-makers. Where involvement with patients and the public has been limited or even tokenistic in the past, there is a growing body of literature on the benefits of meaningful engagement with patients and the public and the impact it has on health and care services (Black et al., 2018; Agyei-Manu et al., 2023; Karlsson and Janssens, 2023).

As a result of such a wide group of users of performance metrics, with their individual needs, the number of performance metrics that are regularly reported on has increased with time. Although a large proportion of metrics may be derived from existing data sources, it is important to consider the data collection burden on those organizations that need to collect the data that feed into these metrics. Healthcare providers play a crucial role, collecting the majority of information needed. From their perspective there are typically two broad categories of performance metrics. Performance metrics providers have to collect, typically dictated by the government, regulator or commissioners ('top-down' metrics), and performance metrics that a provider wants to collect to support their internal performance management and local improvement efforts ('bottom-up' metrics).

Both categories of metrics are collected to monitor and improve healthcare performance. However, how performance is managed can have an impact on how the metrics are collected and reported on. In particular, with top-down metrics that are made publicly available, and may come with policy targets, there may be incentives to present the data in ways that may look more favourable (see the next section on managing performance).

Bottom-up metrics come with their own challenges. As the design of these metrics is typically driven by what information is available in a provider's data warehouse. This may result in a very large (and ever increasing) number of local metrics. Access to too large a set of metrics can result into a lot of time and resource spend in preparing these metrics (e.g. through dashboards) and may result in a loss of focus on what truly matters. Box 22.2 explores the proliferation of quality metrics further.

Box 22.2 The proliferation of quality metrics and dashboards

With the increased availability of data, the number of metrics used to measure quality of care in healthcare systems is also increasing. In the United States for instance, the National Quality Forum maintains a list of approved measures that has increased from 200 in 2005 to 700 measures in 2011, and will likely have increased since (Meyer et al., 2012). Clinicians are ringing alarm bells, arguing that too much of their time is spent on collecting metrics, rather than treating patients (McEvoy, 2015). All these metrics are often presented to healthcare managers and policymakers via dashboards that are growing in size and complexity. Arguably, the volume of metrics being collected may hinder effective monitoring and management or performance.

The proliferation of metrics may be best illustrated by a recent study Perić et al. (2018), bringing together evidence on the health system performance assessment indicators that are used across the 43 member states of the European Union. The study found a total of 2,168 different metrics. Through a series of surveys and expert assessments the authors reduced this number down to 95 metrics that they consider a blueprint for the most relevant headline indicators that can be used to frame and describe performance of healthcare systems in the EU. However, they acknowledge this list needs further refinement and should be seen as a shortlist only.

Learning activity 22.1

Have a look at the six domains of quality (Table 22.1). For your organization, consider what would be important goals or aims for each of these domains.

- What data or information do you already collect that might act as an acceptable performance metric to capture your goals or aims? What are the biggest shortcomings of these metrics?
- If you were to collect this information over a period of time, do you think it would help you better understand performance in your organization? Are there any aspects missing?
- Would colleagues in your organization value the same metrics? Do you think they are meaningful to your patients or customers? What would you want to see if you are on the board of directors for your organization?

Managing performance

With a wide range of performance metrics at our disposal, it is important to consider how we can use these to make a difference and how to manage and improve performance using these metrics. A common approach to managing performance is for policymakers or regulators to set targets for specific metrics.

For instance, it is well established that cancer treatment is most successful in case of early diagnosis and if patients are treated as quickly as possible following diagnosis. As a policymaker you might want to consider how to encourage early diagnosis and treatment. In many countries screening programmes have been introduced to regularly monitor the population for common forms of cancer (e.g. breast cancer). Performance metrics can also be used to set expectations around waiting times, for example, the time it takes from first contact with a GP to diagnosis, and subsequently the waiting time from diagnosis to the start of treatment.

Policymakers are in a position to add targets to metrics, setting an expected level of performance and spurring on improvement against a target where necessary. Policymakers can drive improvement by introducing financial incentives, either by making additional funding available if certain targets are met or by financially penalizing healthcare providers when care provided falls short of an agreed standard.

Rather than setting targets, requiring public reporting on metrics can be another means of managing performance. Setting a national performance metric all healthcare providers in a country or region need to report on can create the incentive to want to perform better or outperform rival providers. These comparisons, or league tables, are quite common and often picked up in journalistic reporting, adding more weight to the accountability of healthcare providers.

Performance metrics can also be used in the evaluation of change initiatives or improvement programmes. There are many different ways to design an evaluation study, but essentially an evaluation would consider relevant performance metrics covering a patient population or period of time where a new model of care has been introduced (intervention group) and compare this with a patient population that received regular care (control group). Provided the intervention and control groups are comparable in most aspects other than the change in care received, the difference in health outcomes between the groups may be considered the impact of the change initiative or improvement programme. Although this may appear straightforward, robust evaluation of differences in performance can be complex. Often it is not possible to draw robust conclusions from a quantitative evaluation study alone, and qualitative insights are necessary to understand what has changed, how this has impacted patients and staff and how to interpret any differences in performance metrics between intervention and control groups (Verhoef and Casebeer, 1997). For instance, when a change initiative causes an increase in admissions to hospitals, quantitative methods may be able to establish this effect and accurately estimate the effect size, but it will give little understanding about why this is happening. The initiative may identify previously unmet need (a good outcome for patients), or it may lower admission thresholds leading to unnecessary admissions (a bad outcome). Qualitative insights, through interviews with patients and clinicians, will help understand what mechanism is at play here.

Using evaluations to consider the impact of a change programme is something that can be done at national level to understand the impact of national policy changes. Equally, local improvement programmes may also benefit from formal evaluation, particularly where a new model of care has been introduced or there has been a step change in the way care is provided.

Performance metrics also play an important role in local improvement programmes that support continuous improvement of the quality of care provided to patients. This is either by providing critical information throughout an improvement cycle (identify, plan, execute, review), or through more sophisticated methods, such as statistical process control (SPC). In SPC a performance metric is monitored over time to establish a trend. Deviations from this trend can then be identified as special cases that either indicate an improvement or deterioration of performance. Qualitative insights will then help understand the cause of the deviation, identifying opportunities to make further improvements to the care provided (either by trying to replicate an improvement or prevent further deterioration of performance) (Dixon-Woods, 2019).

Comparing performance

As outlined above, one of the mechanisms to manage performance is to compare performance metrics of different healthcare providers or systems. Whether comparing performance between organizations or between countries, it is important to be aware of any differences between the metrics themselves. In order to compare performance metrics, their definitions need to be consistent, but we also need to consider differences in data quality, completeness and bias.

Whereas comparing different providers within the same system on a common national metric can provide a helpful comparison, comparing different systems or countries can be more difficult, as illustrated in Box 22.3.

Box 22.3 International comparison of average length of stay

In Box 22.1 we looked at the average length of stay for inpatients in Germany over time. Now we expand that example by comparing Germany to selected other OECD countries. Figure 22.2 shows that although the average length of stay is different across countries, the downward trend in the metric is common across all countries, with the exception of the United States, where the average length of stay increases over the same period.

Before, when considering the German data in isolation, it was difficult to conclude whether the reduction in length of stay was due to gradual improvements in quality of care, or increased pressure to discharge patients because of pressure on the system. Although this data alone is not conclusive, it can be considered as encouraging that the length of stay follows similar trends in other countries.

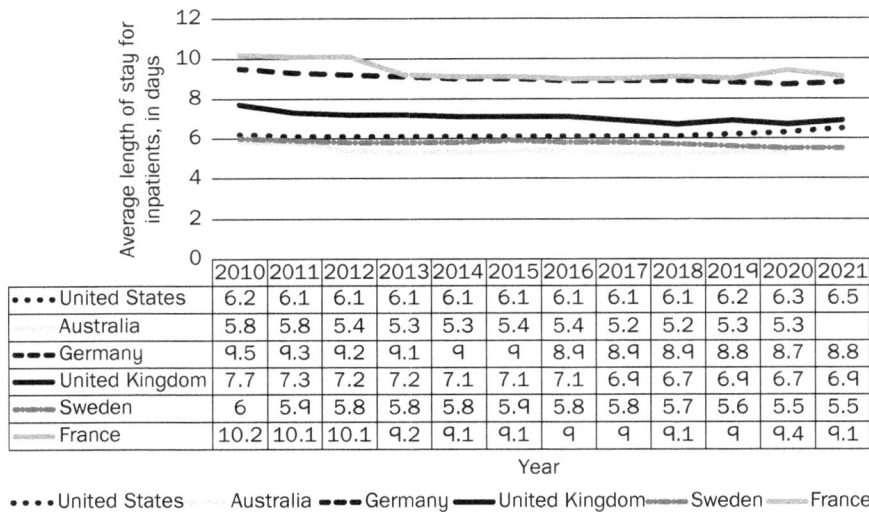

	2010	2011	2012	2013	2014	2015	2016	2017	2018	2019	2020	2021
•••• United States	6.2	6.1	6.1	6.1	6.1	6.1	6.1	6.1	6.1	6.2	6.3	6.5
Australia	5.8	5.8	5.4	5.3	5.3	5.4	5.4	5.2	5.2	5.3	5.3	
▬ ▬ Germany	9.5	9.3	9.2	9.1	9	9	8.9	8.9	8.9	8.8	8.7	8.8
▬▬ United Kingdom	7.7	7.3	7.2	7.2	7.1	7.1	7.1	6.9	6.7	6.9	6.7	6.9
▬▬ Sweden	6	5.9	5.8	5.8	5.8	5.9	5.8	5.8	5.7	5.6	5.5	5.5
▬▬ France	10.2	10.1	10.1	9.2	9.1	9.1	9	9	9.1	9	9.4	9.1

Year

•••• United States ⸻ Australia ▬▬ Germany ▬▬ United Kingdom ▬▬ Sweden ⸻ France

Figure 22.2 Average length of stay (in days) for inpatients in selected OECD countries, over time
Source: OECD (2024b).

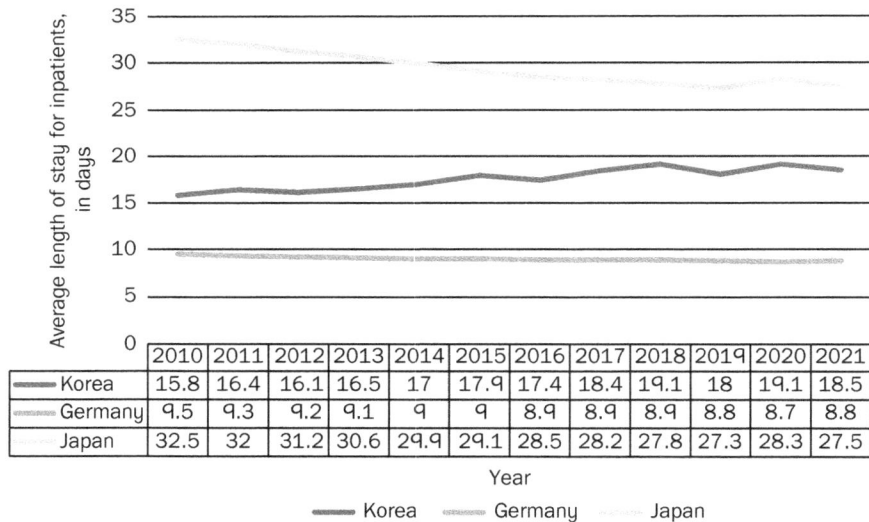

	2010	2011	2012	2013	2014	2015	2016	2017	2018	2019	2020	2021
▬▬ Korea	15.8	16.4	16.1	16.5	17	17.9	17.4	18.4	19.1	18	19.1	18.5
⸻ Germany	9.5	9.3	9.2	9.1	9	9	8.9	8.9	8.9	8.8	8.7	8.8
⸻ Japan	32.5	32	31.2	30.6	29.9	29.1	28.5	28.2	27.8	27.3	28.3	27.5

Year

▬▬ Korea ⸻ Germany ⸻ Japan

Figure 22.3 Average length of stay (in days) for inpatients in selected OECD countries, over time
Source: OECD (2024c).

In order to draw any conclusions from international comparisons (or any comparison for that matter) the different countries' healthcare systems need to be comparable enough to begin with. Figure 22.3 shows that a similar comparison with selected other OECD countries would lead to very different results. Comparing Germany with Korea and Japan makes it almost impossible to draw any conclusions. Where the average length of stay in Germany is 9 days over the period 2010–2021, for Korea this is 18 and for Japan this is even higher at 29. When presented with data like this, it is important to question the validity of the comparison. The most likely explanation for the vast difference in these metrics is that the healthcare systems in these three countries are so fundamentally different as are the definitions used (for example, of what constitutes an inpatient, what facilities are counted as hospitals, etc.) that any comparison would likely be flawed.

When drawing conclusions from performance metrics it is important to be aware of some important statistical concepts. Understanding the difference between correlation and causation and the concept of significance are key to managing performance using metrics.

In statistics, correlation describes the relationship between two metrics. Two metrics that are associated with each other are correlated, but that does not mean that one causes the other (Angrist and Pischke, 2009). For example, alcohol addiction is more common among people who smoke compared with people who do not smoke. However, that does not mean that smoking *causes* people to develop an alcohol addiction. Both smoking and alcohol addiction may be the result of a genetic disposition, socioeconomic factors or lifestyle choices. When analysing the relationship between different performance metrics, in a so-called observational study, it is possible to identify a correlation between metrics, but it is impossible to identify a causal relation.

Causation is where something happens as a direct effect caused by something else (Angrist and Pischke, 2009). For example, if a person drinks alcohol, their blood-alcohol level will increase. In medicine and healthcare causal relationships are very important. A clinician will prescribe medication because it should cure a disease or condition. Establishing any causal relationship is very difficult; maybe a patient's condition would have improved irrespective of the medication prescribed by a clinician; maybe the patient changed a habit, like diet, which had a positive effect on their condition. In healthcare, randomized clinical trials are the gold standard for establishing causal relationships, and quasi-experimental study designs can in some cases also be used (Clarke et al., 2019).

The fact that observational studies using performance metrics can only identify correlations and not causal relations does not mean that you cannot derive valuable insight from the data. It just means that you need to carefully interpret the findings, and not generalize your findings in a way not supported by the data.

When comparing performance metrics between two groups (or two different time periods), and discussing the difference, a statistical term that is commonly used is significance. The difference between two groups is considered statistically significant if the difference observed is not likely to be due to chance. For example, if you measure the blood pressure of a group of patients, there is natural variation in the observations, and the results will not be the same every time. If we now want to compare this group of patients to a second group of patients, to determine if there is a difference in blood pressure, we need to take this variation into account. The difference in average blood pressure between the two groups could be due to chance (the variation in measurement caused the particular observed difference), or the difference could be structural (despite the variation in measurement, blood pressure in one group is always likely to be higher). Where the observed difference between two groups is considered a true difference, this is called a statistically significant difference.

In addition to statistical significance, clinical significance is also very relevant when looking at performance metrics. Something is considered clinically significant if the difference is meaningful in a clinical sense. The difference between two groups can be statistically significant but not clinically significant, for instance, when the difference between two groups is so small that it has no meaningful difference in a clinical sense. Alternatively, due to high variation in the data something may not be statistically significant but still relevant from a clinical perspective. This highlights the importance of carefully interpreting findings when using performance metrics in managing the quality of care offered to patients.

The unintended consequences of performance metrics

When performance metrics are linked to targets there is a risk of unintended consequences that needs to be carefully considered. Performance targets create an incentive to want to do well on a particular metric, especially when the incentive is financial.

Given that performance metrics are often proxies for actual performance, incentives can cause overreliance on the metric itself (Li and Evans, 2022). A healthcare provider may be able to improve the performance on a particular metric without affecting any change on actual performance, or worse, causing the actual quality of care to deteriorate.

Going back to the example of providing timely care in emergency departments. A common metric is the percentage of patients that have been seen (admitted, transferred or discharged) within 4 hours of arriving at the hospital. If a target has been set for this metric with a strong incentive, and a healthcare provider is operating close to the target, there could be a perverse incentive for the provider to focus its efforts on patients that will likely be seen within the 4-hour target. Patients that are already in breach of the 4-hour wait are no longer affecting the metric one way or the other – and could be de-prioritized. This is not in the interest of the patient, and may risk harm to the patient, even though it would lead to better performance against the target that is designed to promote good-quality care. Behaviour like this, that causes performance metrics to improve or look more favourable from the outset without actually improving care, is often referred to as gaming.

Other ways of gaming with performance metrics are through changes to the data collection methods (resulting in the metrics looking more favourable), or changes to the activity that are covered by a certain metric. In England emergency hospital services are provided by Accident and Emergency (A&E) departments. However, most NHS hospitals offer 'Type 1' services (major, consultant-led emergency departments) and/or 'Type 3' services (urgent care centres or minor injury units). Both services are reported through the same national data collection and including in the four-hour target. Achieving this target is easier in a Type 3 A&E, than a Type 1 A&E, and as a result the performance metrics for hospitals providing both services will look more favourable.

When there are strong incentives for healthcare providers to meet certain targets another unintended consequence might be that a disproportionate amount of resource and effort might focus on areas where these metrics apply. Taking focus away from areas of care that are not as closely monitored, but also important in providing good-quality care to patients.

Finally, when policymakers try to effect change through the introduction of metrics and targets it is important that the metrics selected matter and capture the right information. Box 22.4 provides an example where policymakers did not get it right. Even though they introduced a new target, and achieved great adherence to the new target, the actual care received by patients did not change as a result. In this case, it increased the cost of care (through financial incentives) with no benefit to the system or patients.

Box 22.4   Case study – evaluating the named, accountable GP policy for patients aged 75 and over

Evidence suggests that longitudinal continuity of care in general practice, seeing the same GP over time, leads to better outcomes for patients. Patients are better able to manage long-term conditions and become less reliant on emergency hospital use. In order to promote better outcomes for patients, the NHS in England introduced the named, accountable GP policy for patients aged 75 and over in April 2014.

In England, patients are registered with a practice but may be seen by different GPs within the practice. What the new policy aimed for was to have a single, named GP responsible for the care of their elderly patients, and in doing so increase the continuity of care.

Calculating the continuity of care that a patient receives can be complex, and it would make for a complicated metric. So instead, a financial incentive was offered to practices for each patient that has a named GP on their EHR.

An evaluation of the policy was carried out by Barker et al. (2016), using a novel regression discontinuity design, aimed at establishing a causal effect estimate of the new policy on the continuity of care. By comparing patients at either side of the 75 years of age threshold, they were able to establish that the incentive had been effective in increasing the number of patients who had a named, accountable GP on their record, increasing from 3.5 per cent to 79.7 per cent at either side of the threshold. However, no difference was found in the continuity of care received by patients in the first 9 months after the policy had been introduced.

What this case study demonstrates is that although policymakers were keen to improve continuity of care, the policy has not been successful. By selecting a metric that did not reflect the actual aim of the policy well enough, GP practices inadvertently did what was required of them through financial incentives, without impacting the care received by patients.

Learning activity 22.2

Think about conversations with colleagues. Do you compare and contrast performance of your organization to that of similar organizations or competitors nearby? What is your perception of the relative performance of your organization compared with your nearest competitor?

Consider what metrics might be available in the public domain to better understand the actual difference in performance between these two organizations. Write a short report comparing the difference between your organization with that of a nearby competitor or neighbour.

Do you regularly report against a set target? Consider what the consequences would be if you did not meet this target. Consider if you have ever 'gamed' the system in your reporting to reflect an accurate but slightly more positive picture compared with true performance in your area of the organization.

Developing performance metrics that matter

When developing a collection of performance metrics, or a performance management system, it is important to consider what matters most, before considering what data are available. This will help minimize the risk of creating too many metrics, making it difficult to manage performance effectively. Although the process of devising new metrics may be iterative, it will encompass the following steps shown in Figure 22.4.

Aims

Articulating clear aims of what the introduction of performance metrics should achieve is an important starting point. Generally speaking, performance metrics will capture one or more of the domains of quality of care (see Table 22.1), but within these domains it is important to understand what needs to be achieved, or what matters to patients. Patient and public involvement and engagement (PPIE) activity is a great way to engage with those most impacted by healthcare services, learn from their lived experience and understand what aspects of care could be important to improve quality of care (see Chapter 21 for more information on service users' expectations and involvement). Putting patients and the public at the heart of the process at this early stage, gathering a wider range of views, minimizes the risk of being overly focused on processes or efficiency that might be well-represented in existing performance metrics already.

Identify metrics

With a clear set of aims identified, it is time to consider what success would look like, and how this may be measured. It is important not to be limited by what data is already routinely collected, but to consider a wide set of measurements. These could be quantitative in nature (derived from existing data) but can also include qualitative metrics or metrics that may be gathered through surveys (e.g. patient satisfaction surveys).

Data and analysis

The next step is to gather the relevant data required to derive the new metrics that have been identified. Where possible, this data should be re-used from existing data collections. EHRs hold vast amounts of information that, although essential for direct care purposes, may be under-utilized with respect to secondary data uses.

Where new data needs to be collected, either as part of clinical practice or through surveys or interviews, it is important to consider the data collection burden. The data collection burden should not be used as an excuse to not collect new information in favour of existing metrics. Where a new metric has the potential to help understand or lead to improvement in new areas of focus this should be encouraged, but the overall data collection burden is an important factor in being able to operationalize a performance measurement system. Where clinical staff are required to collect information, this may adversely impact on their ability to spend time with patients. Similar consideration should be given to data that is already routinely being collected; if this information is of limited value maybe some data collections can also be stopped.

For more complex metrics, some amount of analysis following the data collection may be required to derive the metric. Although complexity should not be avoided, it is important that whatever metric is being created it remains easy to interpret. Performance metrics should be able to provide insights on a day-to-day basis. If complex analysis is required to understand what drives an observed change in a metric, the level of complexity of that metric might be too high. Conversely, if a metric oversimplifies true performance, or is an aggregate metric trying to encompass too many different aspects of quality at once, the metric will also lose its value.

Reporting

Once the new metrics have been developed, findings against these metrics should be reported. These performance reports can be shared with relevant stakeholders to test out their usefulness and interpretability and assess whether the performance metrics reflect actual performance in line with expectations. Although metrics may in the first instance be created to support management to monitor and improve performance, it is important to test out new metrics with board-level executives, policymakers, healthcare mangers, staff, patients and the public. Seeking relevant feedback from all stakeholders is essential in understanding the effectiveness of a new metric.

Reflection

Upon receiving feedback from all stakeholders, it is important to reflect on that feedback and make any adjustments necessary. It is also important to go back to the original aim of developing the performance metrics in the first place. Does the new metric still capture the intended aim? How does the new metric perform against some of the concepts introduced earlier in this chapter (e.g. data quality, data completeness, bias)?

It is also important to consider at this stage if the performance metrics when in use, particularly if combined with targets and potential incentives, are likely to contribute to a reduction in health inequality or if they inadvertently might worsen inequalities. Reducing health inequalities may be one of the aims in itself, but regardless should be considered when reviewing all performance metrics. One of the common sources in inequalities of health outcomes is inequalities in access to services. This is a fundamental challenge that may be

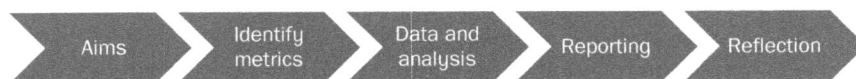

Figure 22.4 Process map for developing new performance metrics

difficult to solve through the use of performance metrics alone. By definition, healthcare providers only have data about users of their service, so patients and the public who struggle accessing services are under-represented in the data.

Each of the stages set out in Figure 22.4 may give cause to take a few steps back, for instance, to go back to the original aims and adjust metrics to make sure they address this aim, or to adjust some of the ambitions around data collection to make sure that gathering the relevant metrics is achievable. At the end of the process, you should have a set of metrics that capture important aspects of quality of care, and that can be meaningfully used to monitor and improve quality of care over time.

It is also important to reflect on what existing performance metrics are already in place. In the case of 'top-down' metrics there may be little scope to make changes, but for the collection of 'bottom-up' metrics, it is worth considering the value of collecting all this information and whether the newly developed performance metrics might replace some of the existing metrics, rather than being collected in addition to what was already there.

Learning activity 22.3

First, identify an area in your organization that you are familiar with, and consider what current reporting requirements exist for this area already. For instance, access and review board papers or minutes of board meetings over the past 12 months to see what performance metrics have been reported to the board.

Now consider what aspects of performance are important to provide good-quality services that are not captured in current reporting. Use Table 22.1 if it is helpful to consider the various domains of quality.

Work through each of the stages outlined in Figure 22.4 to develop a proposed set of metrics that capture performance. Form a task and finish group in your organization, and as a team prepare a report on your proposed metrics using data that are routinely collected in your organization already. Share this with key stakeholders in your organization, gather their views and refine your report.

After you have received feedback from colleagues, consider what, if anything, you would change as a result of this.

Separately, what information do you collect and report on in your day-to-day work that is of limited value to you and your organization? Is this information you could stop collecting?

Bringing it all together

To make sure performance metrics are used as intended, and used well, it is important to bring together the various aspects and performance metrics outlined in this chapter. A concise set of metrics, which are well understood, established with a clear aim in mind, while being mindful of potential pitfalls and unintended consequences, can help healthcare managers better understand and improve the health service they provide. The metrics can provide accountability and support (national) policymakers deliver on their goals, and patients can better understand the quality of care provided to them.

The OECD (2010) outlined seven principles to take into account when using performance metrics, aptly titled 'Handle with care'. These principles provide a helpful summary of this chapter and have been adapted for this book and are outlined in Table 22.3 below.

Table 22.3 Handle with care: seven principles to take into account when using performance metrics

Principle	Explanation
1. Fit for purpose	The choice of performance metrics should only follow a clear definition of its intended purpose. Metrics designed with an external focus (e.g. oversight, accountability) will have different characteristics from those design with an internal focus (e.g. quality improvement). For external use, metrics should be sensitive to safety risks, be sensitive to changes over time and show meaningful differences between services. For internal use, metrics will be more specific to the local setting and signal meaningful difference that warrants investigation and action. Metrics should matter to patients and members of the public.
2. Clear signalling	Metrics should provide a clear signal. Despite improvement over time, the validity of some metrics is often debated. Although some measures are straightforward to collect, such as mortality following discharge from hospital, their value is limited when comparing different hospitals. Crude rates can show lots of differences that are seldom due to differences in quality of care. These rates need to be adjusted for complications, co-morbidities, and other characteristics that are changeable between hospitals and over time.
3. Trustworthiness	The reliability of performance metrics depends on the quality of the metric and the quality of the data they are derived from. This can be a particular concern when metrics are derived from routinely collected data, which have been collected for a different purpose to measuring performance.
4. Beware of single indicators and **5. A chain is only as strong as its weakest link**	Although it is tempting to summarize the quality of care or performance of healthcare providers in a single indicator (e.g. England's Care Quality Commission rates hospitals quality of care as outstanding, good, required improvement or inadequate), these metrics are often an oversimplification of the actual quality of care provided. Care quality has six different domains (see Table 22.1), and most hospitals provide a large range of services, so even a small set of performance indicators might be inadequate at summarizing the quality of care provided.

(continued)

Table 22.3 *(continued)*

Principle	Explanation
6. A league table raises interest but is not always fair	Although interesting to compare different healthcare settings, or even countries, limitations that apply to performance metrics are exacerbated in league tables. A single metric per healthcare provider or country is likely an oversimplification of true performance. Observed differences between providers or countries in performance metrics will most likely be an indication of underlying differences between systems rather than performance. These comparisons can be helpful in understanding trends in data.
7. Be aware of gaming and unintended consequences	Regular (public) reporting of performance metrics can lead to improvements in performance. However, the use of performance metrics, particularly in combination with targets and incentives, can lead to unintended consequences (see Case study in Box 22.4 as an example). Healthcare providers may also overly focus on areas of their service that are regularly measured, and well represented in performance metrics, risking lack of focus in other areas of care.

Source: Adapted from OECD (2010).

Conclusion

This chapter explored what metrics are, and how they may be used to measure performance in healthcare. As proxies for quality of care, they are invaluable in understanding the performance of a healthcare system and can provide important insights in current state of play as well as trends over time. Performance metrics have their shortcomings, and users of performance metrics should be aware of these, particularly when using performance metrics to actively manage quality of care. Decision-makers should also be aware of the potential unintended consequences of using performance metrics, particularly where these are combined with targets and incentives. Finally, the chapter outlined how someone might go about developing new performance metrics, and taking into account challenges that this may bring. Performance metrics have great potential to inform and shape the healthcare we all need and receive. When used well, they will help create a sustainable and equitable healthcare service that will benefit everyone.

Learning resources

OECD Data Explorer: The Organisation for Economic Co-operation and Development (OECD) is an international organization that works to build better policies for better lives. Use their data explorer to find, compare and share the latest OECD data: charts, maps, tables, and related publications [https://data.oecd.org].

HealthData.gov (United States): This site is dedicated to making high-value health data more accessible to entrepreneurs, researchers, and policymakers in the hopes of better health outcomes for all [https://healthdata.gov/].

Statistics Canada – Health statistics: The Health Statistics Branch (HSB) of Statistics Canada is the country's trusted source of timely, accurate and relevant information about the health of Canadians. They provide data and insights about the health of the population, determinants of health and the scope and utilization of Canada's healthcare resources [https://www.statcan.gc.ca/en/subjects-start/health].

NHS England – Digital: The statutory custodian for health and care data for England, serving stakeholders across the UK. We enable the health and social care system to make best use of its data to improve healthcare outcomes, efficiency of services and the impact of research, while safeguarding the privacy of the people whose data we hold [https://digital.nhs.uk/data].

QualityWatch: While many national organizations are monitoring the quality of care, the Nuffield Trust and the Health Foundation believe there is also a need for independent scrutiny by non-statutory bodies. QualityWatch is a joint research programme monitoring how the quality of health and social care is changing over time. They hope it will both augment and inform the work of other statutory national bodies and initiatives in the UK [https://www.nuffieldtrust.org.uk/qualitywatch].

Association of Professional Healthcare Analysts: Their purpose is to raise the profile of and represent the voice of health and care analysts as a recognized and respected industry expert, by providing a professional framework and an established support network [https://www.aphanalysts.org/]

Unintended consequences: Learn more about the unintended consequences of performance management in healthcare from this rapid evidence review. Li, X., Evans, J.M. (2022) Incentivizing performance in health care: a rapid review, typology and qualitative study of unintended consequences, *BMC Health Services Research*, 22: 690 https://doi.org/10.1186/s12913-022-08032-z

Evaluating the impact of healthcare interventions using routine data: Learn more about the use of routine data, and robust observational study designs for real-world evaluation. Clarke, G.M., Conti, S., Wolters, A.T. and Steventon, A. (2019) Evaluating the impact of healthcare interventions using routine data, *British Medical Journal*, 365:l2239. https://doi.org/10.1136/bmj.l2239

References

Agyei-Manu, E., Atkins, N., Lee, B., Rostron, J., Dozier, M., Smith, M. et al. (2023) The benefits, challenges, and best practice for patient and public involvement in evidence synthesis: a systematic review and thematic synthesis, *Health Expectations*, 26: 1436–1452.

Akanbi, M.O., Ocheke, A.N., Agana. P.A., Daniyam, C.A., Agaba, E.I., Okeke, E.N. et al. (2012) Use of electronic health records in sub-Saharan Africa: progress and challenges, *Journal of Medicine in the Tropics*, 14(1): 1–6.

Angrist, J.D. and Pischke, J. (2009) *Mostly Harmless Econometrics. An Empiricist's Companion*. Princeton, NJ: Princeton University Press.

Barker, I., Lloyd, T. and Steventon, A. (2016) Effect of a national requirement to introduce named accountable general practitioners for patients aged 75 or older in England: regression discontinuity analysis of general practice utilisation and continuity of care, *BMJ Open*, 6: e011422.

Black, A., Strain, K., Wallsworth, C., Charlton, S.-G., Chang, W., McNamee, K. et al. (2018) What constitutes meaningful engagement for patients and families as partners on research teams?, *Journal of Health Services Research & Policy*, 23(3):158–167.

Black, D. (1982) Data for management: the Körner Report, *British Medical Journal*, 285: 1227–1228.

Chowdhury, S.R., Das, D.C., Sunna, T.C., Beyene, J. and Hossain, A. (2023) Global and regional prevalence of multimorbidity in the adult population in community settings: a systematic review and meta-analysis, *eClinicalMedicine*, 57: 101860.

Clarke, G.M., Conti, S., Wolters, A.T. and Steventon, A. (2019) Evaluating the impact of healthcare interventions using routine data, *British Medical Journal*, 365: l2239.

Dixon-Woods, M. (2019) Improving quality and safety in healthcare, *Clinical Medicine*, 19: 47–56.

Donabedian, A. (2005) Evaluating the quality of medical care, *The Milbank Quarterly*, 83(4): 691–729.

Health Foundation, The (2020) Contact tracing app threatens to exacerbate unequal risk of COVID-19. [https://www.health.org.uk/news-and-comment/news/contact-tracing-app-threatens-to-exacerbate-unequal-risk-of-covid-19; accessed 3 May 2024].

Institute of Medicine (2001) *Crossing the Quality Chasm: A New Health System for the 21st Century*. Washington (DC: National Academies Press (US).

Karlsson, A.W. and Janssens, A. (2023) Patient and public involvement and engagement (PPIE) in healthcare education and thesis work: the first step towards PPIE knowledgeable healthcare professionals, *BMJ Open*, 13: e067588.

Li, X. and Evans, J.M. (2022) Incentivizing performance in health care: a rapid review, typology and qualitative study of unintended consequences, *BMC Health Services Research*, 22: 690.

Mackway-Jones, K., Marden, J. and Windle, J. (2006) *Emergency Triage* (2nd edn). London: BMJ Publishing Group.

McEvoy, V.R. (2015) Why 'metrics' overload is bad medicine, *Missouri Medicine*, 112(1): 32–33.

Meyer, G.S., Nelson, E.C., Pryor, D.B., James, B., Swenson, S.J., Kaplan, G.S., et al. (2012) More quality measures versus measuring what matters: a call for balance and parsimony, *BMJ Quality & Safety*, 21: 964–968.

NHS England (2018) National Child Measurement Programme, England – 2017/18 School Year. [https://digital.nhs.uk/data-and-information/publications/statistical/national-child-measurement-programme/2017-18-school-year/data-quality---missing-and-imprecise-data; accessed 3 May 2024].

NHS England (2023) 90% of NHS trusts now have electronic patient records. [https://webarchive.nationalarchives.gov.uk/ukgwa/20240106191044/https:/digital.nhs.uk/news/2023/90-of-nhs-trusts-now-have-electronic-patient-records; accessed 21 June 2024].

OECD (2010) *Improving Value in Health Care: Measuring Quality, OECD Health Policy Studies*. Paris: OECD Publishing.

OECD (2024a) Hospital average length of stay by diagnostic categories, Data source: Federal Statistical Office (Germany). [https://data-explorer.oecd.org/; accessed 24 May 2024].

OECD (2024b) Hospital average length of stay by diagnostic categories, Data source: Centers for Disease Control and Prevention/National Center for Health Statistics/National Hospital Discharge Survey Annual Summary, Advance Data from Vital and Health Statistics Summary (United States), Australian Institute of Health and Welfare Hospital Morbidity Database (Australia), Federal Statistical Office (Germany), NHS Digital (United Kingdom), National Board of Health and Welfare (Sweden), Ministère des Solidarités et de la Santé, Drees (France). [https://data-explorer.oecd.org/; accessed 24 May 2024].

OECD (2024c) Hospital average length of stay by diagnostic categories. Data source: Ministry of Health and Welfare, Health Insurance Review & Assessment Service (Korea), Federal Statistical Office (Germany), OECD (Japan). [https://data-explorer.oecd.org/; accessed 24 May 2024].

Perić, N., Hofmarcher, M.M. and Simon, J. (2018) Headline indicators for monitoring the performance of health systems: findings from the european Health Systems_Indicator (euHS_I) survey, *Archives of Public Health*, 76: 32.

Verhoef, M.J. and Casebeer, A.L. (1997) Broadening horizons: integrating quantitative and qualitative research, *Canadian Journal of Infectious Diseases and Medical Microbiology*, 8(2): 65–66.

World Health Organization (2024) Ageing and Health. [https://www.who.int/news-room/fact-sheets/detail/ageing-and-health; accessed 21 June 2024].

Zheng, H. and Jiang, S. (2022) Frequent and diverse use of electronic health records in the United States: a trend analysis of national surveys, *Digital Health*, 8: 20552076221112840.

Conclusions: future challenges for healthcare managers

Simon Moralee and Manbinder Sidhu

Introduction

Since the first edition of this book was published in 2006, much has changed in the world of healthcare management. It was a time of relative growth in UK health services – and more widely and globally, one of optimism about the potential for complex problems to be addressed through a combination of knowledge, expertise, technology and innovation.

This edition arrives at a time of global uncertainty, politically, socially and economically while many of the same issues remain pertinent almost 20 years later: the demographic shift (ageing populations and rising incidence of chronic disease); technological change; changing user and consumer expectations; and rising costs. What has changed is the nature of those factors, as demonstrated, in the context of healthcare, through the new chapters and emerging ideas presented in this book. Politics, policy and the challenge of workforce remain pertinent issues. As does how to manage in primary, acute, integrated, adult social and mental health care. Performance, quality improvement, innovation, priority-setting, health economics and funding also remain highly relevant across all global health systems as policymakers and managers seek increasingly to do more with less. However, we have also seen the increased importance of equality, diversity and inclusion for healthcare managers, how to govern global health in a new geopolitical era, with the aftermath of the pandemic still fresh in the public consciousness and greater focus – and not before time – on issues relating to climate change and sustainability.

This book has attempted to explore the nature of complexity facing healthcare managers, especially in relation to the rapidly changing nature of the conditions in which healthcare is delivered and managed. Healthcare remains an intrinsically political domain in which every citizen has some sort of interest and where managers are just one group of stakeholders within a complex web of actors who influence the development and implementation of health policy and strategy.

In this final chapter, we examine the challenge facing healthcare managers as they seek to deal with the inherent complexity and change within health systems, and we describe the issues that need to be addressed for healthcare management to be truly effective. Akin to the conclusions drawn from the first edition back in 2006, we conclude the book by setting out what this analysis of healthcare management actually means for the task at hand for the modern-day healthcare manager – a manager who needs to be highly competent, compassionate and creative when managing change within a highly complex environment (see Box 23.1).

Box 23.1   Major challenges facing healthcare managers

- Developing the political acumen and astuteness to understand, influence and manage within a contested policy environment.
- Acquiring the skills and capability to manage within and across new organizational and institutional forms, without relying on extant positional powers and relationships.
- Having robust and transparent approaches to making healthcare funding and resource allocation decisions.
- Having sophisticated and sensitive approaches to making decisions about the redesign of services across healthcare systems, including decommissioning longstanding services.
- Understanding and using new approaches to the assessment and prioritization of new health technologies.
- Developing new approaches to the management of chronic disease and long-term conditions, within an ever-changing delivery landscape.
- Having coherent and sophisticated plans for tackling communicable diseases and ensuring proactive, rather than reactive, approaches to nascent and emerging viruses.
- Being able to adopt a range of strategies that enable healthcare funders and providers to work in close partnership with other agencies whose activities impact on health status, with a core focus on social and structural determinants of health.

Setting out the challenges for managers

The book began with a series of chapters relating to some of the fundamental tenets and skills within healthcare management: governance, leadership, quality improvement, equality and diversity, and research and evaluation, before moving on to consider issues around global governance, politics, finance and climate change.

In Chambers' account of governance and leadership (Chapter 2), it was clear that a manager's leadership approach will need to be one that persuades and influences colleagues while setting overall parameters and standards of conduct for teams and organizations – more directive approaches being unlikely to work in such complex and political settings. As the form and functions of healthcare increasingly emphasize the system, place and integration of governance, current models, that are focused on institutions, may be unsuitable. As a consequence, managers will need to adopt a more holistic approach to their understanding of 'health' along with new strategies for addressing multisectoral and highly complex social problems that in turn impact on people's (poor) health.

Furnival's account of quality improvement (Chapter 3) stressed the need for managers to support the building of improvement capability and her chapter outlined a number of tools, techniques and philosophies that help underpin improvement work. Contained within that was a call for healthcare leaders to recognize their roles, behaviours and responsibilities to the wider system and to acknowledge that data and insight are essential but not sufficient for the improvement and transformation of care.

Adab's arguments regarding public health and global inequalities (Chapter 4) set out five core actions for healthcare managers. Starting with developing their own awareness, the chapter urged managers to engage in training and continuing professional development, specifically in the area of skills required for addressing health inequalities; second, monitoring and evaluation of data and involving communities and service users in determining what data is meaningful for change was considered vital to address inequalities; third, it is important to ensure all staff are provided with good-quality work and workforce cultures that support health equity – not just to promote fairness but also to improve productivity, creativity and well-being; fourth, managers should work in partnership with schools, housing, local and regional government, police, charities, third-sector organizations and community groups; and finally, there is a need to advocate for under-represented and marginalized groups, using their positions as experts and trusted professionals to tackle the structural and social determinants of health and illness.

Dunne's overview of equality, diversity and inclusion (Chapter 5) continued a recent, yet long overdue, trend of bringing issues of inequality and inequity into mainstream planning, policy and delivery. Drawing on examples from the UK, Australia, Canada and New Zealand, it set out the variety of approaches being taken for health systems to be more inclusive, ending with a call to action for healthcare managers to practise more inclusively for sound moral and ethical reasons to enhance health and care delivery.

Lamont and Hooper's chapter on research and evaluation (Chapter 6) provided a number of practical insights for healthcare managers in terms of how to search for, select, interpret and use research evidence in their everyday decision-making. They encouraged organizations to promote the use of evidence, as well as creating cultures that actively support tackling some of the complex problems managers face.

In Chapter 7, Thorlby and Exworthy set out the key requirements for healthcare managers operating in politically sensitive healthcare environments. The authors argue that an ability to think through and act upon the broader politics of healthcare management would help managers disentangle the approaches that work to improve care, the level at which problems needed to be solved, along with the most effective ways to work with, rather than against, societal values, all in service to patients who want access to treatments that prolong life and improve the quality of life.

Greer and Wismar's interpretation of governing global health (Chapter 8) called upon healthcare managers to recognize the inherent contradictions and compromises required to manage health at a global level. While the past meant an establishment of the rules and institutions to promote health in a global, capitalist system, the future looks towards promoting health and human rights in a world of rising geopolitical conflict and competition, with new increasingly powerful actors, such as the BRICS (Brazil, Russia, India, China, South Africa) countries and the need to address global health problems, from climate change to healthcare supply chains, not to mention consideration of how global health actors may cooperate when the next, probable, pandemic arrives.

Robinson's chapter on healthcare financing (Chapter 9) encouraged healthcare managers to understand the current funding arrangements within their health systems and at organizational levels. Key to this was the so-called panacea of funding reform, often seen as the mechanism to curb spending to contain costs yet accompanied with a warning that embarking on reform requires consideration of other policy levers outside of changes to funding.

Health economics (Chapter 10) as a discipline can assist managers in making investment (or disinvestment) decisions, alongside an understanding of priority-setting (Chapter 11). As set out by Lewis and Bell, governments and individuals increasingly have to trade-off the cost of healthcare against other important priorities and healthcare managers are frequently faced with demands to get greater value from the resources at their disposal. In demonstrating how countries explored the use of similar economic approaches, albeit in different contexts and often with substantively different types of health system organization, the authors demonstrated that there is no simple solution. As a consequence, healthcare managers would need to understand and make trade-offs between different and competing priorities, using health economics and its associated analytical approaches as tools with which to understand performance and to allocate resources most effectively.

Following on, Williams and Smith (Chapter 11) felt when making decisions about resource allocation and service configuration, managers need to be cognisant of the challenge of how to respond to new and emerging technological advances, about whose efficacy and efficiency data may be initially in short supply, and how to embrace engagement and media strategies, combined with political acumen and change management skills, to realize the benefits of their decisions.

Naylor and Pinto, in Chapter 12, detailed the contribution of health systems towards climate change through use of, for example, anaesthetic gases, transport, procurement, facilities and energy use. Healthcare managers are urged to consider ways in which not only activity can be reduced (prevention, patient empowerment, lean pathways) but also the impact of remaining activities (low-carbon alternatives, operational resource use, such as moving away from reliance on fossil fuels). In practice, this requires implementation of carbon footprinting, life-cycle assessment and triple bottom-line accounting as part of everyday commissioning, contracting, purchasing, planning and delivery of healthcare services.

It is clear managers face new challenges in relation to how the different sectors of healthcare are configured – what might have been traditionally understood as primary, community- or hospital-based care is now much less distinct, as technology increasingly enables the shift of care away from physical settings. In several chapters that focus on specific sectors of healthcare management, it was made clear, first by Sidhu and Smith (Chapter 13), that primary care is becoming more 'fragmented', yet its organization remains vitally important to realizing overall health gain. Some of those main challenges facing healthcare managers include how to enable previously small-scale clinics and practices to form larger networks or organizations and balance the needs and priorities of local professional and community innovation with those of the wider regional and national health system.

Edwards and Vaughan (Chapter 14) outlined how acute care is being redefined by technological advances and workforce skills shortages, along with differential payment mechanisms, with responses including centralization of services, increasing network collaboration and a stronger focus on quality and regulation of acute care. Moreover, with concerted efforts to divert patients away from acute care, there is a resultant impact on primary and community care services. Funding acute care remains a challenge, given resource constraints within and beyond healthcare, and with ageing populations and a continued focus on curative medicine, the focus for managers needs to be in understanding the complexities of the healthcare system and to diagnose the root causes of dysfunctions within it.

The challenge for managers when it comes to integrated care, as outlined by Miller and Stein in Chapter 15, was how to achieve increased working across a greater range of agencies and professions and to understand the parameters, motivations and frustrations of these agencies and professions. Moreover, for integrated care to happen, all stakeholders need to be actively involved in the design, management, implementation and evaluation of any initiatives. To realize integrated care, it needs managers who are able to nurture, lead, coordinate and actively manage; to gain buy-in from policymakers and decision-makers; to engage continuously with people and professionals, stakeholders and communities; and to create, reinforce and adapt a common understanding, language and values according to the needs of the local context.

Fenton and Carr (Chapter 16) encouraged healthcare managers to understand the challenges and complexities associated with mental health, account for social and economic impacts, and respond to social as well as clinical support needs for recovery. Managers need to consider and combat the effects of social and structural discrimination and stigma within and beyond those services and systems, integrating the expertise of those with lived experience to create anti-discriminatory and collaborative approaches, including multisectoral working.

Moreover, Burn and Needham (Chapter 17) stressed the need to understand the interconnectedness between social care and other public service systems. Overseeing services across such systems, managers need to coordinate and work closely with regulatory and quality assurance bodies, dealing with workforce shortages, particularly in rural areas and against a backdrop of alternative employment outside of health and care that offers better pay and conditions. At the heart of this work, managers will need to create a narrative around the value of social care as a career to attract the sorts of high-calibre and committed workers that the sector needs.

The final chapters in this book were all concerned with how managers deliver services. Beginning with consideration of informatics for healthcare (Chapter 18) – probably the area of management where complexity and change converge in the most challenging manner – Taylor explained that changes and developments in informatics pose a range of challenges, not least in relation to how such developments will impact on how healthcare staff work, how services will be delivered and how patients will access the health system. As with most management activity, the people element of this challenge is likely to be the most exacting for managers – how to maximize the benefits of new information technology (IT) and systems. Moreover, managers will need to develop the skills and knowledge to use data, not just in the management of individual patients, but also in running healthcare services at scale and across systems. As we forge forward into a more data-driven world, managers will need to understand how to use data in risk prediction and apply resulting insights to drive improvements across both clinical and managerial decision-making, as well as encouraging its use in changing health behaviour. The advent of greater artificial intelligence (AI), big data and genomics, as well as risks associated with cybersecurity, all need to be areas where healthcare managers gain greater knowledge and specific skills to harness the potential of informatics to improve healthcare.

Chapter 19 introduced readers to the healthcare innovation pathway, where Romanelli and Marjanovic argue there is a need for healthcare managers to support cultures at any level (institutional, organizational, departmental) that prioritize evidence-informed decisions. This is achieved by understanding how research and development translate into commercialization and implementation, recognizing the myriad of actors, such as government, industry stakeholders, workforce and regulators, involved in numerous, intricate processes for assessing new technologies and setting funding priorities.

Palmer's chapter on healthcare workforce (Chapter 20) outlined the many challenges related to training, development, retention and remuneration. Added to this are complex questions related to professional skill mix to deliver care optimally and ensure equitable geographical distribution of the healthcare workforce to meet population needs. Key for healthcare managers is to recognize that, among funding variations, shifting government workforce targets and changes in a competitive global market for valuable healthcare professionals, they need to balance incentives, regulation and workload to ensure that there are the right staff, in the right place, at the right time to deliver care.

In Chapter 21, Ellins and Coldham provided a challenge to healthcare managers with respect to service user perspectives, experience and involvement, presenting a strong case for involving people and communities in the design, implementation and delivery of healthcare services. Managers need to support patients with timely and helpful information about their care, both its substance and the processes by which it is attained, and to collaborate with healthcare professionals to support individuals to practise effective self-management and self-care; this is necessary for sound economic, but also democratic, rights-based and practical reasons. This means going beyond espoused versions of co-production to sharing power in decision-making, which can only come with mutual trust and respect. Managers must not only work with, but be guided by, values and principles that matter to service users, accepting that there are many marginalized and minority groups where structural barriers to meaningful involvement need addressing.

There has been a proliferation of approaches to measuring and managing performance in healthcare in recent years, such as developing 'dashboards', but Chapter 22 by Wolters advised managers to begin with clear quality parameters to inform any set of performance metrics. Such metrics will always be proxies for actual performance and managers will need to have an understanding of data, trends, bias and how different actors – from government, regulators, commissioners/purchasers, providers, clinicians, patients and the public – all have different requirements from these various metrics. A competent healthcare manager will need to be able to understand and compare performance data and metrics in a meaningful way for all those different stakeholders, with the ultimate aim of ensuring they are fit-for-purpose, clear and trustworthy, particularly where these are combined with targets and incentives.

Overall conclusions

As the authors of the first edition remarked, concluding this book appeared a daunting task and with 21 substantive chapters covering so many aspects of healthcare management, this edition confronted a similar challenge. Then, as now, it turns out, the task has not been as difficult as we imagined, for a reading of the totality of the book's contents has revealed a strong and consistent message in relation to the knowledge, skills and behaviours required of healthcare managers across different services, sectors, systems and countries. We have deliberately not attempted to define who or what a healthcare manager is, given the complexity of the context, the changing nature of the task and the degree to which creative and thoughtful responses are required. However, we do attest that the manager needs to be rooted in an ongoing commitment to acquire knowledge and update practical management skills.

In a context of heightened complexity and change – a context that seems set to define healthcare management worldwide for the foreseeable future – healthcare managers need also to attend to a number of other elements of the manager's knowledge and skills base, if they are not just to survive but thrive. Such a 'tool bag' for managers to draw from would include developing trust and credibility – credibility that is concerned not only with acquiring practical skills, such as managing projects, process improvement and resources, but also with the personal integrity that comes from having a well-developed sense of personal awareness and effectiveness, and a commitment to respecting the integrity of colleagues in teams and organizations.

The challenge for the healthcare manager in relation to matching behaviour and management style to specific situations and needs underlines the importance of managers being adaptive and flexible in their practice. Managers need to be able to interpret and make sense of organizations for those with whom they work, acting as both interpreter and 'sensemaker' of organizational pressures. Perhaps one of the most immediately practical and challenging aspects of such management is one that focuses on personal effectiveness and development, asking managers to examine their style of working and to find ways of developing the creativity and reflective practice that is crucial for effective leadership and development.

For managers currently working within health services, each chapter has set out a wealth of evidence-based practical guidance for working in a complex and rapidly changing context. It is clear that managers need to have the skills to set up robust management processes that are both transparent and accountable in an increasingly contested environment, as well as flexible and dynamic. Similarly, when challenged to improve the involvement of service users within the design, delivery and management of services (Chapter 21) or to find new ways of improving the quality and innovation of care (Chapters 3 and 19), this combination of stronger and yet adaptable processes again emerges as a key message for healthcare managers.

In many contexts and countries, the healthcare manager is not considered a popular figure, for they are, as we have seen in this book, charged with making some of the most difficult decisions about healthcare funding, planning and provision. This book continues to be a contribution to the ongoing international effort to develop evidence-based management in healthcare, bringing together the practical challenge of managing health and health services with the wealth of research evidence about what is needed to manage effectively in this complex and changing world.

Nonetheless, this book has sought to add in some small way to the process of developing healthcare management as an international community of professionals dedicated to improving the health and care of people who are often vulnerable and unable to act for themselves within the wider health system and society. This and future editions provide a transition between the founding editors, Kieran Walshe and Judith Smith, to us, as new and aspiring custodians of this seminal contribution to healthcare management. Our thanks go to them, as we are sure it will from the many managers, researchers and readers of this book over the past 20 years who have applied its learning in better informing healthcare management knowledge and practice. Looking to the future and further editions, as new editors, we will endeavour to continue in the vision that they set out.

Index

ACA (*see* Affordable Care Act)
Accountability for Reasonableness (A4R) 237–8
Acheson report 70
Activity-based funding 189
Acute care systems
  changes to hospital system
    development of emergency departments 312,
      315
    in medicine and surgery 312
    overall trends in 312–14
  implications for managers 322–3
  nature and role
    ambulance services 306–7
    hospital levels 304–5
    hospitals 304
    models of ownership 306
  other factors affecting
    digital technology 309–10
    global workforce crisis 310
    payment mechanisms 311
    quality and regulation 311
    rurality of 310
    technological challenges 309
  pressures on 307–8
  responses to challenges and change
    alternative places for first assessment 318
    centralization 316–7
    creating networks of hospitals 317
    diverting patients 318
    governance and autonomy 318
    shifting services to community 319
  unresolved issues/inflection point
    funding for 320
    generalism *vs.* specialism 321–2
    limits of reconfiguration 321
    reductions in hospital beds 320–1
Acute medical units (AMUs) 318
Adult social care
  care diamond 378
  challenges for managers 390–2
  changing approaches to 380–2
  governance of 379–80
  improving quality in 383–5
  interface between social care and health 388–9
  opportunities and challenges 382–3
  policy reform in Japan and Germany 389–90
  strengths-based approaches in 385–6
  structure and scope of, paid care workforce 379

technology and innovation 386–7
  value of hours of 379
Advisory boards 19
Advocacy 75–6
Affiliate organization boards 19
Affirmed gender identity 93
Affordability of care 12
Affordable Care Act (ACA) 412
Ageing population 307
Agency theory 19
AI (*see* Artificial intelligence)
Air pollution 251
AMUs (*see* Acute medical units)
Anglo-Saxon unitary board model 18–19
Anti-racism 92
Arnstein's ladder of participation 474
Artificial intelligence (AI) 414–15
ASEAN (*see* Association of Southeast Asian Nations)
Assigned sex 93
Association of Southeast Asian Nations (ASEAN) 166

Behavioural/cultural theories 64
Black Indigenous People of Colour (BIPOC) 88, 91
Black Report 70
Block payments 209
BMA (*see* British Medical Association)
British Medical Association (BMA) 462
Budget ceilings 228
Bundled-payment funding 190

Carbon emissions
  carbon hot spots identifying 257
  by clinical decisions 256–7
  sources of greenhouse gas emissions 254, 255
  structured engagement with suppliers 254
Carbon footprinting 261
Care Quality Commission (CQC) 383
Capitation funding 189
Capitation systems 213
CFIR (*see* Consolidated framework for implementation
    research)
Change management theory 267
Cisgender (cis) 93
Climate change
  health impacts of 251–2
  public health benefits 252–3
  risks to healthcare delivery 253–4
  sources of greenhouse gas emissions 254, 255

Clinical governance 39
Clinical practice research data link (CPRD) 407
Collective leadership 26
Colonialism 92
Comparative health data 167–8
Comprehensive care 281
Conflict and migration 252
Confounding 125–6
Consolidated framework for implementation research (CFIR) 428
Continuous care 281
Continuous quality improvement (CQI) 38
Contractual models 459
Coordination of care 281
Corporate governance (*see* Institution-level governance)
CPRD (*see* Clinical practice research data link)
CQC (*see* Care Quality Commission)
Cost-effectiveness analysis (CEA) 232–3
Cultural artefacts 341–3
Cybersecurity 415–6

Decision-making, priority setting
    accountability for reasonableness (A4R) 237–8
    cost-effectiveness analysis 232–3
    multi-criteria decision analysis (MCDA) 234
    programme budgeting and marginal analysis (PBMA) 233–4
    public engagement 234–7
Decoupling 170–3
Determinants theory 64
Diagnostic-related groups (DRGs) 311
DICOM® 405
Directory of Open Access Journals (DOAJ) 118
Distributed leadership 26
Diversity 84–5
Diversity, equity and inclusion (DEI) (*see* Equality, diversity and inclusion (EDI)
DRGs (*see* Diagnostic-related groups)
Drift hypothesis 64

Economic Community of West African States (ECOWAS) 166
Economic theory
    adverse selection 207
    competition and choice 219–20
    co-payments 218–19
    creaming 207–8
    diagnosis-related groups (DRG) 215–16
    dumping 208
    externalities 208
    information asymmetry 208
    market failure 208
    moral hazard 208

payer 208
paying for quality 220–1
prices in healthcare
    aggregation of demand 212
    costs of 209–10
    fairness and equity 214
    information asymmetry, consequence of 211
    market mechanisms, use of 213–14
    payment models 212–13
    shadow prices 209
    value in 210
primary care services 216–18
setting currencies and prices 215–16
simplified characterization of markets 207
skimping 208
value (as distinct from cost or price) 208
ECOWAS (*see* Economic Community of West African States)
Education mental health practitioners (EMHPs) 361
EHRs (*see* Electronic health records)
Electronic health records (EHRs) 404, 496
Electronic medical record (EMR) 309
EMHPs (*see* Education mental health practitioners)
EMR (*see* Electronic medical record)
Environmental sustainability
    benefits of climate action 252–3
    effective leaders
        collaborating on 267
        levels of motivation and engagement, strategies for 265
        measuring progress 267–8
        providing visible leadership 263–4
        scaling and spreading 266–7
        training and education for staff 266
        visible leadership 263–5
    examples of 268–70
    impacts of climate change 251–2
    measurement
        carbon foot printing 261
        life-cycle assessment 261
        triple bottom-line accounting 261–2
    at organizational level 255–6
    principles of
        driver diagram 257, 258
        lean pathways 259
        low-carbon alternatives 259–60
        operational resource use 260
        patient empowerment 258–9
        prevention 258
    quality improvement (QI) processes 262–3
    reasons to prioritize 251
    risks to healthcare delivery 253–4
    sources of greenhouse gas emissions 254, 255
    tools and frameworks to 257

Equality, diversity and inclusion (EDI)
  academic definitions 84
  common language and understanding 100
  constructive conversations 101
  discrimination in workplace 84–5
  equality vs.equity 86
  gender, sexuality and identity 93–6
  heteronormative 100–1
  language and terminology 99
  power and privilege
    key points 87
    othering 88–90
    White privilege 87–8
  racism 91–2
  social justice 84
  targeted recruitment initiatives 85
  unconscious bias 100
European Care Strategy 379
European Union's (EU) 167, 168

Familial hypercholesterolemia (FH), cascade model for
    genetic testing 440, 442–3
FAO (*see* Food and Agriculture Organization)
Fee-for-service systems 213
Feminism 95
Food and Agriculture Organization (FAO) 164
Food security 252
Functional integration 340
Fund-pooling 181

Gavi 165
GDP (*see* Gross domestic product)
Gender affirmation surgery/gender reassignment
    surgery 93
Gender dysphoria 93
Gender Recognition Act 93
Gender, sexuality and identity
  feminism 95
  key terms related 93–4
  LGBTQIA+ resource center glossary 93–4
  patriarchy 95–6
  self-identification process 93
General taxation 183–4
Global-based/block funding 188–9
Global health
  climate change 160
  definition of 157–8
  ecosystems and animals 160
  governance in geopolitical era 161–73
  health security 159–60
  terminology in 158–9
  trade and investment law 160
Governance
  and autonomy 318

challenges for
  affordability of care 12
  changing demographics 12
  collaborative forms of leadership 13
  increasing consumer demands 13
  political astuteness 13
  power of the professionals 13
  quality and safety in patient care 12
institution-level governance 14, 18–28
leadership
  collective 26
  distributed 26
  reconciling quality and safety 26
  situational approach to 27–8
  themes and patterns in 28–30
system-level governance 13–17
themes and patterns in 28–30
Gross domestic product (GDP) 180

Health for All 161
Health inequalities
  causes of 64–5
  data gathering and analyzing 65
  definitions of 59–60
  at global level 65–6
  impact of
    economic considerations 69–70
    modifiable inequalities 68
    moral and justice imperatives 68
    social considerations 69
    UN sustainable development goals 70
  implications for practice 60–1
  interventions to tackle
    common themes 71–2
    economic strategies 72–3
    policy reviews and reports 70–1
    resources and summary reviews 73–4
    social interventions 72
  managers role
    advocacy 75–6
    awareness, training and continuous professional
      development 74
    monitoring and evaluation 74–5
    partnership working 75
    workforce diversity 75
  at regional and country level 66–7
  social determinants of health (SDH) 97–9
  structural inequalities and intersectionality 62–3
Healthcare board
  accountability approaches
    effectiveness assessment 24
    markets–hierarchy–networks trichotomy 25
  Anglo-Saxon unitary board model 18
  board of directors 18

Healthcare board (*continued*)
 board of governors 18
 board practices 20–24
 changing and distinctive features of leadership 26–8
 co-operative and mutual traditions 18
 degree of professionalization 18
 failing board, example of 20, 21
 Good Governance Standard for Public Services
  assessment 23–4
 interconnectedness of roles behaviours and
  outcomes 22
 non-profit board members 22
 organization life cycle 18
 political input 18
 principle of co-determination 18
 purpose of 19–21
 realist framework for 20, 21
 Senate model 19
 stability *vs.* transformation/crisis 18
 types of 19
Healthcare funding
 activity-based funding 189
 administrative efficiency 193
 bundled-payment funding 190
 capitation funding 189
 defining terms 179–80
 economic crisis and COVID-19 193–5
 general taxation 183–4
 global-based/block funding 188–9
 healthcare triangle 180–1
 local taxation 184–5
 outcomes-based funding (value-based funding) 190
 out-of-pocket payments 188
 pressures
   health technology assessment (HTA) 196–7
   impacts of climate change 196
   strengthening digital transformation 195
   universal health insurance coverage 196
   workforce investment 195–6
 private healthcare insurance 186–7
 proportion of GDP 191–2
 purchasing activities 181
 revenue collection 181
 revenue generation 181–3
 social health insurance 185–6
 spending on primary care 193
 total health spending, OECD countries 190–1
 type of financing activity 192
Healthcare innovation
 innovation pathway
   commercialization 422, 424–5
   funding for 421–2
   implementation into care delivery 425
   stages of research and development 422, 423

 navigating the innovation journey 440–4
 in practice
   examples of 440–44
   funding 431–3
   information and evidence 435–6
   key influences on 431, 432
   physical and IT infrastructure 437–8
   relationships and networks 436–7
   service user engagement 438–40
   wider policy levers 432
   workforce 434–5
 theoretical and disciplinary perspectives 426–9
   CFIR framework 428
   NASSS framework 428–9
   science, technology 426–7
Healthcare management
 acute care 303–24
 adult social care 377–92
 changing user and consumer expectations 5
 climate change and sustainability 250–70
 demographic challenge 4–5
 economic theory of 206–21
 financial pressures 5
 future challenges for healthcare managers 520–6
 global health 157–76
 governance and leadership 11–30
 healthcare funding 179–99
 healthcare innovation 420–44
 healthcare workforce 450–65
 history of 3
 informatics 401–15
 integrated care 332–46
 measuring, managing healthcare performance 496–516
 mental health 352–68
 organizations 6–8
 primary care 276–96
 politics (*see* politics of healthcare)
 setting and managing priorities for 221–43
 service user perspectives, experiences and involvement 470–88
 technological innovation 5
Healthcare managers
 in acute care 322–3
 adult social care 390–2
 EDI implications for 102–3
 future challenges for 520–6
 positive action and positive discrimination 103
 priority setting 242–3
 research and evaluation 113–27
 understanding politics of health 134
Healthcare organizations
 healthcare process, nature of 7–8
 place of professionals 6
 as a public good 8

role of patients 6–7
Health selection theory 64
Health system efficiency 180
Heatwaves 251
HSPM (*see* Health systems and policy monitor)
Human development index (HDI) score 158

IAPT (*see* Improving access to psychological therapies)
Identity politics 94
ILO (*see* International Labour Organization)
IMF (*see* International Monetary Fund)
IMPACT (*see* Improving adult care together)
Implementation outcomes framework (IOF) 428
Improving adult care together (IMPACT) 385
Inclusion 85
Incremental cost-effectiveness ratio (ICER) 233
Inequality 60
Inequity 60
Informatics
    applying insights to drive improvements 411–3
    controlled clinical terminologies 406
    data into knowledge
        for research 407
        risk prediction in 408–9
        statistical process control (SPC) 410
    development of electronic health records 404–5
    electronic health records, development of 404–5
    future challenges in 414–7
    improvements
        in clinical decision-making 412
        health behaviour 413
        management decision-making 412–3
    information cycle 401–4
    personal health data 406
    standards and interoperability 405–6
    turning data into knowledge 406–11
Information cycle
    across a healthcare system 403–4
    healthcare service 403
    individual patients 401–3
Institute for Healthcare Improvement (IHI) quality
        improvement approach 39, 41
Institution-level governance
    board structures
        accountability approaches 24–26
        board of directors 18
        board of governors 18
        board practices 20–24
        changing and distinctive features of leadership
            26–8
        co-operative and mutual traditions 18
        key variables 18
        principle of co-determination 18
        purpose of 19–21

Senate model 19
    types of 19
    definition of 14
International classification of diseases (ICD) 406
International Labour Organization (ILO) 379
International Monetary Fund (IMF) 164
Integrated care
    definitions of 333
    dimensions of
        challenge for managers 344–5
        normative 341–2
        organizational 336–7
        professional 338–9
        service 343–6
        systemic 334–6
    managing levels of integration 333–46
Integrated care toolbox 345–6
Intersectionality 62–3, 96
Inter-professional education (IPE) 338
Inverse care law 65
IOF (*see* Implementation outcomes framework)
IPE (*see* Inter-professional education)

JMIR (*see* Journal of Medical Internet Research)
Journal of Medical Internet Research (JMIR) 417

Kapiti community health network (KCHN) 288
KCHN (*see* Kapiti community health network)

Lack of precision of data 501
Laissez-faire liberalism 143
Leadership
    collective 26
    distributed 26
    reconciling quality and safety 26
    situational approach to 27–8
    themes and patterns in 28–30
Lean approach
    flow of patients 43
    Virginia Mason Medical Center (VMMC)
        background 44
        example of 44–5
        impact of 45
        partnership with NHS England 45–6
        physician compact 45
Life-cycle assessment (LCA) 261
LMICs (*see* Low-and middle-income countries)
Local taxation 184–5
London School of Hygiene and Tropical Medicine
        (LSHTM) 408
Low-and middle-income countries (LMICs)
    ambulance services 306–7
    first level, district/referral hospitals 304
    hospitals 304

Low-and middle-income countries (LMICs) (*continued*)
    models of ownership 306
    second level, regional/provincial hospitals 305
    third level, national/university hospitals 305
LSHTM (*see* London School of Hygiene and Tropical
    Medicine)

Marmot review 70
Microaggressions 92
Mental health
    architecture of
        case study 360–3
        history of service provision 357–8
        multidisciplinary teams (MDTs) 359
        patient activism 357–8
        peer support and the recovery approach 360
        treatment in relation to spectrum 359
    defining terms 353–4
    management
        future of 367–8
        measuring systems 366–7
        service users and patients involvement 364
        tackling racism 364–6
    management in 363–8
    social determinants of 354–7
Mental health gap action programme (mhGAP) 367
Mental health support teams (MHSTs) 361
mhGAP (*see* Mental health gap action programme)
MHSTs (*see* Mental health support teams)
Multilateral organizations
    Food and Agriculture Organization (FAO) 164
    Gavi 165
    International Monetary Fund (IMF) 164
    The pandemic treaty 162–3
    President's Emergency Plan for AIDS Relief
        (PEPFAR) programme 166
    United Nations Office for Project Services (UNOPS)
        163–4
    World Bank 165
    World Health Organization (WHO)
        budget 161
        global health agendas 161
        The pandemic treaty 162–3
        technical outputs 162
    World Trade Organization (WTO) 164
Multi-criteria decision analysis (MCDA) 234
Multimorbidity, patient-related factors 307–8

NASSS (*see* Non-adoption, abandonment, scale-up,
    spread, and sustainability)
National Institute of Health and Care Excellence
    (NICE) 117–8
Newcastle University Hospitals (NUH) 255
NHS Blood and Transplant (NHSBT) 440, 443–4
NICE (*see* National institute for health and care
    excellence)

Non-adoption, abandonment, scale-up, spread, and
    sustainability (NASSS) 291, 428
Normative integration 341–2

OECD (*see* Organisation for economic co-operation and
    development)
OHP (*see* Our health partnership)
OLAP (*see* Online analytical processing)
Online analytical processing (OLAP) 412
Organisation for economic co-operation and
        development (OECD)
    challenges for healthcare governance 12
    changes to hospital systems 312
    funding for acute care 320
    healthcare financing 188
    impact of inequalities 69
    institution-level governance 14
    international comparison 508
    management of primary care 278
    performance metrics 501
    politics and society 3
    workforce planning 454
Organizational integration 336–7
Othering
    expressions of power 89–90
    slavery 88–9
    social construction 88–9
Our health partnership (OHP) 285
Outcomes-based funding (value-based funding) 190
Out-of-pocket payments 188
Outsourced training 457

The pandemic treaty 162–3
Parent boards 19
Path dependency concept 147–8
Patient-reported experience measures (PREMs) 366
Patient-reported outcome measures (PROMs) 366
Patriarchy 95–6
People's Republic of China (PRC) 169
Performance metrics
    articulating clear aims of 512
    average length of stay 500–1
    common challenges with
        bias 502
        changes over time 502
        lack of precision 501
        missing data 501–2
    data and analysis 513
    different users of
        clinicians 504
        commissioners/purchasers of care 503–4
        governments 503
        healthcare providers and managers 504
        patients and the public 504–5
        regulators 503
    identify metrics 512

managing healthcare performance
    comparing performance 507–10
    evaluation study 506–7
    unintended consequences of 510–12
process map for developing 512, 514
proxy for actual performance 498–9
reflection 514–15
reporting 513
seven principles to 515–16
six domains of care quality 498, 499
trends over time 499–501
waiting times 498
Personal health data 406
Person-centred approaches 381
Policymaking
    micro-politics 148–9
    path dependency concept 147–8
    political institutions role 146–7
Politics of healthcare
    costs of healthcare 135–6
    important for healthcare managers 134
    policymaking 146–9
    structural interest theory
        management consultancies role 142
        medical organizations, attributes of
            139–40
        patients and citizens, role of 142–3
        profession 138
        role of professional organizations 138–9
        stakeholders importance 142
        state, central role 136–8
        stewardship and governance 137–8
    triple aim concept 135
varieties/types of health care systems 143–6
Power and privilege
    key points 87
    othering 88–90
        expressions of power 89–90
        slavery 88–9
        social construction 88–9
    White privilege 87–8
PREMs (*see* Patient-reported experience measures)
President's Emergency Plan for AIDS Relief
    (PEPFAR) programme 166
Prices in healthcare
    aggregation of demand 212
    costs of 209–10
    fairness and equity 214
    information asymmetry, consequence of 211
    market mechanisms, use of 213–14
    payment models 212–13
    shadow prices 209
    value in 210
Primary healthcare
    in health system 278

within health systems
    community health organizations 286–7
    corporate chains 284–5
    independent practices 289–90
    organizations of 284
    patient registration 282–3
    primary care gatekeeping 283–4
    provider networks 287–8
    public health-based primary care 289
    super-partnerships/independent physician
        associations 285
management task
    coordinating a wide range of services 290–1
    embracing technology and self-care 293–4
    ensuring equitable access 291–2
    local health system, collaborating 292–3
    service provision 280–2
    strategic planning and management 294
    stronger and more extensive planning 294
nature and role of
    categorization of core activities 280
    management of primary care 278
    organizational models of 278–80
    policy focus and implementation 277
    Starfield's four Cs 281
organizations 278–80
Primary prevention 60
Primordial prevention 59
Priority setting
    decision-making
        accountability for reasonableness (A4R) 237–8
        cost-effectiveness analysis 232–3
        multi-criteria decision analysis (MCDA) 234
        programme budgeting and marginal analysis
            (PBMA) 233–4
        public engagement 234–7
    drivers of demand 228
    ethical precepts 230–2
    forms of rationing 228–9
    healthcare managers messages 242–3
    implementation 240–2
    politics 238–40
    technocracy 229–30
Private healthcare insurance 186–7
Process management 42–3
Professional integration 338–9
Programme budgeting and marginal analysis (PBMA)
    233–4
PROMs (*see* Patient-reported outcome measures)
Public health (*see also* Health inequalities)

Quality-adjusted life years gained (QALYs) 233
Quality improvement (QI)
    Agile approach 41–2
    care-specific improvement 38

Quality improvement (QI) (*continued*)
  common approaches for 39, 40
  core challenges to organizing 48
  definitions of 36, 37
  fundamental commonalities
    flow of patients 43
    Lean at Virginia Mason Medical Center (VMMC) 44–6
    people role 43
    process view 42–3
    role of customer 43
    variation 43
  Institute for Healthcare Improvement (IHI) 39, 41
  measurement mechanisms 47
  patient safety 41
  performance improvement, categories of 37, 38
  Plan Do Study Act improvement cycles 42

Racial trauma 91
Racism 91–2
RE-AIM (*see* Reach, effectiveness, adoption, implementation and maintenance)
Regional international organizations
  Association of Southeast Asian Nations (ASEAN) 166
  comparative health data 167–8
  Economic Community of West African States (ECOWAS) 166
  European Union's (EU) 167
  Shanghai Cooperation Organisation (SCO) 166
  Southern Common Market 166
Research and evaluation
  evidence to support decisions
    case study 115–6
    Directory of Open Access Journals (DOAJ) 118
    Medline 117
    PubMed database 116
    twelve-hour nursing shifts 119–20
  evidence-informed organizations 120–2
  planning evaluations
    aims of improvement 123
    confounding 125–6
    level of investment 125
    logic model 123–4
    mortality and morbidity, maternity services 124–5
    quantitative study designs 126–7
Resource dependency theory 19
Retention 457–9
Revenue generation 181–3

Same-day emergency care (SDEC) 318
SDEC (*see* Same-day emergency care)
Secondary prevention 60
Senate model 19
Service integration 343–4

Service users
  Arnstein's ladder of participation 473, 474
  assessing involvement 486–8
  collaborative relationships, healthcare professionals 478–9
  community involvement 471–3
  definitions 470–1
  different levels and types of involvement 475
  effective self-management and self-care 479
  involvement in planning, delivering, improving services
    co-production 480–2
    in strategic decisions 482–3
  levels of involvement 474
  person-centred care a reality 483–4
  person-centred organizations 485–6
  priorities of 476
  timely and helpful information 476–8
  Triangle of Care 475
Shadow prices 209
Shanghai Cooperation Organisation (SCO) 166
Shifting dietary behaviours 252
Six Sigma approach 43
Slavery 88–9
Sleepio 440–1
SNOMED (*see* Systematics Nomenclature of Medicine)
Social causation 64
Social construction 88–9
Social determinants of health (SDH)
  dimensions for assessing inequalities 97
  indigenous health strategies 98
  mental health, disability and stigma 355–7
  role of epidemiology 355
  social environment role 355
  voices of lived experience 101
Social health insurance 185–6
Social justice 84
Southern common market 166
SPC (*see* Statistical process control)
Stakeholder theory 19
Statistical process control (SPC) 507
Stewardship theory 19
Storms and flooding 251–2
Structural/materialist theories 64
Subsidiary boards 19
Sustainable development goals (SDGs) 355
Sustainability in quality improvement (SusQI) 262
System-level governance
  accountability arrangements 13–14
  COVID-19 pandemic management 14–17
  markets, hierarchies and networks 13
  performance monitoring 13–14
  priority setting 13–14
Systemic integration 334–6
Systematics Nomenclature of Medicine (SNOMED) 406

TAVI (*see* Transcatheter aortic valve implantation)
Technocracy 229–30
Tertiary prevention 60
THREAT (*see* Tracking healthcare ransomware events and traits)
Total Quality Management (TQM) 38
Tracking healthcare ransomware events and traits (THREAT) 415
Transcatheter aortic valve implantation (TAVI) 309
Triple bottom-line accounting 261–2

UK Equality Act 85
United Nations Office for Project Services (UNOPS) 163–4
UN Convention on the Rights of Persons with Disabilities (UNCRPD) 356
UNCRPD (*see* UN Convention on the Rights of Persons with Disabilities)

Vector-borne diseases 251
Virginia Mason Production System (VMPS) 44–5

Water shortages 252
Workforce
  distribution within health services 463–5
  managing the supply, healthcare workers international migration 456–7
  pay, rewards and employment models 459–61
  retention of staff 457–9
  training 454–6
  workforce planning 452–3
  rebalancing the mix of professions 461–3
  size of 451–2
Workforce planning of 453
World Bank 165
World Health Organization (WHO) 251
  approaches to social care 380
  budget 161
  controlled clinical terminologies 406
  funding for acute care 320
  global health agendas 161
  global healthcare workforce 451
  health impacts of climate change 251
  managing levels of integration 333
  The pandemic treaty 162–3
  primary care role and importance 277
  risk prediction 408
  social determinants of mental health 355
  sustainable healthcare initiatives 268
  technical outputs 162
The Welsh board model 19
World Trade Organization (WTO) 164
White privilege 87–8

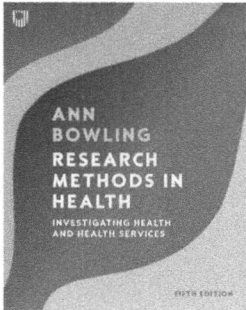

Research Methods in Health:
Investigating Health and Health Services

Ann Bowling

Fifth Edition

ISBN: 9780335250929 (Paperback)
eISBN: 9780335250936

2023

This bestselling book provides an accessible introduction to the concepts and practicalities of multi-disciplinary research methods in health and health services. The new edition has updated and expanded coverage of:

- **International examples, terms and approaches**
- **Epidemiology and methods of tracing epidemics**
- **Evaluation and assessment of health services**
- **Health services research and audit, including data generation**
- **Methods of evaluating patients' perspectives**
- **Measuring quality of life outcomes**
- **Health economics methods and applications**
- **Quantitative and qualitative research**

Core processes and methodologies such as social research, mixed methods, literature reviewing and critical appraisal, secondary data analysis and evidence-based practice will be covered in detail. The book also looks at the following key areas of health research:

- **Health needs**
- **Morbidity and mortality trends and rates**
- **Costing health services**
- **Sampling for survey research**
- **Cross-sectional and longitudinal survey design**
- **Experimental methods and techniques of group assignment**
- **Questionnaire design**
- **Interviewing techniques**
- **Coding and analysis of quantitative data**
- **Methods and analysis of qualitative observational studies**
- **Unstructured interviewing**

The book is grounded in the author's career as a researcher on health and health service issues, and the valuable experience this has provided in meeting the challenges of research on people and organisations in real life settings.

OPEN UNIVERSITY PRESS
McGraw Hill

www.mheducation.co.uk

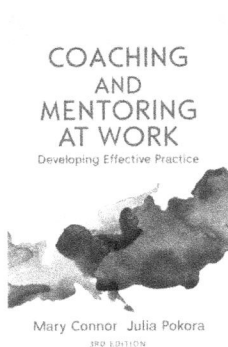

Coaching and Mentoring at Work:
Developing Effective Practice

Mary P. Connor, Julia B. Pokora

Third edition

ISBN: 9780335226924 (Paperback)
eISBN: 9780335226931

2017

The third edition of this popular, practical and authoritative book has been revised and updated, with two new chapters. It is aimed at coaches, mentors and clients and features:

- **Nine key principles of effective coaching and mentoring, showing how to apply them**
- **Discussion of differences between coaching and mentoring across different contexts and sectors**
- **Ideas about how to be an effective coach or mentor and how to be an effective client**
- **Self-development checklists and prompts, and a wealth of interactive case material**
- **New chapter on useful approaches and models**
- **The Skilled Helper model and how to apply it to coaching and mentoring**
- **A range of tried and tested tools and techniques**
- **Ethical issues, reflective practice and supervision**
- **New chapter in which coaches and mentors share experiences from Business, Health, Education & the Public Sector**

www.mheducation.co.uk

OPEN UNIVERSITY PRESS
McGraw Hill

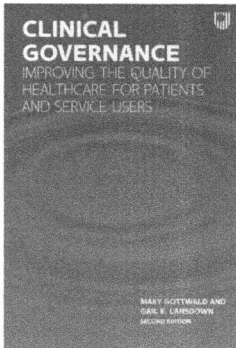

Clinical Governance:
Improving the Quality of Healthcare of Patients
and Service Users

Mary Gottwald, Gail E. Lansdown

Second Edition

ISBN: 9780335251049 (Paperback)
eISBN: 9780335251056

2021

The new edition of this key text offers an accessible guide to clinical governance across a range of healthcare settings. Designed to help students, practitioners, and professionals deliver quality care to patients and to improve overall patient experience, this new edition is packed with practical insight into how individuals can contribute to clinical governance.

Grounded in the application of clinical governance, this text benefits from thorough worked examples of common causality diagrams; up to date consideration of high profile clinical governance case studies; reflective activities as well as tips and real experiences to help readers apply the theory to practice.

This is the go-to book for students, practitioners and professionals across health and allied health disciplines including mental health nursing, midwifery, physiotherapy and occupational therapy.

www.mheducation.co.uk

OPEN UNIVERSITY PRESS
McGraw Hill

www.ingramcontent.com/pod-product-compliance
Lightning Source LLC
Chambersburg PA
CBHW081216220326
41598CB00037B/6795